Handbook
of
Tremor
Disorders

NEUROLOGICAL DISEASE AND THERAPY

Series Editor

WILLIAM C. KOLLER

Department of Neurology
University of Kansas Medical Center
Kansas City, Kansas

Handbook
of
Tremor
Disorders

edited by

Leslie J. Findley
Regional Centre for Neurology and Neurosurgery
Oldchurch Hospital
and Harold Wood Hospitals
Romford, Essex
and Institute of Neurology
London, England

William C. Koller
University of Kansas Medical Center
Kansas City, Kansas

Marcel Dekker, Inc.   **New York • Basel • Hong Kong**

Library of Congress Cataloging-in-Publication Data

Handbook of tremor disorders / edited by Leslie J. Findley, William C. Koller.
    p.   cm. — (Neurological disease and therapy; v. 30)
    Includes bibliographical references and index.
    ISBN 0-8247-8859-1 (alk. paper)
    1. Tremor. I. Findley, Leslie J. II. Koller, William C. III. Series: Neurological disease and therapy; 30.
    [DNLM: 1. Tremor—physiopathology. 2. Tremor—etiology.
3. Tremor—diagnosis. W1 NE33LD v.30 1994 / WL 340 H2367 1994]
RC376.5.H36 1995
616.8'4—dc20
DNLM/DLC
for Library of Congress   94-28740
                                                      CIP

The publisher offers discounts on this book when ordered in bulk quantities. For more information, write to Special Sales/Professional Marketing at the address below.

This book is printed on acid-free paper.

MARCEL DEKKER, INC.
270 Madison Avenue, New York, New York 10016

Current printing (last digit):
10 9 8 7 6 5 4 3 2 1

Printed in the United States of America

Series Introduction

The *Handbook of Tremor Disorders* addresses a very common neurological syndrome. Tremor looks simple in its rhythmicity but, in fact, is a most complex physiological event. The opening chapter discusses the definition and classification of tremor. Several chapters discuss its central and peripheral components and further elucidate its basic physiological mechanisms. Others discuss in detail neurophysiological techniques in distinguishing tremors as well as both the central and peripheral mechanisms involved in tremor genesis. The entity of essential tremor is covered in great detail, as are the physiological, pathological, and neurochemical bases of essential tremor and the relationship of essential tremor to other movement disorders. Other areas discussed are pharmacological and surgical treatment of essential tremor; tremors seen in Parkinson's disease and other parkinsonian states, such as MPTP-induced parkinsonism, and the medical and surgical treatment of parkinsonian tremor; and cerebellar, primary orthostatic; primary writing, and other types of tremor. The relationship of trauma to tremor, as well as the relationship of tremor to other movement disorders, such as dystonia and Parkinson's disease; tremor due to stroke and other lesions of the nervous system; tremors related to specific body parts, such as head and vocal tremor; and the entity of psychogenic tremor, which is commonly seen in clinical practice, are also addressed.

The *Handbook of Tremor Disorders* is in keeping with other books in the series that provide both basic science information and detailed clinical approaches to a common neurological problem. The physician will be well served by this reference source when dealing with the differential diagnosis of patients with tremor disorders.

WILLIAM C. KOLLER

Preface

The last three decades have seen an exponential growth in interest in movement disorders. This was originally stimulated by an increase in understanding of the pathophysiology of Parkinson's disease and the introduction of pharmacological treatments. More recently, there has been increasing interest in the other tremulous disorders.

Tremor represents the most common movement disorder met within clinical practice. It may be seen as an interesting physiological phenomenon, which is present in all living organisms. It can also be seen as a symptom of underlying dysfunction of the nervous system, or as a disease in its own right, such as "essential tremor."

This volume brings together the views of both basic and clinical scientists reviewing current concepts of basic mechanisms of tremor, through to the practical problems of differential diagnosis and clinical management. It is not meant to be a complete review of the field of tremor, but rather to emphasize current areas of basic scientific and clinical interest.

New biological techniques for investigating tremor are discussed, as well as the more traditional modes of clinical observation and pathophysiological correlation.

Apart from academic curiosity and satisfaction, the end point of clinical research must be the benefit of the sufferer. Patients in the United States and in Europe have shown increasing dissatisfaction with the lack of suitable treatments available for the management of such common disorders as essential tremor. The concern has been reflected in the growth of the International Tremor Foundation both in the United States and, lately, in Europe. This organization, which is patient oriented, promotes research activities in all aspects of tremulous disorders and provides support services for patients with symptomatic tremors.

We intended this volume to be a valuable addition to the literature for those working in the field of tremor, and provocative and interesting to those clinicians and scientists whose work will bring them into contact with patients who have tremulous disorders.

LESLIE J. FINDLEY
WILLIAM C. KOLLER

Contents

Contributors

Michael Bacher   Department of Neurology, University of Tübingen, Tübingen, Germany

Peter Bain, M.A., M.R.C.P.   Department of Neurology, Radcliffe Infirmary, Oxford, England

N. Bathien, M.D., D.Sc.   Department of Neurology, Centre R. Garcin–CHSA, Paris, France

A. T. Birmingham, B.Sc., M.B., B.S., M.R.C.S., L.R.C.   Professor of Pharmacology, Department of Physiology and Pharmacology, Medical School, Queen's Medical Centre, University of Nottingham, Nottingham, England

Andrew Blitzer, M.D., D.D.S.   Professor of Clinical Otolaryngology and Acting Chairman, Department of Otolaryngology, College of Physicians and Surgeons, Columbia University, New York, New York

Mitchell F. Brin, M.D.   Assistant Professor, Department of Neurology, College of Physicians and Surgeons, Columbia University, New York, New York

Thomas C. Britton, M.D.   MRC Human Movement and Balance Unit, Institute of Neurology, National Hospital for Neurology and Neurosurgery, Queen Square, London, England

David J. Brooks, M.D.   Professor, MRC Cyclotron Unit, Hammersmith Hospital, London, England

David Buckwell, B.Eng.   Computer Officer, Section of Neuro-Otology, MRC Human Movement and Balance Unit, Institute of Neurology, National Hospital for Neurology and Neurosurgery, Queen Square, London, England

Karen Busenbark, R.N., B.S.N.   Nurse Clinician, Department of Neurology, University of Kansas Medical Center, Kansas City, Kansas

Stefano Calzetti, M.D.   Associate Professor, Institute of Neurology, University of Parma, Parma, Italy

J. D. Cole, M.D.   Wessex Neurological Centre, Southampton General Hospital, Southampton, England

Terry G. Curran, M.D., F.R.C.P.(c)   Movement Disorder Clinic, Department of Neurology, Vernon Jubilee Hospital, Vernon, British Columbia, Canada

Mahlon R. DeLong, M.D.   Timmie Professor and Chairman, Department of Neurology, Emory University School of Medicine, Atlanta, Georgia

G. Deuschl, M.D.   Neurologische Klinik, University of Freiburg, Freiburg, Germany

Richard M. Dubinsky, M.D.   Associate Professor, Department of Neurology, University of Kansas Medical Center, Kansas City, Kansas

Rodger J. Elble, M.D., Ph.D.   Director and Interim Chairman, Department of Neurology, and the Center for Alzheimer Disease and Related Disorders, Southern Illinois University School of Medicine, Springfield, Illinois

Leslie J. Findley, T.D., M.D., F.R.C.P.   Consultant Neurologist, Regional Centre for Neurology and Neurosurgery, Oldchurch Hospital and Harold Wood Hospitals, Romford, Essex, and Honorary Senior Lecturer, Institute of Neurology, London, England

H. Genger   Neurologische Klinik, University of Freiburg, Freiburg, Germany

Marc S. Goldman, M.D.   Chief Resident, Department of Neurosurgery, Mayo Clinic, Rochester, Minnesota

Michael A. Gresty, Ph.D.   Senior Scientist and Section Head (Neuro-Otology), MRC Human Movement and Balance Unit, Institute of Neurology, National Hospital for Neurology and Neurosurgery, Queen Square, London, England

Kurt J. Hopfensperger, M.D.   Movement Disorder Fellow, Department of Neurology, University of Kansas Medical Center, Kansas City, Kansas

Joseph Jankovic, M.D.   Professor of Neurology and Director of Parkinson's Disease Center and Movement Disorders Clinic, Department of Neurology, Baylor College of Medicine, Houston, Texas

James Kelly, M.D. Care of the Elderly, Erne Hospital, Enniskillen, Northern Ireland

Patrick J. Kelly, M.D. Department of Neurosurgery, Mayo Clinic, Rochester, Minnesota

William C. Koller, M.D., Ph.D. Professor and Chairman, Department of Neurology, and Professor of Pharmacology, University of Kansas Medical Center, Kansas City, Kansas

Martin Lakie, Ph.D. Senior Lecturer, Applied Physiology Research Group, University of Birmingham, Birmingham, England

Yves Lamarre, M.D., Ph.D. Professor, Department of Physiology, Faculté de Médecine, University of Montreal, Montreal, Quebec, Canada

Anthony E. Lang, M.D., F.R.C.P.(c) Director, Morton and Gloria Shulman Movement Disorders Centre, and Associate Professor, Department of Medicine (Neurology), The Toronto Hospital, University of Toronto, Toronto, Ontario, Canada

J. William Langston, M.D. President, The Parkinson's Institute, Sunnyvale, California

Peter A. LeWitt, M.D. Professor of Neurology, Wayne State University School of Medicine and Clinical Neuroscience Center, West Bloomfield, Michigan

Rodolfo Llinás, M.D., Ph.D. Chairman and Professor, Department of Physiology/ Biophysics, New York University Medical Center, New York, New York

C. H. Lücking, M.D. Professor, Neurologische Klinik, University of Freiburg, Freiburg, Germany

I. A. Macdonald, B.Sc., Ph.D. Professor of Metabolic Physiology, Department of Physiology and Pharmacology, Medical School, Queen's Medical Centre, University of Nottingham, Nottingham, England

Concepció Marin, M.D. Department of Neurology, Hospital Clinic I Provincial Barcelona, University of Barcelona, Barcelona, Spain

Paul McCullagh Lecturer, Department of Mental Health, The Queen's University of Belfast, Belfast, Northern Ireland

Steven L. Moon, M.D., M.Ph. Department of Neurology, University of Kansas Medical Center, Kansas City, Kansas

Stuart Mossman Consultant Neurologist, Department of Neurology, Wellington Hospital, Wellington South, New Zealand

Rajesh Pahwa, M.D. Assistant Professor, Department of Neurology, University of Kansas Medical Center, Kansas City, Kansas

Denis Paré, Ph.D.   Research Scientist, Department of Physiology, University Laval, Quebec, Canada

Emilio Perucca, M.D., Ph.D.   Associate Professor, Clinical Pharmacology Unit, University of Pavia, Pavia, Italy

Ali H. Rajput, M.B.B.S., M.S.C.(Neurol), F.R.C.P.C.   Professor of Neurology, Department of Medicine, University of Saskatchewan, Saskatoon, Saskatchewan, Canada

P. Rondot, M.D.   Professor, Department of Neurology, Centre R. Garcin–CHSA, Paris, France

J. C. Rothwell, M.D.   MRC Human Movement and Balance Unit, Institute of Neurology, National Hospital for Neurology and Neurosurgery, Queen Square, London, England

Erich Scholz, M.D.   Department of Neurology, University of Tübingen, Tübingen, Germany

Carlos Singer, M.D.   Assistant Professor, Department of Neurology, University of Miami School of Medicine, Miami, Florida

Ian Stewart Smith, M.A., M.R.C.P.   Department of Clinical Neurophysiology, Leeds General Infirmary, Leeds, England

Celia Stewart, Ph.D.   Assistant Professor, Department of Speech–Language Pathology and Audiology, New York University, and Instructor, Neurology Department, Columbia University, New York, New York

Albrecht Struppler   Professor Emeritus of Neurology and Clinical Neurophysiology, Motor Research Unit, Klinikum rechts der Isar, Munich, Germany

Hugh McA. Taggart   Senior Lecturer, Department of Geriatric Medicine, The Queen's University of Belfast, Belfast, Northern Ireland

James W. Tetrud, M.D.   Medical Director, Clinical Center for Parkinson's Disease and Movement Disorders, The Parkinson's Institute, Sunnyvale, California

P. D. Thompson, M.B., Ph.D., F.R.A.C.P.   Honorary Senior Lecturer and Consultant Neurologist, Institute of Neurology, National Hospital for Neurology and Neurosurgery, Queen Square, London, England

Eduardo S. Tolosa, M.D.   Professor, Department of Neurology, Hospital Clinic I Provincial Barcelona, University of Barcelona, Barcelona, Spain

Jerrold L. Vitek   Assistant Professor, Department of Neurology, Emory University School of Medicine, Atlanta, Georgia

E. Geoffrey Walsh, M.D., F.R.C.P., F.R.S.E. Honorary Neurophysiological Specialist, Lothian Health Board, Department of Physiology, University of Edinburgh, Edinburgh, Scotland

William J. Weiner, M.D. Professor of Neurology and Director, Movement Disorder Centre, Department of Neurology, University of Miami School of Medicine, Miami, Florida

Thomas Wichmann, M.D. Resident, Department of Neurology, Emory University School of Medicine, Atlanta, Georgia

R. Zimmermann Neurologische Klinik, University of Freiburg, Freiburg, Germany

Definitions and Behavioral Classifications

Leslie J. Findley
Regional Centre for Neurology and Neurosurgery
Oldchurch Hospital and Harold Wood Hospitals
Romford, Essex
and Institute of Neurology
London, England

William C. Koller
University of Kansas Medical Center
Kansas City, Kansas

I. DEFINITIONS

Although in the last 20 years there has been an exponential increase in the clinical and research interest in movement disorders in general, and tremor in particular, there is still confusion over certain terms referring to the phenomenology of tremor. Unless there is some common agreement on definitions, progress in research and clinical communication will be hampered.

Following an initial meeting of the Tremor Investigation Group (TRIG) in Houston, Texas, in December 1990, a series of working definitions were proposed. It was hoped that these definitions could be amended in the light of experience and feedback from experienced workers.

The following definitions have been proposed:

Tremor: A rhythmical involuntary oscillatory movement of the body part. [Small-amplitude tremors may be detectable only by sensitive recording devices.]

Rest tremor: Tremor occurring when muscles are not voluntarily activated. [In the rest position, the body part is completely supported against gravity. Some forms of rest tremor may be mimicked be segmental myoclonus, which may be distinguished electrophysiologically.]

Action tremor: Any tremor occurring on voluntary contraction of muscle. This includes postural, kinetic, and isometric tremor.

Postural tremor: Tremor present while voluntarily maintaining position against gravity. [This assumes voluntary or purposive activation of muscle is necessary for the maintenance of position. It is recognized that postural tremor may appear or become exacerbated in specific, usually visually guided, tasks. The presence or exacerbation of tremor in this situation may be called *position-specific postural tremor*.]

Kinetic tremor: Tremor during any form of movement. [The pronounced exacerbation of kinetic tremor toward the end of goal-directed movement, has been commonly referred to as intention or terminal tremor. It is recognized that kinetic tremor may appear or become exacerbated in specific activities. The presence or exacerbation of tremor in this situation is called *task-specific kinetic tremor* (i.e., tremors occurring during the performance of highly specific, skilled movement, including occupational tremors and primary writing tremor).]

Isometric tremor: Tremor occurring as a result of muscle contraction against a rigid stationary object.

Tone: The resistance encountered by the examiner when the limb of other body part is moved passively about a joint.

Rigidity: A sustained enhancement of resistance throughout the range of passive movement about a joint.

Cogwheel phenomenon: Rhythmic, repetitive alteration in resistance during passive movement about a joint.

Froment's Sign: (Signe de Froment); 1). A rhythmical resistance to passive movement of a limb about a joint that can be detected specifically when there is a voluntary action of another body part. [This phenomenon may be seen in a wide variety of tremulous disorders including essential tremor and Parkinson's disease. It is appreciated that the definition of Froment's sign adapted above, is different from the original description, but has become the most common and practical method of eliciting this sign.]

Reinforced tone: An increase in resistance during passive movement about a joint induced by voluntary activity in a noncontiguous body segment.

Dystonia: A syndrome dominated by sustained muscle contractions, frequently causing twisting and repetitive movement or abnormal postures.

Dystonic tremor: Tremor in a body part affected by dystonia.

Rhythmic myoclonus: Intermittent brief muscle jerks, irregular or rhythmic, arising in the central nervous system. [Rhythmic myoclonus can be distinguished from tremor only when the driving muscle contractions are impulsive, so that there are pauses between the individual jerks.]

II. PROPOSED CLASSIFICATION OF ESSENTIAL TREMOR

With the current state of knowledge, the presence of essential tremor (ET) refers to a phenomenological criterion. It is not a function of disability, pathophysiology, or heredity.

A. Definite Essential Tremor

1. Inclusions

1. *Tremor*: Bilateral postural tremor with or without kinetic tremor, involving hands or forearms, that is visible and persistent. [Tremor of other body parts may be present in addition to upper limb tremor. Bilateral postural tremor may be asymmetric. Tremor is reported by patient to be persistent although the amplitude may fluctuate. Tremor may or may not produce disability.]
2. *Duration*: Relatively long-standing (i.e., longer than 5 years).

2. Exclusions

1. Other abnormal neurological signs. [With the exception of the presence of tremor and Froment's sign, the full neurological examination should be normal for age.]
2. Presence of known causes of enhanced physiological tremor.
3. Concurrent or recent exposure to tremorogenic drugs or the presence of a drug withdrawal state. [Many drugs acting on the central nervous system can produce tremor as a side effect. In humans, drug-induced tremor is most often in the form of action tremor. Subjects should be drug-free for a period exceeding the known biological effect of the agent.]
4. Direct or indirect trauma to the nervous system within 3 months preceding the onset of tremor. [This includes head injury (direct or indirect), and peripheral injury, if the anatomical distribution of injury is the same as that of the tremor.]
5. Historial or clinical evidence of psychogenic origins of tremor. [The definition of psychogenic tremor is itself open to debate. Clinical features that may suggest this are unphysiological variations (>1 Hz) in tremor frequency, unusual and inconsistent behavioral characteristics, and spontaneous remissions. Psychiatric or social factors (multiple somatizations, secondary gain, litigation or compensation pending) may support the diagnosis of psychogenic tremor (2).
6. Convincing evidence of sudden onset or evidence of stepwise deterioration.

B. Probable Essential Tremor

1. Inclusions

1. Tremor: The same as those for definite essential tremor. [Tremor may be confined to body parts other than hands. These may include head and postural tremor of the legs. However, abnormal posture of the head would suggest the presence of dystonic head tremor.]
2. Duration: Longer than 3 years.

2. Exclusions

1. The same for definite essential tremor.

2. Primary orthostatic tremor (isolated, high-frequency (14–18 Hz) bilaterally synchronous tremor of lower limbs on standing; 3,4).
3. Isolated voice tremor. (Because of the clinical difficulty of separating essential tremor of the voice from the speech disturbances of laryngeal dystonia and other dystonias of the vocal apparatus).
4. Isolated position-specific or task-specific tremors, including occupational tremors and primary writing tremor.
5. Isolated tongue or chin tremor.

C. Possible Essential Tremor

1. Inclusions

1. Type I
   a. Subjects who satisfy the criteria of definite or probable essential tremor, but exhibit other recognizable neurological disorders, such as parkinsonism, dystonia, myoclonus, peripheral neuropathy, or restless leg syndrome.
   b. Subjects who satisfy the criteria of definite or probable essential tremor, but exhibit other neurological signs of uncertain significance not sufficient to make the diagnosis of a recognizable neurological disorder. Such signs may include mild extrapyramidal features, such as hypomimia, decreased arm swing, or mild bradykinesia.
2. Type II
   a. Monosymptomatic and isolated tremors of uncertain relation to essential tremor. This includes position-specific and task-specific tremors, such as occupational tremors, primary writing tremor, primary orthostatic tremor (as defined in the foregoing), isolated voice tremor, isolated postural leg tremor, and unilateral postural hand tremor.

2. Exclusions

The exclusions are the same as items 2–4 under Definite Essential Tremor (see Sect. II.A).

A further form of classification could be whether the tremor is familial or presumed sporadic.

MEMBERS OF TREMOR INVESTIGATION GROUP (TRIG)

M. Brinn (USA)	W. C. Koller (USA)
R. Eble (USA)	T. Lang (Canada)
L. J. Findley (UK)	P. Lewitt (USA)
J. Jankovic (USA)	Ali Rajput (Canada)

REFERENCES

1. Froment J, Gardere H. La rigidite et la rue dentee parkinsoniene s'effacent au repos. Rev Neurol 1926; 1:52–53.
2. Koller WC, Lang A, Vetere-Overfield B, et al. Psychogenic tremors. Neurology 1989; 39:1094–1099.
3. Heilman KM. Orthostatic tremor. Arch Neurol 1984; 41:880–881.
4. Thompson PD, Rothwell JC, Day BL, et al. The physiology of orthostatic tremor Arch. Neurol 1986; 43:584–587.

Role of Intrinsic Neuronal Oscillations and Network Ensembles in the Genesis of Normal and Pathological Tremors

Rodolfo Llinás
New York University Medical Center
New York, New York

Denis Paré
University Laval
Quebec, Canada

I. INTRODUCTION

It is now clear from basic and clinical studies that normal and pathological tremors are multifactorial emerging properties involving both central and peripheral factors (1). Indeed, tremor emerges from the dynamic interactions between multiple synaptically coupled neuronal systems and the physical properties of the external somatic effectors (2). In this context, the present chapter hopes to reveal new information concerning the properties of the thalamocortical and olivocerebellar networks, which are most likely to contribute to the generation of the synchronized neuronal activity underlying normal and abnormal tremor.

Phenomenologically, tremor is an involuntary rhythmic movement of a body part, having a relatively fixed frequency and amplitude, over a reasonable period. On the basis of their appearance, tremors have been classified in two broad groups (3): (1) tremors appearing at rest in fully supported limbs, and (2) tremors occurring during motor activity (movement and posture). In what will follow, we will address resting tremor, as in Parkinson's disease; and action tremors, the so-called physiological tremor, which relates to abnormalities of the olivocerebellar system.

II. PARKINSONIAN TREMOR

A. General Phenomenology

Together with rigidity, bradykinesia, and postural instability, resting tremors constitute the defining features of Parkinson's disease (4). The classic resting tremor is a 4- to 5-Hz oscillation, primarily affecting the distal portion of the upper limb. Although the lower limbs and the proximal portion of the upper limbs are occasionally involved, the head and trunk are usually spared. In many cases, one or more muscle groups beat at different frequencies. Moreover, dissociations between the two sides of the body, as well as between lower and upper extremities, have been reported (5,6). As implied by its name, the resting tremor diminishes or disappears before or at the onset of movement and results from the reciprocal activation of antagonistic muscle groups (7). Like most forms of tremors, it disappears during sleep.

Parkinson's disease is believed to result from the degeneration of the nigrostriatal pathway and ensuing reduction in striatal dopamine levels (8). However, the various parkinsonian symptoms react differentially to dopamine replacement therapy, thus suggesting that more subtle interactions may be involved. In particular, levodopa (L-dopa) proved less effective in controlling the resting tremor than in control of rigidity and bradykinesia. Moreover, in spite of their side effects and limited effectiveness, muscarinic antagonists are currently the drug of choice in treating resting tremor.

B. Central Origin of the Parkinsonian Resting Tremor

A wide variety of experimental findings and clinical observations indicate that the parkinsonian resting tremor is generated by a central oscillator. First, the resting tremor is not abolished by sectioning of the dorsal roots, thus indicating that it does not reflect only the action of spinal reflex loops (9,10). Second, in contrast with tremor of peripheral origin, it is difficult to reset the parkinsonian tremor by mechanical perturbations. Moreover, in these cases, the phase shift lasts for only a few cycles (11,12). Third, microneurographic recordings of Ia muscle spindle afferents demonstrated that the pattern of spindle discharges during resting tremor is similar to that observed during voluntary alternating movements. This finding suggests that the parkinsonian resting tremor results from the involuntary activation of a motor program of central origin (13).

This view, however, is not new, as the resting tremor has been known to be abolished by localized lesions of the motor cortex (14,15), the ventrolateral part of the thalamus (16), or the internal segment of the globus pallidus (GPi; 17). In addition, this conclusion was strengthened by the presence of tremor-related single-unit activity in the ventral complex of the thalamus of parkinsonian patients (18–20).

C. Identification of the Central Structures Involved in the Genesis of the Resting Tremor

Although it has been claimed that the nuclear boundaries of the human ventral thalamic complex can be easily identified (18,20–22), the optimal site of effective tremor blockade by thalamotomy is still controversial. This is partly because histological controls are rarely performed. Moreover, their interpretation is complicated by the fact that the diameter of the lesions increases with time (23). According to the current view, the most effective lesion site for alleviation of the resting tremor is the inferolateral limit of the ventral thalamic complex (22,24,25), a region named "nucleus ventralis intermedius" (Vim) in the terminology of Schaltenbrand and Bailey (26). To understand why lesions of the Vim are effective in abolishing the resting tremor, we will briefly review the anatomy of the ventral thalamic complex (see Sect. II.C.1) and correlate the connectivity of its nuclear components with the tremor-related activity of the constitutive cells, as recorded in parkinsonian patients undergoing stereotaxic surgery (see Sect. II.C.2).

1. The Ventral Thalamic Complex: Nuclear Systematization and Hodology

The ventral thalamic complex comprises five interdigitated nuclei, each receiving distinct subcortical inputs (27). The most caudally located nucleus of the ventral thalamic complex, the ventral posterior (VP) nucleus, is divided into a medial segment (VPM) and a lateral segment (VPL), which receive trigeminal and medial lemniscal inputs, respectively. The VP nucleus is composed of a main central region of neurons responsive to cutaneous stimuli surrounded by a thin (0.3- to 0.5-mm) layer of cells responding to stimulation of deep tissues (28,29).

Rostral to the VP nucleus is the VL nucleus which, on hodological grounds, was divided into two subnuclei: a posterior nucleus (VLp), receiving a massive projection from the deep cerebellar nuclei (30); and an anterior nucleus (VLa), the specific subcortical input of which is a GABAergic pathway (31,32) arising in the GPi (33,34). In the systematization of Schaltenbrand and Bailey (26), the VLa is termed ventrooralis anterior and the VLp is termed Vim.

Ventromedial to the VP and VL nuclei is the ventral medial (VM) complex whose main component receives a GABAergic input from the substantia nigra pars reticulata (SNr; 35). The most anterior nucleus of the ventral complex is the ventral anterior nucleus. Because the connections of this nucleus are poorly understood (27), it will not be discussed further.

The specific subcortical inputs terminating in these various nuclei are paralleled by a distinct pattern of cortical projections. For instance, the VLp and VLa project to the motor (36,37) and premotor cortices (37,38), respectively, whereas the VM projects more diffusely to frontal and medial cortical areas (39,40). Finally, the VP complex projects to the somatosensory cortex (37).

Because the main subcortical input of the Vim originates in the deep cerebellar nuclei (30), a system that does not display pathological signs in Parkinson's disease, it is likely that the effectiveness of Vim lesions in alleviating the resting tremor results from the destruction of a pathway coursing through the Vim and ending in a neighboring nucleus. Since Parkinson's disease affects primarily the basal ganglia, it seems reasonable to suspect that Vim lesions interrupt thalamo-petal fibers arising in the GPi or the SNr, the two main output stations of the striatum. Support for this contention comes from the analysis of tremor-related activities recorded from the ventral thalamic area of parkinsonian patients under-going stereotaxic surgery.

2. *Tremor-Related Activities of Ventral Thalamic Neurons*

Since the initial discovery by Guiot and collaborators (16) of ventral thalamic neurons discharging rhythmically in phase with the resting tremor, numerous studies have been performed to develop criteria for the accurate placement of neurosurgical lesions. Unfortunately, the interpretation of these studies is compli-cated by the poor quality of many recordings (for notable exceptions, see 24,41). Moreover, the time base of most oscilloscopic traces does not permit an adequate assessment of the tremor-related discharge patterns. Finally, no histological controls could be performed to confirm the location of the recorded units.

Nevertheless, three types of neurons where distinguished in the ventral thalamic complex.

a. *Units that Do Not Display Tremor-Related Activity.*   Included in this group of cells are posteriorly located neurons responding to light touch, more rostral cells responsive to deep somesthetic stimuli or active during some motor events, and unresponsive neurons disseminated throughout the ventral thalamic complex (20,24,42–44).

b. *Tremor-Related Units Responsive to Somesthetic Stimuli or Active During Voluntary Movements.*   These presumed Vim cells displayed rhythmic spike trains of varying duration in relation to the resting tremor. Moreover, voluntary movements disrupted their tremor-related activity (25,45–47). In light of the electrophysiological and anatomical evidence reviewed in Section II.C.1, it is probable that these neurons were located in the shell portion of the VP nucleus or in the VLp nucleus.

c. *Tremor-Related Cells Unresponsive to Peripheral Stimuli.*   These cells were unresponsive to somesthetic stimuli, and their discharge was not modified by passive and voluntary movements. They discharged rhythmically at the frequency of the resting tremor, even when the resting tremor ceased. These cells were located rostrodorsally to the neurons of the second class in an area that seems to overlap with the VLa nucleus (47,48).

On the whole, VLp neurons seem to discharge short tremor-related bursts of three to four spikes at 100–300 Hz (49). In contrast, VP neurons responsive to deep stimuli discharged low-frequency tremor-related spike trains lasting up to 200 ms (20,49). Finally, VLa neurons appear to discharge brief, high-frequency (200–300 Hz) bursts of four to eight spikes (48,50). Interestingly, a proportion of the thalamic neurons recorded rostrodorsally to the VP nucleus, in a primate model of the parkinsonian state, discharged high-frequency spike bursts similar to those displayed by VLa neurons. Moreover, this rhythmic activity resisted curarization (51) and rhyzotomy (52).

It is important to emphasize that the rhythmic discharges of VP and VLp cells in phase with the resting tremor is no proof of their involvement in the genesis of the tremor. Indeed, in intact experimental animals, some VLp cells discharge in relation to the activation of particular muscle groups, whereas VP neurons are responsive to deep stimuli (53,54). In other words, the tremor-related activity of these cells could simply reflect normal sensory feedback or efferent copy.

Much more significant is the discovery of VLa units that were rhythmically active at the frequency of the tremor, but were unresponsive to sensory stimulation and unaffected by voluntary movements. The persistence of this rhythmic activity when the tremor ceases establishes that these unitary activities do not reflect a sensory feedback, nor an efferent copy. Other findings point to the VLa nucleus as a crucial link in the genesis of the resting tremor observed in parkinsonian patients. First, the main subcortical input to the VLa originates in the GPi, the lesion of which abolishes the parkinsonian resting tremor. Second, the VLa nucleus projects to the premotor cortex (see Sect. II.C.1) and, thus, is in a strategic position to influence motor execution. Finally, Bertrand and collaborators, after an extensive review of their cases of thalamotomy, have concluded that the destruction of pallidothalamic fibers explains the effectiveness of the lesions placed at the *inferior border* of the Vim in abolishing the tremor (55).

D. In Search of the Mechanisms Responsible for the Genesis of the Parkinsonian Resting Tremor

The evidence reviewed so far points to the pallidothalamic pathway as a crucial link in the genesis of the resting tremor. However, it does not address the question of the mechanisms underlying tremor genesis.

1. Consequences of Dopaminergic Loss for the Activity of the Internal Globus Pallidus Neurons

The first issue to be reviewed concerns to the consequences of dopamine (DA) loss for the activity of the basal ganglia. Although the effects of DA on striatal neurons are still poorly understood (56,57), some insight can be gained by comparing the activity of neurons recorded from the internal and external segments of the GP in normal and parkinsonian monkeys following the administration of the neurotoxin 1-methyl-4-phenyl-1,2,3,6-tetrahydropyridine (MPTP; 58,59) or lesion of the ventromedial tegmentum (60). The firing rate of GPi cells were up to 50% higher in the parkinsonian models. Moreover, the tonic discharge characteristic of GPi neurons in normal animals was transformed in a 12- to 15-Hz burst–silence pattern which was uncorrelated with the resting tremor. The GPe neurons also displayed a burst–silence discharge pattern, but their overall frequency of discharge decreased dramatically.

When one considers that DA probably has inhibitory effects on GABAergic striatal neurons (56,57), it is unclear how DA loss could result in an increase in the discharge rate of GPi neurons. A possible explanation is that it is mediated indirectly, by an increase in the excitatory input from the subthalamic nucleus to the GPi (61), consequently, to the inhibition of the GABAergic cells of the GPe, which exert an inhibitory effect on the latter nucleus (62). In agreement with this interpretation, Bergman et al. (63) have reported that subthalamic lesions abolish the major parkinsonian symptoms in MPTP-treated monkeys.

Considering that GPi stimulation evokes inhibitory postsynaptic potentials in VLa neurons (64,65), it is not obvious how a 12- to 15-Hz inhibitory input could elicit a 3- to 6-Hz burst discharge in these neurons. The solution to this quandary relates to the intrinsic membrane properties of dorsal thalamic neurons.

2. Intrinsic Membrane Properties of Dorsal Thalamic Neurons

The intrinsic membrane properties of dorsal thalamic neurons, their ionic dependency, and their pharmacology were initially described in the in vitro brain slice preparation (66–68). These and other experiments performed in vivo showed that the firing mode of thalamocortical neurons varies with their membrane potential (66–69). As shown in Figure 1, depolarizing pulses applied at a depolarized membrane potential evoke a tonic discharge lasting the duration of the pulse, whereas from a hyperpolarized level (-65 mV and more), it evokes a brief (30-ms), high-frequency (250–400 Hz) burst of fast sodium-dependent action potentials riding on a slow calcium-mediated spike (66,67). This low-threshold calcium conductance is inactive at the resting potential, deinactivated by membrane hyperpolarization, and activated at the break of the hyperpolarization or in response to a depolarization applied during the hyperpolarization (66,67). As first described in the inferior olive (70,71), the low-threshold calcium conductance is also time-dependent.

On the basis of these findings, it was proposed that the intrinsic activity of thalamic neurons, specifically, the rebound low-threshold response, was probably responsible for the parkinsonian resting tremor (2).

Another important feature of thalamocortical neurons is that they are endowed with a powerful hyperpolarization-activated, time-dependent cation current

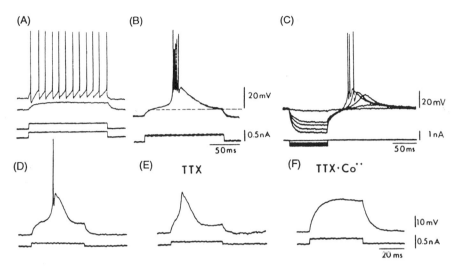

Figure 1 Intrinsic membrane properties of dorsal thalamic neurons. (A) Subthreshold depolarization of the cell at resting level produces, after a DC depolarization, repetitive firing of the cell during the same current pulse. (B) After DC hyperpolarization, similar current pulses as in A produce a single high-frequency burst. (C) Rebound burst response after hyperpolarizing pulses of different amplitudes. (D) Slow all-or-none response generating a fast spike, from a cell held at a slightly hyperpolarized membrane potential. (E) After blockage of sodium conductance with tetrodotoxin (TTX), the fast-action potential is blocked, but the slow response remains unchanged. (F) Addition of $COCl_2$ to the bathing solution completely abolishes the slow response seen in E, even when the current pulse is increased in amplitude by 2.5 times. (From Ref. 68.)

termed I_h. As a result, hyperpolarization of thalamocortical cells elicits a strong time-dependent inward rectification that displaces the membrane potential toward resting values (72,73). Moreover, the interaction between the I_h, the low-threshold calcium conductance, and the calcium-dependent potassium conductance ($g_{K(Ca)}$), can evoke slow oscillations of 0.5–4 Hz both in vitro (74) and in vivo (75,76).

3. Transformation of the 12- to 15-Hertz Inhibitory GPi Input Into the Rhythmic 3- to 6-Hertz Tremor-Related Bursting of VLa Neurons

We would like to propose two possible mechanisms for the transformation of the abnormal 12- to 15-Hz inhibitory input arising in the GPi into a series of high-frequency burst discharged rhythmically by VLa neurons at a frequency of 3–6 Hz. The first was formulated elsewhere (77) and is based on the hysteretic capabilities conferred to thalamocortical neurons by the properties of the low-threshold calcium conductance (Fig. 2A). When a train of short, repetitive, hyperpolarizing pulses, mimicking a series of rhythmic inhibitory postsynaptic

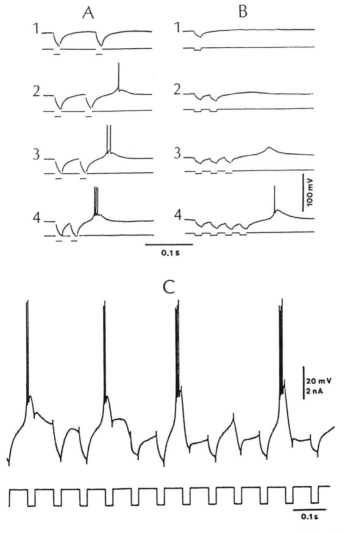

Figure 2 Time dependent deinactivation of the low-threshold calcium conductance in dorsal thalamic neurons. Progressive deinactivation of the low-threshold calcium conductance by (A) decreasing the duration of the interval between to short-lasting hyperpolarizing pulses and by (B) the injection of subthreshold hyperpolarizing pulses. (C) Frequency transformation of rhythmic hyperpolarizations by dorsal thalamic neurons. Response of a cat ventral lateral thalamic neuron to a train of hyperpolarizing pulses delivered at a frequency of 12 Hz. Note the rhythmic occurrence of low-threshold spikes at 4 Hz. (From Ref. 77.)

potentials (IPSPs) is imposed on a thalamic neuron, the train of hyperpolarizing pulses is temporally integrated and transformed into discrete low-threshold calcium spikes occurring at a lower frequency. This point is illustrated in Figure 2B where hyperpolarizing current pulses were delivered at a frequency of 10–12.5 Hz, whereas the resulting low-threshold calcium spikes (and superimposed high-

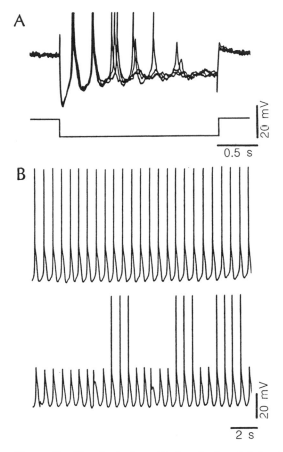

Figure 3 Slow intrinsic oscillations in dorsal thalamic neurons. In (A) the injection of a 1.5-nA hyperpolarizing pulse elicited a stereotyped oscillation. Action potentials are truncated. (B) illustrates a slow (0.5-Hz) spontaneous oscillations in an intracellularly recorded dorsal thalamic neuron deprived of cortical afferents. Note that this oscillation is not dependent on the presence of action potentials, since the oscillation persisted in spite of the fact that some low-threshold rebound spike were subthreshold for action potential generation. (From Ref. 75.)

frequency burst of sodium-dependent action potentials) occurred at a frequency of 2.5–4.5 Hz.

The other possible mechanism of frequency transformation involves the interplay between the low-threshold calcium conductance and the I_h (74–76). According to this second view (Fig. 3), the inhibitory input arising in the GPi would bring the membrane potential of thalamic neurons to the activation range of the I_h, which would produce a rapid depolarization, thereby activating a rebound calcium spike. The ensuing calcium entry would activate the $g_{K(Ca)}$ and, in conjunction with the rhythmic train of IPSPs arising in the GPi, would bring the membrane potential to the activation range of the I_h.

The result of this frequency transformation would be transmitted by VLa axons to the premotor cortex and, then, through corticocortical connections, to the motor cortex. The precise timing required to produce alternating contractions in antagonistic muscles is probably not the reflection of synchronized bursting in alternating pools of VLa neurons. Rather, the parkinsonian tremor probably reflects the involuntary running of a motor program normally used to produce rapid voluntary alternating movements (78). The neuronal network(s) underlying this motor program could be located anywhere from the premotor cortex to the spinal cord. The persistence of VLa bursting discharges after cessation of the tremor (during voluntary movements or sleep) underscores the dependence of tremor genesis on the functional state of the structures sustaining this motor program.

III. INVOLVEMENT OF THE OLIVOCEREBELLAR SYSTEM IN THE GENESIS OF PHYSIOLOGICAL TREMOR

The physiological tremor is a normal small-amplitude 9- to 12-Hz oscillatory movement that can be accentuated by several factors, such as stress and fatigue. It is observed during maintained posture and, to a lesser extent, during movement execution. As pointed out by Marsden (3), the physiological tremor reflects the interacting influence of a variety of factors, including the passive vibration of body tissues induced by the mechanical activity of the heart, the inertia and resonance of the musculoskeletal system, the synchronizing influence of spindle afferents, the recruitment and firing rate of motoneurons, and such. Although they are sometimes neglected, supraspinal influences are very important in the generation of physiological tremor (2). For instance, it has been reported by Sutton and Sykes (79) that removal of visual cues during posture *diminishes* markedly the physiological tremor of subjects instructed to maintain a constant force to a joystick. Moreover, unilateral damage to the cerebellum abolishes physiological tremor, as may be seen in the outstretched hand (3).

In this section, we will present recently obtained evidence arguing for the involvement of the olivocerebellar system in the genesis of the physiological tremor.

A. Intrinsic Membrane Properties of Inferior Olive Neurons: Biophysical Properties of a Timing Signal Generator

The role of the inferior olive (IO) in the synchronization of cerebellar activities is rooted in two fundamental characteristics. First, IO neurons are electrotonically coupled (80). Second, IO cells are endowed with a variety of voltage-dependent ionic conductances, the distribution and kinetics of which allow them to behave as single-cell oscillators (70,71,81). As shown in Figure 4, the firing of IO cells studied in an in vitro slice preparation is characterized by an initial fast-rising action potential that is prolonged to 10–15 ms by an after-depolarization. This after-depolarizing plateau is followed by a long-lasting after-hyperpolarization, which is usually terminated by an active rebound potential arising at negative membrane potentials, and that can again activate the cell.

Ionic substitution experiments (70) and analysis of extracellular field potentials (71) allowed the identification of the ionic conductances underlying this peculiar electrorhythmicity and the determination of their distribution (see Fig. 4). These experiments revealed that the conventional somatic sodium action potential elicits a dendritic depolarization that results in the opening of the high-threshold calcium conductance. The ensuing calcium entry generates, through the activation of a $g_{K(Ca)}$, a profound hyperpolarization lasting 80–100 ms. As the hyperpolarization diminishes, the low-threshold calcium conductance is activated, thereby generating a rebound action potential, which may initiate another cycle. The resulting 10-Hz membrane potential oscillations can be enhanced by application of harmaline through a dual effect: hyperpolarization of IO neurons and potentiation of the low-threshold calcium conductance.

In pharmacologically untreated slices, intracellular recordings of cell pairs revealed the presence of synchronous oscillations in IO neuronal ensemble (81,82). These quasisinusoidal oscillations appeared to be generated by sub-threshold properties of IO neurons. In fact, this ensemble oscillation was not altered by direct activation of a particular cell. This observation suggests that very little current flows between IO cells and that the electrical coupling between them acts as a low-pass filter (83). Yet, this current flow is sufficient to maintain a uniform oscillation in the different neurons of a given slice.

B. Transmission of Inferior Olive Oscillatory Events to the Cerebellum

The IO axons project to the contralateral cerebellar cortex where they synapse on Purkinje cells (84), after emitting a collateral ending in the cerebellar nuclei; namely, the fastigial, interpositus, and dentate nuclei (85,86). That the climbing fiber system is an afferent pathway in its own right was shown in a series of experiments based on intracellular recordings of Purkinje cells performed in vivo. These experiments demonstrated that harmaline produces a cyclic activation of the

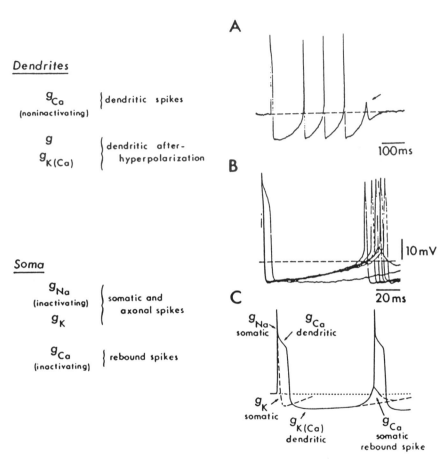

Figure 4 Ionic conductances underlying the oscillatory properties of IO neurons. The left panel describes the distribution of ionic conductances for dendrites and soma. The right panel shows the oscillatory properties of a single IO cell recorded intracellularly in vitro following harmaline administration. In (A), note that the first action potential is longer-lasting and is followed by a more prolonged after-hyperpolarization. The subsequent action potentials are generated at an interval of approximately 100 ms. (B) depicts a superposition of 15 spikes occurring during an oscillatory train. (C) illustrates the ionic conductances responsible for the different components of the oscillatory response. (From Ref. 2.)

climbing fiber system through a direct effect on IO cells. These results were confirmed in the isolated brainstem–cerebellum preparation and in the isolated guinea pig brain maintained in vitro. In these latter experiments, IO stimulation evoked excitatory postsynaptic potential (EPSP)–IPSP sequences or isolated IPSPs in intracellularly recorded neurons of the cerebellar nuclei (87). A rebound burst of action potentials was often seen in cerebellar nucleus neurons at the termination of the IPSPs (87). Moreover, the enhancement of IO oscillatory activities by harmaline administration produced rhythmic 10-Hz IPSPs in cells of the deep cerebellar nuclei (Fig. 5).

That the oscillatory activity of the IO can propagate to several levels of the neuroaxis was demonstrated by simultaneous recordings of the electrical activity in the IO, cerebellum, thalamus, and sensorimotor cortex, before and after harmaline administration (deCurtis and Llinás, unpublished observations). Following harmaline administration, the electrical activity in these regions had a similar dominant frequency, about 8–10 Hz, thereby showing that the rhythmic activity of the IO is transferred along cerebellothalamocortical pathways. In agreement with these findings, experiments performed in vivo by de Montigny and Lamarre (88) and Llinás and Volkind (89) have shown that the harmaline-

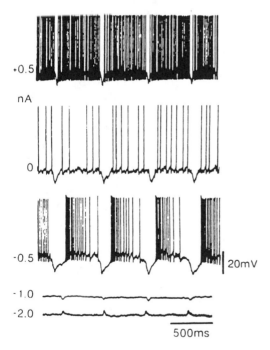

Figure 5 Effect of harmaline on cerebellar nuclear neurons in the isolated brainstem cerebellum preparation. Addition of harmaline (5 mg/ml) to the arterial perfusate generated rhythmic IPSPs, which were studied at different membrane potential by intracellular current injection. At depolarized levels, the sustained discharge of the cell was rhythmically interrupted by the IPSPs. At slightly hyperpolarized levels, the IPSPs were followed by a rebound spike burst. Further hyperpolarization abolished the rebound potential and eventually reversed the IPSPs. (From Ref. 87.)

enhanced IO oscillations can also be transmitted to the bulbar reticular formation, the vestibular nuclei, and spinal motoneurons themselves.

C. Spatiotemporal Organization of the Climbing Fiber System Seen Through Multiple Simultaneous Purkinje Cell Recordings

To study the reflection of IO activities at the cerebellar cortical level, a technique allowing the simultaneous recording of multiple Purkinje cells was developed (90,91). It is based on the independent positioning of glass micropipettes with a robotic arm; this technique now allows one to simultaneously record up to 96 Purkinje cells (92). Purkinje cells are recorded extracellularly at a depth of 150 μm and are physiologically identified by the complex spikes characteristic of climbing fiber activation.

Cross-correlation studies of the complex spike activity recorded in these experiments revealed that climbing fiber activation elicits a virtually synchronous activation in a large number of Purkinje cells. Over a certain region of the folium, Purkinje cells tend to discharge within 1 ms of each other. Moreover, the degree of correlation between Purkinje cells was higher for cells aligned in the rostrocaudal axis (Fig. 6); therefore, suggesting that neighboring electrotonically coupled IO cells project to the cerebellar cortex in well-defined rostrocaudal bands (90), as suggested by anatomical and physiological findings (93).

The crucial role played by the gap junctions coupling neighboring IO cells in the synchronization of Purkinje cell bands was confirmed by studying the activation of Purkinje cells following surface stimulation of the cerebellar cortex (90), taking advantage of the so-called olivary reflex (84). Because the antidromic invasion of IO cells and subsequent spread of activation within the IO survives abolition of synaptic transmission (70), the IO reflex was used to map the distribution of the climbing fibers originating from coupled IO cells. In agreement with the results of the cross-correlation analysis of spontaneous complex spike activity, it was found that antidromic activation of climbing fibers is followed by a synchronous return volley in rostrocaudal bands of Purkinje cells (90).

D. GABAergic Control of the Electrotonic Coupling Between Inferior Olive Cells

Following the discovery of gap junctions and their occurrence at well-defined sites, the IO glomerulus, it was proposed that this structure could be the site of dynamic modulations of electrotonic coupling by dendritic shunting (94). It is now known that the dendritic spines, through which IO cells are electrotonically coupled, receive a GABAergic input from the deep cerebellar nuclei (95–97) and a non-GABAergic innervation from the mesodiencephalic junction (95,98,99). To

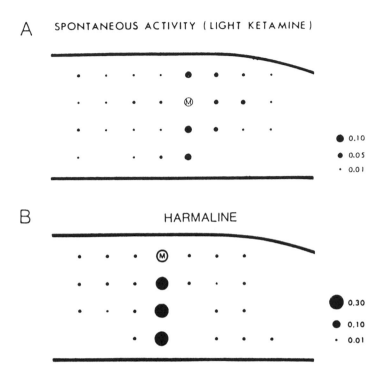

Figure 6   Cross-correlation of spontaneously occurring fiber activation (CFA) of Purkinje cells over a folium. The correlation coefficient between the CFA of a master Purkinje cell (M) and 27 other Purkinje cells recorded in a rectangular matrix (4 × 8) as indicated by the location of the dots in (A) and (B). Electrodes were individually placed at a 250-μm distance from each other. The correlation coefficient is indicated by the area of the circle at each recording sites (see calibration to the right). Hatched area shows the location of a vessel that prevented recording from all 32 electrodes. (B) The correlation coefficient between CFAs of Purkinje cells after administration of harmaline. Note the increased correlation and the preservation of the spatial organization of the cross-correlation that is seen in control experiments (A). (From Ref. 127.)

determine if the rostrocaudal organization of climbing fiber activation reflects a fixed anatomical property of the IO, or is a manifestation of the dynamic control of IO coupling by extraolivary afferents, experiments were designed to block the action of the GABAergic synapses ending on the IO glomeruli (100).

To this end, local pressure injections of the GABAergic blockers bicuculline and picrotoxin were performed in the IO. Their effect on the synchronization of Purkinje cell activity was then determined in the contralateral cerebellar hemisphere. Following these injections (Fig. 7), the rostrocaudal bands of correlated

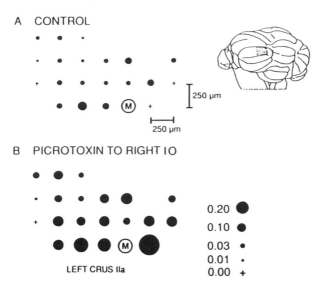

A   CONTROL

250 μm

250 μm

B   PICROTOXIN TO RIGHT IO

0.20 ●
0.10 ●
0.03 •
0.01 ·
LEFT CRUS IIa   0.00 +

Figure 7   Effect of local injection of picrotoxin in the contralateral IO on the degree of cross-correlation between CFAs of Purkinje cells located in Crus IIa folium. (A) Control and (B) following picrotoxin injection. See legend of preceding figure for details. (From Ref. 103.)

complex spike activity were abolished, and the synchronization of Purkinje cells discharges encompassed most of the area recorded by the multiple electrode matrix. In agreement with the anatomical data indicating that the GABAergic input ending on the dendritic spines of IO neurons originates from the deep cerebellar nuclei, identical results were obtained following damage to the contralateral cerebellar nuclei (101).

E.   Relation Between Inferior Olive Oscillatory Events and the Physiological Tremor

The abolition of the physiological tremor following lesions of the cerebellum (3) suggests that the rhythmic activity of the olivocerebellar system might be involved in the genesis of this tremor. To study the implication of the olivocerebellar system in this form of action tremor, the timing of complex spike activity relative to the tremorlike 10-Hz vibrissal movements was studied in the rat (92). This motor event was chosen because the vibrissa constitute a load-change free motor event where the movement can be unambiguously determined.

The cycle of vibrissal vibration was preceded by climbing fiber activation of a

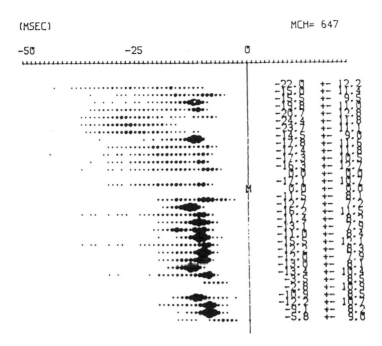

Figure 8 Relationship between vibrissal movements and the onset of complex spike activity in 29 Purkinje cells. The position of each dot represent the time of onset of the spike relative to the onset of vibrissal movement (0 ms). The diameter of the dots is proportional to the number of times it fired at that interval. A total of 647 vibrissal movements were used for this figure. The mean and standard deviation of the onset time of the activity of each cell is shown on the right. (From Ref. 103.)

significant proportion of Purkinje cells (Fig. 8). In the raster display of Figure 8, each line illustrates the complex spike activity of a particular Purkinje cell relative to the onset of a vibrissal cycle. The size of the circles is proportional to the number of times a Purkinje cell fired a complex spike at a particular interval, relative to the onset of movement. These results illustrate clearly that a number of Purkinje cells discharged complex spikes in a consistent manner 15–25 ms before the movement. In agreement with these results, Semba et al. (102) have shown that damage to the IO impairs the 10-Hz vibrissal movement.

These results imply that the intrinsic properties of IO neurons and their electrotonic coupling contribute to generate a distributed oscillatory event involving an important proportion of Purkinje cells. Furthermore, this oscillatory event is translated in a timing signal used in motor control (2,103).

IV. INVOLVEMENT OF THE OLIVOCEREBELLAR AND THALAMOCORTICAL SYSTEMS IN PATHOLOGICAL ACTION TREMORS AND RELATED PHENOMENA

On the basis of their appearance, pathological action tremors are usually divided in two main classes (3): tremors occurring during maintained posture; and those appearing during the initiation, performance, or termination of actual movements. These tremors rarely appear in isolation and often coexist to various degrees in the same subjects. To complicate the matter further, the different tremors have been linked to various pathological conditions affecting one or more functional systems.

In the discussion that follows, we will consider some conditions that give rise to action tremors and attempt to relate given structural lesions to the known oscillatory properties of the olivocerebellar and thalamocortical systems.

A. Palatal Myoclonus: Synchronized Internal Olive Oscillations Resulting from Lesions of the Dentate Nucleus

The term *palatal myoclonus* refers to involuntary rhythmic 1- to 3-Hz movements of the soft palate and larynx. It can occur in isolation or be accompanied by similar movements of the mouth, face, eyes, and tongue. In these cases, the muscle contractions are time-locked in the different body parts (104). Involvement of other skeletal muscles occurs occasionally.

In a recent review of the cases published in the literature since the end of the 19th century, Deuschl et al. (105) distinguished two forms of palatal myoclonus. In cases of *essential palatal myoclonus*, autopsy fails to reveal signs of structural lesions, and the involuntary movements are susceptible to sleep, anesthesia, and coma. In contrast, *symptomatic palatal myoclonus* is resistant to sleep, and autopsy usually reveals a hypertrophy of IO neurons associated with a fibrillary gliosis (106,107). These morphological changes at the IO level appear to result from a lesion of the pathway linking the contralateral dentate nucleus to the IO (108,109). In support of this contention, a topographical relation was found between the location of the degenerative changes in the IO and contralateral dentate nucleus (108).

Because of these autopsy findings and of the fixed phase relation between the involuntary muscular contractions characterizing palatal myoclonus, it has been proposed that the IO is the central pacemaker in this condition (110). The evidence presented in Section III supports these early intuitions. First, by virtue of their intrinsic membrane properties (70,71) and of the gap junctions coupling them (80), IO cells are able to generate synchronized oscillations that can be transmitted to the cerebellar cortex through olivocerebellar axons (90,91). Second, the degree of electrotonic coupling between IO neurons is controlled by a GABAergic input, arising in the deep cerebellar nuclei. Abolition of this inhibitory control by dentate lesions or local application of GABAergic antagonists induces synchronous complex spike firing in distant Purkinje cells spread over a large area of the cerebellar cortex (100,101).

These results imply that the pathological changes observed at the IO level in palatal myoclonus do not reflect transneuronal degeneration, but hypersynchronous activity of IO neurons, as a result of a decrease in dentate inhibition. In agreement with this suggestion, a recent positron emission tomography (PET) study revealed that the glucose uptake of IO neurons is increased in symptomatic palatal myoclonus (111). Moreover, electron microscopic observations revealed expanded cisternal profiles (112) and increased mitochondria (113). Finally, the variety of afferents ending on IO cells should prevent transneuronal degeneration of IO cells following removal of the inhibitory dentate input (112).

The precise pathways through which the result of IO hypersynchronous oscillatory activities are transmitted to brainstem motoneurons are unknown. The cerebelloreticular and cerebellovestibular pathways are probably involved.

B. Cerebellar Action Tremors

Because the structural lesions present in most of the conditions associated with cerebellar action tremors usually involve several nervous structures, the pathophysiology of this type of tremors is poorly understood. In addition to trying to localize the structural alterations responsible for this disorder, it is crucial to determine if we are dealing with an abnormal central oscillator, or simply with the consequence of motor discoordination. In the latter event, the so-called action tremors would represent reflex attempts at correcting dysmetric movements. Here, the tremorlike movements would be difficult to distinguish from true tremor, because the maximal speed for movement correction may be quite close to tremor frequency (2). A strong argument in favor of the involvement of a central oscillator is the abolition of the tremor by a central lesion.

On the basis of their appearance, Marsden (3) has distinguished three forms of cerebellar tremors: kinetic or intention tremor, tremor occurring during maintained posture, and titubation. To our knowledge, the only type of cerebellar tremor for which there is convincing evidence of the involvement of a central generator is the kinetic or intention tremor.

1. Kinetic Tremor

The kinetic type tremor appears during movements and increases in amplitude as the movement reaches its goal. The severity of this 3- to 5-Hz tremor varies from a low-amplitude tremor, appearing at the termination of the movement, to large-amplitude oscillations, present when the subject attempts to adopt a posture. Because this form of tremor is observed in a variety of conditions, it is unclear if these diverse manifestations reflect different degrees of the same physiological aberration, or of altogether different mechanisms. Therefore, we will consider only the mildest forms of kinetic tremor.

Although the phase of the kinetic tremor can be reset by peripheral inputs (114), it persists deafferentation of the affected limb (115). However, the main argument in favor of the involvement of a central generator in the genesis of the kinetic tremor, is that it is abolished by lesions of the Vim nucleus (116). It is commonly believed that the kinetic tremor results from a lesion of the main neocerebellar output because a similar tremor can be produced in primates by interrupting the cerebellodentothalamic pathway (117,118). There are some clinicopathological observations consistent with this explanation (119).

2. Functional Consequences of the Removal of the Cerebellar Input for Thalamic Operations

Intracellular recordings in vivo suggest that the cerebellothalamic input (see Sect. II.C.1) exerts a tonic depolarizing influence on recipient thalamic cells (75,76). Indeed, the spontaneous activity of cat VL neurons, the cat equivalent of the human Vim, is characterized by the repetitive occurrence (20–70 Hz) of fast prepotentials (FPPs) which occasionally trigger fast sodium spikes. Stimulation of the deep cerebellar nuclei elicits short-latency FPPs of identical amplitude and time course, thereby suggesting that these tonically occurring FPPs reflect the constant synaptic bombardment of VL neurons by dentatothalamic axons.

Removal of this tonic depolarizing input probably produces a profound hyperpolarization of the thalamic neurons normally receiving this input. In agreement with this suggestion, removal of an important excitatory input, such as the corticothalamic fibers, provokes a membrane hyperpolarization that brings the membrane potential of thalamic neurons in the activation range of the I_h. As a result, the interplay between the I_h, the low-threshold calcium conductance and the calcium-dependent potassium conductance generates 0.5- to 4-Hz oscillations (74–76; see Sect. II.D.3). It is likely that the interruption of the cerebellothalamic pathway has a similar effect on the thalamic neurons normally receiving this input.

The propensity of Vim thalamic neurons to generate slow intrinsic oscillations as a result of this lesion is probably reinforced by the synaptic organization of the thalamocortical network. Indeed, the dorsal thalamus is reciprocally connected with the reticularis (RE) thalamic nucleus, a thin (0.5-mm) sheet of GABAergic neurons (120) surrounding the dorsal thalamus. The connections between the dorsal thalamus and the RE nucleus are organized in such a way that particular districts of the RE nucleus are related to specific sectors of the dorsal thalamus (121,122). Moreover, there are reciprocal connections between the dorsal thalamus and the cerebral cortex, with corticothalamic axons contacting the various cell types present in the thalamus: RE neurons, relay cells, and interneurons (27).

The insertion of intrinsically oscillating Vim neurons in this recurrent synaptic network probably tends to synchronize their activity into a rhythmic population

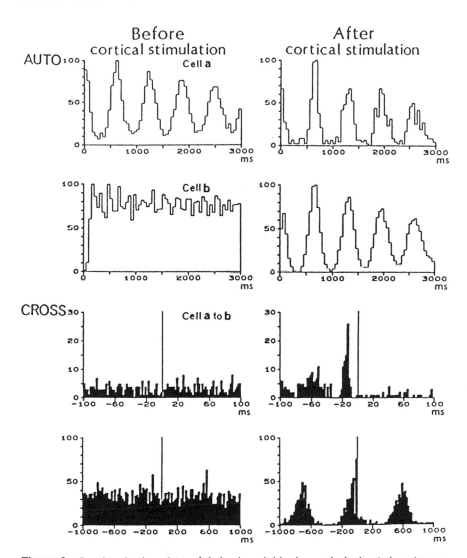

Figure 9 Synchronization of dorsal thalamic activities by cortical stimulation. Autocorrelogram (top) and cross-correlogram (bottom) of two simultaneously recorded ventral lateral thalamic neurons (cell a and b) before (left) and after (right) cortical stimulation. Two different bins were used to compute the cross-correlograms (2 ms and 20 ms). Before cortical stimulation, cell a was rhythmically active, whereas cell b was not. After cortical stimulation, cell b became rhythmically active at the same frequency as cell a (1.6 Hz). The cross-correlogram revealed that the firing of cell a preceded that of cell b by about 10–20 ms. (From Ref. 76.)

network probably tends to synchronize their activity into a rhythmic population event. This phenomenon was demonstrated recently in pairs of dorsal thalamic neurons, the discharge of which was initially uncorrelated (76). Following the application of a few electrical stimuli to the cerebral cortex, their discharge became synchronized (Fig. 9). We can only speculate about the sequence of events leading to the synchronization of slowly oscillating thalamic cells. The ability of RE neurons to generate IPSPs in Vim neurons is probably central to this phenomenon. A likely mechanism is that random Vim burst discharges, transmitted through thalamo-RE and thalamocortico-RE pathways, lead to the activation of several RE neurons. As a result, the GABAergic RE cells generate IPSPs in a subpopulation of Vim cells. The combined influence of this IPSP and of the intrinsic hyperpolarization generated by $g_{K(Ca)}$ will, at the termination of the hyperpolarization, tend to produce a synchronous burst discharge in a number of cells through the activation of the low-threshold conductance. Repetition of this sequence of events will progressively synchronize the oscillatory activity of more and more Vim neurons.

The result of this synchronizing process will be transmitted to the motor cortex along Vim axons (see Sect. II.C.1). The translation of this slow rhythmic activity into motor commands only during voluntary movements probably reflects the exclusive involvement of this circuit in the production of voluntary movements.

V. TREMOR AS A WINDOW TO NORMAL BRAIN FUNCTION

Central to the genesis of the tremors discussed in the foregoing is the ability of IO and thalamic neurons to generate intrinsic membrane oscillations. Intracellular studies performed in recent years indicate that the capability of neurons to behave as oscillators or resonators is not a particular property of these neuronal types, but an ubiquitous feature of central mammalian neurons (123,124).

One clue to the functional significance of this prevalent feature comes from the realization that these individual neuronal oscillators are inserted into complex synaptic networks that tend to synchronize their activity into coherent population events. The implications of this phenomenon are twofold. First, this synchronization constitutes an energetically efficient means to control the functional state of all the neurons belonging to a particular neuronal system. The importance of achieving accurate control over a large number of functionally related cells is that brain functions, such as movement execution, necessitates the coordination of multiple parallel neuronal operations, both within and between different neuronal systems.

Second, the synchronization of individual neuronal oscillators into a global population event generates a timing signal that can be used to synchronize the activity of multiple parallel neuronal systems into a coordinated process. Evidence for the use of a time-signal generator in the coordination of motor operations comes from the work of Travis (125) and Goodman and Kelso (126) who showed a systematic relation between the phase of the physiological tremor and movement initiation. For instance, upward movements were found to be initiated during the ascending phase of the physiological tremor. These results suggest that the nervous system uses intrinsic oscillations to reduce the amount of energy required to produce movements and to coordinate the activity of the multiple neuronal systems involved in motor control.

ACKNOWLEDGMENTS

This work was supported by NIH grant NS13742. Denis Paré was a postdoctoral fellow supported by the Medical Research Council of Canada.

REFERENCES

1. Findley LJ, Capildeu R. Movement Disorders: Tremor. London: Macmillan Press, 1984:493.
2. Llinás R. Rebound excitation as the physiological basis for tremor: a biophysical study of the oscillatory properties of mammalian central neurons in vitro. In: Findley LJ, Capiledo R, eds. Movement Disorders: Tremor. London: Macmillan Press, 1984: 165–182.
3. Marsden CD. Origins of normal and pathological tremor. In: Findley LJ, Capiledo R, eds. Movement Disorders: Tremor. London: Macmillan Press, 1984:37–84.
4. Adams RD, Victor M. Principles of Neurology. New York: McGraw-Hill, 1984: 1094.
5. Bishop GH, Clare MH, Price J. Pattern of tremors in normal and pathological conditions. J Appl Physiol 1948; 1:123.
6. Schwab RS, Cobb S. Simultaneous electromyograms and electroencephalograms in paralysis agitans. J Neurophysiol 1939; 2:36.
7. Rondot P, Bathien N. Pathophysiology of parkinsonian tremor. In: Desmedt JE, ed. Progress in Clinical Neurophysiology. Vol. 5: Physiological Tremor, Pathological Tremor and Clonus. Basel: S. Karger, 1978:138–149.
8. Hornykiewicz O. Metabolism of brain dopamine in human parkinsonism: neurochemical and clinical aspects. In: Costa E, Cote LJ, Yahr MD, eds. Biochemistry and Pharmacology of the Basal Ganglia. New York: Raven Press, 1966:171–185.
9. Leriche R. Radiocotomie cervicale pour un tremblement parkinsonien. Lyon Med 1914; 122:1075–1076.
10. Pollock LJ, Davis L. Muscle tone in parkinsonian states. Arch Neurol Psychiatry 1930; 23:303–319.
11. Lee RG, Stein RB. Resetting of tremor by mechanical perturbations: a comparison of essential tremor and parkinsonian tremor. Ann Neurol 1981; 10:523–531.
12. Teravainen H, Evarts E, Calne DB. Effects of kinesthetic inputs on parkinsonian tremor. In: Poirier LJ, Sourkes TL, Bedard PJ, eds. Advances in Neurology, Vol. 24. New York: Raven, 1979:161–173.

13. Hagbarth KE. Muscle spindle discharge patterns in tremor and clonus. In: Findley LJ, Capildeo R, eds. Movement Disorders: Tremor. London: Macmillan Press, 1984: 157–164.
14. Bucy PC, Case TJ. Tremor: physiologic mechanism and abolition by surgical means. Arch. Neurol Psychiatry 1949; 41:721–746.
15. Klemme RM. Surgical treatment of dystonia, paralysis agitans and athetosis. Arch Neurol Psychiatry 1940; 44:926.
16. Guiot G, Brion S, Fardeau M, Bettaieb A, Molina P. Dyskinésie volitionelle d'attitude supprimée par la coagulation thalamo-capsulaire. Rev Neurol 1960; 102: 220–229.
17. Houdart R, Mamo H. Résultats lointains de la coagulation pallidale dans les syndromes parkinsoniens. Neurochirurgie 1964; 10; 455–462.
18. Albe-Fessard D, Arfel G, Guiot G. Activités électriques caractéristiques de quelques structures cérébrales chez l'homme. Ann Chir 1963; 17:1185–1214.
19. Guiot G, Hardy J, Albe FD, Délimitation précise des structures sous-corticales et identification de noyaux thalamiques chez l'homme par l'électrophysiologie stéréotaxique. Neurochirurgia 1962; 5:1–18.
20. Jasper HH, Bertrand G. Thalamic units involved in somatic sensation and voluntary and involuntary movements in man. In: Purpura DP, Yahr MD, eds. The Thalamus. New York: Columbia University Press, 1966:365–390.
21. Bertrand G, Jasper HH. Microelectrode recording of unit activity in the human thalamus. Confin Neurol 1965; 26:205–208.
22. Fukamachi A, Ohye C, Narabayashi H. Delineation of the thalamic nuclei with a microelectrode in stereotaxic surgery for parkinsonism and cerebral palsy. J Neurosurg 1973; 39:214–225.
23. Reichert T. Stereotaxic surgery for treatment of Parkinson's syndrome. Prog Neurol Surg 1973; 5:1–78.
24. Jasper HH. Recording from microelectrodes in stereotactic surgery for Parkinson's disease. J Neurosurg 1966; 24:219–221.
25. Ohye C, Narabayashi H. Physiological study of presumed ventralis intermedius neurons in the human thalamus. J Neurosurg 1979; 50:290–297.
26. Schaltenbrand G, Bailey P. Introduction to Stereotaxis With an Atlas of the Human Brain. New York: Grune & Stratton, 1959:356.
27. Jones EG. The Thalamus. New York: Plenum Press, 1985:708.
28. Poggio GF, Mountcastsle VB. The functional properties of ventrobasal thalamic neurons studied in unanesthetized monkeys. J Neurophysiol 1963; 26:775–806.
29. Jones EG, Friedman DP. Projection pattern of functional components of thalamic ventrobasal complex in monkey somatosensory cortex. J Neurophysiol 1982; 48: 521–544.
30. Asanuma C, Thach WT, Jones EG. Distribution of cerebellar terminations and their relation to other afferent terminations in the ventral lateral thalamic region of the monkey. Brain Res 1983; 286:237–65.
31. Kultas-Ilinsky K, Ribak CE, Peterson GM, Oertel WH. A description of the GABAergic neurons and axon terminals in the motor nuclei of the cat thalamus. J Neurosci 1985; 5:1346–1369.

32. Penney JB, Young AB. GABA as the pallidothalamic transmitter: implications for basal ganglia function. Brain Res 1981; 207:195–199.

33. Kuo JS, Carpenter MB. organization of pallidothalamic projections in the rhesus monkey. J Comp Neurol 1973; 151:201–236.

34. Parent A, DeBellefeuille L. Organization of efferent projects from the internal segment of the globus pallidus in primate as revealed fluorescence retrograde labeling method. Brain Res 1982; 245:201–213.

35. Beckstead RM, Domesik VB, Nauta WJH. Efferent connections of the substantia nigra and ventral tegmental area in the rat. Brain Res 1979; 175:191–217.

36. Asanuma C, Thach WT, Jones EG. Cytoarchitectonic delineation of the ventral lateral thalamic region in the monkey. Brain Res 1983; 286:219–35.

37. Jones EG, Wise SP, Coulter JD. Differential thalamic relationship of sensory motor and parietal cortical fields in monkeys. J Comp Neurol 1979; 183:833–882.

38. Tracey DJ, Asanuma C, Jones EG, Porter R. Thalamic relay to motor cortex: afferent pathways from brainstem, cerebellum and spinal cord in monkeys. J Neurophysiol 1980; 44:532–554.

39. Herkenham M. The afferent and efferent connections of the ventromedial thalamic nucleus in the rat. J Comp Neurol 1979; 183:487–518.

40. Glenn LL, Hada J, Roy JP, Deschênes M, Steriade M. Anterograde tracer and field potential analysis of the neocortical layer. Neuroscience 1982; 7:1861–1877.

41. Lenz FA, Kwan HC, Dostrovsky JO, Tasker RR, Murphy JT, Lenz YE. Single unit analysis of the human ventral thalamic nuclear group. Brain 1990; 113:1795–1821.

42. Bates JAV. The significance of tremor phasic units in the human thalamus. In: Gillingham FJ, Donaldson IML, eds. Third Symposium on Parkinson's Disease. Edinburgh: Churchill Livingstone, 1969:251–259.

43. Crowell RM, Perret E, Siegfried J, Villoz JP. "Movement units" and "tremor phasic units" in the human thalamus. Brain Res 1968; 11:481–488.

44. Donaldson I. The properties of some human thalamic units. Brain 1973; 96: 419–440.

45. Lenz FA, Tasker RR, Kwan HC, et al. Single unit analysis of the ventral thalamic nuclear group: correlation of thalamic "tremor cells" with the 3–6 Hz component of parkinsonian tremor. J Neurosci 1988; 8:754–764.

46. Raeva S. Localization in human thalamus of units triggered during "verbal commands," voluntary movements and tremor. Electroencephalogr Clin Neurophysiol 1986; 63:160–173.

47. Velasco F, Molina NP. Electrophysiological topography of the human diencephalon. J Neurosurg 1973; 38:204–214.

48. Hardy J, Bertrand C, Martinez N. Activités cellulaires thalamiques liées au tremblement parkinsonien. Neurochirurgie 1964; 10:449–457.

49. Albe-Fessard D, Guiot G, Lamarre Y, Arfel G. Activation of thalamocortical projections related to tremorogenic processes. In: Purpura DP, Yahr MD, eds. The Thalamus. New York: Columbia University Press, 1966:237–249.

50. Bertrand C, Martinez SN, Hardy J, Molina-Negro P, Velasco F. Stereotaxic surgery for parkinsonism. Neurol Surg 1973; 5:79–112.

51. Lamarre Y, Joffroy AJ. Thalamic unit activity in monkey with experimental tremor. In: Barbeau A, McDowell FH, eds. L-Dopa and Parkinsonism. Philadelphia: FA Davis, 1970:163–170.

52. Lamarre Y. Tremorogenic mechanisms in primates. Adv Neurol 1975; 10:23–34.

53. Macpherson JM, Rasmusson DD, Murphy JT. Activities of neurons in "motor" thalamus during control of limb movement in the primate. J Neurophysiol 1980; 44: 11–28.

54. Strick PL. Activity of ventrolateral thalamic neurons during arm movement. J Neurophysiol 1976; 39:1032–1044.

55. Bertrand C. Localization of lesions. J Neurosurg 1966; 24:446–448.

56. Nicoll RA, Malenka RC, Kauer JA. Functional comparison of neurotransmitter receptor subtypes in mammalian central nervous system. Physiol Rev 1990; 70:513–565.

57. Siggins GR, Gruol DL. Mechanisms of transmitter action in the vertebrate central nervous system. In: Mountcastle VB, Bloom FE, eds. Handbook of Physiology, Sect. 1, Vol. 4. Bethesda: American Physiological Society, 1986:1–114.

58. Filion M, Boucher R, Bédard P. Globus pallidus unit activity in the monkey during the induction of parkinsonism by 1-methyl-4-phenyl-1,2,3,6-tetrahydropyridine (MPTP). Soc Neurosci Abstr 1985; 11:1160.

59. Miller WC, DeLong MR. Altered tonic activity of neurones in the globus pallidus and subthalamic nucleus in the primate MPTP model of parkinsonism. In: Carpenter MS, Jayaraman A, eds. The Basal Ganglia II. Advances in Behaviour Biology. New York: Plenum Press, 1987:415–427.

60. Filion M. Effects of interruption of the nigrostriatal pathway and of dopaminergic agents on the spontaneous activity of globus pallidus neurons in the awake monkey. Brain Res 1979; 178:425–441.

61. DeVito JL, Anderson ME, Walsh KE. A horseradish peroxidase study of afferent connections of the globus pallidus in *Macaca mulatta*. Exp Brain Res 1980; 38: 65–73.

62. Kita H, Chang HT, Kitai ST. Pallidal inputs to subthalamus: intracellular analysis. Brain Res 1983; 264:255–265.

63. Bergman H, Wichmann T, DeLong M. Reversal of experimental parkinsonism by lesions of the subthalamic nucleus. Science 1990; 249:1436–1438.

64. Yamamoto T, Hassler R, Huber C, Wagner A, Sasaki K. Electrophysiologic studies on the pallido- and cerebellothalamic projections in squirrel monkeys. Exp Brain Res 1983; 51:77–87.

65. Yamamoto T, Noda T, Miyata M, Nishimura Y. Electrophysiological and morphological studies on thalamic neurons receiving entopedunculo- and cerebellothalamic projections in the cat. Brain Res 1984; 301:231–242.

66. Jahnsen H, Llinás R. Electrophysiological properties of guinea pig thalamic neurones: an in vitro study. J Physiol (Lond) 1984; 349:205–226.

67. Jahnsen H, Llinás R. Ionic basis for the electroresponsiveness and oscillatory properties of guinea-pig thalamic neurons in vitro. J Physiol (Lond) 1984; 349: 227–248.

68. Llinás R, Jahnsen H. Electrophysiology of mammalian thalamic neurones in vitro. Nature 1982; 297:406–408.

69. Deschênes M, Paradis M, Roy JP, Steriade M. Electrophysiology of neurons of lateral thalamic nuclei in cat: resting properties and burst discharges. J Neurophysiol 1984; 51:1196–1219.
70. Llinás R, Yarom Y. Electrophysiology of mammalian inferior olivary neurones in vitro. Different types of voltage-dependent ionic conductances. J Physiol (Lond) 1981; 315:549–567.
71. Llinás R, Yarom Y. Properties and distribution of ionic conductances generating electroresponsiveness of mammalian inferior olivary neurones in vitro. J Physiol (Lond) 1981; 315:569–584.
72. Crunelli V, Kelly JS, Leresche N, Pirchio M. The ventral and dorsal lateral geniculate nucleus of the rat: intracellular recordings in vitro. J Physiol (Lond) 1987; 384:587–601.
73. McCormick DA, Pape HC. Acetylcholine inhibits identified interneurones in the cat lateral geniculate nucleus. Nature 1988; 334:246–248.
74. McCormick DA, Pape HC. Properties of a hyperpolarization-activated cation current and its role in rhythmic oscillation in thalamic relay neurons. J Physiol (Lond) 1990; 431:291–318.
75. CurróDossi R, Nunez A, Steriade M. Electrophysiology of a slow (0.5–4 Hz) intrinsic oscillation of cat thalamocortical neurones in vivo. J Physiol (Lond) 1992; 447:215–234.
76. Steriade M, CurróDossi R, Nunez A. Network modulation of a slow intrinsic oscillation of cat thalamocortical neurons implicated in sleep delta waves: cortically induced synchronization and brainstem cholinergic suppression. J Neurosci 1991; 11:3200–3217.
77. Paré D, CurróDossi R, Steriade M. Neuronal basis of the parkinsonian resting tremor: a hypothesis and its implications for treatment. Neuroscience 1990; 35: 217–226.
78. Alberts WW. A simple view of parkinsonian tremor. Electrical stimulation of cortex adjacent to the rolandic fissure in awake man. Brain Res 1972; 44:357–369.
79. Sutton GG, Sykes K. The effect of withdrawal of visual presentation of errors upon the frequency spectrum of tremor in a manual task. J Physiol (Lond) 1967; 190: 281–293.
80. Llinás R, Baker R, Sotelo C. Electrotonic coupling between neurons in cat inferior olive. J Neurophysiol 1974; 37:560–571.
81. Llinás R, Yarom Y. Oscillatory properties of guinea-pig inferior olivary neurons and their pharmacological modulation: an in vitro study. J Physiol (Lond) 1986; 376:163–182.
82. Benardo LS, Foster RE. Oscillatory behavior in inferior olive neurons: mechanism, modulation, cell aggregates. Brain Res Bull 1986; 17:773–784.
83. Bennett MVL. Electrical transmission: a functional analysis and comparison to chemical transmission. In: Kandel E, ed. Handbook of Physiology. Vol 1. Cellular Biology of Neurons. Baltimore: Williams & Wilkins, 1977:357–416.
84. Eccles JC, Llinás R, Sasaki K. The excitatory synaptic action of climbing fibers on the Purkinje cells of the cerebellum. J Physiol (Lond) 1966; 182:268–296.
85. Bloedel JR, Courville J. Cerebellar afferent systems. In: Brookhart JM, Mountcastle

VB, eds. Handbook of Physiology Sect 1: The Nervous System. Bethesda: American Physiological Society. 1981:735–830.

86. Courville J, Augustine JR, Martel P. Projections from the inferior olive to the cerebellar nuclei in the cat demonstrated by retrograde transport of horseradish peroxidase. Brain Res 1977; 130:405–419.

87. Llinás R, Mühlethaler M. An electrophysiological study of the in vitro perfused brainstem/cerebellum of adult guinea pig. J Physiol (Lond) 1988; 404:215–240.

88. de Montigny C, Lamarre Y. Rhythmic activity induced by harmaline in the olivo-cerebello-bulbar system of the cat. Brain Res 1973; 53:81–95.

89. Llinás R, Volkind RA. The olivocerebellar system: functional properties as revealed by harmaline-induced tremor. Exp Brain Res 1973; 18:69–87.

90. Llinás R, Sasaki K. The functional organization of the olivocerebellar system as examined by multiple Purkinje cell recordings. Eur J Neurosci 1989; 1:587–602.

91. Sasaki K, Bower JM, Llinás R. Multiple Purkinje cell recording in rodent cerebellar cortex. Eur J Neurosci 1989; 1:572–586.

92. Fukuda M, Yamamoto T, Llinás R. Simultaneous recordings from Purkinje cells of different folia in the rat cerebellum and their relation to movement. Soc Neurosci Abstr 1987; 13:536.

93. Oscarsson O. Functional organization of olivary projection to the cerebellar anterior lobe. In: Courville J, de Montigny C, Lamarre Y, eds. The Inferior Olivary Nucleus: Anatomy and Physiology. New York: Raven Press, 1980:279–289.

94. Llinás R. Bodwitch lecture: motor aspects of cerebellar control. Physiologist 1974; 17:19–46.

95. de Zeeuw CI, Holstege JC, Calkoen F, Ruigrok TJH, Voogd J. A new combination of WGA-HRP anterograde tracing and GABA-immunocytochemistry applied to afferents of the cat inferior olive at the ultrastructural level. Brain Res 1988; 447:369–375.

96. Nelson B, Barmack NH, Mugnaini E. A GABAergic cerebello-olivary projection in the rat. Soc Neurosci Abstr 1984; 10:539.

97. Tolbert DL, Massopust LC, Murphy MG, Young PA. The anatomical organization of the cerebello-olivary projection in the cat. J Comp Neurol 1976; 170:525–544.

98. de Zeeuw CI, Holstege JC, Ruigrok TJH, Voogd J. An ultrastructural sturdy of the GABAergic, the cerebellar and the mesodiencephalic innervation of the cat medial accessory olive: anterograde tracing combined with immunocytochemistry. J Comp Neurol 1989; 284:12–35.

99. Onodera S. Olivary projections from the mesodiencephalic structures in the cat studied by means of axonal transport of horseradish peroxidase and tritiated amino acids. J Comp Neurol 1984; 227:37–49.

100. Lang E, Chou M, Sugihara I, Llinás R. Intraolivary injection of picrotoxin causes reorganization of complex spike activity. Soc Neurosci Abstr 1989; 15:179.

101. Lang E, Sugihara I, Llinás R. Lesions of cerebellar nuclei, but not of mesencephalic structures alters the spatial pattern of complex spike synchronicity as demonstrated by multiple electrode recordings. Soc Neurosci Abstr 1990; 16:894.

102. Semba K, Komisaruk BR. Neural substrates of two different rhythmical vibrissal movements in the rat. Neuroscience 1984; 12:761–774.

103. Llinás R. The noncontinuous nature of movement execution. In: Humphrey DR,

Freund HJ, eds. Motor Control: Concepts and Issues. New York: John Wiley & Sons, 1991:223–242.

104. Lapresle J. Palatal myoclonus. Adv. Neurol 1986; 43:265–273.

105. Deuschl G, Mischke G, Schenk Z, Schulte-Montig J, Lucking CH. Symptomatic and essential rhythmic palatal myoclonus. Brain 1990; 113:1645–1672.

106. Aberfeld DC. The hypertrophic degeneration of the olives. Acta Neurol Scand 1966; 42:296–306.

107. Gauthier JC, Blackwood W. Enlargement of the inferior olivary nucleus in association with lesions of the central tegmental tract of dentate nucleus. Brain 1961; 84:341–361.

108. Lapresle J. Correspondance somatotopique, secteur par secteur, des dégénérescences de l'olive bulbaire consécutives à des lésions limitées du noyau dentelé control-latéral: étude des observations anatomiques. Rev Neurol 1965; 113:439–448.

109. Lapresle J, Ben Hamida M. Contribution à la connaissance de la voie dento-olivaire: étude anatomique de deux cas de dégénérescence hypertrophique de l'olive bulbaire secondaire à un ramollissement limité de la calotte mésencéphalique. Presse Med 1968; 76:1226–1230.

110. Tielles JO. Les myoclonies vélo-palatines. Considérations anatomiques et physiopathologiques. Rev Neurol 1968; 119:165–171.

111. Dubinsky RM, Hallett M. Palatal myoclonus and facial involvement in other types of myoclonus. Adv Neurol 1988; 49:263–278.

112. Barron KD, Dentinger MP, Koeppen AH. Fine structure of neurons of the hypertrophied human inferior olive. J Neuropathol Exp Neurol 1982; 41:186–203.

113. Vuia O. Aspects morphologiques (optiques et ultrastructuraux) de l'hypertrophie de l'olive bulbaire. Rev Neurol 1976; 132:51–61.

114. Villis T, Hore J. Effects of changes in mechanical state of limb on cerebellar intention tremor. J Neurophysiol 1977; 40:1214–1224.

115. Gillman S, Carr D. Hollenberg J. Kinematic effects of deafferentation and cerebellar ablation. Brain 1976; 99:311–330.

116. Narabayashi H. Surgical approach to tremor. In: Marsden CD, Fahn S, eds. Movement Disorders. London: Butterworths, 1982; 292–299.

117. Brooks VB, Kozlovskaya IB, Atkin A, Horvath FE, Uno M. Effects of cooling dentate nucleus on tracking-task performance in monkeys. J Neurophysiol 1973; 36: 974–995.

118. Growdon H, Chambers WW, Liu CN. An experimental dyskinesia in the rhesus monkey. Brain 1967; 90:603–632.

119. Fahn S. Cerebellar tremor: clinical aspects. In: Findley LJ, Capildeo R, eds. Movement Disorders: Tremor. London: Macmillan Press 1984:355–363.

120. Houser CR, Vaughn JE, Barber RP, Roberts E. GABA neurons is the major cell type of the nucleus reticularis thalami. Brain Res 1980; 200:341–354.

121. Jones EG. Some aspects of the organization of the thalamic reticular complex. J Comp Neurol 1975; 162:285–308.

122. Steriade M, Parent A, Hada J. Thalamic projections of nucleus reticularis thalami of cat: a study using retrograde transport of horseradish peroxidase and fluorescent tracers. J Comp Neurol 1984; 229:531–547.

123. Llinás R. The intrinsic electrophysiological properties of mammalian neurons: insights into central nervous system function. Science 1988; 242:1654–1664.
124. Llinás R. Intrinsic electrical properties of mammalian neurons and CNS function. In: Fidia Research Foundation Neuroscience Award Lectures. New York: Raven, 1990:173–192.
125. Travis CE. The relation of voluntary movement to tremors. J Exp Psychol 1929; 12: 515–524.
126. Goodman D, Kelso JAS. Exploring the functional significance of physiological tremor: a biospectroscopic approach. Exp Brain Res 1983; 49:419–431.
127. Sasaki K. Bower JM, Llinás R. Multiple Purkinje cell recording in rodent cerebellar cortex. Eur J Neurosci 1989; 1:572–586.

3

Current Concepts of Basal Ganglia Neurophysiology Relative to Tremorgenesis

Jerrold L. Vitek, Thomas Wichmann, and Mahlon R. DeLong

Emory University School of Medicine
Atlanta, Georgia

I. INTRODUCTION

The basal ganglia have long been implicated in the development of tremor by virtue of their role in the pathogenesis of Parkinson's disease. The precise role of these nuclei in tremor has generally been considered as indirect, rather than direct, as in biasing other structures (e.g., the thalamus) that are presumed to be more directly involved in the oscillatory mechanisms. However, recent findings suggest a more direct role. In this article, we will review earlier studies, as well as the newer findings on the role of the basal ganglia in tremor.

The involvement of the basal ganglia in the pathogenesis of tremor should be considered within the framework of the functional anatomy of these structures and in the context of both the extrinsic and intrinsic connectivity. It has become increasingly clear that the basal ganglia should be viewed as components of several larger corticosubcortical pathways, which also involve the thalamus. One of these pathways is the basal ganglia–thalamocortical "motor" circuit (Fig. 1). This circuit appears to subserve the normal motor functions of the basal ganglia. It is strongly implicated in the pathophysiology of both hypo- and hyperkinetic movement disorders and may have particular importance in the development of tremor. It takes origin from pre- and postcentral sensorimotor areas and engages specific portions of the putamen, the external and the internal segment of the globus pallidus (GPe, GPi, respectively), the pars reticulata of the substantia nigra

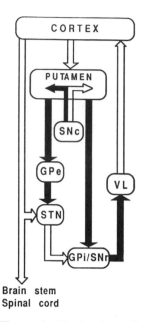

Figure 1 The basal ganglia–thalamocortical motor circuit.

(SNpr), the subthalamic nucleus (STN), and the ventrolateral thalamus (VL), and appears to return to the same precentral motor fields. Cortical motor fields project not only to the striatum, which is traditionally viewed as the major input structure of the basal ganglia, but also to the STN. The GPi and SNpr give rise to the major basal ganglia efferents, and project mainly to the VL thalamus.

The intrinsic connections of the basal ganglia are organized as two basic circuits: a "direct" pathway from striatum to GPi, and an "indirect" pathway from striatum to GPi through GPe and STN. Output from GPi–SNpr tonically inhibits thalamocortical neurons [in nucleus ventralis lateralis, pars oralis (VLo), and nucleus ventralis anterior (VA)], thereby modulating motor activity. The dopaminergic nigrostriatal and nigropallidal projections as well as serotonergic inputs from the raphe appear to modulate activity in the basal ganglia components of the motor circuit.

Several animal models of tremor have been used to investigate the involvement of the basal ganglia in the development of tremor. The results from these studies may not necessarily be directly applicable to tremor in humans. For instance, tremor induced by brainstem lesions in animals has been taken as a model for parkinsonian tremor (49,68). However, such lesions involve pathways that may not be involved in Parkinson's disease. Likewise, the current 1-methyl-4-phenyl-1,2,3,6-tetrahydropyridine (MPTP) model of "parkinsonian" tremor in monkeys, to date the most specific animal model for the human disorder, has some limitations. Tremor in this model occurs much less frequently than other parkinsonian signs. Furthermore, the tremor is primarily postural, rather than resting, and the pattern of dopamine depletion in the basal ganglia is different from that seen in humans (67,76). The pathophysiological basis of tremor induced by other drugs (e.g., harmaline) is even more difficult to assess, since these drugs have widespread effects on different parts of the brain.

Even given these limitations, significant progress has been made over the last years that allows a more accurate assessment of the role of the basal ganglia in tremor than was previously possible. In this discussion we will first review studies on the effects of lesions that either produce or alleviate tremor, then consider the potential tremor-inducing role of neurotransmitter alterations in the basal ganglia, and finally present the results of investigations of the neuronal activity of the basal ganglia–thalamocortical circuitry.

II. ABLATION STUDIES

A. Lesions Inducing Tremor

Tremor can be produced by midbrain lesions that involve the nigrostriatal pathway. However, to induce tremor, these lesions must also include cerebellothalamic and rubroolivary pathways (49,68). Isolated lesions of the substantia nigra or the dopaminergic nigrostriatal tract are not sufficient to induce tremor in experimental animals (21). In accordance with this, tremor following MPTP treatment, which is a relatively specific toxin for dopaminergic nigrostriatal cells, is generally considered to be the least consistent parkinsonian sign in the MPTP model (56).

Interestingly, the expression of tremor after exposure to MPTP seems to be species-dependent. Although experimental application of MPTP to African green monkeys (2,71,75) or inadvertent consumption of MPTP in humans (7,20,48) leads to tremor in a high percentage of cases, other primates seem to be much less affected. Some of this variability may be explained by differences in the vulnerability of dopaminergic fibers in different parts of the basal ganglia. Thus, although the most prominent biochemical abnormality in parkinsonian patients is certainly the dopamine loss in the striatum, dopamine deficiency in GP may also play a significant role in tremor (4). Recently, a more severe dopaminergic deficit in GPi was demonstrated in humans relative to that found in macaque monkeys treated with MPTP (76). Species differences may also be explained by differential involvement of nondopaminergic midbrain nuclei after MPTP treatment (26,29).

B. Lesions Abolishing Tremor

There is abundant evidence to suggest that lesions appropriately placed in GPi abolish parkinsonian tremor. This evidence comes almost exclusively from clinical studies in parkinsonian patients. Since Meyers first described the alleviation of parkinsonian tremor following section of pallidofugal fibers in 1942 (55), it has become increasingly clear that surgical interruption of pallidal outflow, either by disruption of pallidal efferents or by lesions of GPi, can produce lasting relief of tremor (13,34,37,39,46,62,78,79). Svennilson et al. (79) provided one of the most elegant and best-controlled studies on the effects of pallidotomy on parkinsonian signs. Patients were followed for at least 1 year and some for over 5 years with 67/81 obtaining lasting relief from tremor following selective pallidotomy. By systemically varying the location and size of the lesion, the lesion parameters could be optimized so that 19 of the last 20 patients (95%) had long-lasting relief from tremor. The optimal target was the ventroposterior portion of GPi, an area that was later defined as being a component of the basal ganglia–thalamocortical motor circuit.

The report of Svennilson and colleagues appears to have been largely unnoticed, since surgeons began to target the VL thalamus in the belief that lesioning this structure was safer and possibly a more effective means of treating parkinsonian tremor (5,37). Because of this and the introduction of levodopa (L-dopa) therapy in the early 1960s, pallidotomies became less popular and have been rarely used in the treatment for parkinsonian tremor. However, in a recent study, Laitinen et al. (47) confirmed Svennilson's view that ventroposterior medial pallidotomy alleviates all parkinsonian signs, including tremor.

Independently of the work in humans, it was recently shown that lesions of the STN in MPTP-treated green monkeys reduce tremor significantly (2). This study, as well as earlier metabolic (18,57,70,73), pharmacological (64,65), and anatomical studies (28), cast particular emphasis on the involvement of activity changes in the "indirect" pathway of the basal ganglia thalamocortical motor circuit in the development of parkinsonian tremor. In parkinsonian animals, neurons in the STN are tonically and phasically overactive. This, in turn, leads to increased excitation of GPi, eventually resulting in overinhibition of thalamocortical neurons. According to this scheme, reduction of GPi output, either by lesions of GPi or by reducing the excitatory drive on GPi from the STN, would ameliorate parkinsonian signs, including tremor.

Interestingly, a few earlier studies in both humans and monkeys indicate that pallidotomy can also be eeffective in abolishing cerebellar tremor. Obrador and Dierssen (63) reported that pallidotomy could abolish cerebellar intention tremor in humans, and Carpenter et al. showed that cerebellar tremor in monkeys induced by lesions of the deep cerebellar nuclei could also be abolished by pallidal lesions (9). One possible explanation for this may be that pallido- and cerebellothalamic circuits are functionally overlapping at the thalamic or cortical level. Thus, tremor may, at times, occur as a result of the combined involvement of both pallidal and cerebellar circuits. This suggestion gains further support from the observation (described earlier) that tremor resulting from midbrain lesions in monkeys must interrupt both nigrostriatal and cerbellothalamic pathways. In a general sense, it is suggested that the expression of cerebellar and perhaps even parkinsonian tremor, may depend on the interaction between basal ganglia and cerebellar circuitry.

III. NEUROPHARMACOLOGICAL STUDIES

Most major neurotransmitters in the basal ganglia have been implicated in tremorgenesis. Among these, dopamine has received the most attention, owing to its prominent role in the pathogenesis of parkinsonism.

A. Dopamine

A role for dopamine in tremor is supported by the finding that a decrease of striatal dopamine is necessary for tremor production after mesencephalic lesions in monkeys (31,33,69), and that this type of tremor is alleviated by treatment with L-dopa (1,31–33) or dopamine receptor agonists (66). The finding that MPTP induces tremor is further support for a role of dopamine loss in tremor development. The MPTP-induced tremor is probably, in large part, due to striatal dopamine loss, because the most prominent histological abnormality in MPTP-treated monkeys is damage to the dopaminergic nigrostriatal pathway (6). Conceivably, dopamine loss in the pallidum or the STN may also play a role in the pathogenesis of tremor.

Similar results have been obtained in parkinsonian patients, in whom tremor responds to prolonged treatment with high doses of L-dopa (14–16,30,85). However, a significant percentage of patients with Parkinson's disease do not develop tremor, despite the presence of the other major signs of striatal dopamine deficiency (42). It is also generally acknowledged, that L-dopa treatment in parkinsonian patients is not as effective against tremor as it is against akinesia or rigidity. Thus, more widespread damage to nondopaminergic midbrain nuclei may be required for tremor to develop in parkinsonian patients (4,41).

B. Serotonin

The functional relation between serotonin and the development of tremor is not well established. Both decreases and increases of serotonin levels in the striatum have been implicated. Thus, in monkeys, tremor was demonstrated to result from mesencephalic lesions that reduce serotonin synthesis and storage in the striatum (68,69,77). The tremor after these brainstem lesions can be reversed by treatment with the serotonin precursor 5-hydroxytryptophane (33). Similarly, rats with lesions of the (serotonergic) raphe nuclei, reducing the striatal serotonin content, also develop tremor (35,45). On the other hand, increasing the striatal serotonin content with intracaudate injections of serotonin in rats also induces tremor, which can be blocked by serotonin receptor antagonists (53), and systemic injections of the tremorgenic substance N-carbamoyl-2(2,6-dichlorophenyl) acetamide hydrochloride (LON-954) specifically increase the serotonin concentration in the striatum (58) coincident with the induction of tremor. The relevance of these studies for the development of parkinsonian tremor in humans is unclear. Although in parkinsonian patients the serotonin content of several brain regions, including the striatum, is reduced (3), drug-induced changes in the availability of serotonin have either no effect or even worsen the tremor (10,36,82).

C. Acetylcholine

Local injections of muscarinic agonists into various basal ganglia structures can induce tremor. Thus, intracaudate injections of muscarinic agonists, or of the cholinesterase inhibitor physostigmine, produce tremor of high frequency (10–20 Hz) in cats (11,12), rats (17,22,44), and monkeys (59). Local injections of muscarinic agonists into the globus pallidus or the substantia nigra may also produce tremor (12,27,59), which is decreased after subsequent lesions of the striatum, or the GP in rats (12).

Given these findings, tremor induced by muscarinic agonists in rodents has been widely used in the development of new drug therapies for parkinsonian tremor. In fact, anticholinergic drugs are highly effective in the treatment of tremor in parkinsonian patients. However, there is as yet no direct evidence that overactivity of cholinergic neurons in the basal ganglia is indeed causally involved in the development of tremor in man.

IV. NEUROPHYSIOLOGICAL STUDIES

On neurophysiological grounds, a role for the basal ganglia in tremorgenesis can be considered in the framework of two nonexclusive models: (1) the central oscillator, and (2) the peripheral feedback models. According to the former, tremor originates from a group of bursting neurons in the thalamus or possibly the basal ganglia. According to the latter, tremor results from the instability of long loop reflexes. In resting tremor, these may involve or be influenced by parts of the motor circuit of the basal ganglia.

A. Central Oscillatory Model

Brainstem lesions involving the substantia nigra frequently induce bursting activity in GPi neurons in monkeys, with bursts typically occurring at a frequency of 12–15 Hz (23). A similar bursting pattern in GPi neurons has also been described by Miller and DeLong (74) and Filion and Tremblay (24,50) in MPTP-treated monkeys. Interestingly, in these studies, the 12- to 15-Hz bursts were observed in animals that did not manifest tremor. However, in Filion's studies, a second bursting pattern at a lower frequency (5–8 Hz) was observed, occurring in animals only when these animals manifested tremor. In the earlier study, prolonged administration of haloperidol or reserpine in intact animals produced irregular bursting at higher frequencies, whereas injections of dopamine agonists in lesioned animals abolished tremor and silenced GPi bursting. Bursts of spikes *synchronous with tremor* have been recorded in MPTP-treated monkeys, both in the STN (Fig. 2) and in GPi (24,25,50,83). Tremblay et al. (81) also observed that, after striatal microstimulation, GPi neurons frequently developed oscillatory responses at frequencies close to that of the spontaneous tremor displayed at other occasions by the same animals. Similar bursting patterns were also obtained by intracellular recordings from GP in brain slices from adult guinea pigs when these cells were depolarized from a hyperpolarized membrane potential (60).

Although tremor may directly result from oscillatory activity originating in the basal ganglia, which is then transmitted through the basal ganglia–thalamocortical circuit, it is also possible that changes in the *tonic* inhibitory output from GPi to the thalamus may induce oscillations in thalamocortical neurons. Miller and DeLong (74), and Filion et al. (25) observed that tonic activity in GPi is increased in parkinsonian monkeys treated with MPTP. This increased inhibitory basal ganglia output may lead to hyperpolarization of thalamic cells in VLo, which may, in turn, induce oscillatory activity (8). The proposal that GABAergic inputs to the thalamus from SNpr and pallidum are burst- and oscillation-promoting systems is partly derived from previous observations in in vitro slice recordings in guinea pig thalamus, examining the effect of hyperpolarization on the oscillatory properties of these cells (40,51,52). Membrane hyperpolarization leads to deinactivation of low-threshold calcium channels that induces rebound excitation and, thereby, promotes oscillatory activity. In addition, periodic bursting in the reticular thalamus during moments of immobility, when combined with the condition of hyperpolarization of thalamocortical projection neurons, may also enhance the tendency for rhythmic oscillation of these thalamocortical neurons. Such bursting activity in VLo may lead to oscillations in the motor cortex, by virtue of direct thalamocortical projects or, indirectly, through projections to other cortical areas, such as the SMA (19,38,43,54,61,72,84). In addition, the oscillatory activity in the reticularis or VLo could affect the population synchrony of other thalamic areas such as nucleus ventralis posterolateralis, pars oralis (VPLo), the cerebellar-receiving area of the thalamus. This may help to explain why tremor induced by midbrain lesions requires damage to nigrostriatal as well as to cerebellothalamic pathways. Such midbrain lesions would lead to hyperpolarization of both VLo and VPLo neurons, since the inhibition to VLo is increased and the excitation to VPLo is decreased. Thus, both areas would be hyperpolarized and, consequently, prone to develop oscillatory activity. Oscillatory tendencies in VPLo could interact with the basal ganglia thalamocortical circuit through overlapping neuronal circuities at the cortical level or by population synchrony at a local circuit neuron level in the thalamus. It may be that such an interaction is necessary for the overt manifestations of tremor.

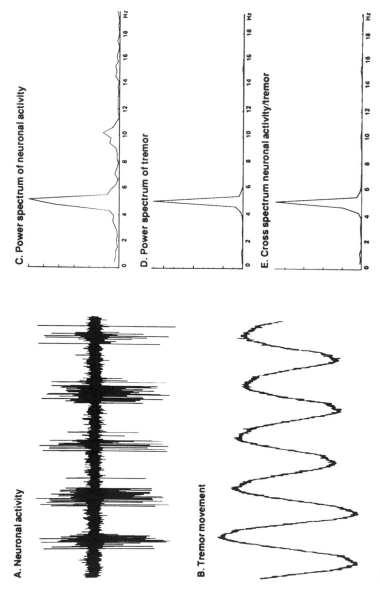

Figure 2 Bursts of spikes in the STN synchronous with tremor in MPTP-treated monkeys.

B. Peripheral Feedback Model

Supportive evidence for the peripheral feedback model comes from studies that have revealed an increase in the M2 component of long-loop reflexes in patients with Parkinson's disease (80). A relation between the increased gain in long-loop reflexes and basal ganglia dysfunction has been suggested by comparable studies in monkeys rendered parkinsonian with MPTP (25,74,81). These studies have demonstrated an increase in gain in the basal ganglia thalamocortical motor circuit in relation to passive limb movement. Thus, a greater percentage of GPi neurons responds to passive manipulations of the limbs, and phasic neuronal responses to GPi to torque perturbations or passive manipulation are increased in magnitude and duration. Pallidal neurons, which had been highly specific in their response properties in normal animals, were far less specific following treatment with MPTP, responding to movements of more than one joint in multiple directions, sometimes on both sides of the body. In these high-gain circuits internal oscillations may develop, which may contribute to the development of tremor.

V. SUMMARY AND CONCLUSIONS

The importance of the basal ganglia in the development of tremor is suggested by ablation experiments, as well as neuropharmacological and neurophysiological studies. The basal ganglia are particularly implicated in the pathogenesis of parkinsonian tremor. Unlike other parkinsonian signs, the development of tremor may require damage to both dopaminergic and nondopaminergic systems. Components of the basal ganglia may act themselves as oscillators, or changes in the tonic activity levels of neurons in the basal ganglia may promote oscillation(s) in the thalamus. Changes in the basal ganglia function may result in increased gain in long-loop reflexes, which may also lead to oscillatory activity.

REFERENCES

1. Battista AF, Nakatani S, Goldstein M. The effects of DL dopa on harmaline induced tremor and on resting tremor in monkeys with tegmental lesions. Confin Neurol 1969; 32:332–340.
2. Bergman H, Wichmann T, DeLong MR. Reversal of experimental parkinsonism by lesions of the subthalamic nucleus. Science 1990; 249:1436–1438.
3. Bernheimer H, Birkmayer W, Hornykiewicz O. Verteilung des 5-hydroxytryptamins (serotonin) im Gehirn des Menschen und sein Verhalten bei Patienten mit Parkinson-Syndrom. Klin Wochenschr 1961; 39:1056–1059.
4. Bernheimer H, Birkmayer W, Hornykiewicz O, Jellinger K, Seitelberger F. Brain dopamine and the syndromes of Parkinson and Huntington. J Neurol Sci 1973; 20: 415–455.

5. Bravo GJ, Cooper IS. A clinical and radiological correlation of the lesions produced by chemopallidectomy and thalamectomy. J Neurol Neurosurg Psychiatry 1959; 22: 1–10.

6. Burns RS, Chiueh CC, Markey SP, Ebert MH, Jacobowitz DM, Koppin IJ. A primate model of parkinsonism: selective destruction of dopaminergic neurons in the pars compacta of the substantia nigra by N-methyl-4-phenyl-1,2,3,6-tetrahydropyridine. Proc Natl Acad Sci USA 1983; 80:4546–4550.

7. Burns RS, LeWitt PA, Ebert MH, Pakkenberg H, Kopin I. The clinical syndrome of striatal dopamine deficiency. N Engl J Med 1985; 312(22):1418–1421.

8. Buzsaki G, Smith A, Berger S, Fisher LJ, Gage FH. Petit mal epilepsy and parkinsonian tremor: hypothesis of a common pacemaker. Neuroscience 1990; 36: 1–14.

9. Carpenter MB, Glinsman W, Fabrega H. Effects of secondary pallidal and striatal lesions upon cerebellar dyskinesia. Neurology 1958; 8:352–358.

10. Chase TN, Ng LKY, Watanabe AM. Parkinson's disease: modification by 5-hydroxy-tryptophan. Neurology 1972; 22:479–484.

11. Connor JD, Rossi GV, Baker WW. Analysis of the tremor induced by injection of cholinergic agents into the caudate nucleus. Int J Neuropharmacol 1966; 5:207–216.

12. Connor JD, Rossi GV, Baker WW. Characteristics of tremor in cats following injections of carbachol into the caudate nucleus. Exp Neurol 1966; 14:371–382.

13. Cooper IS, Poloukhine N. The globus pallidus as a surgical target. J Am Geriatr Soc 1956; 4:1182–1207.

14. Cotzias GC, Papavasiliou PS, Gellene R. Modification of parkinsonism—chronic treatment with L-dopa. N Engl J Med 1969; 280:337–345.

15. Cotzias GC, Papavasiliou PS, Gellene R, Aronson RB. Parkinsonism and dopa. Trans Am Assoc Physicians 1968; 81:171–183.

16. Cotzias GC, Van Woert MH, Schiffer LM. Aromatic amino acids and modification of parkinsonism. N Engl J Med 1967; 276:374–379.

17. Cox B, Potkonjak D. An investigation of the tremorgenic effects of oxotremorine and tremorine after stereotaxic injection into rat brain. Int J Neuropharmacol 1969; 8:291–297.

18. Crossman AR, Mitchell IJ, Sambrook MA. Regional brain uptake of 2-deoxyglucose in N-methyl-4-phenyl-1,2,3,6-tetrahydropyridine (MPTP)-induced parkinsonism in the macaque monkey. Neuropharmacology 1985; 24:587–591.

19. Darian-Smith C, Darian-Smith I, Cheema SS. Thalamic projections to sensorimotor cortex in the macaque monkey: use of multiple retrograde fluorescent tracers. J Comp Neurol 1990; 299:17–46.

20. Davis GC, Williams AC, Markey SP, et al. Chronic parkinsonism secondary to intra-venous injection of meperidine analogues. Psychiatry Res 1979; 1:249–254.

21. DeLong MR, Georgopoulos AP. Motor functions of the basal ganglia. In: Brookhart JM, Mountcastle VB, Brooks VB, Geiger SR, eds. Handbook of Physiology: The Nervous System Motor Control. Bethesda: American Physiological Society, 1981; 1017–1061.

22. Dill RE, Nickey WM, Little MD. Dyskinesias in rats following chemical stimulation of the neostriatum. Tex Rep Biol Med 1968; 26:101–106.

23. Filion M. Effects of interruption of the nigrostriatal pathway and of dopaminergic agents on the spontaneous activity of globus pallidus neurons in the awake monkey. Brain Res 1979; 178:425–441.

24. Filion M, Tremblay L. Abnormal spontaneous activity of globus pallidus neurons in monkeys with MPTP-induced parkinsonism. Brain Res 1991; 547:142–151.

25. Filion M, Tremblay L, Bedard PJ. Abnormal influences of passive limb movement on the activity of globus pallidus neurons in parkinsonian monkeys. Brain Res 1988; 444: 165–176.

26. Forno LS, Langston JW, DeLanney LE, Irwin I, Ricaurte GA. Locus ceruleus lesions and eosinophilic inclusions in MPTP-treated monkeys. Ann Neurol 1986; 20: 449–455.

27. George R, Haslett WL, Jenden DJ. A cholinergic mechanism in the brainstem reticular formation: induction of paradoxical sleep. Int J Neuropharmacol 1964; 3:541–552.

28. Gerfen CR, Engber TM, Mahan LC, et al. D_1 and D_2 dopamine receptor-regulated gene expression of striatonigral and striatopallidal neurons. Science 1990; 250:1429–1432.

29. German DC, Dubach M, Askari S, Speciale SG, Bowdens DM. 1-Methyl-4-phenyl-1,2,3,6-tetrahydropyridine-induced parkinsonian syndrome in *Macaca fascicularis*: which midbrain dopaminergic neurons are lost? Neuroscience 1988; 24(1):161–174.

30. Godwin-Austen RB, Frears CC, Tomlinson EB, and Kok HWL. Effects of L-dopa in Parkinson's disease. Lancet 1969; 1:165–168.

31. Goldstein M, Anagnoste B, Battista AF, and Ogawa M. Monkeys with nigrostriatal lesions: effects of monoaminergic drugs. Pharmacol Ther 1976; 2:97–103.

32. Goldstein M, Anagnoste B, Battista AF, Owen WS, Nakatani S. Studies of amines in the striatum in monkeys with nigral lesions. J Neurochem 1969; 16:645–653.

33. Goldstein M, Battista AF, Nakatani S, Anagnoste B. The effects of centrally acting drugs on tremor in monkeys with mesencephalic lesions. Proc Natl Acad Sci USA 1969; 63:1113–1116.

34. Guiot G. Le treatment des syndromes parkinsoniens par la destruction du pallidum interne. Neurochirurgie 1958; 1:94–98.

35. Gumulka W, Ramirez del Angel A, Samanin R, Valzelli L. Lesion of substantia nigra: biochemical and behavioral effects in rats. Eur J Pharmacol 1970; 10:79–82.

36. Hall CD, Weiss EA, Morris CE, Prange AJ. Rapid deterioration in patients with parkinsonism following tryptophan–pyridoxine administration. Neurology 1972; 22: 231–237.

37. Hassler R, Reichert T, Mundinger F, Umbach W, Gangleberger JA. Physiological observations in stereotaxic operations in extrapyramidal motor disturbances. Brain 1960; 83:337–350.

38. Holsapple JW, Preston JB, Strick PL. The origin of thalamic inputs to the "hand" representation in the primary motor cortex. J Neurosci 1991;

39. Horne DJ. Sensorimotor control in parkinsonism. J Neurol Neurosurg Psychiatry 1973; 36:742–746.

40. Jahnsen H, Llinás R. Electrophysiological properties of guinea-pig thalamic neurones: an in vitro study. J Physiol 1984; 349:205–226.

41. Jellinger K. Overview of morphological changes in Parkinson's disease. Adv Neurol 1987; 45:1–18.
42. Jenner P, Marsden CD. neurochemical basis of parkinsonian tremor. In: Findley LJ, Capildeo R, eds. Movement Disorders: Tremor. New York: Oxford University Press, 1984:305–319.
43. Kievit J, Kuypers HGJM. Organization of the thalamo-cortical connexions to the frontal lobe in the rhesus monkey. Exp Brain Res 1977; 29:299–322.
44. Kjell F, Ungerstedt U. Studies on the cholinergic and dopaminergic innervation of the neostriatum with the help of intraneostriatal injections of drugs. Pharmacol Ther 1976; 2:29–36.
45. Kostowski W, Giacalone E, Garattini S, Valzelli L. Studies on behavioural and biochemical changes in rats after lesion of midbrain raphe. Eur J Pharmacol 1968; 4:371–376.
46. Laitinen LB. Brain targets in surgery for Parkinson's disease. J Neurosurg 1985; 62:349–351.
47. Laitinen LB, Hariz MI. Pallidal surgery abolishes all parkinsonian symptoms. Mov Disord 1990; 5:82.
48. Langstron JW, Ballard P. Chronic parkinsonism in humans due to a product of meperidine-analog systhesis. Science 1983; 219:979–980.
49. LaRochelle L, Bedard P, Boucher R, Poirier LJ. The rubro-olivo-cerebello-rubral loop and postural tremor in the monkey. J Neurol Sci 1970; 11:53–64.
50. Lidsky TI, Buchwald NA, Hull CD, Levine MS. Pallidal and entopeduncular single unit activity in cats during drinking. Electroencephalogr Clin Neurophysiol 1975; 39: 79–84.
51. Llinás R, Jahnsen H. Electrophysiology of mammalian thalamic neurones in vitro. Nature 1982; 29:406–408.
52. Llinás RR. The intrinsic electrophysiological properties of mammalian neurons: insights into central nervous system function. Science 1988; 242:1654–1664.
53. Malseed RT, Baker WW. Analysis of tremogenic effects of intracaudate serotonin. Proc Soc Exp Biol Med 1973; 143:1088–1093.
54. Matelli M, Luppino G, Fogassi L, Rizzolatti G. Thalamic input to inferior area 6 and area 4 in the macaque monkey. J Comp Neurol 1989; 280:468–488.
55. Meyers R. The modification of alternating tremors, rigidity and festination by surgery of the basal ganglia. Assoc Nerv Ment Dis 1942; 20:602–665.
56. Miller WC, DeLong MR. Altered tonic activity of neurons in the globus pallidus and subthalamic nucleus in the primate MPTP model of parkinsonism. In: Carpenter MB, Jayaraman A, eds. The Basal Ganglia II. New York: Plenum Press, 1987; 415–427.
57. Mitchell IJ, Clarke CE, Boyce S, et al. Neural mechanisms underlying parkinsonian symptoms based upon regional uptake of 2-deoxyglucose in monkeys exposed to 1-methyl-4-phenyl-1,2,3,6-tetrahydropyridine. Neuroscience 1989; 32:213–226.
58. Mohanakumar KP, Ganguly DK. Tremorogenesis by LON-954 [N-carbamoyl-2(2,6-dichlorophenyl) acetamidine hydrochloride]: evidence for the involvement of 5-hydroxytryptamine. Brain Res Bull 1989; 22:191–195.
59. Murphey DL, Dill RE. Chemical stimulation of discrete brain loci as a method of producing dyskinesia models in primates. Exp Neurol 1972; 34:244–254.

60. Nambu A, Llinás R. Electrophysiology of the globus pallidus neurons: an in vitro study in guinea pig brain slices. Soc Neurosci Abstr 1990; 180.8:(Abstract).

61. Nambu A, Yoshida S, Jinnai K. Projection on the motor cortex of thalamic neurons with pallidal input in the monkey. Exp Brain Res 1988; 71:658–662.

62. Narabayashi H. Procaine oil blocking of the globus pallidus for the treatment of rigidity and tremor of parkinsonism. Psychiat Neurol Jpn 1954; 56:471–495.

63. Obrador S, Dierssen G. Observations on the treatment of intentional and postural tremor by subcortical stereotaxic lesions. Confin Neurol 1965; 26:250–253.

64. Pan HS, Frey KA, Young AB, Penney JR Jr. Changes in [^{3}H]muscimol binding in substantia nigra, entopeduncular nucleus, globus pallidus and thalamus after striatal lesions as demonstrated by quantitative receptor autoradiography. J Neurosci 1983; 3:1189–1198.

65. Pan HS, Penney JB, Young AB. gamma-aminobutyric acid and benzodiazepine receptor changes induced by unilateral 6-hydroxydopamine lesions of the median forebrain bundle. J Neurochem 1985; 45:1396–1404.

66. Pechadre JC, LaRochelle L, Poirier LJ. Parkinsonian akinesia, rigidity and tremor in the monkey. Histopathological and neuropharmacological study. J Neurosci 1976; 28: 147–157.

67. Pifl C, Bertel O, Schingnitz G, Hornykiewicz O. Extrastriatal dopamine in symptomatic and asymptomatic rhesus monkeys treated with 1-methyl-4-phenyl-1,2,3,6-tetrahydropyridine (MPTP). Neurochem Int 1990; 17:263–270.

68. Poirier LJ. Experimental and histological study of midbrain dyskinesias. J Neurophysiol 1960; 23:534–551.

69. Poirier LJ, Sourkes TL, Bouvier G, Boucher R, Carabin S. Striatal amines, experimental tremor and the effect of harmaline in the monkey. Brain 1966; 89:37–55.

70. Porrino LJ, Burns RS, Crane AM, Palombo E, Kopin IJ, Sokoloff L. Changes in local cerebral glucose utilization associated with Parkinson's syndrome induced by 1-methyl-4-phenyl-1,2,3,6-tetrahydropyridine (MPTP) in the primate. Life Sci 1987; 40: 1657–1664.

71. Redmond DE, Roth RH, Elsworth JD, Sladek RJ Jr, Collier TJ, Deutch AY. Fetal neuronal grafts in monkeys given methylphenyltetrahydropyridine. Lancet 1986; 1: 1125–1127.

72. Schell GR, Strick PL. The origin of thalamic inputs to the arcuate premotor and supplementary motor areas. J Neurosci 1984; 4:539–560.

73. Schwartzman RJ, Alexander GM, Ferraro TN, Grothusen JR, Stahl SM. Cerebral metabolism of parkinsonian primates 21 days after MPTP. Exp Neurol 1988; 102: 307–313.

74. Schwarz R, Hokelt T, Fuxe K, Jonsson G, Goldstein M, Tereniius L. Ibotenic acid-induced neuronal degeneration: a morphological and neurochemical study. Exp Brain Res 1979; 37:199–216.

75. Sladek JR Jr, Redmond DE Jr, Collier TJ, et al. Transplantation of fetal dopamine neurons in primate brain reverses MPTP induced parkinsonism. In: Seil FJ, Herbert E, Carlson BM, eds. Progress in Brain Research. New York: Elsevier Science Publishers, 1987:309–323.

76. Smith MG, Schneider JS. Immunohistochemical study of the pallidal complex in

symptomatic and asymptomatic MPTP-treated monkeys, normal human, and Parkinson's disease patients [abstr]. Neuroscience 1990; 16:428.

77. Sourkes TL, Poirier LJ. Neurochemical bases of tremor and other disorders of movement. Can Med Assoc J 1966; 94:43–60.

78. Spiegel EA, Wycis HT. Ansotomy in paralysis agitans. Arch Neurol Psychiatry 1954; 71:598–614.

79. Svennilson E, Torvik A, Lowe R, Leksell L. Treatment of parkinsonism by stereotactic thermolesions in the pallidal region. A clinical evaluation of 81 cases. Acta Psychiat Neurol Scand 1960; 35:358–377.

80. Tatton WG, Lee RG. Evidence for abnormal long-loop reflexes in rigid parkinsonian patients. Brain Res 1975; 100:671–676.

81. Tremblay L, Filion M, Bedard PJ. Responses of pallidal neurons to striatal stimulation in monkeys with MPTP-induced parkinsonism. Brain Res 1989; 498:17–33.

82. Van Woert MH, Ambani LM, Levine RJ. Clinical effects of *para*-chlorophenylalanine in Parkinson's disease. Dis Nerv Syst 1972; 777–780.

83. Wichmann T, Bergman H, DeLong MR. Increased neuronal activity in the subthalamic nucleus of MPTP treated monkeys. Mov Disord 1990; 5(suppl 1):78.

84. Wiesendanger R, Wiesendanger M. The thalamic connections with medial area 6 (supplementary motor cortex) in the monkey (*Macaca fascicularis*). Exp Brain Res 1985; 59:91–104.

85. Yahr MD, Duvoisin RC. Drug therapy of parkinsonism. N Engl J Med 1972; 287:20–24.

4

Mechanisms of Physiological Tremor and Relationship to Essential Tremor

Rodger J. Elble
Southern Illinois University School of Medicine
Springfield, Illinois

I. INTRODUCTION

Many authors have hypothesized that essential tremor emerges from a pathological change in the mechanisms of physiological tremor (1). Until recently, this hypothesis was based largely on the relatively benign nature of essential tremor in many patients, the lack of other neurological signs in most patients, and the similarities in frequency content of both tremors. Recent physiological studies have clarified the mechanistic components of both tremors and have thereby provided more rigorous criteria for comparing these two forms of tremor. These studies are now reviewed. In addition, a hypothetical relation between physiological tremor and essential tremor is stated more precisely to facilitate the design of future studies.

II. MECHANICAL COMPONENT OF PHYSIOLOGICAL TREMOR

The body is a mechanical structure, with inertial, viscous, and elastic properties. The viscosity of most bodily parts (e.g., the limbs) is not so great that it prevents oscillation in response to an exogenous or endogenous force. The passive mechanical oscillations that result from such disturbances constitute the principal rhythmic component of physiological tremor, which is frequently referred to as the mechanical resonant component (2–4).

Mechanical oscillations have a frequency that is directly proportional to the square root of the stiffness of the limb (5) and inversely proportional to the square root of the limb inertia (4). Therefore, the frequency of mechanical tremor is decreased when inertial loads are attached to a limb, and the frequency of oscillation is increased by the addition of spring loads (Fig. 1; 3,6–9).

The frequency range of physiological tremor is traditionally defined as 8–12 Hz. However, this definition ignores the relation between the frequency of physiological tremor and the mechanical properties of the bodily part from which the tremor is measured. Normal elbow tremor has a frequency of 3–5 Hz (10),

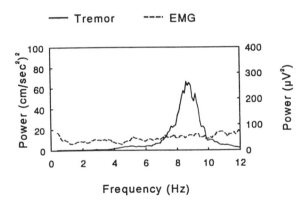

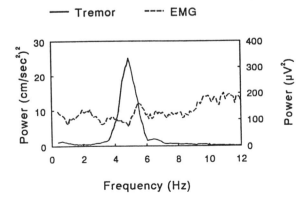

Figure 1   Autospectra of normal wrist tremor, recorded with a miniature accelerometer, and of rectified-filtered EMG from the extensor carpi radialis brevis. As in all normal adults, wrist tremor had a spectra peak at 7–10 Hz, but the EMG spectrum was statistically flat, reflecting the lack of motor unit entrainment. Mass loading reduced the frequency of tremor.

wrist tremor 8–12 Hz (2), metacarpophalangeal joint tremor 17–30 Hz (4), and ocular tremor 35–40 Hz (11). The frequency of physiological tremor is not confined to 8–12 Hz.

The passive mechanical properties of a limb (or other bodily part) are a source of oscillation only when the limb is subjected to external or internal forcing. The ejection of blood at cardiac systole provides a significant forcing to the entire body, creating oscillations that are occasionally visible to the naked eye (e.g., the dangling foot of a man sitting with his legs crossed). These cardioballistic oscillations account for most of physiological tremor at rest, but they account for 40% or less of physiological postural tremor (2,12–18).

The irregularities of subtetanic motor unit firing produce an additional source of mechanical forcing. The subtetanic firing and fluctuating recruitment of motoneurons that are near threshold produce the greatest fluctuations in muscular force (19). Schafer and co-workers (20) were the first to emphasize this source of tremor, which was later rigorously demonstrated by others (19,21–23). Depending on the rhythmicity of the motor units (24), irregularities in motor unit firing produce a fairly broad-frequency forcing that combines with cardioballistics to drive the limb at its natural frequency.

Irregularities in motor unit firing also produce irregular fluctuations in force and displacement, particularly at frequencies from 0 to 4 Hz. Irregularities above 4 Hz are attentuated by the low-pass filtering properties of skeletal muscle (25–27). The aperiodic 0- to 4-Hz fluctuations in force and displacement may exceed the rhythmic components of physiological tremor, depending on the conditions under which the tremor is measured (7,21,28,29).

III. STRETCH REFLEX OSCILLATION IN PHYSIOLOGICAL TREMOR

Muscle spindles are exquisitely sensitive to small oscillations in muscle length (30). Hagbarth and Young (31) demonstrated that the passive mechanical oscillations of physiological tremor are associated with rhythmic modulation of spindle activity, but reflex-induced modulation of the electromyogram (EMG) occurs only when physiological tremor is enhanced by fatigue or by drugs (3,8,9,32). The timing of spindle and EMG discharge relative to some limb oscillations is such that the stretch reflex may promote tremor, rather than impede it (32). This reflex-induced enhancement of mechanical oscillation is referred to as enhanced physiological tremor. Because the mechanical component of physiological tremor can lead to reflex-induced modulation of motor unit activity, Stiles recommended that the principal rhythmic component of physiological tremor be referred to as mechanical reflex tremor, not mechanical tremor (9,33).

The use of this terminology is not meant to emphasize or imply reflex instability. Because of its low gain, the stretch reflex becomes an unstable source of oscillation only in combination with extraordinary mechanical loads or unusual reflex enhancement (34–40). Fatigue- and drug-induced enhancement of mechanical reflex oscillations (i.e., enhanced physiological tremor) requires an intact stretch reflex (41).

IV. THE 8- TO 12-Hz COMPONENT OF PHYSIOLOGICAL TREMOR

The second rhythmic component of physiological tremor, called the 8- to 12-Hz tremor, is readily demonstrable in a minority of normal adults. In contrast with the mechanical reflex component, inertial and spring loads have little effect on the frequency of the 8- to 12-Hz tremor (2,7,42,43). The frequency of the 8- to 12-Hz tremor also bears no relation to the length of reflex arc. Travis and Hunter found evidence of motor unit entrainment at 8–12 Hz in EMG of the tongue and forearm (44). Thomas and Whitney found 8- to 12-Hz tremor in postural sway (45), and Mori recorded 8- to 12-Hz bursts of EMG from the soleus (46). The 8- to 12-Hz tremor has also been recorded from biceps brachii (10), extensor digitorum communis (47), and intrinsic hand muscles (28).

Under normal circumstances, the 8- to 12-Hz tremor is associated with motor unit entrainment, whereas the mechanical reflex component is not, even though the mechanical reflex component is much larger (Fig. 2; 2,6,47). Individual motor units, firing at mean frequencies of 10–22 spikes per second, are synchronously modulated at 8–12 Hz (47). The mechanical reflex oscillation, by contrast, is associated with no entrainment or modulation of motor units unless its amplitude is increased greatly by fatigue (2,8,9,31), by mechanical perturbations (42), or by drugs (32,48).

Although stretch reflex instability has been proposed as a mechanism for the 8- to 12-Hz tremor (49,50), studies of human stretch reflex dynamics did not support this hypothesis (37,51). This hypothesis is also incompatible with the lack of any relation between the frequency of this tremor and the length of reflex arc.

As reviewed by Elble and Koller (52), existing experimental data are most compatible with the notion that the 8- to 12-Hz tremor is primarily the result of an oscillating system of neurons located with the central nervous system (CNS). According to this hypothesis, the underlying 8- to 12-Hz rhythm is determined primarily by properties that are intrinsic to the putative central oscillator, but the amplitude of 8- to 12-Hz tremor may be governed by both central and peripheral factors. The stretch reflex may oscillate in response to this tremor, but this tremor is not produced by reflex instability per se.

V. MECHANISTIC PROPERTIES OF ESSENTIAL TREMOR

The frequency range of essential tremor is 4–12 Hz and, therefore, includes the frequencies of most physiological and pathological tremors (1,6). My analysis of 44 patients revealed a strong negative correlation between tremor frequency and amplitude (Fig. 3), whereas patient age had little additional bearing on the

No Added Mass

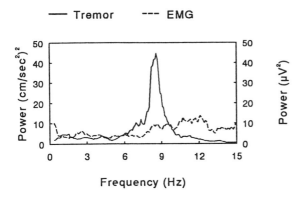

500 gm Added Mass

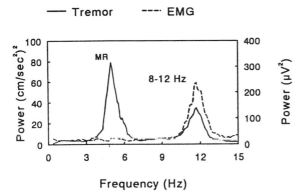

Figure 2 Wrist tremor and extensor digitorum communis EMG autospectra recorded with and without mass loading from a normal adult with a prominent 8- to 12-Hz component of physiological tremor. With no mechanical loading, the mechanical reflex (MR) and 8- to 12-Hz tremors merged into a single spectral peak, but these two tremors were clearly separated by inertial loading. The 8- to 12-Hz spectral peak in the rectified-filtered EMG was most apparent during mechanical loading. The mechanical reflex tremor had no corresponding EMG spectral peak, even though the amplitude of the mechanical reflex tremor was much larger than the 8- to 12-Hz oscillation.

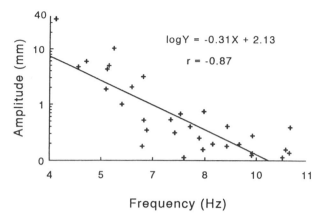

Figure 3   The amplitude of essential tremor, recorded from the wrists of 44 patients, bore a logarithmic relation to tremor frequency. Tremor amplitude was measured with an accelerometer, as described by Elble (6). Tremor frequency was determined using spectral analysis of rectified-filtered EMG, recorded from the forearm during 500-g loading.

frequency of tremor (6). The inverse relation between tremor amplitude and frequency was confirmed by Calzetti and co-workers in a study of 59 patients (53). The full range of tremor frequencies (i.e., 4–12 Hz) is commonly encountered across members of the same family, illustrating the futility of classifying essential tremor solely on the basis of frequency.

As in physiological tremor, experiments using spring and inertial loading have revealed that essential tremor of the wrist has two rhythmic components, mechanical reflex and a frequency-invariant component, ranging from 4 to 12 Hz (Fig. 4; 6,7,42). The frequency-invariant component is associated with abnormal entrainment of motor unit discharges, the sine qua non of essential tremor. The mechanical reflex component of essential tremor does not differ from that found in physiological tremor (6). The frequency-invariant component is the fundamental abnormality of essential tremor and is, hereafter, referred to as essential tremor. The frequency of essential tremor bears no relation to the length of the reflex arc (Fig. 5; 6,54,55).

The frequency-invariance of essential tremor in response to mechanical loading is not absolute. The frequency of essential tremor may exhibit changes of 1 Hz or less in response to mechanical loads (see Fig. 4; 6,7). Furthermore, essential tremor may become entrained by an enhanced mechanical reflex oscillation if the frequency of the mechanical reflex oscillation is near the frequency of essential tremor or its harmonics (52).

Qualitatively, there are no features that distinguish the 8- to 12- Hz physiological tremor from mild, high-frequency essential tremor (6). Mild essential tremor

No Added Mass

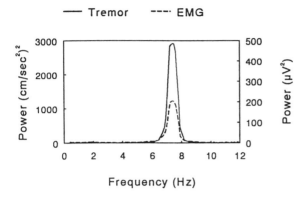

500 gm Added Mass

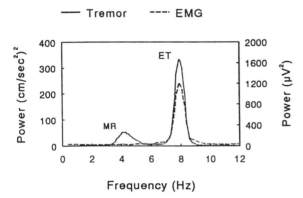

Figure 4 Wrist tremor and extensor carpi radialis brevis EMG autospectra recorded with and without mass loading from a patient with essential tremor. Note that the mechanical reflex (MR) tremor and frequency-invariant essential tremor (ET) responded to inertial loading in a manner that was qualitatively identical with the response of the MR and 8- to 12-Hz tremors in normal adults (see Fig. 2). The 8.0-Hz essential tremor was associated with a prominent spectral peak in the forearm EMG spectrum, reflecting the entrained motor unit modulation. Note how the frequency of the EMG spectral peak paradoxically increased slightly during inertial loading. This is characteristic of ET and of the 8- to 12-Hz physiological tremor (6).

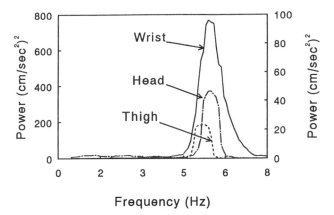

Figure 5 Autospectra of essential tremor recorded from the head (right *y*-axis) and from the wrist and thigh (left-*y*-axis) of a man with familial tremor. Thigh (hip) tremor was recorded with an accelerometer taped to the medial surface of the left knee. The patient was sitting in a chair with both feet on the floor and with both hips abducted and externally rotated a few degrees. Head tremor was recorded with an accelerometer on the left temple. The frequencies of these tremors differed by less than 0.3 Hz.

of the wrist generally has a frequency of 7–12 Hz, but its amplitude and associated motor unit entrainment are greater than the 8- to 12-Hz tremor of normal adults. The firing patterns of individual motor units in essential tremor are similar to the patterns observed in the 8- to 12-Hz physiological tremor: synchronous modulation of motor units at the frequency of tremor, irrespective of mean firing frequency (56).

From these observations, I have postulated that the 8- to 12-Hz component of physiological tremor is a forme fruste of essential tremor, and that essential tremor and the 8- to 12-Hz physiological tremor originate from the same central neuronal oscillator(s). According to this hypothesis, essential tremor begins as an abnormal enhancement of the 8- to 12-Hz component of physiological tremor. As essential tremor worsens, its frequency decreases, resulting in a negative logarithmic relation between the amplitude and frequency of tremor. Existing data are compatible with this hypothesis, but a longitudinal study is needed to confirm it.

VI. CAVEATS AND BENEFITS OF THE PHYSIOLOGICAL CHARACTERIZATION OF TREMOR

Great methodological care must be taken to demonstrate the phenomena discussed in this review. The details of the methodology are discussed elsewhere (52). Of particular importance is the restriction of motion to one joint. The popular method of recording tremor with an accelerometer on the hand while the entire upper extremity is extended horizontally can provide a measure of disability, but the accelerometer signal will not be an accurate measurement of wrist tremor. Tremor from proximal and distal joints are recorded in this manner, and the accelerometer signal may reflect only the dominant source of oscillation (2). The frequency of essential tremor and of the 8- to 12-Hz physiological tremor is measured most consistently by performing spectral analysis on rectified-filtered EMG that is recorded during inertial loading (see Figs. 2 and 4).

Physiological studies cannot define the underlying disfunction of a disease. In discussions of physiological studies, the principal argument frequently converges on the issue of whether essential tremor is generated by oscillation in the stretch reflex or in a centrally located network of neurons. These two mechanisms are not mutually exclusive. Even if essential tremor is produced by a central oscillator, this oscillation must be expressed through the neuromuscular machinery of the stretch reflex and limb mechanics (52). The stretch reflex and limb mechanics must play a role in governing the clinical expression of any tremor, and no physiological method has been able to isolate these peripheral factors from putative central mechanisms (i.e., oscillators). Reflex pathways could augment or promote oscillation in a central neuronal network, alter the frequency of oscillation through entrainment, and reset or entrain the rhythm of tremor. All of these phenomena have been observed in studies of essential tremor (52).

These limitations of physiological studies not withstanding, the proposed relation between essential tremor and the 8- to 12-Hz component of physiological tremor is an attractive and testable hypothesis. This hypothesis agrees nicely with existing animal models of essential tremor, and it emphasizes the importance of studying the dynamics of the oscillator once it is identified. Given the negative logarithmic relation between tremor amplitude and frequency (see Fig. 4), a therapeutic change in tremor frequency from 5 to 10 Hz would theoretically produce a 35-fold reduction in tremor amplitude. Similarly, modification of stretch reflex dynamics or limb mechanics could also have logarithmic effects on tremor amplitude.

Finally, further physiological characterization of essential tremor is important for establishing a database that will assist investigators in the development of accurate animal models and in the identification of pathology in postmortem studies. Given the monosymptomatic nature of essential tremor in most patients and the few existing nondiagnostic postmortem studies (57), the underlying pathology is certainly subtle and probably involves pathological alteration of physiological oscillation within the motor system.

ACKNOWLEDGMENTS

This work has been supported by NS20973 from the National Institute of Neurological Disorders and Stroke and by Biomedical Research Grant S07-RR05843 from the National Institutes of Health.

REFERENCES

1. Marshall J. Observations on essential tremor. J Neurol Neurosurg Psychiatry 1962; 25:122–125.
2. Elble RJ, Randall JE. Mechanistic components of normal hand tremor. Electroencephalogr Clin Neurophysiol 1978; 44:72–82.
3. Lakie M, Walsh EG, Wright GW. Passive mechanical properties of the wrist and physiological tremor. J Neurol Neurosurg Psychiatry 1986; 49:669–676.
4. Stiles RN, Randall JE. Mechanical factors in human tremor frequency. J Appl Physiol 1967; 23:324–330.
5. Robson JG. The effect of loading on the frequency of muscle tremor. J Physiol (Lond) 1959; 149:29P–30P.
6. Elble RJ. Physiologic and essential tremor. Neurology 1986; 36:225–231.
7. Hömberg V, Hefter H, Reiners K, Freund H-J. Differential effects of changes in mechanical limb properties on physiological and pathological tremor. J Neurol Neurosurg Psychiatry 1987; 50:568–579.
8. Stiles RN. Frequency and displacement amplitude relations for normal hand tremor. J Appl Physiol 1976; 40:44–54.
9. Stiles RN. Mechanical and neural feedback factors in postural hand tremor of normal subjects. J Neurophysiol 1980; 44:40–59.
10. Fox JR, Randall JE. Relationship between forearm tremor and the biceps electromyogram. J Appl Physiol 1970; 29:103–108.
11. Bengi H, Thomas JG. Studies on human ocular tremor. In: Kenedi RM, ed. Perspectives in Biomedical Engineering. Baltimore: University Park Press, 1973: 281–292.
12. Brumlik J. On the nature of normal tremor. Neurology 1962; 12:159–179.
13. Brumlik J, Yap C-B. Normal Tremor: A Comparative Study. Springfield, IL: Charles C. Thomas, 1970:3–15.
14. Van Buskirk C, Fink RA. Physiological tremor: an experimental study. Neurology 1962; 12:361–370.
15. Van Buskirk C, Wolbarsht ML, Stecher K. The non-nervous causes of normal physiologic tremor. Neurology 1966; 16:217–220.
16. Yap CB, Boshes B. The frequency and pattern of normal tremor. Electroencephalogr Clin Neurophysiol 1967; 22:197–203.
17. Carrie JRG, Bickford RG. Cardiovascular factors in limb tremor. Neurology 1969; 19:116–127.
18. Marsden CD, Meadows JC, Lange GW, Watson RS. The role of the ballistocardiac impulse in the genesis of physiological tremor. Brain 1969; 92:647–662.
19. Freund H-J. Motor unit and muscle activity in voluntary motor control. Physiol Rev 1983; 63:387–436.
20. Schafer EA, Canney HEL, Tunstall JO. On the rhythm of muscular response to volitional impulses in man. J Physiol (Lond) 1886; 7:111–117.
21. Allum JHJ, Dietz V, Freund H-J. Neuronal mechanisms underlying physiological tremor. J Neurophysiol 1978; 41:557–571.
22. Dietz V, Bischofberger E, Wita C, Freund H-J. Correlation between the discharges of

two simultaneously recorded motor units and physiological tremor. Electroencephalogr Clin Neurophysiol 1976; 40:97–105.

23. Marshall J, Walsh EG. Physiological tremor. J Neurol Neurosurg Psychiatry 1956; 19:260–267.

24. Christakos CN, Lal S. Lumped and population stochastic models of skeletal muscle: implications and predictions. Biol Cybern 1980; 36:73–85.

25. Partridge LD. Signal-handling characteristics of load-moving skeletal muscle. Am J Physiol 1966; 210:1178–1191.

26. Rosenthal NP, McKean TA, Roberts WJ, Terzuolo CA. Frequency analysis of stretch reflex and its main subsystems in triceps surae muscles of the cat. J Neurophysiol 1970; 33:713–749.

27. Stein RB. Peripheral control of movement. Physiol Rev 1974; 54:215–243.

28. Stephans JA, Taylor A. The effect of visual feedback on physiological muscle tremor. Electroencephalogr Clin Neurophysiol 1974; 36:457–464.

29. Sutton GG, Sykes K. The effect of withdrawal of visual presentation of errors upon the frequency spectrum of tremor in a manual task. J Physiol (Lond) 1967; 190:281–293.

30. Matthews PBC. Muscle spindles: their messages and their fusimotor supply. In: Brooks VB, ed. Handbook of Physiology: The Nervous System, Motor Control. Baltimore: Williams & Wilkins, 1981:189–228.

31. Hagbarth K-E, Young RR. Participation of the stretch reflex in human physiological tremor. Brain 1979; 102:509–526.

32. Young RR, Hagbarth K-E. Physiological tremor enhanced by maneuvers affecting the segmental stretch reflex. J Neurol Neurosurg Psychiatry 1980; 43:248–256.

33. Stiles RN. Lightly damped hand oscillations: acceleration-related feedback and system damping. J Neurophysiol 1983; 50:327–343.

34. Brown TIH, Rack PM, Ross HF. Forces generated at the thumb interphalangeal joint during imposed sinusoidal movements. J Physiol (Lond) 1982; 332:69–85.

35. Brown TIH, Rack PM, Ross HF. Electromyographic responses to imposed sinusoidal movements of the human thumb. J Physiol (Lond) 1982; 332:87–99.

36. Brown TIH, Rack PM, Ross HF. A range of different stretch reflex responses in the human thumb. J Physiol (Lond) 1982; 332:101–112.

37. Brown TIH, Rack PMH, Ross HF. Different types of tremor in the human thumb. J Physiol (Lond) 1982; 332:113–123.

38. Rack PMH. Limitations of somatosensory feedback in control of posture and movement. In: Brooks VB, ed. Handbook of Physiology: The Nervous System, Motor Control. Baltimore: Williams & Wilkins, 1981:229–256.

39. Rack PMH, Ross HF, Thilmann AF. The ankle stretch reflexes in normal and spastic subjects: the response to sinusoidal movement. Brain 1984; 107:637–654.

40. Zahalak GI, Cannon SC. Predictions of the existence, frequency, and amplitude of physiological tremor in normal man based on measured frequency-response characteristics. J Biomech Eng 1983; 105:249–257.

41. Sanes JN. Absence of enhanced physiological tremor in patients without muscle or cutaneous afferents. J Neurol Neurosurg Psychiatry 1985; 48:645–649.

42. Elble RJ, Higgins C, Moody CJ. Stretch reflex oscillations and essential tremor. J Neurol Neurosurg Psychiatry 1987; 50:691–698.

43. Matthews PBC, Muir RB. Comparison of electromyogram spectra with force spectra during human elbow tremor. J Physiol (Lond) 1980; 302:427–441.
44. Travis LE, Hunter TA. Muscular rhythms and action-currents. Am J Physiol 1927; 81: 355–359.
45. Thomas DP, Whitney RJ. Postural movements during normal standing in man. J Anat 1959; 93:524–539.
46. Mori S. Discharge patterns of soleus motor units with associated changes in force exerted by foot during quiet stance in man. J Neurophysiol 1973; 36:458–471.
47. Elble RJ, Randall JE. Motor-unit activity responsible for 8- to 12-Hz component of human physiological finger tremor. J Neurophysiol 1976; 39:370–383.
48. Logigian EL, Wierzbicka MM, Bruyninckx F, Wiegner AW, Shahani BT, Young RR. Motor unit synchronization in physiologic, enhanced physiologic, and voluntary tremor in man. Ann Neurol 1988; 23:242–250.
49. Halliday AM, Redfearn JWT. An analysis of the frequencies of finger tremor in healthy subjects. J Physiol (Lond) 1956; 134:600–611.
50. Lippold OCJ. Oscillation in the stretch reflex arc and the origin of the rhythmical 8–12 c/s component of physiological tremor. J Physiol (Lond) 1970; 206:359–382.
51. Agarwal GC, Gottlieb GL. Oscillation of the human ankle joint in response to applied sinusoidal torque on the foot. J Physiol (Lond) 1977; 268:151–176.
52. Elble RJ, Koller WC. Tremor. Baltimore: Johns Hopkins University Press, 1990: 10–89.
53. Calzetti S, Baratti M, Gresty M, Findley L. Frequency/amplitude characteristics of postural tremor of the hands in a population of patients with bilateral essential tremor; implications for the classification and mechanism of essential tremor. J Neurol Neurosurg Psychiatry 1987; 50:561–567.
54. Dueschl G, Lucking CH, Schenck E. Essential tremor: electrophysiological and pharmacological evidence for a subdivision. J Neurol Neurosurg Psychiatry 1987; 50:1435–1441.
55. Biary N, Koller WC. Essential tongue tremor. Mov Disord 1987; 2:25–29.
56. Young RR, Shahani BT. Analysis of single motor unit discharge patterns in different types of tremor. In: Cobb WA, Van Duijn H, eds. Contemporary Clinical Neurophysiology. Amsterdam: Elsevier, 1978:527–528.
57. Herskovits E, Blackwood W. Essential (familial, hereditary) tremor: a case report. J Neurol Neurosurg Psychiatry 1969; 32:509–511.

5

Physiological Finger Tremor in Medical Students and Others

E. Geoffrey Walsh
University of Edinburgh
Edinburgh, Scotland

I. INTRODUCTION

In teaching the rudiments of a neurological examination to medical students I have repeatedly noticed that, although most are steady, a significant minority show substantial finger tremor. Conspicuous instability in otherwise healthy people is referred to as *essential tremor*. Its prevalence is subject to debate. One study, from the Mayo Clinic, gave the incidence as 23.7:100,000 population (1). These figures are evidently a gross underestimate, in view of the results described later. There appear to have been no measurements of tremor in a normal population to ascertain the range to be expected and, accordingly, essential tremor has not been defined quantitatively. It was initially assumed that the medical students, being young, presumably healthy, and from good backgrounds, would be a representative normal population. As will be seen, however, when comparisons were made with other populations, they were exceptional. As some of the students had high levels of tremor, several factors that were thought to be significant have been investigated.

II. METHODS

A silicon chip accelerometer (ICS 3021) was fixed by a Velcro strap to the middle finger of the right hand to record vertical motion. For the investigation the person raised his or her fingers to a horizontal position, with the palm supported. The device incorporated a tiny mass supported on strain gauges; as the finger moved the resistance of the strain gauges changed, this unbalanced a bridge circuit. The signal was rectified, and in the instrument used for all of the investigations, except where otherwise stated, components above 12 Hz were removed by a fifth-order low-pass filter, whereas those below 7 Hz were removed by a 80-db/octave high-pass elliptical filter. The waveform was amplified, rectified, and integrated over a 5-s period. The mean output of the tremorometer was displayed on a digital meter. A delay circuit was arranged so that the integration started 3 s after the finger was raised, to avoid the initial instability during positioning. For some observations, a similar instrument was used, but the frequency reponse was wide, being flat within 1 db between 2 and 30 Hz. This was referred to as the *broad-band* tremorometer. Other observations were made isometrically. The person was instructed to press down with a force of 5 N with the middle finger on a RS Components (2 kg) load cell. Visual feedback of the mean force was displayed to the subject on a dampened analog meter. The signals were filtered to pass only components between 7 and 12 Hz, rectified and integrated, as in the main instrument. The large low-frequency fluctuations so prominent in the unfiltered output were thus excluded. In each observation, four measurements were made in succession, and the mean was calculated, the procedure thus took about 2 min.

Except where otherwise stated, tremor levels in the different groups were compared by Wilcoxon rank sum test and changes over time were tested by Wilcoxon signed rank tests. Kendall rank correlation was used to test for association between tremor and other quantitative measurements. Estimates and confidence intervals (CI) for percentage changes were calculated by the use of the *t*-distribution applied to the logarithms of the tremor values.

III. RESULTS

A. Tremor Levels in Edinburgh and Glasgow Medical Students

A histogram giving the distribution of tremor amplitudes in first-year medical students is shown in Figure 1. There is no significant difference between the results for the students in the two cities; the observations were made during practical classes. The results for our students were thus presumably not influenced by the positions on the staff of those involved in the testing (EGW and GWW). Tremor is just visible above about 50 cm $s^{-1} s^{-1}$ and conspicuous above, 100 cm $s^{-1} s^{-1}$. The instrument could record tremor below the levels of visibility. It is evident that the values were skew-distributed, most subjects had little tremor, but in a few tremor was striking. Plotted logarithmically the distributions are sensibly normal and unimodal; there was no suggestion of two populations: the tremulous and the stable (Fig. 2). The data were analyzed according to sex. There was no difference in the Edinburgh students, but in the Glasgow students, the men had significantly

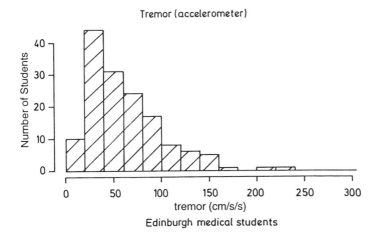

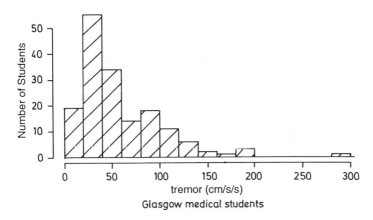

Figure 1 Histograms of tremor levels in Edinburgh and Glasgow medical students. The distribution is similar, and both are heavily skewed. Most have relatively little tremor, but a few shake conspicuously. One entry, for a value of 530 in an Edinburgh medical student, is not shown for reasons of scale.

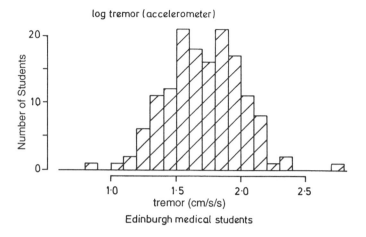

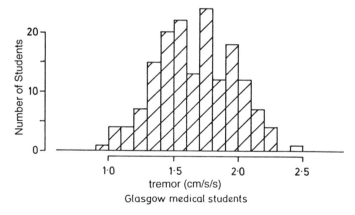

Figure 2 The same data as Figure 1 plotted on a logarithmic scale; the distribution is now sensibly normal.

more than the women, the median being 36 for the women and 53 for the men ($p <$ 0.01). I have no explanation for this difference. There was no relation with handedness.

B. Reproducibility

The Edinburgh medical students were tested on two occasions, in the autumn in their first term and in the following spring (Fig. 3). The results were in broad agreement. The correlation coefficient was 0.63 ($p < 0.001$). In addition 14

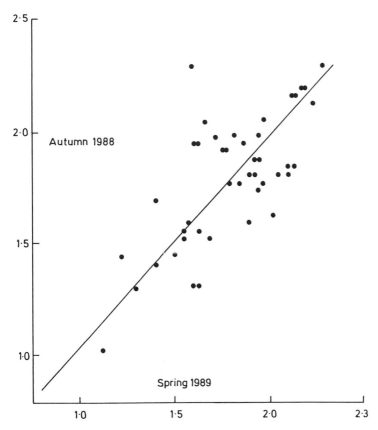

Figure 3 Log tremor value data from Edinburgh medical students obtained on two occasions with a 3-month interval. There is a clear correlation between the two sets of data.

students at the Napier Polytechnic working for their Bachelor of Science in biological sciences were tested twice, once in December 1989, and again in May 1990. A correlation coefficient of 0.83 was obtained between the two sets of data ($p < 0.001$). In general, subjects with high values on one occasion are likely to have high values when tested again, whereas those with low values initially are likely to be low subsequently.

Diurnal variations were not studied. One report describes such changes, but they were small and perhaps of doubtful statistical significance (2).

We tested two subjects several times over a period of more than a month. The results are shown in Figure 4. The person who had the higher initial tremor remained at a higher level throughout. There was a significant decrease in tremor levels during the course of the observation, a correlation coefficient of -0.70

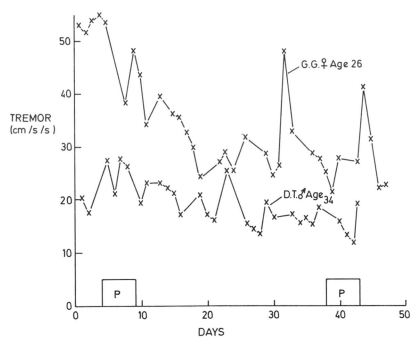

Figure 4 Tremor levels in two subjects to show variations in successive determinations. The overall drop as time goes by is statistically significant (see text). It was not likely to be due to increasing familiarity with the procedure, as both subjects were laboratory technicians. It may have related to a change of limb temperature, as the observations were made in October and November with the onset of winter. It is known that cooling reduces tremor (3). The days indicated (P) refer to the menstrual periods of the woman, there would appear to be no relation to the values recorded.

being obtained for the man, and -0.73 for the woman, over the period. Both changes were highly significant ($p < 0.001$). There was thus substantial variation, but this was much less than the differences between different persons.

C. Comparison of Tremor Levels in Medical and Other Students Doing the Same Courses

At Glasgow University, first-year medical, dental, science, and nursing students have a core curriculum doing the same practical experiments in the same laboratory, with the same demonstrators. The tremor values are given in Table 1. The median for the dental students is marginally higher than that for the Edinburgh

Table 1 Tremor in Glasgow Physiology Students
(cm s^{-1} s^{-1})

	n	Median	Range	Difference vs Edinburgh medicals[a]
Dental	23	54	21–106	NS
Medical	164	47	9–282	NS
Science	78	41	14–177	$p < 0.05$
Nursing	16	35	13–88	$p < 0.05$

[a]NS, not significant.

medical students (see later), but the difference is not significant. The science and nursing students have less.

In honors physiology in Edinburgh, some students are medical doing an intercalated year, whereas others are in the science faculty. For six medical students the mean log tremor was 1.77, SD 0.14, that for seven science students 1.60, SD 0.15. From the Students t-test, the difference was significant ($p < 0.05$).

D. Comparison of Edinburgh Medical Students with Other Lay Populations

Initial studies and the data already described suggested that the levels of tremor in medical students might not be characteristic of the population as a whole. Accordingly, observations were made on a considerable number of persons with a wide range of skills and occupations. The results are shown in Table 2. Because of the skew nature of the distribution of amplitudes, we have used the median as an indicator. It will be seen that the median for the Edinburgh medical students is unusually high.

E. Comparison of Edinburgh Medical Students with Members of Religious Groups

Measurements were made of tremor levels in several persons who were affiliated with religious organizations. The results are shown in Table 3. The median for the Edinburgh medical students (see Table 2) was higher than that of any of these groups.

F. Comparison with Other Procedures for Estimating Tremor Levels

With practice, I found that by observing the fingers beforehand, I could predict with reasonable certainty the general level of the results that the instrument would display. In 13 firemen and 21 laboratory workers I compared the figures obtained

Table 2 Tremor Levels (cm s^{-1} s^{-1}) in Medical Students and Others[a]

Group	n	Median	Range	Details
Edinburgh medical students	149	52	7–530	1st year 1988
Edinburgh veterinary students	46	50	10–273	1st year 1989
Trainee general practitioners	23	50	14–140	Attending postgraduate lectures
Polytechnic students	64	49	14–406	Science and management studies
Music students	39	47	14–388	Edinburgh University
Glasgow medical students	164	47	10–282	1st year 1989
Consultant orthopaedic surgeons	14	45	28–88	Princess Margaret Rose Hospital
St. Andrews medical students	102	42	9–353	1st year 1989
University cleaners	17	40	8–174	Work in Edinburgh Medical School
Prospective medical students	32	40	15–208	Visiting
Business consultants	18	40	9–131	Advisers to unemployed
Pharmacy workers	33	40	12–120	Edinburgh Royal Infirmary
Glasgow police	44	40	11–166	Attending sick parade
Dundee medical students	76	40	9–150	1st year 1989
Trainee teachers	38	38	13–156	Moray House
Schoolchildren	70	38	9–95	Attending University open day
Electronic factory employees	40	37	15–143	Hughes microelectronics
2H science students	30	36	18–161	2nd year physiology, Edinburgh
Established general practitioners	20	35	19–112	Attending postgraduate lectures
Bank of Scotland staff	54	35	11–150	Training school
Air cadets	24	34	10–172	University air squadron
SAGA holidaymakers	36	34	12–201	Health and fitness week, Dundee
Edinburgh firemen	46	34	14–110	McDonald Road Station
Advocates	28	34	14–75	Parliament House
Journalists	49	33	11–111	Scotsman and Evening News
Art students	16	32	16–65	Silversmith course
Security staff	24	31	10–65	Royal Museum of Scotland
Eye surgeons	30	29	11–74	Edinburgh and Glasgow
Ethicon employees	61	27	11–173	Surgical suture factory
Marksmen	34	27	8–67	Includes some Olympic standard

Table 2 Continued

Group	n	Median	Range	Details
University staff	20	27	15–95	Academic, technical, secretarial
Foreign language students	24	27	2–115	Institute of Applied Languages
Meditators	27	27	7–122	Transcendental
Museum staff	23	26	10–77	Designers and curators
Students of humanities	14	26	18–60	Edinburgh University
Wheelchair shooters	9	25	15–72	Paraplegic and amputees

[a]Ranked in descending order according to values for median.

with the standard and the broad-band tremorometers (Fig. 5). The correlation coefficient was 0.9, and this was highly significant ($p < 0.001$). Naturally, the instrument with the wider bandwidth gave higher values. A comparison was also made between results with the standard instrument and the isometric method. One hundred thirty-three medical students were tested. The correlation coefficient was 0.30 ($p < 0.001$). The data described are thus not likely to be critically dependent on the design of the instrumentation.

G. Thyroid Hormone Levels

Students take blood for their practical work. With their permission the level of certain thyroid hormones was estimated, analyses were arranged by Dr. G. Beckett (Dept. of Clinical Chemistry). In 34 students the levels of thyrotropin (TSH), free throxine (FR_4), and triiodothyronine (T_3) did not correlate with tremor levels.

Table 3 Tremor Levels (cm s^{-1} s^{-1}) in Members of Religious Organizations[a]

Group	n	Median	Range	Details
Young Unitarians	16	43	13–107	Weekend group
Church of Scotland Ministers	27	34	15–123	Commissioners at General Assembly, 1990
Seventh Day Adventists	19	34	11–77	At a communal meal
Quakers	28	34	10–62	After Sunday meeting
Lay Catholics	29	32	19–116	University chaplaincy
Nuns	11	32	18–67	Teachers
Muslims	17	31	16–141	Students in Potter Row Mosque
Buddhists	26	23	8.5–74	Samye Ling Tibetan Centre
Brahma Kumaris	13	22	11–124	Prayer and Meditation Group

[a]Ranked in descending order according to values for median.

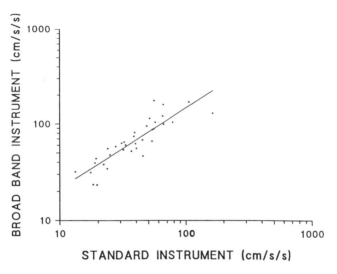

Figure 5   Data comparing results using the standard instrument with filtering with those of an instrument having a flat frequency response over a wide range. The data are clearly correlated.

H.   Fine Work

I wondered if people doing fine work had less tremor than others. The students at the Edinburgh College of Art had low, but not particularly low, values (see Table 2). The sample was from the silversmith class. The group of "eye surgeons" were not all engaged in major eye surgery, some were opthalmologists, but all had occasion to remove foreign bodies from the cornea. Their values, although not high, were not especially low. A more useful comparison was the "electronic factory employees" (Hughes Microelectronics, Glenrothes, Fife). Twenty-one subjects were employed on fine work involving the freehand attachment of connections to silicon chips under the microscope, whereas 19 were clerical and administrative staff nearby. There were no differences between the two groups. A similar comparison was possible with the Ethicon employees. This firm manufactures surgical sutures, and operatives insert the sutures into the needles freehand under magnification. The 31 people engaged in this fine work had values that did not differ significantly from the 30 office workers tested at the same factory.

It is unlikely that a person with a very high tremor level would be employed in very dextrous work, but a postgraduate music student with a level of 388 cm $s^{-1}s^{-1}$ played the piano for us in a highly accomplished way. On playing stringed musical instruments a form of voluntarily induced tremor is used to produce vibrato (4).

I. Consideration of Smoking, Coffee, Bronchodilators, Alcohol, and Heredity

The Edinburgh medical students were asked about their smoking habits. Only a few smoked, and smoking habits did not correlate with tremor levels. We also asked for volunteers among the university staff. The 25 subjects abstained from smoking for at least an hour before the tests and then smoked two king-sized, special filter Benson & Hedges cigarettes. Immediately after the second cigarette, tremor increased significantly ($p < 0.05$); the 95% confidence limits were -1 to $+37\%$; 15 min later the control level was again reached.

We also inquired by questionnaire about the students' intake of dietary substances conaining xanthines and, from the data, estimated the daily intake of caffeine, theobromine, and theophylline. There was no correlation between these values and the tremor levels. We sought volunteer students from the Faculty of Arts and measured their tremor, they then drank 2 cups of coffee and the measurements were repeated 40 min later, the presumed time of peak absorption. Nescafe was used, the estimated caffeine intake being 270 mg. There was no significant change in tremor level. The confidence limits were -13 to $+32\%$.

Very few of the students took bronchodilator drugs, which through their β-adrenergic agonist properties, are known to increase tremor. The students taking these drugs did not have particularly high values.

The levels of alcohol intake were ascertained by questionnaire and found to be a little below those reported for a population of medical students in London (5). There was no discernible relation between intake and tremor level. We inquired about a family history of essential tremor and of parkinsonism; again, no relations were established.

J. Vegetarianism

It is a common belief that eating red meat in excess is associated with a somewhat wild personality. I wondered accordingly whether there would be a difference between vegetarians and nonvegetarians in their tremor levels. The Seventh Day Adventists were all vegetarians, their median (34 cm $s^{-1}s^{-1}$) was neither particularly high nor low, but the Buddhists and the Brahma Kumaris groups, also wholly vegetarian, had the lowest values in the whole survey. Of 97 students interviewed, in the class of 1989, 9 were vegetarians (there were no vegans), but there was no significant differences in tremor levels. My investigations on this aspect of tremor are thus inconclusive, but further study might be worthwhile.

K. Age

Tremor was measured in a population of fit elderly persons, most of whom were on a "Saga" holiday in Dundee. The mean age was 67 (range 50–90). The values were in no way exceptional (see Table 2).

L. Influence of Exercise

Exercise is commonly believed to increase tremor. Accordingly, two experiments were undertaken in the practical class, exercising either the muscles of the arm being tested or the legs. In one procedure the subjects squeezed a Harpenden dynamometer (British Indicators Ltd.) with the right hand using maximal, or one-third maximal, strength every 3 s for 2 min. In the second, the person pedaled on a bicycle ergometer as vigorously as possible for 2 min. Measurements were made beforehand, and observations made immediately after, or 5 min, after stopping. The results are shown in Table 4. It will be seen that there were significant increases, but the alterations even with vigorous activity was much less than the variation found between different subjects (see Table 2).

At a reading party at the Firbush Field Centre, Loch Tay, 12 students spent 3 h canoeing on 16 occasions. There was no significant change in tremor.

Anecdotally, people speak of a tremor following exercise. This may arise from unusually strenuous eccentric work during which the muscles although active are lengthening under a load. There is no reason to suppose that variations of physical activity account for the variability of the medical student's tremor.

M. An Increase with Flying

Observations were made on 17 trainee pilots with the East Lowlands Universities Air Squadron. The median during a resting period was 34, that immediately after landing 58 cm $s^{-1}s^{-}$. The difference was highly significant ($p < 0.001$). There was thus a 58% increase after the flight. The 95% confidence limit for the increase was 29–95%. The light aircraft used were "Bulldogs." Increases have also been reported in commercial pilots flying intercontinental airliners (6). Changes were also recorded using the isometric method; a table of the results has been published elsewhere (7).

Table 4 Effects of Exercise on Tremor in Medical Students

Limb	Strength of exercise	Waiting time before measurement	n	Estimated percentage increase in tremor	95% confidence interval (%)
Forearm	⅓ maximal	None	42	+24	+8, +42
Forearm	Maximal	None	31	+25	+9, +44
Forearm	Maximal	5 min	14	+9	−12, +35
Leg	Maximal	None	44	+49	+25, +78
Leg	Maximal	5 min	11	+32	+20, +46

Table 5 Tremor in Male Medical Students Studying in Edinburgh

	n	Median (cm s^{-1} s^{-1})	>100 (cm s^{-1} s^{-1})
Scottish	44	58	2%
English	33	70	13%

N. An Increase with Rappelling (Abseiling)

Volunteers who had never rappelled before undertook this activity down the six-story "Crest" hotel. Measurements were made immediately beforehand, and immediately after, in 12 subjects. The median before was 55 cm s^{-1} s^{-1} (range 20–159). Afterward the median was 119 cm s^{-1} s^{-1} (range 41–197). The increase was highly significant ($p < 0.01$).

O. Relation with Site of Domicile

The data for the Edinburgh medical students were analyzed according to the home addresses. Most were from Scotland or England. There was no difference between the women, but the English men had unusually high values (Table 5). The number with high values was particularly striking (> 100 cm s^{-1} s^{-1}).

IV. DISCUSSION

In some earlier work, the distinction between wrist tremor and finger tremor has not been clear. If the forearm is supported and a transducer placed on a finger, the results will be compounded of motion at the wrist as well as that at the fingers. Because of the difference in the radius of gyration, a linear accelerometer, the type virtually always employed, would be especially sensitive to wrist tremor. Studies of wrist tremor have uncovered a passive resonance at about 8 Hz, even in anesthetized, paralyzed patients (8). This was attributed to the inertia of the hand interacting with the stiffness of the musculature. Muscles have short-range stiffness and show properties that are demonstrably thixotropic (9). The prominence of wrist tremor may well be affected by the degree of thixotropy. A suggestion that this is so comes from the easily made observation that physiological tremor is enhanced for a few seconds following a movement when thixotropic stiffness is reduced and when, presumably, greater active muscular contraction is needed to hold a given posture.

In the present study, motion at the wrist was excluded by supporting the palm to see more clearly the effects of nervous factors. Preliminary experiments showed that finger resonance occurs at considerably higher frequencies. The influence of high frequencies, and of low-frequency instability, was reduced by the filtering system used. Accordingly, the effect of passive tissue properties were expected to be minimal. In the event, as described in a foregoing paragraph, we came to believe that the general nature of the results did not depend at all critically on the particular instrumentation.

We considered several factors that might explain the wide variability of finger tremor in our students. Thyroid hormone levels, smoking, coffee, bronchodilators, alcohol, heredity, and exercise did not appear to have substantial weight. It seems highly improbable that any of these potential causes account for the large differences, nearly 100-fold, that we have found in our students.

It is a common human experience that powerful emotions, including fear, can give rise to shaking, and there are plentiful references to this both in the Bible and in Shakespeare, and clinicians have long spoken of an "anxiety tremor." The medical course is intense and prolonged, with numerous examinations and tests. After qualification there is hospital work, and later, problems of finding suitable employment. Our students, in general, represent a group of the population who drive themselves hard to achieve difficult goals. Value judgments on the merits or otherwise of particular levels of tremor may be misplaced. Perhaps very placid people have low values, whereas higher levels may be a reflection of more "get up and go," but such psychological speculations would require careful study to establish their validity; this seems never to have been undertaken. We believe that the high levels of tremor in the English men merits further consideration. It is known that homesickness is common in first-year university students (10). The English students in Edinburgh are mostly farther, many much farther, from home than their Scottish peers. The entry to veterinary colleges is also highly competitive, and those students also have high values. There is evidence of an unusually high level of compulsiveness in people seeking careers in medicine (11,12). A recent monograph has dealt with stress in health professionals (13).

It might be that first-year medicine is the most stressful part of the medical course. However, an assessment of stress in fourth-year medical students, using the general health questionnaire, showed that 31% were emotionally disturbed (14). Furthermore, years on, the trainee general practitioners, too, had high levels of tremor. Whether or not students with very high values should be dissuaded from seeking a career in surgery is outside the scope of this paper. Finally, it would be surprising if populations and persons who differed in the way described did not differ also in other physiological and biochemical parameters.

V. SUMMARY

Tremor has been measured with an accelerometer on an outstretched finger, the mean output over a 5-s period being ascertained in over 2500 persons. Edinburgh medical students showed wide variation among different subjects, and the levels were skew-distributed, with a minority having high values. A comparison with a considerable number of persons, with widely differing skills, occupations, and affiliations, showed that the Edinburgh medical students had unusually high levels of tremor. Correlations were not established with levels of thyroid hormones, smoking habits, coffee intake, the use of bronchodilators, alcohol intake, or heredity. Vigorous exercise of the arm or legs gave rise to a significant increase of tremor, but the variation was much smaller than that between different persons. The levels were increased by flying a light aircraft and by rappelling down the side of a hotel. The English male medical students at Edinburgh had exceptionally high values.

ACKNOWLEDGMENTS

My thanks are due to the many persons who volunteered for these studies and, particularly, to the members of the various organizations who facilitated the work. Dr. R. H. Baxendale kindly arranged for tests to be carried out in the Institute of Physiology, Glasgow. My grateful thanks are due to Dr. Neil Powers and Mr. G. W. Wright for practical help, to Dr. R. A. Elton for much useful statistical advice and Dr. A. S. Davies and Dr. M. H. Draper for useful discussions.

REFERENCES

1. Rajput A, Offord KP, Beard CM, Kurland LT. Essential tremor in Rochester, Minnesota: a 45 year study. J Neurol Neurosurg Psychiatry 1984; 47:466–470.
2. Tyrer PJ, Bond AJ. Diurnal variation in physiological tremor. Electroencephalogr Clin Neurophysiol 1974; 37:35–40.
3. Lakie, M, Walsh EG, Arblaster LA, Villagra, F, Roberts RC. Limb temperature and human tremors. J Neurol Neurosurg Psychiatry 1994; 57:35–42.
4. Schlapp M. Observations on a voluntary tremor—violinist's vibrato. Q J Exp Physiol 1973; 58:357–368.
5. Collier DJ, Beales ILP. Drinking among medical students: a questionnaire survey. Br Med J 1989; 299:19–22.
6. Nicholson AN, Hill LE, Borland RG, Ferres HM. Activity of the nervous system during the let-down, approach and landing: a study of short duration high work load. Clin Aviation Aerospace Med 1970; 41:436–446.
7. Cyster D, Elton R, Lakie M, Powers N, Walsh EG, Wright GW. Tremor in aviators. J Physiol 1989; 413:29P.
8. Lakie M, Walsh EG, Wright GW. Passive mechanical properties of the wrist and physiological tremor. J Neurol Neurosurg Psychiatry 1986; 49:669–676.
9. Lakie M, Walsh EG, Wright GW. Resonance at the wrist demonstrated by the use of a torque motor: an instrumental analysis of muscle tone in man. J Physiol 1984; 353: 265–285.

10. Fisher S, Hood B. The stress of transition to university: a longitudinal study of psychologial disturbance, absent-mindedness and vulnerability to homesickness. Br J Psychol 1987; 78;425–441.
11. Lloyd C, Gartrell NK. Psychiatric symptoms in medical students. Compr Psychiatry 1984; 25:552–565.
12. Gabbard GO. The role of compulsiveness in the normal physician. JAMA 1985; 254: 2926–2929.
13. Payne R, Firth-Cozens J. Stress in Health Professionals. Chichester: John Wiley & Sons, 1987.
14. Firth J. Levels and sources of stress in medical students. Br Med J 1986; 292:1177–1180.

6

Are Neurophysiological Techniques Useful in Differentiating Tremor?

Peter Bain
Radcliffe Infirmary
Oxford, England

I. INTRODUCTION

The accurate diagnosis of tremor is of fundamental importance to both patients and clinicians because assessment of prognosis and treatment selection depend on tremor type. For instance, a patient with benign tremulous Parkinson's disease might be treated with L-dopa, whereas another patient with an action tremor of the limbs might be given primidone (if the underlying disease was believed to be essential tremor). Furthermore, the correct classification of each patient's tremor is vital to the success of therapeutic trials and to genetic, family, and epidemiological studies.

Currently, clinicians favor the classification of tremor into rest and action varieties, the latter being subdivided into postural, kinetic, intention, and task-specific types (Table 1); or according to the etiology of the underlying diseases with which a particular tremor type is associated (Table 2). Although these approaches have been widely adopted, in practice, clinicians experience difficulties in establishing whether a tremulous limb is truly at rest or is activated and also in distinguishing the intention and kinetic components of tremor, particularly if a postural component is also present. What different clinicians mean by intention tremor is also questionable: recently, four neurologists, all of whom had a special interest in movement disorders, were asked to classify the upper limb tremors of 20 video-taped patients. Before the assessments, all four neurologists agreed to define kinetic and intention tremor as illustrated in Figure 1. The results,

Table 1 Classification of Tremor by Appearance

1. Rest
2. Action
A. Postural
B. Movement (kinetic or intention)
C. Task-specific

which were analyzed using Cohen's kappa coefficient (1,2) for interrater reliability, showed that there was very poor agreement among the assessors concerning which of the patients had kinetic or intention tremor and even less agreement on the severity of these two components of tremor.

A further flaw in the traditional classification of tremor is the underlying implication that the cause of a rest tremor is different from that of a postural or movement tremor. For example, in Parkinson's disease, is the mechanism underlying rest tremor different from that causing postural tremor, or different from that underlying benign tremulous Parkinson's disease? Does midbrain (rubral) tremor, with its rest, postural, and movement components, involve three separate mechanisms? Are the postural tremors seen in peripheral neuropathy, essential tremor, and idiopathic torsion dystonia really different, or are they generated in an identical fashion? These questions are manifestations of a more fundamental one, which is: are all pathological tremors the expressions of a single functional defect in a complex nonlinear oscillator–generator system, their apparent differences being the effect of disorders elsewhere, or do different tremors represent defects in different oscillatory systems, or defects at different sites within the same system?

Table 2 Classification of Tremor by Etiology

1. Physiological and enhanced physiological
2. Parkinson's disease and causes of parkinsonism
3. Essential (familial and sporadic)
4. Dystonic
a. Primary (idiopathic and hereditary torsion dystonia)
b. Secondary causes of dystonia (e.g., Wilson's disease)
5. Neuropathic
6. Midbrain ("rubral")
7. Cerebellar
8. Drug-induced
9. Functional

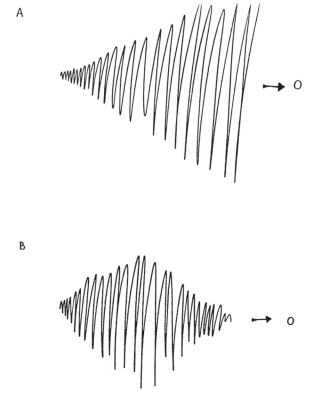

Figure 1 Neurologists' perceptions of (A) intention tremor; increasing in amplitude as a limb approaches an object O; and (B) kinetic tremor. In practice differentiating these profiles is difficult with little interobserver agreement (see text).

Could tremor be similar to "pyramidal" weakness?, which can be caused by a multitude of disease processes causing lesions at a plethora of sites, yet usually produces the same characteristic signs: hypertonia, hyperreflexia, clonus, and extensor plantar responses. Answering this question is complicated by the absence of any consistent pathological lesion in postmortem and radiographic studies of essential tremor and the paucity of postmortem studies of tremor in general. This leaves the etiological classification of tremor heavily dependent on clinical criteria and open to idiosyncratic interpretation. Similar difficulties arise from insufficient knowledge about the genetics of essential tremor and torsion dystonia. For example, do patients with task-specific tremor on writing (but no tremor at rest or with posture) have a forme fruste of essential tremor, a variant of writer's cramp (focal dystonia), or an entirely separate condition?

Resolution of these problems will depend on further insights obtained from neurophysiological, genetic, and pathological studies.

It is with these difficulties in mind that this account of how neurophysiological techniques may help differentiate tremor is given.

II. NEUROPHYSIOLOGICAL TECHNIQUES USED TO DIFFERENTIATE TREMOR

1. Accelerometry
2. Electromyography (EMG)
   a. Surface recordings (polymyography)
   b. Single motor unit studies
3. Peripheral nerve conduction studies
4. Resetting tremor
5. Reciprocal inhibition of the H-reflex
6. Stretch reflexes
7. Voluntary ballistic movements
8. Positron emission tomography (PET)

A. Accelerometry

Accelerometry was introduced by Agate et al., in 1956, and has been used ubiquitously since then to measure tremor frequency and amplitude. It is a simple, reliable, and convenient technique that is widely employed in therapeutic trials, although its validity for this purpose is questionable. The results of accelerometry are usually displayed as either power spectra, in which acceleration power $(m/s^2)^2$ of a tremor is plotted against its frequency (Hz), or as simple spectra [acceleration (m/s^2) against frequency (Hz)]. Modern accelerometers having a sensitivity of $0.01 \text{ mV cm}^{-1} \text{ s}^{-2}$.

The observation that individual types of tremor, such as the rest tremor of Parkinson's disease or the action tremor observed in some cerebellar lesions, have relatively constant frequencies was made by Gordon Holmes in 1904. He suggested that the frequency of a tremor was specific to its pathophysiological origin (3). Accelerometry has shown that this view contains an element of truth, in that certain tremor frequencies are characteristic of various diseases (Table 3). However, in practice, these frequencies overlap considerably, making differentiation of tremor types by frequency alone hazardous. Further complexity occurs because the frequency of tremor varies with the site of measurement. Typically, the frequency of upper limb tremor will be slightly faster the more distally it is measured, and the frequencies of lower limb and head tremor will be lower than that in the upper limbs of a subject. Age is also a factor; the 8- to 12-Hz component

Table 3 Characteristic Frequencies of Various Types of Tremor

Type of tremor	Typical frequency in the upper limb (Hz)[a]
Cerebellar intention	3–4
Parkinson's disease (rest)	3–6
(postural)	4–8
Essential	4–10
Dystonic	4–10
Neuropathic	4–6
Physiological	8–12
Primary orthostatic	16

[a]Measured with an accelerometer placed over the dorsum of the hand between the second and third metacarpal.

of physiological tremor observed in the fingers of young adults occurs at lower frequencies in children and the elderly (4).

Despite the drawbacks, accelerometry can be useful in suggesting that within an individual two apparently different tremors have a common origin. A good example of this is shown in Figure 2, which illustrates a curious phenomenon: this patient had primary writing tremor affecting his right (dominant) hand, but not his left. He had no postural tremor in either hand, but on writing with his left hand (which was not affected), he developed a tremor in his relaxed right hand. The frequencies of his primary writing tremor and the tremor in his right hand induced by writing with his left were identical (5.63 Hz), suggesting a common mechanism.

B. Electromyographic Studies

1. Surface Recordings

In EMG pairs of silver–silver chloride electrodes are arranged approximately 2 cm apart over the muscles involved in generating a tremor. The impedance of the skin is reduced by skin abrasion and electrode gel. The signal from the electrodes is then subjected to high-impedance differential amplification before recording. Multiple muscles can be sampled simultaneously.

Motor unit synchronization is readily detectable as bursts of activity separated by relative silence in the EMG records of the involved muscles. This synchronicity is characteristic of all the pathological tremors and enhanced physiological tremor, but not normal, low-amplitude, physiological tremor (5). The segregation of the EMG into bursts can be analyzed, and the frequency, amplitude, and width of the burst can be measured. Once again, the frequency of the EMG bursts is relatively

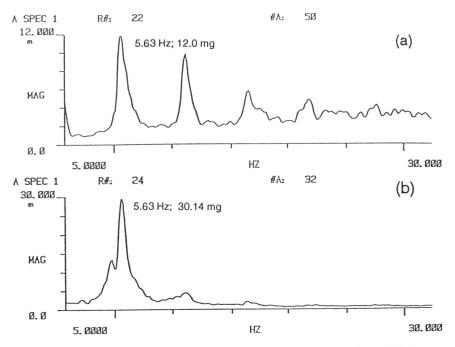

Figure 2   Power spectra from a patient with primary writing tremor: (a) A 5.63-Hz peak in the patient's right hand on writing with the right hand; (b) a peak at exactly the same frequency (5.63 Hz) in the same patient's right hand when writing with the left hand. This did not occur when the left hand performed other tasks, such as drawing an Archimedes' spiral.

unhelpful in distinguishing various types of tremor. The one exception to this is primary orthostatic tremor: a rare condition in which unsteadiness, resulting from tremulous lower limbs, occurs when standing rather than walking (6). This distinctive clinical picture [apparently first described by Pazzaglia et al. (7)] is associated with 16-Hz rhythmic EMG activity in the musculature of a weight-bearing limb (Fig. 3). Symptomatic amelioration can be obtained in some cases with clonazepam (6).

The relation of the EMG bursts in agonist–antagonist muscle pairs has been studied. In patients with dystonic posturing of a tremulous limb (or head) the EMG records typically show cocontraction of the agonist–antagonist muscles when an abnormal posture occurs and either coactivation or alternating patterns of the EMG bursts during tremor. Furthermore, because of the interplay between EMG bursts producing tremor and those producing a muscle spasm (altered posture), the variability in the EMG burst duration appears to be much greater in patients with dystonia than those with other causes of tremor (Fig. 4). Surface EMG studies can also be helpful in determining which muscles are primarily responsible for producing a specific tremor and can help target treatment. For instance, if the right sternocleidomastoid and splenius capitis were excessively active in a tremulous spasmodic torticollis, these muscles could be injected with botulinum toxin.

2. Single Motor Unit Studies

Single motor unit discharges can be recorded by inserting concentric needle electrodes into the muscles involved in tremorgenesis. This technique can be used to determine the firing rate of individual motor units, the synchronization of units within one muscle, and the synchrony and coherence of tremor in homologous muscle groups of the arms or legs.

In normal subjects, a moderate tonic contraction results in motor unit discharges of about 10–15 Hz. In patients with Parkinson's disease (PD) or essential tremor (ET), the motor units fire in bursts of up to 50 Hz, which are not sustained, but are grossly grouped within each tremor cycle. In both ET and PD there is a further tendency for the discharges from individual motor units to synchronize over a shorter time span. The relations between this short-term synchrony and that responsible for the EMG bursts in tremor have yet to be elucidated.

Single-unit studies have shown a difference in the recruitment order of motor units within each tremor burst in PD and ET. Patients with PD have a normal order of recruitment, whereas those with ET have a disrupted pattern (5,8).

In primary orthostatic tremor cross-correlation techniques have shown that the timing of activation of the motor units (in each tremor cycle) are highly synchronized in the homologous muscle groups of the legs (6), this does not appear to be true of essential tremor.

C. Peripheral Nerve Conduction Studies

Postural tremor is seen in some patients, but not others, with acute or chronic idiopathic demyelinating polyneuropathies and IgM paraproteinemic neuropathies. The reason some patients with these conditions become tremulous, whereas others with equally severe neuropathies do not, is ill understood. Postural tremor is also associated with hereditary motor–sensory neuropathies [for example, the Roussy–Levy (9) and Dejerine Sottas syndromes (10,11)].

Tremor can be the presenting symptom in paraproteinemic neuropathies and predate the onset of paresthesia or weakness by several years. Consequently, areflexic patients presenting with postural tremor should have their peripheral nerve conduction velocities measured. Typically median and ulnar nerve motor conduction velocities are reduced to between 10 and 25 m/s. As central motor conduction latencies are normal in these conditions, an alternative (screening) test is to measure the latencies to the hand muscles (abductor pollicis brevis or first dorsal interosseous) in response to magnetic cortical stimulation; if these are

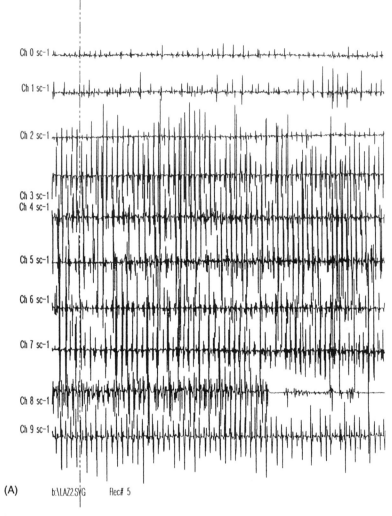

Ch 0 sc-1

Ch 1 sc-1

Ch 2 sc-1

Ch 3 sc-1
Ch 4 sc-1

Ch 5 sc-1

Ch 6 sc-1

Ch 7 sc-1

Ch 8 sc-1

Ch 9 sc-1

(A)   b:\LAZ2.SVG   Rec# 5

Figure 3 A 4 second polymyographic recording from a patient with primary orthostatic tremor: (A) A 16-Hz rhythmic EMG activity when the patient was standing with both arms held out in front of the body; (B) the disappearance of rhythmic activity when the patient was lifted off his feet. Channels 0, 2, 4, 6 (right) and 1, 3, 5, 7 (left) quadriceps femoris, hamstrings, tibialis anterior, and gastrocnemius, respectively; channel 8, right splenius capitis; channel 9, right anterior deltoid muscles.

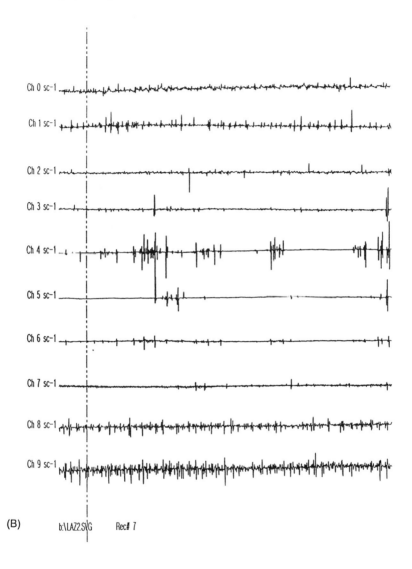

(B)   b:\LAZ2.SVG   Rec# 7

prolonged (to more than 25 ms in an adult) formal nerve conduction studies should
be performed.

D. Resetting Tremor

Attempts have been made to differentiate tremors by using various stimuli to alter
the phase of a tremor (12–19) relative to the phase before the stimulus. Originally
conceived as a method of determining how susceptible a tremor generator is to

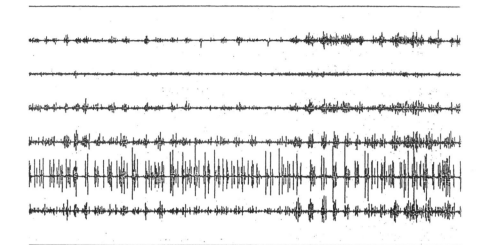

Figure 4 An 8 second polymyogram from a patient with idiopathic torsion dystonia showing an irregular tremor (at a frequency of about 4 Hz) with the characteristic variation in the EMG burst duration that typifies "dystonic" tremor. Channels 1; biceps; 2, triceps; 3, wrist flexors; 4, wrist extensors; 5, abductor pollicis brevis; 6, adductor digiti minimi.

peripheral inputs (mechanical wrist perturbations or median nerve shocks), the technique has stumbled because of methodological intricacies that have led to conflicting reports. However, once the size of the stimulus is standardized relative to tremor amplitude, there appears to be little discriminatory power in this technique. The degree to which any tremor is reset is more a function of the ratio of stimulus size to tremor amplitude than to the underlying disease process. Recently, magnetic cortical stimulation has been used instead of peripheral perturbations, but the results appear to be equally nondiscriminatory.

E. Reciprocal Inhibition of the H-Reflex

It is now apparent that one of the manifestations of hereditary torsion dystonia is postural tremor alone (20–23). A problem then arises in distinguishing these patients from those with essential tremor. One potential method for doing this is by examining the effect of radial nerve stimulation on the ipsilateral median nerve H-reflex. In patients with dystonia, an abnormal reciprocal relationship has been found in which there is a reduction in the extent of later-phase (presynaptic) inhibition compared with normal controls. This abnormal relationship may occur in patients with dystonia, even if a limb is not symptomatic, but it is not known to occur in essential tremor. Similarly, abnormalities in the H-reflex recovery curve have been described in idiopathic torsion dystonia, but not in essential tremor (24). This technique may help resolve the controversy over the nature of primary writing tremor (25–33), which some consider a variant of essential tremor (28,30,32) and others as a variant of writer's cramp (focal dystonia; 29,31–33).

F. Stretch Reflexes

Abnormalities in the stretch reflexes of patients with Parkinson's disease or neuropathic and dystonic tremor have been described, but are unlikely to provide a useful way to distinguish tremor types, although an attempt to subcategorize essential tremor on the basis of electrically elicited reflex aberrations has been made (34).

The forearm short- and long-latency stretch reflexes are delayed, but present, in neuropathic tremor. In patients with Parkinson's disease, enhancement of the long-latency stretch reflexes has been consistently found (35–39), although not in some tremulous patients (35). In dystonia, the long latency stretch reflexes have been reported to be of normal amplitude, but are prolonged compared with control subjects (38), and overflow of the reflex response, from the muscle being stretched, to normally uninvolved muscles has been observed (40). In essential tremor, the forearm stretch reflexes have been reported to be normal (5), although followed by an underdamped oscillation, and when using an electrical method of eliciting long-latency reflexes, two types of response have been observed that are said to correlate with different pharmacological responses: one group had normal responses and had cocontracting tremor that improved with propranolol. The second group had enhanced long-latency responses and alternating tremor that responded better to primidone than to β-adrenergic blockade (34). These observations, if reproducible, shed some light on the heterogeneous pharmacological behavior of essential tremor.

G. Voluntary Ballistic Movements

Measuring the speed of voluntary ballistic movements does not probe into the origins of tremor directly, but does provide a useful way of detecting and quantifying bradykinesia in a tremulous limb. There are certain methodological problems caused by the fact that normally large movements produce faster maximum speeds than small ones. However, if a target is used, the movement is not truly ballistic, but if the movement is not targeted, standardization is tricky. In practice targets at several distances are usually employed, but even then, it may still be difficult to measure velocity over a small distance if the patient has a large amplitude tremor. Despite this drawback, patients with essential tremor perform voluntary ballistic movements at normal speeds, those with neuropathic tremor appear to have normal maximum speeds, but an abnormal velocity profile and may be dysmetric, whereas patients with parkinsonism are expected to be slow.

Table 4 The Neurophysiological Characteristics of Some Postural Tremors

Type of tremor	EMG pattern in agonist–antagonist muscles	EMG burst width in forearm flexors (ms)	Velocity of voluntary ballistic movements	Reciprocal inhibition of H-reflex	Stretch reflex responses	Results of PET scan studies	Motor nerve conduction velocity
Essential	Cocontracting or alternating	50–175	Normal	Normal	Normal responses to mechanical stretch. Enhanced long latency response to electrical stimulation if EMG shows an alternating pattern (34).	Cerebellar activation	Normal
Dystonic	Cocontracting or alternating	Variable 50–1000+	Normal	Reduced presynaptic inhibition	Prolonged duration of long-latency response.	Unknown	Normal
Neuropathic	Cocontracting or alternating	75–300	Normal maximum velocity, but may be dysmetric	Delayed or absent H-reflexes	Delayed short- and long-latency responses.	Cerebellar activation	Slow typically (10–25 m/s)
Parkinson's disease	Cocontracting or alternating	Usually <100	Slow	Inconclusive although abnormalities have been reported (24)	Enlarged long-latency response in some patients.	Reduced uptake of ^{18}-F dopa into the putamen	Normal

Consequently, the technique is useful in unmasking subclinical bradykinesia or confirming the presence of mild bradykinesia in patients with benign tremulous Parkinson's disease and, thus, helps distinguish it from essential tremor.

H. Positron Emission Tomography

Positron emission tomography (PET) might help differentiate different types of tremor in two ways. First, it might be possible to distinguish essential tremor from benign tremulous Parkinson's disease if subsequent data confirm that the reduced rate of ^{18}F-dopa uptake in the putamen, which is characteristic of Parkinson's disease (41), does not happen in essential tremor. Second, by using O^{15}-labelled carbon dioxide, it is possible to determine (with careful paradigm and patient selection) changes in regional cerebral blood flow that occur when different types of tremor happen. The regional increases in cerebral blood flow are believed to be produced by locally enhanced neuronal activity. Early work has suggested that the cerebellum is abnormally activated in essential tremor (42). Whether this applies to other forms of tremor remains to be seen. The results of future studies should be intriguing.

III. CONCLUSION

Neurophysiological techniques can help the clinician differentiate tremor to some extent. Nerve conduction studies ought to be routinely considered when areflexic patients present with postural limb tremor. As neuropathy and dystonia can mimic essential tremor, careful consideration should be given to excluding these conditions before the diagnosis of essential tremor is made. To equate postural tremor with essential tremor is clearly incorrect, and I suspect some examples of "severe essential tremor" in the literature in fact describe dystonia. Perhaps some of the previous series detailing the characteristics of essential tremor are also similarly contaminated. Subtle differences in the EMG patterns, stretch reflexes, speed of voluntary ballistic movements, and the effect of reciprocal inhibition of the H-reflex can be of some help in distinguishing tremors. The main neurophysiological characteristics of various causes of postural tremor are summarized in Table 4.

Several problem areas remain, not least being the problem of distinguishing physiological or enhanced physiological tremor from early (fine) essential tremor. Currently, there is no accepted way of doing this.

REFERENCES

1. Francis DA, Bain PG, Swan AV, Hughes RAC. An assessment of disability rating scales used in multiple sclerosis. Arch Neurol 1991; 41:499–301.
2. Landis JR, Koch GG. The measurement of observer agreement for categorical data. Biometrics 1977; 3:159–173.

3. Holmes G. On certain tremors in organic cerebral lesions. Brain 1904; 27:360–375.
4. Marshall J. Tremor. In: Vinken PJ, Bruyn GW, eds. Handbook of Clinical Neurology. Amsterdam: Elsiever North-Holland, 1970:809–825.
5. Rothwell JC, Kachi T, Thompson PD, Day BL, Marsden CD. Physiological investigations of parkinsonian rest tremor and benign essential tremor. In: Benecke R, Conrad B, Marsden CD, eds. Motor Disturbances I. London: Academic Press, 1987:1–17.
6. Britton TC, Thompson PD, Van der Kamp W, Rothwell JC, Day BL, Marsden CD. Primary orthostatic tremor: further observations in five cases. J Neurol 1992; 239: 209–217.
7. Pazzaglia P, Sabattini L, Lugaresi E. Su di singulare disturbo della stazione evetta (osservazione de tre casi). Riv Freniatria 1970; 96:450–459.
8. Young RR, Hagbarth KE. Physiological tremor enhanced by manoeuvres affecting the segmental stretch reflex. J Neurol Neurosurg Psychiatry 1980; 43:248–256.
9. Roussy G, Levy G. Sept cas d'une maladie familiale particulière—troubles de la marche, pieds bots et arreflexie tendineuse generalisee avec accessoirement legere maladresse des main. Rev Neurol 1926; 2:427–450.
10. Dejerine J, Sottas H. Sur la nevrite interstitielle, hypertorphique et progressive de l'enfance. C R Soc Biol (Paris) 1893; 45:63–96.
11. Salisachs P. Charcot–Marie–Tooth disease associated with "essential tremor." Report of 7 cases and review of the literature. J Neurol Sci 1976; 28:17–40.
12. Lippold OCJ. Oscillation in the stretch reflex arc and the origin of the rhythmical 8–12 c/s component of physiological tremor. J Physiol 1970; 206:359–382.
13. Lee RG, Stein RB. Resetting of tremor by mechanical perturbations: a comparison of essential tremor and parkinsonian tremor. Ann Neurol 1981; 10:523–531.
14. Elble RJ, Higgins C, Moody CJ. Stretch reflex oscillations and essential tremor. Neurol Neurosurg Psychiatry 1987; 50:691–698.
15. Gresty MA, Findley LJ. Definition, analysis and genesis of tremor. In: Findley LJ, Capildeo R, eds. Movement Disorders: Tremor. London: Macmillan Press, 1984:15–26.
16. Marsden CD. The pathophysiology of movement disorders. Neurol Clin 1984; 2: 435–459.
17. Marsden CD. The origins of normal and pathological tremor. In: Findley LJ, Capildeo R, eds. Movement Disorders: Tremor. London: Macmillan Press, 1984:37–84.
18. Rack PMH, Ross HF, Thilmann AF. The ankle stretch reflexes in normal and spastic subjects. The response to sinusoidal movement. Brain 1984; 107:637–754.
19. Rack PMH, Ross HF. The role of reflexes in the resting tremor of Parkinson's disease. Brain 1986; 109:115–141.
20. Fletcher NA, Harding AE, Marsden CD. A genetic study of idiopathic torsion dystonia in the United Kingdom. Brain 1990; 113:379–395.
21. Bundey S, Harrison MJG, Marsden CD. A genetic study of torsion dystonia. J Med Genet 1975; 12:12–19.
22. Cohen LG, Hallett M, Sudarsky L. A single family with writer's cramp, essential tremor and primary writing tremor. Move Disord 1987; 2:109–116.
23. Forsgren L, Holmgren G, Almay BGL, Drugge U. Autosomal dominant torsion dystonia in a Swedish family. In: Fahn S, Marsden CD, Calne DB, eds. Dystonia 2. Adv Neurol 1988; 50:83–92.

24. Panizza M, Lelli S, Nilsson J, Hallett M. H-reflex recovery curve and reciprocal inhibition of H-reflex in different kinds of dystonia. Neurology 1990; 40:824–828.

25. Rothwell JC, Traub MM, Marsden CD. Primary writing tremor. J Neurol Neurosurg Psychiatry 1979; 42:1106–1114.

26. Klawans HL, Glantz R, Tanner CM, Goetz CG. Primary writing tremor: a selective action tremor. Neurology 1982; 32:203–206.

27. Ohye C, Miyazaki M, Hirai T, Shibazaki T, Hakashima H, Nagaseki Y. Primary writing tremor treated by stereotactic selective thalamotomy. J Neurol Neurosurg Psychiatry 1982; 45:988–997.

28. Kachi T, Rothwell JC, Cowan JMA, Marsden CD. Writing tremor: its relationship to benign essential tremor. J Neurol Neurosurg Psychiatry 1985; 48:545–550.

29. Ravits J, Hallett M, Baker M, Wilkins D. Primary writing tremor and myoclonic writer's cramp. Neurology 1985; 35:1387–1391.

30. Koller WC, Martyn B. Writing tremor: its relationship to essential tremor. J Neurol Neurosurg Psychiatry 1986; 49:220.

31. Elble RJ, Moody C, Higgins C. Primary writing tremor. Neurology 1987; 37(suppl 1):283.

32. Rosenbaum R, Jankovic J. Focal task-specific tremor and dystonia: categorization of occupational movement disorders. Neurology 988; 38:522–527.

33. Elble RJ, Moody C, Higgins C. Primary writing tremor: a form of focal dystonia? Mov Dis 1990; 5:118–126.

34. Deuschl J, Lucking CH, Schenk E. Essential tremor: electrophysiology and pharmacological evidence for a subdivision. J Neurol Neurosurg Psychiatry 1987; 50: 1435–1441.

35. Tatton WG, Lee RG. Evidence for abnormal long-loop reflexes in rigid parkinsonian patients. Brain Res 1975; 100:671–676.

36. Mortimer JA, Webster DD. Relationships between quantitative measures of rigidity and tremor and the electromyographic responses to load perturbations in oscillated normal subjects and Parkinson patients. Prog Clin Neurophysiol 1978; 4:342–360.

37. Rothwell JC, Obeso JA, Traub MM, Marsden CD. The behaviour of the long-latency stretch reflex in patients with Parkinson's disease. J Neurol Neurosurg Psychiatry 1983; 46:35–44.

38. Tatton WG, Bedingham W, Verrier MC, Blair RDG. Characteristic alterations in responses to imposed wrist displacements in parkinsonian rigidity and dystonia musculorum deformans. Can J Neurol Sci 1984; 11:281–287.

39. Cody FWJ, MacDermott N, Mathew PBC, Richardson HC. Observations on the genesis of the stretch reflex in Parkinson's disease. Brain 1986; 109:229–249.

40. Rothwell JC, Obeso JA, Day BL, Marsden CD. The pathophysiology of dystonias. Adv Neurol 1983; 39:851–864.

41. Leenders KL, Salmon EP, Tyrrell PJ, et al. Brain L-[^{18}F]-6-flurodopa and [^{11}C]-nomifensine uptake in patients with Parkinson's disease and healthy volunteers. J Cereb Blood Flow Metab 1989; 9:S722.

42. Colebatch JG, Findley LJ, Frackowiak RSJ, Marsden CD, Brooks DJ. Preliminary report: activation of the cerebellum in essential tremor. Lancet 1990; 336:1028–30.

7

Central and Peripheral Mechanisms in Tremorgenesis

Thomas C. Britton
Institute of Neurology
National Hospital for Neurology and Neurosurgery
London, England

I. INTRODUCTION

Two hypothetical models of tremor generation can be envisaged. In one model, tremor results from oscillation in an unstable peripheral stretch reflex loop. In the other model, tremor is generated by a central autonomous oscillator that drives the motoneuron pool independently of any sensory feedback from the limb. These two mechanisms are not mutually exclusive, and their relative importance in the generation and maintenance of different pathological tremors has been the subject of much tremor research. The purpose of this chapter is to review this work and to assess how useful the models are to the understanding of pathological tremors.

II. METHODS OF TESTING THE MODELS

Testing these models in humans has proved difficult. The anatomical pathways responsible for tremors remain unknown, and most studies, of necessity, are noninvasive. Several different approaches have been taken and are described in the following. All approaches have their limitations, and none can precisely separate the role of central or peripheral mechanisms in any tremor. Most of the approaches assess the dependence of tremor on sensory input from the limb, rather than examining central or peripheral mechanisms directly.

A.   Removal of Sensory Input From Limb

Tremors that persist following removal of sensory input must, by definition, be of central origin. This has been the basis for several studies in which sensory input from a limb has been removed by surgical deafferentation (1–3) or local anesthesia (4). However, two conditions must be satisfied by such studies before it can be concluded that central mechanisms are of primary importance to the generation of tremor. First, it must be established that the limb is totally deafferented. Second, the tremor before and after removal of sensory input must be the same.

Limb tremors that are abolished by anesthetizing selected muscles (5) are not necessarily of peripheral origin. The abolition of tremor in such circumstances merely reveals the importance of sensory input to the tremor generator, not its location. Removal of sensory input might abolish tremor by interrupting an unstable peripheral stretch reflex loop or by removing tonic inputs to a central autonomous oscillator (6).

B.   Behavioral Studies

Behavioral studies have been the most common method of probing the mechanisms responsible for pathological tremors. Although the basic principle behind such studies is relatively easy to understand, the interpretation of the results is, in practice, extremely problematic. Behavioral studies may be divided into two types: those that study the response of tremors to changes in sensory feedback from the limb, and those that study the response to direct brain stimulation.

1.   Response to Changes in Sensory Feedback

It should be relatively easy to distinguish between tremors that conformed to one or other hypothetical tremor model. Changing or altering the sensory feedback from the limb should influence the rhythm of tremor produced by a peripheral reflex mechanism, but should have no effect on tremor produced by a central autonomous oscillator. A variety of techniques have been employed to change sensory feedback, including (1) inertial loading (7–10), (2) brief mechanical perturbations (10–14), (3) electrical peripheral nerve stimuli (15–18), and (4) externally applied rhythmic torques (19,20) and displacements (7).

However, the application of these techniques to common pathological tremors has generally been unrewarding (see later discussion). There are two theoretical reasons for this. First, the method assumes that a tremor produced by a peripheral reflex mechanism would respond to a change in sensory feedback in a simple and predictable way. This assumption is almost certainly false because of the non-linearities in the peripheral feedback loop that must exist for tremor (produced by a peripheral mechanism alone) to reach a stable amplitude (7). If two or more peripheral feedback loops were to interact with each other (21), the response of peripherally generated tremors to changes in sensory feedback would be even more difficult to predict (7). Second, the method assumes that tremors produced by central oscillators would be unaffected by changing sensory feedback. This assumption is also likely to be flawed by multiple interconnections within the nervous system: wherever a central oscillator was located, it would almost certainly be influenced to some extent by sensory input from the tremoring limb.

The interpretation of the results of all behavioral studies is, therefore, difficult. It cannot be inferred that a tremor, the rhythm of which is influenced by changes in sensory feedback from the limb, is primarily of peripheral origin, since tremors of central origin may also be influenced by changes in sensory feedback. Neither can it be inferred that a tremor that is unaffected by changes in sensory feedback is primarily of central origin, since nonlinear peripheral feedback loops may also appear unaffected by changes in sensory feedback.

2. Direct Brain Stimulation

An alternative approach has been to study the response of tremors to direct stimulation of the brain, either by electrical stimulation of the exposed motor cortex at operation (22), or transcranially by the use of a magnetic stimulator (23). However, modulation of tremor rhythm by motor cortex stimuli does not necessarily imply the presence of central mechanisms. Peripheral reflex mechanisms could be influenced either by the effect of motor cortex stimulation on spinal motoneuron excitability (the spinal motoneuron must be part of any peripheral reflex loop), or by the production of a short-latency electromyographic (EMG) response altering sensory feedback from the limb. Thus, direct brain stimulation cannot provide conclusive evidence for a central tremor generator.

C. Recording of Muscle Spindle Activity

Microneurography allows direct examination of muscle spindle activity (24). By observing muscle spindle firing in relation to the tremor cycle and by calculating the loop delay for the stretch reflex arc, it is possible to assess whether muscle spindle activity could contribute (by positive-feedback of the stretch reflex) to the tremor. However, failure to find evidence that the stretch reflex operates in a particular tremor does not exclude the possibility that other peripheral reflex mechanisms contribute to the tremor. The facts that the amplitudes and latencies of short- and long-latency stretch reflexes are normal in essential tremor (10,20), and that they do not correlate with tremor frequency in parkinsonian tremor (25), suggest that these particular peripheral reflex pathways are not the origin of essential or parkinsonian tremor.

III. APPLICATION OF TECHNIQUES TO TREMORS

The following methods have been applied to a number of common pathological tremors. Some studies have employed a single method to examine one type of pathological tremor: the interpretation of the findings in these studies is necessarily limited for the reasons given in the foregoing. Other investigators have compared the response of two or more types of tremor with similar stimuli. Comparative studies are potentially more interesting, since they may uncover differences between tremors that may indicate that their mechanisms differ (without having to specify what the exact mechanisms are). However, it is important to ensure that similar paradigms are used when examining the different tremors and that due account is taken of tremor and perturbation size where appropriate.

A. Removal of Sensory Input From the Limb

Parkinsonian tremor is reported to persist following dorsal root section (1–3). However, from the limited information available about these cases, it is not certain that the tremor after dorsal root section was the same as that before: although a tremor was present after dorsal root section, it was noted to be different in nature, being more irregular in amplitude and frequency. Parkinsonian tremor is also reported to persist after the administration of intramuscular anesthetic sufficient to abolish the stretch reflex (4). However, other peripheral reflex loops may have been responsible for the persistence of tremor in this case. These studies, therefore, cannot be taken as evidence that central mechanisms are of primary importance in parkinsonian tremor.

Dystonic tremor is reported to be abolished by intramuscular anesthetic to selected muscles of the limb (5). Such studies emphasize the importance of peripheral sensory input from the limb to the maintenance of tremor, but do not establish that peripheral mechanisms are of primary importance in the generation of tremor. There are no reports of dorsal root section or of local anesthetic blocks in patients with essential tremor.

B. Behavioral Studies

1. Response to Changes in Sensory Feedback

a. *Inertial Loading.*   Inertial loading alters sensory feedback from the limb by reducing the rate at which the limb can move. Inertial loading should slow the frequency of peripherally generated tremors that depend on the stretch reflex and the mechanical properties of the limb (i.e., a mechanical reflex loop). In contrast, the rhythm of a tremor produced by a central autonomous oscillator should not be affected by inertial loading (but its amplitude might be reduced). The effect of inertial loading has been examined in essential tremor (8,9), parkinsonian rest tremor (7), and parkinsonian postural tremor (9). The dominant frequency of both essential tremor (8,9) and parkinsonian postural tremor (9) is unaffected by inertial loading, suggesting that neither type of tremor depends primarily on mechanical reflex mechanisms. However, the frequency of parkinsonian rest tremor may occasionally be reduced by inertial loading (7), indicating that the generator responsible for parkinsonian rest tremor may sometimes be influenced by altering the limb mechanics.

b. *Mechanical Perturbations.* Several studies have examined the response of pathological tremors to brief mechanical perturbations (10–14). All of these studies have concentrated on how such stimuli influence tremor phase: some have assessed phase modulation by examination of single or averaged trials, whereas others have derived a resetting index based on the timing of the rhythmic EMG bursts before and after the perturbation. Despite the increasing sophistication of the method, the results have been inconsistent. Brief mechanical perturbations are reported to reset the phase of parkinsonian tremors in some studies (11,12), but not in others (13). Some have found resetting of essential tremor (13), whereas others have not (12).

There are two main reasons for these apparently contradictory results. First, the extent to which brief mechanical perturbations modulate tremors depends critically on the size of the perturbation in relation to the size of the on-going tremor (14). Second, some studies have been performed on parkinsonian rest tremor (11,13), whereas others have been on parkinsonian postural tremor (12,14). This may be important, since parkinsonian rest and postural tremors are thought to have different pathophysiological origins (26).

What conclusions can be drawn from these studies? Parkinsonian postural tremor and essential tremor behave similarly to appropriately scaled mechanical perturbations (14). It remains possible that parkinsonian rest tremor may be less susceptible than essential tremor to brief mechanical perturbations (13), but a study using perturbations appropriately scaled to the size of the tremor has not been performed.

c. *Electrical Peripheral Nerve Stimulation.* Supramaximal electrical stimulation of peripheral nerves modulates the phase of parkinsonian rest tremor (15–17), parkinsonian postural tremor (17,18), and essential tremor (17,18). After a direct motor response in the respective forearm muscle, there is a period of EMG suppression that lasts 100–200 ms before the rhythmic EMG bursts of tremor reappear. In parkinsonian postural tremor and essential tremor, the duration of EMG suppression is directly related to the tremor period (18), and the two types of tremor behave similarly. In parkinsonian rest tremor, it has been suggested that the period of EMG suppression is fixed at about 200 ms (17), but all the patients in this study had low-frequency tremors.

One observation that has not previously been emphasized is that distal nerve stimulation can modulate limb tremor more proximally. Mones and Weiss (16) found that stimulation of the median nerve at the wrist altered the timing of rhythmic EMG bursts in the forearm muscles of patients with parkinsonian rest tremor. A tremor model consisting of only a single peripheral reflex loop could not explain this result: either peripheral reflex loops must interact (7,21), or the peripheral nerve stimulus must influence the central oscillator responsible for the tremor.

    d. *Rhythmic Torques or Displacements.* The interactions of tremor with external sinusoidal forcings have been examined in parkinsonian rest tremor (7,19) and essential tremor (20). The basis for these studies is that nonlinear oscillators (in contrast with linear oscillators) may be entrained by sinusoidal forcing at frequencies different from their spontaneous frequency, provided that the forcing frequency lies within the zone of entrainment of the oscillator and that the forcing is sufficiently large. Tremors that depend primarily on (nonlinear) peripheral reflex mechanisms, therefore, should be entrainable by external forcings. In practice it has proved difficult to entrain either essential tremor (20) or parkinsonian rest tremor (19) using sinusoidal torques at frequencies different from their spontaneous frequencies: the occurrence of "beating" in these studies has been taken as evidence in favor of a central autonomous oscillator, although similar behavior may, in certain circumstances, be observed with sinusoidal forcing of nonlinear oscillators (27). Rack and Ross found that it was possible to entrain the tremor of some patients with Parkinson's disease using sinusoidal displacements (7), suggesting that afferent activity from the limb is important to the maintenance of tremor in a proportion of patients.

2. Direct Brain Stimulation

Electrical stimulation of the exposed motor cortex with single cathodal pulses can reset the phase of parkinsonian rest tremor (22), and transcranial magnetic stimulation over the motor cortex can phase-modulate parkinsonian postural tremor (23) and essential tremor (23,28). Successful modulation was always associated with a short-latency motor response following cortical stimulation. These results indicate that the motor cortex, or its output pathways, are closely related to the mechanisms responsible for tremor, but they do not reveal the location of these mechanisms. The possibility that the effect occurred at a spinal motoneuron level or by peripheral pathways cannot be excluded.

C. Recording of Muscle Spindle Activity

Muscle spindle activity has been recorded in parkinsonian rest tremor (24). Spindles active twice during each tremor cycle: while the muscle was shortening, and while it was lengthening. This is similar to that in voluntary oscillatory movements (29) and indicates alpha–gamma coactivation during muscle shortening. It suggests that the conventional stretch reflex is not of primary importance in the generation of parkinsonian rest tremor. No similar study has been reported in essential tremor.

IV. CONCLUSIONS

The hypothetical concept that tremors are due to central autonomous generators, or to instability in peripheral reflex loops, has been a spur to numerous studies, but as yet the anatomical basis of the common pathological tremors remains unknown. Physiological studies do not suggest a primary role for the conventional stretch reflex in the generation of parkinsonian rest or postural tremors or in essential tremor. Nevertheless, afferent activity from the tremoring limb is important and probably interacts with other oscillatory mechanisms. The location of these other oscillatory mechanisms remains uncertain and cannot be determined by current physiological methods.

REFERENCES

1. Leriche R. Radiocotomie cerricale pour un tremblement parkinsonism. Lyon Med 1914; 122:1075–1076.
2. Foerster O. Zur analyse und pathophysiologie der striären bewegungsstörungen. Z Gesamte Neurol Psychiatr 1921; 73:1–169.
3. Pollock LJ, Davis L. Muscle tone in parkinsonian states. Arch Neurol Psychiatry 1930; 23:303–319.
4. Walshe FMR. Observations on the nature of muscular rigidity of paralysis agitans, and its relationship to tremor. Brain 1924; 47:159–177.
5. Rondot P, Korn H, Scherrer J. Suppression of an entire limb tremor by anesthetising a selective muscular group. Arch Neurol 1968; 19:421–429.
6. Elble RJ, Koller WC. Tremor. Baltimore: Johns Hopkins University Press, 1990.
7. Rack PMH, Ross HF. The role of reflexes in the resting tremor of Parkinson's disease. Brain 1986; 109:115–141.
8. Elble RJ. Physiologic and essential tremor. Neurology 1986; 36:225–231.
9. Hömberg V, Hefter H, Reiners K, Freund H-J. Differential effects of changes in mechanical limb properties on physiological and pathological tremor. J Neurol Neurosurg Psychiatry 1987; 50:568–579.
10. Elble RJ, Higgins C, Moody CJ. Stretch reflex oscillations and essential tremor. J Neurol Neurosurg Psychiatry 1987; 50:691–698.
11. Gybels JM. The neural mechanism of parkinsonian tremor. Brussels: Arscia, 1963: 68–70.
12. Teräväinen H, Evarts E, Calne D. Effects of kinesthetic inputs on parkinsonian tremor. Adv Neurol 1979; 24:161–173.
13. Lee RG, Stein RB. Resetting of tremor by mechanical perturbations: a comparison of essential tremor and parkinsonian tremor. Ann Neurol 1981; 10:523–531.
14. Britton TC, Thompson PD, Day BL, Rothwell JC, Findley LJ, Marsden CD. "Resetting" of postural tremors at the wrist with mechanical stretches in Parkinson's disease, essential tremor and normal subjects mimicking tremor. Ann Neurol 1992; (in press).
15. Hufschmidt H-J. Proprioceptive origin of parkinsonian tremor. Nature 1963; 200: 367–368.

16. Mones RJ, Weiss AH. The response of tremor of patients with parkinsonism to peripheral nerve stimulation. J Neurol Neurosurg Psychiatry 1969; 32:512–518.
17. Bathien N, Rondot P, Toma S. Inhibition and synchronisation of tremor induced by a muscle twitch. J Neurol Neurosurg Psychiatry 1980; 43:713–718.
18. Britton TC, Thompson PD, Day BL, Rothwell JC, Findley LJ, Marsden CD. Modulation of postural tremors at the wrist by supramaximal median nerve shocks in essential tremor, Parkinson's disease and normal subjects mimicking tremor. (In preparation).
19. Walsh EG. Beats produced between a rhythmic force and the resting tremor of parkinsonism. J Neurol Neurosurg Psychiatry 1979; 42:89–94.
20. Marsden CD, Obeso JA, Rothwell JC. Benign essential tremor is not a single entity. In: Yahr MD, ed. Current Concepts of Parkinson's Disease and Related Disorders. Amsterdam: Exerpta Medica, 1983:31–46.
21. Marsden CD, Merton PA, Morton HB. Human postural responses. Brain 1981; 104: 513–534.
22. Alberts WW, Libet B, Wright EW, Feinstein B. Physiological mechanisms of tremor and rigidity in parkinsonism. Confin Neurol 1965; 26:318–327.
23. Britton TC, Day BL, Findley LJ, Marsden CD, Rothwell JC, Thompson PD. Effects of magnetic brain stimulation on wrist tremor in patients with Parkinson's disease. J Physiol 1991; 438:214P.
24. Hagbarth KE, Wallin G, Lofstedt L, Aquilonius SM. Muscle spindle activity in alternating tremor of parkinsonism and in clonus. J Neurol Neurosurg Psychiatry 1975; 38:636–641.
25. Mortimer JA, Webster DD. Evidence for a quantitative association between EMG stretch responses and parkinsonian rigidity. Brain Res 1979; 162:169–173.
26. Findley LJ, Gresty MA, Halmagyi GM. Tremor, the cogwheel phenomenon and clonus in Parkinson's disease. J Neurol Neurosurg Psychiatry 1981; 44:534–546.
27. Stein RB, Lee RG. Tremor and clonus. In: Handbook of Physiology. Sect 1, Vol 2, part 1. Baltimore: Williams & Wilkins, 1981:325–343.
28. Britton TC, Thompson PD, Day BL, Rothwell JC, Findley LJ, Marsden CD. Modulation of postural wrist tremors by magnetic stimulation of the motor cortex in Parkinson's disease, essential tremor and normal subjects mimicking tremor. (In preparation).
29. Hagbarth KE, Wallin G, Lofstedt L. Muscle spindle activity in man during fast alternating movements. J Neurol Neurosurg Psychiatry 1975; 38:625–635.

8

Central Mechanisms of Experimental Tremor and Their Clinical Relevance

Yves Lamarre
University of Montreal
Montreal, Quebec, Canada

I. INTRODUCTION

This chapter will review briefly our work on the central mechanisms responsible for different types of experimental tremor and their relevance to clinical tremor. By using a variety of experimental approaches, we have been able to distinguish three types of experimental tremor and to characterize their neural mechanisms. Under the influence of harmaline, the olivocerebellar system generates a fine tremor at 8–12 Hz, which has the characteristics of either normal or enhanced physiological tremor. This system can also generate a coarser tremor at 6–8 Hz following harmaline and lesion of some cerebellar efferents. This tremor has features of what is called essential tremor in humans. One other type of tremor at 3–6 Hz, similar to parkinsonian tremor, appears to involve a different mechanism, which lies at the thalamocortical level.

II. OLIVOCEREBELLAR TREMOR

Following the pioneering work of Poirier and his collaborators (1), we have discovered that some β-carbolines, such as harmaline, harmine, and ibogaline, produce rhythmic and synchronized activation in the olivocerebellar system at a frequency corresponding to the natural oscillatory tendency of the olivary neurons (2). This drug-induced activity, in normal animals, produces a fast and fine muscle tremor, the frequency of which tends to be higher in smaller animals (e.g., mice: 15–20 Hz; monkeys: 8–11 Hz). In the cat, repetitive electrical stimulation of the cerebellum showed that the optimal frequency of harmaline tremor is between 8 and 12 Hz (3). Most of the time this tremor occurs synchronously in antagonistic muscles. In the cat, where a major part of the cerebellar output is directed toward the brain stem, the tremorgenic activity from the cerebellar nuclei is transmitted to segmental levels mainly by the reticulo- and vestibulospinal pathways to produce rhythmic coactivation of alpha and gamma motoneurons (4,5). In monkeys, the tremorgenic impulses must also be transmitted to the segmental levels by the well-developed cerebellothalamocorticospinal route. This olivocerebellar tremor does not require the integrity of the peripheral loop to manifest itself, since muscle paralysis and limb deafferentation by section of the dorsal roots does not prevent the rhythmic activation of motoneurons (6).

When harmaline is injected in monkeys having partial lesion of the cerebellar output (nuclei or cerebellar peduncles), the characteristics of the tremor induced in the arm corresponding to the side of the lesion are greatly modified. The tremor is coarser, slower (usually about 6–7 Hz instead of 8–11 Hz) and often organized reciprocally in antagonistic muscles. It shows a strong postural component and is sometimes exaggerated during phasic movements. The tremor induced in the opposite arm is not modified. This slower tremor, observed only in lesioned monkeys injected with harmaline, was also found to be generated by the olivocerebellar system. This was based on the results of numerous experiments involving recordings and lesions in the brainstem and cerebellum (7). We would like to put forward the hypothesis that such changes in the harmaline tremor characteristics occur when the inferior olive is deprived of its γ-aminobutyric acid (GABA)ergic input from the cerebellar nuclei. This system is identified (G) in Figure 1, which summarizes the tremorgenic pathways involved in the olivocerebellar tremor.

A. Possible Mechanisms of Action of Harmaline on the Olivocerebellar System

That local application of harmaline in the inferior olive (8,9) induces rhythmic activity in the olivocerebellar system, strongly suggests that the drug has as direct action on the inferior olivary neurons themselves. The precise mechanism by which the drug enhances rhythmic discharges in the inferior olivary complex still remains uncertain. The increased, synchronized, rhythmic activity induced by harmaline could be due to a facilitation of the pacemakerlike behavior of individual inferior olivary cells and to an increased electrotonic coupling between the cells. There is evidence that harmaline does, indeed, facilitate the oscillatory behavior of inferior olivary cells by increasing the rebound Ca^{2+} conductance at the soma membrane (10), an effect that is antagonized by octanol (11). On the other hand, repeated treatment with harmaline results in the development of tolerance (12,13). This phenomenon is illustrated in Figure 2. Such observations suggest that the drug may act at a receptor-binding site. Harmaline is a β-carboline alkaloid and,

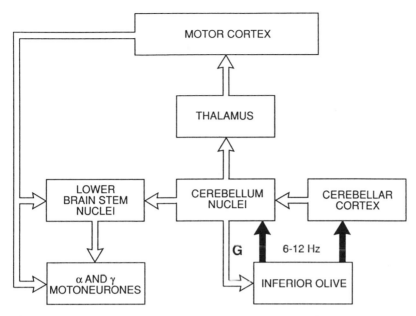

Figure 1 Tremorgenic structures and their interconnections presumably responsible for physiological and essential types of tremor. Lesion of the GABAergic nucleoolivary system (G) may increase coupling between olivary cells and lower the frequency of the inferior olivary oscillator (see text for further explanation).

as a group, β-carbolines are inverse agonists of the benzodiazepine-binding site associated with the $GABA_A$ receptor complex (14).

There is evidence that the tremorgenic effects of β-carbolines may be mediated by an interaction at the benzodiazepine receptor level (15,16) and that it can be antagonized by diazepam (17–19). However, in the rat and in the cat, diazepam blocks harmaline-induced tremor, mainly by an action at the level of the spinal cord, rather than at the inferior olive (17,18), although in the rabbit, some short-duration blocking effect was seen in the inferior olive (18). In a recent paper, Deecher et al. reported an interaction of harmane (an analogue of harmaline) with the GABA receptor–ionophore complex, but no interaction of harmaline or ibogaine (20). Their binding studies were done on whole brain bovine or rat tissue homogenates. These results and those obtained with diazepam may indicate that the benzodiazepine-binding sites in the inferior olive have characteristics different from those of the receptors in other parts of the brain. This issue cannot be clarified until the benzodiazepine–GABA receptor complex in the inferior olive itself has been fully characterized pharmacologically.

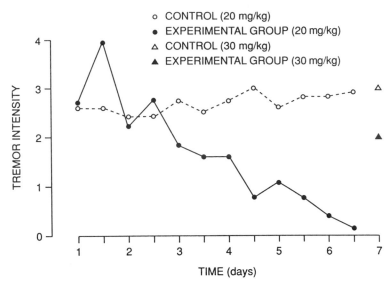

Figure 2 Effect of repeated injections of harmaline in the rat. The same group of four rats (closed circles) were injected twice a day (10 AM and 2 PM) with harmaline (20 mg/kg, iv), and the intensity of the resulting tremor was compared with different control groups (open circles). The second injection produced some enhancement of the tremor. However, the following injections were less and less effective, until no tremor was seen after 6 days. The tremor reappeared when the dose of harmaline was increased to 30 mg/kg (filled triangles). (Modified from Ref. 12.)

The GABAergic fibers originating from the cerebellar nuclei appear to establish synapses in the vicinity of gap junctions (21–23), thereby giving credit to the notion that this system could modulate the electrical coupling between individual inferior olivary neurons (24). This is supported by the results of Figure 3, illustrating the effect of microiontophorectic application of GABA on the rhythmic activity induced by harmaline in the inferior olive of the cat. γ-Aminobutyric acid clearly depresses only the larger spikes associated with each burst of rhythmic activity. One interpretation of these results is that GABA reduces coupling of the cells closest to the pipette and isolates it from the rest of the ensemble of synchronously firing neurons.

That harmaline has an inverse agonist effect on GABAergic synaptic transmission could increase the electrotonic coupling by reducing the current shunt induced by GABA in the vicinity of the junctional membrane (25). Another hypothesis is that the modulation of electrotonic coupling by GABAergic transmission could also be mediated by physiologically relevant local intracellular pH modification near the junctional membrane. Gap junctional conductance can

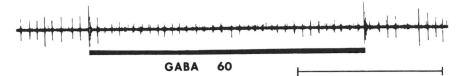

GABA 60

Figure 3 Effect of microiontophoretic injection of GABA on the rhythmic activity induced by harmaline (5 mg/kg, iv) in the inferior olive of the unanesthetized and decerebrated cat. GABA clearly depressed only the largest extracellular spikes associated with each burst of rhythmic activity. The black bar indicates the period of 60-nA GABA application. The horizontal calibration is 5 s. (From Ref. 8.)

display a steep fall with intracellular acidification, on the order of 0.1 pH units (26). Since the anion channel gated by the $GABA_A$ receptor has a significant permeability to HCO_3^- (27) and induces, at least in crayfish muscle, an intracellular acidification (28) and, in the turtle cerebellum (29), an extracellular alkaline shift, such a mechanism may represent another way by which GABA synaptic activity could reduce electrotonic coupling between inferior olivary cells. If this were true, the inverse agonist action of harmaline could produce a local intracellular alkaline shift near the gap that would cause increased junctional conductance.

B. Relevance to Human Tremor

We believe that physiological and essential tremors in humans are generated by the olivocerebellar system and that the mechanisms of these tremors are similar, if not identical, to the ones discussed here. The effect of small amount of ethanol in reducing essential tremor in humans is a well-documented fact (30,31). Ethanol also antagonizes harmaline tremor (32,33). This action of ethanol could well be mediated by the GABAergic control of junctional conductance in the inferior olive, since ethanol and other short-chained alcohols potentiate GABA-mediated neurotransmission in the central nervous system (34–36). Also alcohols, such as heptanol and octanol, have been used routinely to reduce electrotonic coupling in a variety of coupled cell systems (37–39).

Figure 4, taken from Sinclair et al. (32), illustrates the effect of intravenous infusion of ethanol on the intervals between rhythmic complex spikes induced by harmaline. The essential finding is that ethanol does not modify the basic oscillatory pattern of the complex spikes, but elicits failures of discharge on one or more cycles, as revealed by the appearance of several harmonics of the first mode (see Fig. 4C). This kind of effect of ethanol could well be explained by a reduced coupling between inferior olivary cells. The effectiveness of octanol against harmaline-induced tremor has been attributed to the block of the low-threshold calcium channel in inferior olive cells (11). However, the possibility that octanol

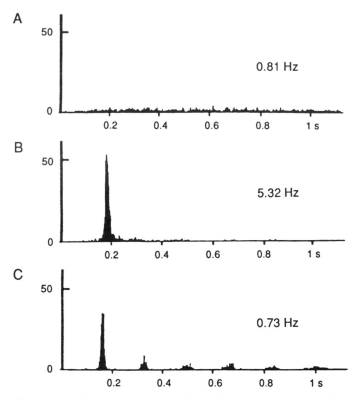

Figure 4   Effects of ethanol on the harmaline-induced rhythmic climbing fiber activity in the rat cerebellar cortex. Each histogram represents the interval distribution between complex spikes: (A) before drug treatment, (B) after harmaline (5 mg/kg, iv), and (C), following ethanol (1.5 g/kg, iv). The mean frequency of the complex spikes ($N = 1000$) during construction of each histogram is indicated on the right side of each histogram. Note that ethanol lowers the mean frequency without altering the fundamental oscillatory period (compare B with C). (From Ref. 32.)

also acts by reducing electrotonic coupling between inferior olivary cells has not been ruled out.

Essential tremor in humans can display a wide range of frequencies (4–12 Hz) (31,40), covering the spectrum from enhanced physiological tremor to classic benign and severe essential tremor (41). Harmaline-induced tremor can also manifest itself in this frequency range under certain conditions. Indeed, small progressive doses of barbiturates can reduce the frequency of tremor in the cat from 10–12 Hz down to about 4 Hz before being completely blocked (6,42). This is illustrated in Figure 5. Again, this effect could be linked to an action of barbiturates on the $GABA_A$ receptor controlling junctional conductance (14,43).

In humans, the frequency of essential tremor tends to be lower (4–7 Hz), and its amplitude tends to be larger in advanced cases than in early tremor (7–10 Hz) (31,44). In normal monkeys, harmaline tremor is similar to early essential tremor, with frequencies in the 8- to 12-Hz range. However, partial lesion of the lateral cerebellar nuclei or of the superior cerebellar peduncle increases the amplitude of harmaline tremor and lowers its frequency (6–7 Hz) on the side of the lesion (45).

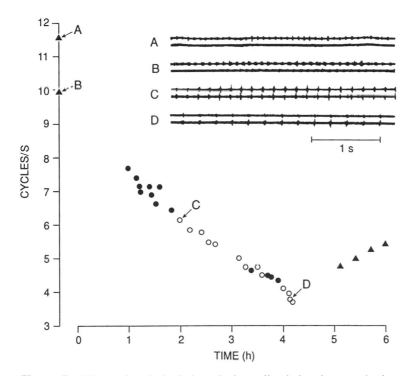

Figure 5 Effects of methohexital on the harmaline-induced tremor in the cat. (A–D) EMG recordings from hamstring (top trace) and quadriceps (bottom trace) muscles. Before decerebration, the tremor frequency was 11.6 Hz (triangle A); 2 h after decerebration the frequency had dropped to 10 Hz (triangle B). The origin on the abcissa represents the time of injection of 9 mg of methohexital (iv), which was followed by additional doses of 1 mg (closed circles) or 2 mg (open circles). The tremor frequency decreased progressively to 3.6 Hz before disappearing after a total cumulative dose of 51 mg of barbiturates administered over a period of about 4 h. This was followed by a gradual recovery of the tremor (closed triangles). The EMG traces correspond to the points identified on the plot (A–D). (From Ref. 42.)

This could be the result of the lesion of the GABAergic projections from the cerebellar nuclei to the inferior olive (23) and the consequent increase in the number of olivary cells firing in synchrony (46).

Propranolol has beneficial effects in some patients with essential tremor (47). The mechanism of action for this effect of the drug is still disputed, but it is worth mentioning that harmine tremor was also antagonized by L-propranolol (48). Primidone is another drug that can be of benefit in essential tremor (31). It seems that this effect could be mainly by phenobarbitone, one of the drug's active metabolites (49). The blocking effect of barbiturates has been documented on harmaline tremor (see Fig. 5) had so has the interaction of phenobarbitone on the benzodiazepine receptors (14).

There does not seem to be any specific brain structural abnormality related to the occurrence of essential tremor (50). In accordance with the hypothesis of an interaction of harmaline with the benzodiazepine receptors in the inferior olive, one could raise the possibility that some β-carboline derivatives may be present in the brain of patients with essential tremor. Such "endogenous ligands" could act specifically in the inferior olive as inhibitors of benzodiazepine receptor binding and disturb the normal GABAergic control of the olivocerebellar activity. This idea finds some support in the fact that β-carboline derivatives have been identified in the urine of human subjects after a load of ethanol (51). Similar investigations in patients with essential tremor might well be worth carrying out.

If essential tremor in humans is generated by abnormal activity in the olivo-cerebellar system, why can this tremor be abolished, like parkinsonian tremor, by thalamotomy (52–54)? In the cat, where the influence of the cerebellobulbar systems predominate, tremorgenic impulses are mediated to the segmental levels by mainly the reticulospinal and vestibulospinal pathways. In the monkey, and presumably also in humans, the influence of the cerebellothalamocortical pathways is more important and is probably more involved in the transmission of tremorgenic impulses from the cerebellum to the spinal levels. Indeed, thalamic recordings in the monkey revealed sustained rhythmic unit activity in-phase with the fast harmaline-induced tremor (8–12 Hz) in the contralateral upper limb (55), an activity that is not abolished by motor cortex cooling. Rhythmic activity linked to the tremor beats were also recorded in the lateral thalamus of patients with essential tremor (56).

III. PARKINSONIAN TREMOR AT 4–6 HERTZ

Following electrolytic lesion in the ventromedian tegmentum or treatment with neurotoxic agents, such as 1-methyl-4-phenyl-1,2,3,6-tetrahydropyridine (MPTP), in monkeys, one can observe a spontaneous tremor, at 4–6 Hz, that closely resembles the classic rest tremor seen in parkinsonian patients. This tremor persists unchanged after complete ablation of the cerebellum (including the deep nuclei), a procedure that produces secondary degeneration of the inferior olivary neurons (7). Thus, this tremor cannot be generated by the olivocerebellar system, presumably responsible for the physiological and essential types of tremor. The results of numerous lesion and recording experiments led us to believe that this experimental parkinsonianlike tremor is generated at diencephalic levels (57).

In the thalamus and in the motor cortex (area 4), rhythmic activity was recorded in-phase with the peripheral tremor in monkeys with deafferented limb and total cerebellectomy. The precise mechanisms responsible for such abnormal rhythmic activity in the thalamocortical circuitry has not yet been elucidated. Contrary to the inferior olivary cells, which always display an oscillatory mode of activity, neurons in the ventrolateral thalamus can function in two different modes of activity: (1) a rhythmic, bursting-firing mode, during which thalamocortical transmission is impaired; and (2) a tonic, desynchronized-firing mode, with high-fidelity transmission (58–61). Because of the difference seen in the amplitude and shape of the extracellular spikes during the two modes of activity, we had suggested a different spike-generating mechanism for rhythmic-bursting and for tonic, desynchronized firing (60,62). These mechanisms have now been studied extensively, and rhythmic bursting of thalamocortical cells appears to involve at least some processes similar to the ones described for the inferior olive (61).

Thus, ventrolateral thalamic neurons can behave as oscillators, with rhythmic-bursting activity at the frequency of about 3–5 Hz. This rhythmic activity is always concomitant with a behavioral state of relaxation (motor rest and decreased vigilance). The slightest arousal of the animal arrests bursting, which is replaced by more or less continuous firing of isolated spikes at a frequency of about 10–30 Hz. This is contrary to the inferior olivary neurons that always behave as oscillators, irrespective of the behavioral state of the animal.

In monkeys with parkinsonianlike tremor following brainstem lesions, presumably involving dopaminergic fibers, many thalamic cells are found that discharge in a rhythmic-bursting fashion at 3–5 Hz, irrespective of the state of vigilance of the animal. Thus, these cells always behave as oscillators, more like inferior olivary cells (57). How midbrain tegmentum lesion (or MPTP neurotoxic lesion) can induce such sustained rhythmic abnormal activity remains unknown. Recent evidence suggests that the subthalamic nucleus may be involved by producing overinhibition of thalamocortical circuits by the pallidothalamic system (63). Since cooling of the motor cortex can stop this tremor, along with the associated thalamic activity (55), this raises the possibility that corticothalamic or cortico-subthalamic circuits might also be involved in the generation or maintenance of tremorgenic activity (3).

With these facts in mind, it is of interest to ask: What is the direct effect of harmaline on the ventrolateral thalamic activity? In the olivocerebellar system, harmaline exaggerates and synchronizes rhythmic activity. In the thalamus, however, harmaline blocks the episodes of 3- to 5-Hz rhythmic bursting, which appear to be replaced by episodes of high-frequency firing (up to 70 Hz). These prolonged bursts of high-frequency firing resemble the pattern of activity seen in the ventrolateral thalamus during paradoxical sleep (59). Between these episodes of high-frequency firing, the activity resembles the normal 10- to 30-Hz tonic firing seen during arousal without the drug. This effect of harmaline on the activity in the thalamus of a normal awake monkey is shown in Figure 6. This cell was recorded before and after the injection of harmaline. Records A were obtained at a time when the effect of the drug was vanishing (2 h after the injection), whereas records B were obtained at the peak of the effect (20 min after the injection). The typical spindling at 25–30 Hz that harmaline induces in the motor cortex (lower traces) can also be seen to occur synchronously in the thalamic records, and this is more pronounced when the effect of the drug is maximal (see Fig. 6B). The abrupt onset of high frequency firing in B is concomitant with the abolition of the 25- to 30-Hz oscillations in both the cortex and thalamus. In A, when the drug has minimal effect, the episodes of 25- to 30-Hz oscillations alternate with episodes of slow cortical waves associated with rhythmic thalamic bursting at 4–6 Hz, similar to the activity seen before the injection of the drug.

Synchronized 30-Hz oscillations were observed in the sensorimotor cortex of awake monkeys, particularly in association with the performance of motor tasks requiring a high level of attention and dexterity (64). Hence, harmaline seems to be able to enhance this type of oscillatory activity in the thalamocortical system and to possibly increase the level of attentive responsiveness. However, harmaline also prevents the occurrence of normal episodes of reduced attention and responsiveness characterized by slow thalamic rhythmic bursting. This is replaced by

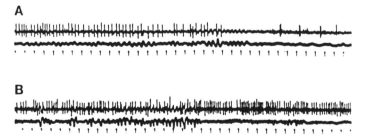

Figure 6 Effect of harmaline (5 mg/kg, im) on the neuronal activity in the ventrolateral thalamus (VLO) of a normal, awake monkey. (A) and (B) show the activity of a single unit (top trace) with the motor cortex electrocorticogram underneath. (A) Alternation of episodes of tonic firing at about 25 Hz with episodes of rhythmic bursting at 4.5–5 Hz associated with cortical slow waves. (B) Activity of the same cell 20 min after the injection of harmaline. The episodes of rhythmic bursting are replaced by periods of sustained high-frequency firing. The time marker interval is 100 ms.

episodes of high-frequency firing that could characterize a state of increased attentiveness, but reduced responsiveness, to external stimuli because of the concomitant blocking of coherent rhythmic oscillations in the thalamocortical system. This state of activity could well be related to the well-known hallucinogenic properties of harmaline (65), and it is also quite consistent with the hypotheses elegantly elaborated by Llinás (66).

On the other hand, in monkeys with brainstem lesions and parkinsonianlike tremor, harmaline can also exaggerate the abnormal 3- to 5-Hz rhythmic thalamic bursting (57), as it does to the normal 8- to 10-Hz rhythmic activity in the inferior olive. Thus, harmaline seems to have different effects on the activity of some thalamic cells, depending on the integrity of the control exerted by the basal ganglia on the thalamocortical circuitry. Figure 7 summarizes the tremorgenic pathways presumably involved in the parkinsonian-type tremor.

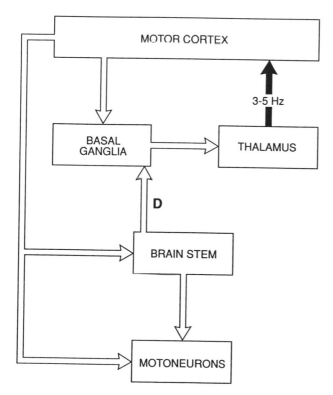

Figure 7 Tremorgenic structures and pathways presumably involved in the generation of parkinsonian-type tremor. Lesion of the dopaminergic striatonigral system (D) is thought to be responsible for the appearance of abnormal rhythmic activity at the diencephalic level.

IV. SUMMARY AND CONCLUSION

We have summarized our hypotheses in discussing two central oscillatory mechanisms responsible for different types of tremor. The efferent pathways of these two tremor generators (thalamocortical and olivocerebellar) likely overlap at the brainstem and thalamic levels. In the normal situation, the olivocerebellar system can generate a fine, physiological tremor at 8–10 Hz that could serve some timing functions in motor control (67). Harmaline exaggerates this tremor, producing something similar to what is called enhanced physiological tremor in humans (68). With partial cerebellar lesion involving the GABAergic nucleoolivary fibers (see G in Fig. 1), the olivocerebellar system, deprived of its GABAergic-controlling input, generates a coarser and slower tremor (6–7 Hz) that has characteristics similar to essential tremor in humans. Harmaline also exaggerates this abnormal tremor. The rhythmic activity of the inferior olivary system can reach the spinal motoneurons by both the cerebellobulbar systems and the cerebellothalamocortical systems. The latter being prevalent in primates, this could explain why essential tremor can sometimes be alleviated by thalamotomy.

With an intact dopaminergic system (see D in Fig. 7) and normal striatopallidal control of the thalamocortical activity, harmaline does not induce or exaggerate intrinsic rhythmic activity at the diencephalic level, but rather, converts episodes of normal rhythmic bursting seen during relaxation into episodes of very high-frequency activity, similar to what is seen in paradoxical sleep.

Following brainstem lesions (presumably involving, among others, the dopaminergic systems), sustained abnormal rhythmic activity at the diencephalic levels may produce a spontaneous parkinsonianlike tremor at 3–5 Hz. In this instance, harmaline will enhance this type of tremor and will also activate the olivocerebellar system, producing tremor at higher frequencies (8–10 or 6–7 Hz, depending on the integrity of the cerebelloolivary GABAergic system). Both tremor frequencies could then be recorded in the same muscle, as was indeed observed in monkeys (7) and humans (69,70). Furthermore, total lesion of the cerebellar output will abolish only the higher-frequency olivocerebellar tremor, leaving intact the slower parkinsonianlike tremor (7).

Some of these hypotheses are admittedly quite speculative. However, it is our belief that they may stimulate new research that could lead to a better understanding of the physiopathology of tremors in humans and help in the search for more specific and efficient therapies.

ACKNOWLEDGMENTS

This work was supported by the Medical Research Council of Canada. Yves Lamarre is a member of the MRC Group in Neurological Sciences at the University of Montreal.

REFERENCES

1. Poirier LJ, Sourkes TL, Bouvier G, Boucher R, Carabin S. Striatal amines, experimental tremor and the effect of harmaline in the monkey. Brain 1966; 89:37–52.
2. Lamarre Y, de Montigny C, Dumont M, Weiss M. Harmaline-induced rhythmic activity of cerebellar and lower brain stem neurons. Brain Res 1971; 32:246–250.
3. Lamarre Y, Joffroy AJ, Dumont M, de Montigny C, Grou F, Lund JP. Central mechanisms of tremor in some feline and primate models. Can J Neurol Sci 1975; 2: 227–233.
4. de Montigny C, Lamarre Y. Rhythmic activity induced by harmaline in the olivo-cerebello-bulbar system of the cat. Brain Res 1973; 53:81–95.
5. Lamarre Y, Weiss M. Harmaline-induced rhythmic activity of alpha and gamma motoneurons in the cat. Brain Res 1973; 63:430–434.
6. Lamarre Y, Mercier LA. Neurophysiological studies of harmaline-induced tremor in the cat. Can J Physiol Pharmacol 1971; 49:1049–1058.
7. Lamarre Y, Dumont M. Activity of cerebellar and lower brain stem neurons in monkeys with harmaline-induced tremor. In: Goldsmith EI, Moor-Jankowski J, eds. Medical Primatology. Basel: S Karger, 1972:274–281.
8. Lamarre Y, Puil E. Induction of rhythmic activity by harmaline. Can J Physiol Pharmacol 1974; 52:905–908.
9. de Montigny C, Lamarre Y. Effects produced by local applications of harmaline in the inferior olive. Can J Physiol Pharmacol 1975; 53:845–849.
10. Llinás R, Yarom Y. Oscillatory properties of guinea-pig inferior olivary neurones and their pharmacological modulation: an in vitro study. J Physiol 1986; 376:163–182.
11. Sinton CM, Krosser BI, Walton KD, Llinás RR. The effectiveness of different isomers of octanol as blockers of harmaline-induced tremor. Pflugers Arch 1989; 414:31–36.
12. Busby L. Tremblements induits par l'harmaline: mécanisme et tentatives d'antagonisme. MSc dissertation, University of Montréal, Montreal, Quebec, Canada, 1978.
13. Lutes J, Lorden J, Beales M, Oltmans G. Tolerance to the tremorogenic effects of harmaline: evidence for altered olivocerebellar function. Neuropharmacology 1988; 27:849–855.
14. Polc P, Bonettei EP, Schaffner R, Haefely W. A three-state model of the benzodiazepine receptor explains the interactions between the benzodiazepine antagonist Ro 15-1788, benzodiazepine tranquilizers, β-carbolines, and phenobarbitone. Naunyn Schmiedebergs Arch Pharmacol 1982; 321:260–264.
15. Robertson H. Harmaline-induced tremor: the benzodiazepine receptor as a site of action. Eur J Pharmacol 1980; 67:129–132.
16. Mao CC, Guidotti A, Costa E. Inhibition by diazepam of the tremor and the increase of cerebellar cGMP content elicited by harmaline. Brain Res 1975; 83:516–519.
17. Busby L, Lamarre Y. Effect of diazepam on the neuronal rhythmic activity and tremor induced by harmaline. In: Courville J, de Montigny C, Lamarre Y, eds. The Inferior Olivary Nucleus: Anatomy and Physiology. New York: Raven Press, 1980:315–320.
18. Mariani J, Delhaye-Bouchaud N. Effect of diazepam on the spontaneous and harmaline induced electrical activity of Purkinje cells in the cerebellum of the rat and the rabbit. Neuropharmacology 1978; 17:45–51.

19. Pranzatelli MR, Snodgrass SR. Harmala alkaloids and related β-carbolines: a myoclonic model and antimyoclonic drugs. Exp Neurol 1987; 96:703–719.

20. Deecher DC, Teitler M, Soderlund DM, Bornmann WG, Kuehne ME, Glick SC. Mechanisms of action of ibogaine and harmaline congeners based on radioligand binding studies. Brain Res 1992; 571:242–247.

21. Sotelo C, Gotow T, Wassef M. Localization of glutamic acid decarboxylase-immunoreactive axon terminals in the inferior olive of the rat, with special emphasis on anatomical relations between GABAergic synapses and dendrodendritic gap junctions. J Comp Neurol 1986; 252:32–50.

22. deZeeuw CI, Holstege JC, Ruigrok TJH, Voogd J. Ultrastructural study of the GABAergic, cerebellar, and mesodiencephalic innervation of the cat medial accessory olive: anterograde tracing combined with immunocytochemistry. J Comp Neurol 1989; 284:12–35.

23. Fredette BJ, Mugnaini E. The GABAergic cerebello-olivary projection in the rat. Anat Embryol 1991; 184:225–243.

24. Llinás R. Electrophysiological properties of the olivocerebellar system. In: Strata PG, ed. The Olivocerebellar System in Motor Control. Berlin: Springer-Verlag, 1989: 201–208.

25. Spira ME, Bennett MV. Synaptic control of electrotonic coupling between neurons. Brain Res 1972; 37:294–300.

26. Spray DC, Harris AL, Bennett MV. Gap junctional conductance is a simple and sensitive function of intracellular pH. Science 1981; 211:712–715.

27. Bormann J, Hamill OP, Sakmann B. Mechanism of anion permeation through channels gated by glycine and gamma-aminobutyric acid in mouse cultured spinal neurones. J Physiol 1987; 385:243–286.

28. Kaila K, Voipio J. Postsynaptic fall in intracellular pH induced by GABA-activated bicarbonate conductance. Nature 1987; 330:163–165.

29. Chen JC, Chesler M. A bicarbonate-dependent increase in extracellular pH mediated by $GABA_A$ receptors in turtle cerebellum. Neurosci Lett 1990; 116:130–135.

30. Growdon JH, Shahani BT, Young RR. The effect of alcohol on essential tremor. Neurology 1975; 25:259–262.

31. Findley LJ, Koller WC. Essential tremor: a review. Neurology 1987; 37:1194–1197.

32. Sinclair JG, Lo GF, Harris DP. Ethanol effects on the olivocerebellar system. Can J Physiol Pharmacol 1982; 60:610–614.

33. Rappaport MS, Gentry RT, Schneider DR, Dole VP. Ethanol effects on harmaline-induced tremor and increase of cerebellar cyclic GMP. Life Sci 1984; 34:49–56.

34. Nestoros JN. Ethanol specifically potentiates GABA-mediated neurotransmission in feline cerebral cortex. Science 1980; 209:708–710.

35. Celentano JJ, Gibbs TT, Farb DH. Ethanol potentiates GABA- and glycine-induced chloride currents in chick spinal cord neurons. Brain Res 1988; 455:377–380.

36. Suzdak PD, Schwartz RD, Skolnick P, Paul SM. Alcohols stimulate γ-aminobutyric acid receptor-mediated chloride uptake in brain vesicles: correlation with intoxication potency. Brain Res 1988; 444:340–350.

37. Johnston MF, Simon SA, Ramon F. Interaction of anaesthetics with electrical synapses. Nature 1980; 286:498–500.

38. Spray DC, White RL, Mazet F, Bennett MV. Regulation of gap junctional conductance. Am J Physiol 1985; 248:753–764.

39. Williamson R. Electrical coupling between secondary haircells in the statocyst of the squid *Alloteuthis subula*. Brain Res 1989; 486:67–72.

40. Salisachs P, Findley LJ. Problems in the differential diagnosis of essential tremor. In: Findley LJ, Capildeo R, eds. Movement Disorders: Tremor. London: Macmillan Press, 1984:219–224.

41. Marsden CD. Origins of normal and pathological tremor. In: Findley LJ, Capildeo R, eds. Movement Disorders: Tremor. London: Macmillan Press, 1984:37–84.

42. Lamarre Y, Mercier LA. Etude neurophysiologique du tremblement à l'harmaline chez le chat. Rev Can Biol 1972; 31:181–191.

43. Olsen RW. GABA–benzodiazepine–barbiturate receptor interactions. J Neurochem 1981; 37:1–13.

44. Elble RJ. Physiologic and essential tremor. Neurology 1986; 36:225–231.

45. Lamarre Y. Cerebro-cerebellar mechanisms involved in experimental tremor. In: Massion J, Sasaki K, eds. Cerebro-Cerebellar Interactions. Amsterdam: Elsevier North-Holland Biomedical Press, 1979:249–259.

46. Llinás R, Sasaki K. The functional organization of the olivo-cerebellar system as examined by multiple Purkinje cell recordings. Eur J Neurosci 1989; 1:587–602.

47. Wilson JF, Marshall RW, Richens A. Essential tremor: treatment with beta-adrenoceptor blocking drugs. In: Findley LJ, Capildeo R, eds. Movement Disorders: Tremor. London: Macmillan Press, 1984:245–260.

48. Kulkarni SK, Kaul PN. Modification by *levo*-propranolol of tremors induced by harmine in mice. Experientia 1979; 35:1627–1628.

49. Procaccianti G, Martinelli P, Barruzi A, Pazzaglia P, Lugaresi E. Benign familial tremor treated with primidone. Br Med J 1981; 283:558.

50. Hersovits E, Blackwood W. Essential (familial, hereditary) tremor. A case report. J Neurol Neurosurg Psychiatry 1969; 32:509–511.

51. Rommelspacher H, Strauss S, Lindermann J. Excretion of tetrahydroharmane and harmane in the urine of man and rat after a load with ethanol. FEBS Lett 1980; 109: 209–212.

52. Angel RW, Aguilar JA, Hofmann WW. Action tremor and thalamotomy. Electroencephalogr Clin Neurophysiol 1979; 26:53–61.

53. Narabayashi H, Ohye C. Importance of microstereoencephalotomy for tremor alleviation. Appl Neurophysiol 1980; 43:222–227.

54. Andrew J. Surgery for involuntary movements. Br J Hosp Med 1981; 26:522–528.

55. Jasper H, Lamarre Y, Joffroy AJ. The effect of local cooling of the motor cortex upon experimental Parkinson-like tremor, shivering, voluntary movements, and thalamic unit activity in the monkey. In: Frigyesi T, Rinvik E, Yahr MD, eds. Corticothalamic Projections and Sensorimotor Activities. New-York: Raven Press, 1972:461–473.

56. Ohye C, Hirai T, Miyazaki M, Shbazaki T, Nakajima H. Vim thalamotomy for the treatment of various kinds of tremor. Appl Neurophysiol 1982; 45:275–280.

57. Lamarre Y, Joffroy AJ. Experimental tremor in monkey: activity of thalamic and precentral cortical neurons in the absence of peripheral feedback. Neurol 1979; 24: 109–122.

58. Filion M, Lamarre Y, Cordeau JP. Neuronal discharges of the ventrolateral nucleus of the thalamus during sleep and wakefulness in the cat. II. Evoked activity. Exp Brain Res 1971; 12:499–508.

59. Lamarre Y, Filion M, Cordeau JP. Neuronal discharges of the ventrolateral nucleus of the thalamus during sleep and wakefulness in the cat. I. Spontaneous activity. Exp Brain Res 1971; 12:480–498.

60. Joffroy AJ, Lamarre Y. Single cell activity in the ventral lateral thalamus of the unanesthetized monkey. Exp Neurol 1974; 42:1–16.

61. Steriade M, Llinás R. The functional states of the thalamus and the associated neuronal interplay. Physiol Rev 1988; 68:649–742.

62. Lamarre Y, Joffroy AJ. Rhythmic bursting of unit potentials in the ventrolateral thalamus of the monkey. In: Frigyesi T, Rinvik E, Yahr MD, eds. Corticothalamic Projections and Sensorimotor Activities. New-York: Raven Press, 1972:273–278.

63. Bergman H, Wichmann T, DeLong MR. Reversal of experimental parkinsonism by lesions of the subthalamic nucleus. Science 1990; 249:1436–1437.

64. Murthy VN, Fetz EE. Synchronized 25–35 Hz oscillations in sensorimotor cortex of awake monkeys. Soc Neurosci Abstr 1991; 17:310.

65. Narajo C. Psychotherapeutic possibilities of new fantasy-enhancing drugs. Clin Toxicol 1969; 2:209–224.

66. Llinás RR, Paré D. Of dreaming and wakefulness. Neuroscience 1991; 44:521–535.

67. Llinás R. The noncontinuous nature of movement execution. In: Humphrey DR, Freund HJ, eds. Motor Control: Concepts and Issues. New York: John Wiley & Sons, 1991:223–242.

68. Young RR. Physiological and enhanced physiological tremor. In: Findley LJ, Capildeo R, eds. Movement Disorders: Tremor. London: Macmillan Press, 1984:127–134.

69. Lance JW, Schwab RS, Peterson EA. Action tremor and the cogwheel phenomenon in Parkinson's disease. Brain 1963; 86:95–110.

70. Shahani BT, Young RR. Physiological and pharmacological aids in the differential diagnosis of tremor. J Neurol Neurosurg Psychiatry 1976; 39:772–783.

9

Adrenoceptors in Tremor Mechanisms

A. T. Birmingham and I. A. Macdonald
Medical School
Queen's Medical Centre
University of Nottingham
Nottingham, England

I. INTRODUCTION

It is a common observation that the amplitude of physiological finger tremor is increased in states of anger, fright, anxiety, and mental stress (1–3).

In normal volunteers, the effect of stress can readily be demonstrated. Figure 1 shows a record of heart rate and of right-hand tremor (measured with a small accelerometer taped to the middle finger) (4), before and during a period of stress. The stress was caused by the manikin test in which rapid decisions are required at a speed designed to induce stress. It is clear that both the heart rate (by about 30 beats per minute; BPM) and tremor [a doubling of root mean square (RMS) amplitude] were increased during the 2-min period of stress. The effect on the frequency spectrum, as a mean from six subjects, is shown in Figure 2; the tremor reverted to normal after the period of stress (5).

The first comprehensive investigation of tremor in relation to the roles of the sympathetic nervous system and of circulating catecholamines was reported in the now classic paper of Marsden et al. in 1967 (6). They showed convincingly that intravenous infusions of epinephrine (adrenaline) or isoproterenol (isoprenaline) increased the amplitude of finger tremor, and that the increase was reduced by the β-adrenoceptor blocker propranolol. From comparisons of the results from intravenous or intra-arterial infusions of epinephrine, norepinephrine, and propranolol, they concluded that the receptors involved in the increase in tremor were β-adrenoceptors located in the forearm muscles.

With the advent of sensitive methods for the measurement of catecholamines in

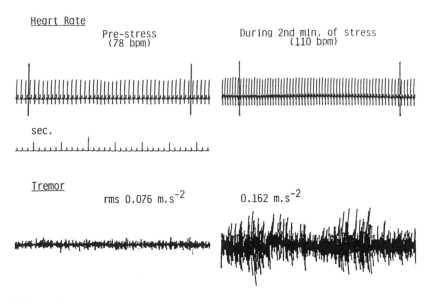

Figure 1 Effect of mental stress on heart rate (top) and finger tremor (bottom). (From Ref. 5.)

blood (7) it became clear that the doses of epinephrine used in the earlier studies would have resulted in plasma epinephrine concentrations much higher than those likely to be encountered in physiological situations. Nevertheless, when epinephrine was infused in doses that produced plasma concentrations within the physiological range (see Sect. II.A) of those associated with, for example, severe exercise, there was a clear increase in tremor with an infusion of 50 ng kg^{-1} min^{-1}, with the threshold seeming to be at 10 ng kg^{-1} min^{-1} (8).

In the same way, it can be shown that it is not necessary to use the higher concentrations of isoproterenol used in earlier studies (6,9,10) to demonstrate an effect on tremor. An investigation by Mansell et al. (11) of several effects of infusions of low doses of isoproterenol, extended downward the range of concentrations below those reported in earlier studies and established that isoproterenol, at 5 ng kg^{-1} min^{-1} was about the threshold for a detectable increase in tremor. The well-established greater potency of isoproterenol was confirmed by noting that an infusion of 15 ng kg^{-1} min^{-1} produced about the same amount of increase in tremor as that of epinephrine at 50 ng kg^{-1} min^{-1} in another six subjects.

The question of the subtype of β-adrenoceptor involved in muscle tremor has been addressed many times by different groups of workers, both in relation to physiological tremor and to essential tremor. The availability over the years of a range of β-adrenoceptor antagonists to include cardioselective and nonselective

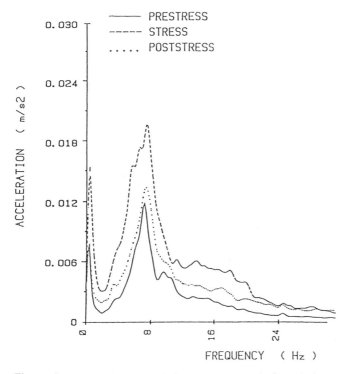

PRESTRESS
STRESS
POSTSTRESS

Figure 2 Group mean ($n = 6$) frequency spectra before, during, and after mental stress. (From Ref. 5.)

groups (and, more recently, some relatively β_2-selective antagonists) has mainly led to the conclusion that, at least in the periphery, the subtype is β_2.

Further evidence for believing that the β_2-adrenoceptor subtype is the main one involved in tremor came with the development of more selective agonists for the management of bronchospasm. Investigation of tremor as a side effect in asthmatic patients and studies in normal volunteers with albuterol (salbutamol), terbutaline, clenbuterol, and other β_2-agonists, all have indicated the preponderance of effects at muscle β_2-adrenoceptors. Watson and Richens made accelerometer measurements of finger tremor in normal volunteers to demonstrate significant increases in tremor produced by oral albuterol and by terbutaline (12). Patients become tolerant to the tremor-producing effect of β_2-agonists; this phenomenon was demonstrated quantitatively in normal volunteers by Basran et al. (13), when they used cumulative doses of intravenous albuterol to provoke tremor before and during 2 weeks of twice-daily oral dosing with clenbuterol, a relatively long-acting β_2-agonist. The tremor-provoking effect of albuterol declined over the 14 days from a mean maximum increase of 170% before clenbuterol to a mean maximum increase of only 28% on the 14th day of clenbuterol treatment. Two weeks after stopping clenbuterol dosing, the response to albuterol challenge was back to preclenbuterol levels. These findings were interpreted to be in keeping with the widely studied phenomenon of β-adrenoceptor desensitization or down-regulation observed in many tissues.

Measurements of the effects of β-adrenoceptor blockers of different degrees of relative β_1- and β_2-adrenoceptor antagonist potency, in acute (14) and chronic (15,16) studies, emphasized the β_2-adrenoceptor classification of receptors associated with tremor, but did not exclude some involvement of β_1-adrenoceptors. Some effect of β_1-selective compounds has been demonstrated with metoprolol and atenolol in essential tremor (17,18). The relative lipophilicity of the compound appears to be a factor in determining effectiveness against tremor; betaxolol (liphophilic) was more effective than atenolol (hydrophilic) in reducing finger tremor in healthy volunteers when given in doses equally effective against exercise heartrate (19). The β-adrenoceptor blockers cover a wide range, from the hydrophilic atenolol to the lipophilic drugs, such as propranolol (19a,20). These differences have implications for their ability to cross the blood–brain barrier and to penetrate deeper tissue compartments. Abila et al. used a closely argued discussion of the time courses of effects on the heart and on tremor of β-adreno-ceptor blockers of differing lipophilicity to suggest that some deeper compartment in muscle, such as the muscle spindles, is also a site for β-adrenoceptors involved in tremor mechanisms (14).

Further evidence for a greater role for β_2- than for β_1-adrenoceptors in tremor came when relatively selective β_2-antagonists became available. Cleeves and Findley showed that a dose of a hydrophilic β_2-antagonist (LI 32-468), which had no effect on heart rate, significantly reduced essential tremor (21). When the β_2-selective antagonist ICI-118,551 was given orally (150 mg daily for 7 days) to ten patients with essential tremor, it was as effective as propranolol (120 mg daily) in reducing tremor, but unlike propranolol it produced only a small reduction in exercise heart rate (22).

II. PLASMA CATECHOLAMINES AND TREMOR

The advent of more sensitive and reliable techniques for measuring the plasma concentrations of norepinephrine and epinephrine have enabled the identification of a more widespread physiological role for these catecholamines. Most of the norepinephrine found in plasma is the result of spillover from sympathetic neuroeffector junctions. Thus, plasma norepinephrine mainly provides a qualitative index of the activity of the sympathetic nervous system. However, the epinephrine in plasma is derived from the adrenal medulla, and its plasma concentration is directly related to adrenal medullary secretory activity.

Under normal, supine resting conditions, plasma epinephrine concentrations are usually less than 0.5 nmol/L, whereas the level can rise to 5 nmol/L in hypoglycemia, 10 nmol/L in severe exercise, and over 50 nmol/L after a myocardial infarction. One of the major factors complicating studies of the relation between plasma epinephrine concentration and functional changes is the marked extraction of epinephrine that occurs in peripheral tissues. This extraction process is a combination of both neuronal and extraneuronal uptake of epinephrine, together with some metabolism, and can result in the removal of more than 50% of the epinephrine present in arterial blood. Thus, care needs to be taken in comparing possible thresholds for effects of epinephrine on tremor, depending on whether arterial or venous concentrations are measured. It is now generally considered to be preferable to use arterialized venous blood to equate with arterial blood (23).

A. Plasma Epinephrine Thresholds for Physiological Responses

The first study of plasma epinephrine thresholds for physiological effects was performed by Clutter et al. (24). They measured venous epinephrine concentrations and observed the threshold for increases in heart rate was 0.3–0.6 nmol/L, for a rise in systolic blood pressure 0.4–0.7 nmol/L, and for a fall in diastolic blood pressure 0.8–1.1 nmol/L. Subsequently, Sjöstrom et al. (25) measured arterialized venous epinephrine levels and found the changes in blood pressure occurred at lower concentrations, approximately 0.6 nmol/L, equivalent to 0.4 nmol/L in venous blood.

Fellows ct al. attempted to identify the plasma epinephrine threshold for stimulating finger tremor (8). Infusion of 10 ng epinephrine per kilogram body weight per minute intravenously for 30 min raised venous epinephrine concentration to 0.77 nmol/L (four times baseline level) but had no effect on finger tremor, compared with the control condition. By contrast, infusion of 50 ng epinephrine per kilogram per minute (raising venous epinephrine to 2.3 nmol/L) increased finger tremor by 340%. Subsequent investigation has revealed that infusion of epinephrine at 25 ng kg^{-1} min^{-1} caused a 50% increase in finger tremor, and raised the arterialized plasma epinephrine level to approximately 1.8 nmol/L. If one assumes the venous epinephrine level of 0.77 nmol/L, which failed to stimulate tremor, is equivalent to an approximate arterial concentration of 1.1 nmol/L, the arterial plasma epinephrine threshold for increasing tremor would appear to be about 1.5 nmol/L. This is substantially above the plasma thresholds for effects on heart rate, blood pressure, and limb blood flow. The plasma epinephrine threshold for the stimulation of finger tremor is exceeded during moderate hypoglycemia, moderate to severe exercise, or severe stress. We have confirmed the observation of Warren et al. that patients with essential tremor have higher resting levels of venous plasma epinephrine than normal control subjects (Table 1; 26)

Table 1 Plasma Norepinephrine and Epinephrine (nmol/L) and Finger Tremor (m s^{-2}) Measured Supine and After Standing for 10 Min

	Normal controls (n = 10, age range 28–54 yr)			Essential tremor patients (no treatment) (n = 8 or 9, age range 26–76 yr)		
	Norepinephrine	Epinephrine	Tremor	Norepinephrine	Epinephrine	Tremor
Supine	0.85 ± 0.01	0.08 ± 0.01	0.08 ± 0.02	2.03[a] ± 0.46	0.18[b] ± 0.02	0.78 ± 0.36
Standing	2.11 ± 0.38	0.14 ± 0.02	0.10 ± 0.01	3.14 ± 0.55	0.23 ± 0.02	1.26 ± 0.92
Change	+1.26[c] ± 0.33	+0.06[c] ± 0.02	+0.034 ± 0.01 (6–11-Hz band)	+1.35[c] ± 0.23	+0.03 ± 0.02	+0.48 ± 0.6

Source: Sankarayya R, Eves H, Jones R, Macdonald IA, Wharrad HJ, Birmingham AT. Unpublished results.

	Normal control patients (n = 10, age range 16–69 yr)			Essential tremor patients (off treatment) (n = 10, age range 19–75 yr)		
	Norepinephrine	Epinephrine	Tremor	Norepinephrine	Epinephrine	Tremor
Supine	2.1 ± 0.22	0.19 ± 0.02		2.4 ± 0.25	0.43[a] ± 0.04	
Standing	3.3 ± 0.25	0.23 ± 0.03		3.1 ± 0.35	0.48[a] ± 0.04	
Change	+1.2	+0.04		+0.7	+0.05	

[a]Significantly higher than normal control ($p < 0.005$)
[b]Significantly higher than normal control ($p < 0.001$)
[c]Significant increase on standing ($p < 0.02$)
Source: Adapted from Ref. 26.

From our studies on epinephrine thresholds for increase in tremor, referred to earlier, it seems unlikely that the raised basal levels found in essential tremor are sufficient alone to account for the tremor increase. Use of the plasma norepinephrine as a marker of sympathetic activity, indicated that our group of essential tremor patients had a higher basal level than that of the controls; the increase provoked by changing from a supine to a standing position was similar in both groups. In considering the possibility that β-adrenoceptor responsiveness may be increased in patients with essential tremor, Kilfeather et al. investigated the β-adrenoceptors of blood lymphocytes (27). When they compared the lymphocytes from normal controls with those from patients with essential tremor, they found no significant differences in responsiveness to isoproterenol-induced cAMP activity, nor in ligand-binding results for β-adrenoceptor affinity or density. They concluded that a general defect in responsiveness of the receptor system was not involved in the pathogenesis of essential tremor.

B. Hypoglycemia

Tremor has always been considered one of the classic signs and symptoms of hypoglycemia; until recently, it was usually assessed by observation, or on the basis of subjective reporting by the patient. This could have caused some confusion, as some patients describe shaking or trembling during hypoglycemia, which is not necessarily the same as tremor. For example, the increase in cardiac output that occurs in hypoglycemia, and the palpitations that patients describe, could contribute to the shaking or trembling sensation.

The first objective measurements of tremor during hypoglycemia were made by Heller et al. (28). They infused both insulin and glucose into diabetic and nondiabetic subjects to produce stable hypoglycemia at two glucose concentrations, 3.2 and 2.5 mmol/L, maintaining each for 30 min. The mild hypoglycemia (3.2 mmol/L) produced only a small rise in plasma epinephrine in the nondiabetic subjects and had no significant effect on tremor. In these nondiabetic subjects, more marked hypoglycemia (glucose at 2.5 mmol/L) increased plasma epinephrine concentration to 2.71 nmol/L and caused a 180% increase in finger tremor. The 15 diabetic patients were divided into two categories, the 4 who were aware of being hypoglycemic when their blood glucose level was 2.5 mmol/L, and the 11 who were not aware of being hypoglycemic at this level. (This phenomenon of unawareness of mild to moderate hypoglycemia is relatively common in patients with insulin-dependent diabetes). The patients aware of hypoglycemia had marked increases in epinephrine and in finger tremor, whereas the other 11 patients had very small epinephrine responses and no increase in tremor when their blood glucose value was 2.5 mmol/L (Fig. 3). When all diabetic and nondiabetic subjects were considered together, there was a significant correlation between the rise in epinephrine and the increase in finger tremor (Fig. 4), although

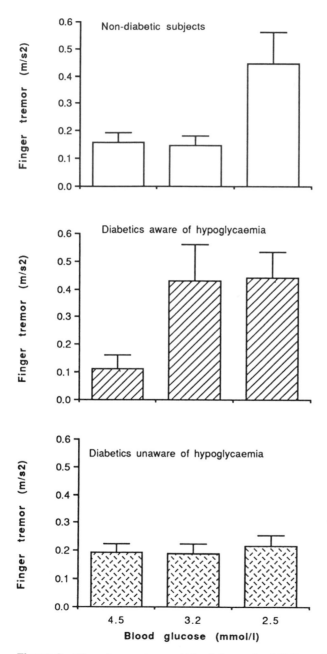

Figure 3 Finger tremor at normal blood glucose level (4.5 mmol/L), mild (3.2), and moderate (2.5) hypoglycemia in 10 nondiabetic and 15 diabetic subjects. Four of the diabetic subjects were aware of the moderate hypoglycemia, 11 were not. Values are means ± SEM.

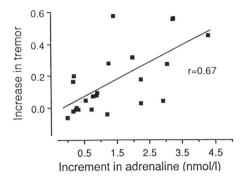

Figure 4 Relation between increase in plasma epinephrine and increase in finger tremor (ms^{-2}) during moderate hypoglycemia (glucose level 2.5 mmol/L) in nondiabetic ($n = 8$) and diabetic ($n = 15$) subjects.

the correlation coefficient of 0.67 indicates that there were other factors contributing to the tremor response.

The tremor seen during insulin-induced hypoglycemia in nondiabetic subjects was prevented by a 1-week treatment with propranolol (160 mg daily), even though such treatment was accompanied by a marked increase in plasma epinephrine levels (Table 2). Similar treatment with metoprolol (100 mg CR daily) or atenolol (100 mg daily) did not reduce the tremor response to hypoglycemia. However, both of these β_1-selective antagonists led to enhanced plasma epinephrine levels during hypoglycemia (see Table 2), and one might have expected the higher epinephrine levels to produce a larger tremor response. Thus, it seems likely that these β_1-antagonists do slightly reduce tremor during hypoglycemia (29).

Table 2 Plasma Epinephrine (nmol/L) and Finger Tremor (ms^{-2}) During Hypoglycemia: Effects of β-Adrenoceptor Antagonists

	Saline	Propranolol	Metoprolol	Atenolol
Plasma Epinephrine				
Baseline	0.30	0.39	0.30	0.30
Hypoglycemia	2.17	6.18[a]	3.79[b]	4.70[b]
Tremor				
Baseline	0.198	0.180	0.184	0.170
Hypoglycemia	0.356	0.160[a]	0.273	0.315

[a]Significantly different from saline, metoprolol, and atenolol: $p < 0.01$.
[b]Significantly different from saline: $p < 0.01$.
Source: Ref. 29.

It is widely believed that alcohol consumption reduces tremor, although there is little objective evidence to support this belief. Growdon et al. reported a rapid, marked reduction in tremor after the ingestion of alcohol in patients with essential tremor (30). This was in contrast with the relative lack of effect of alcohol infused into a brachial artery on hand tremor in the same patients. However, there were no objective studies of the effects of alcohol on subjects with normal tremor until a recent study of the effects of alcohol on tremor during hypoglycemia also provided the opportunity to assess the effects at normal blood glucose levels (31). In both diabetic and nondiabetic subjects, finger tremor was reduced 20 min after the ingestion of alcohol (0.75 g/kg body weight), when blood glucose was maintained at a normal level, but the differences were not statistically significant.

The subsequent induction of hypoglycemia was accompanied by lower levels of finger tremor in the presence of alcohol than in the control experiment (Table 3), which was statistically significant in both groups. Plasma epinephrine concentrations during hypoglycemia were not significantly different on the two occasions (nondiabetic subjects: control 1.70, alcohol 1.55 nmol/L; diabetic subjects: control 1.65, alcohol 1.80 nmol/L). Thus, it is likely that the reduction of tremor during hypoglycemia in the presence of alcohol is due to direct effects of alcohol or its metabolites within the muscle, rather than through any reduction in adrenal medullary response.

C. Caffeine and Starvation

Caffeine was thought for a long time to be capable of stimulating tremor owing to its inhibition of phosphodiesterase, its stimulation of catecholamine release, and through its direct effects on muscle. However, with normal levels of caffeine intake, the concentrations achieved are usually below those needed to inhibit phosphodiesterase, and the main effects of caffeine are probably through antagonism at adenosine receptors. Nevertheless, it was widely believed that caffeine

Table 3 Effects of Alcohol and Hypoglycemia on Finger Tremor (ms^{-2})

	Nondiabetic		Diabetic	
	Alcohol	Control	Alcohol	Control
Baseline	0.18	0.17	0.18	0.16
After alcohol	0.14	0.17	0.15	0.17
Hypoglycemia	0.26[a]	0.40[a]	0.23[a]	0.31[a]

[a]Significantly different: $p < 0.05$.
Source: Ref. 31.

intake stimulates tremor. This was shown not to be so by Wharrad et al. (32), when subjects consumed, as three 150 mg doses, 450 mg caffeine per day for 2 days, or no caffeine, and tremor was measured 1.5–2 h after the final dose. When subjects consumed their normal diet, there was no effect of caffeine on finger tremor. These subjects also underwent two periods of starvation for 48 h (with sodium and potassium supplementation to prevent confounding changes in extracellular fluid volume), consuming caffeine during one period and placebo during the other. Starvation itself had no significant effect on tremor, but the combination of starvation and caffeine intake did produce a significant rise in postural hand tremor compared with the level recorded in the fed state with no caffeine intake. As starvation is thought to lead to a reduction in sympathetic nervous system activity and leads to increased sensitivity of cardiovascular and metabolic responses to infused epinephrine (33), it seems likely that normal doses of caffeine will stimulate tremor only in subjects whose catecholamine sensitivity is enhanced. However, the study by Wharrad et al. (32) provides no information on the mechanisms underlying this effect of caffeine on tremor, and under normal conditions there was no effect at all.

III. SYMPATHETIC NERVOUS SYSTEM

There have been no studies of the plasma norepinephrine threshold concentration for increasing tremor. However, studies with other variables have revealed that the threshold for norepinephrine-stimulated effects is a plasma concentration of 5–10 nmol/L (compared with basal levels of 0.5–2.5 nmol/L), up to ten times higher than the threshold epinephrine concentration (34,35).

A. Orthostasis

Movement from the supine to the upright position produces a marked hydrostatic stress on the cardiovascular system, requiring baroreflex-mediated alterations in cardiac function and vascular resistance to maintain arterial blood pressure. The efferent pathways of these reflexes include activation of the sympathetic nervous system—which is reflected in an approximate doubling of plasma norepinephrine concentration. However, the norepinephrine concentrations do not normally exceed the thresholds for cardiovascular effect, and so are more likely to be a marker of increased sympathetic nerve activity, rather than being primarily responsible for initiating the cardiovascular changes. Under normal circumstances, the plasma epinephrine response to moving to an upright position is small; the increase above baseline being approximately 50%, giving arterial plasma epinephrine concentrations of 0.5–0.75 nmol/L. Thus, given these relatively low plasma catecholamine concentrations in the upright position (compared with hypoglycemia), it is intriguing that there is an increase in finger tremor; both young and elderly subjects showed an increase in finger tremor of 30–50% when being tilted toward the upright position. In the young subjects, the effect was maximal by the time the subjects were tilted to 25° head-up (36), whereas in the elderly subjects, the maximum effect was noted at 45° head-up tilt (37). In both groups, these increased levels of tremor were then maintained as the subjects were moved to the upright position.

B. Food Intake

There is good evidence that food ingestion, especially meals with a high carbohydrate content, activates the sympathetic nervous system. This can be demonstrated by increases in plasma norepinephrine, in the appearance rate of norepinephrine in the plasma (spillover from sympathetic neuroeffector junctions) after a mixed meal (38), and by increases in the sympathetic nerve-firing rate after ingestion of oral glucose (39). The rise in plasma norepinephrine is small (25–50% of basal levels), and there is little if any change in plasma epinephrine after food. However, a high-carbohydrate meal was accompanied by a significant increase in resting finger tremor in the supine position in young (36), but not in elderly (37) subjects.

Thus, in both conditions (standing and food ingestion), when there is evidence of sympathetic nervous system activation, there is also an increase in finger tremor that cannot always be readily explained by direct effects of circulating catecholamines. The possibility that the sympathetic nervous system may have direct effects on tremor requires further study. It may be relevant that muscle spindles, which play a part in tremor generation, have been shown in animal muscle to have a sympathetic innervation and to increase in sensitivity when exposed to epinephrine (40). Hodgson et al. used vibration of the Achilles tendon to activate muscle spindles in the calf muscles of human subjects to show that epinephrine infusion increased the sensitivity of muscle spindles (41).

REFERENCES

1. Graham JDP. Static tremor in anxiety states. J Neurol Neurosurg Psychiatry 1945; 8:57–60.
2. Redfearn JWT. Frequency analysis of physiological and neurotic tremor. J Neurol Neurosurg Psychiatry 1957; 20:302–303.
3. Tyrer P, Lader MH. Tremor in acute and chronic anxiety. Arch Gen Psychiatry 1974; 31:506–510.
4. Birmingham AT, Wharrad HJ, Williams EJ, Wilson CG. Accelerometric measurement of finger tremor: analysis of the analogue signal. J Physiol 1984; 361:12P.
5. Wharrad HJ. The measurement of finger tremor in man. Ph.D. dissertation, University of Nottingham, England, 1982:170–172.
6. Marsden CD, Foley TH, Owen DAL, McAllister RG. Peripheral β-adrenergic receptors concerned with tremor. Clin Sci 1967; 33:53–65.

7. Macdonald IA, Lake DM. An improved technique for extracting catecholamines from biological fluids. J Neurosci Methods 1985; 13:239–248.

8. Fellows IW, Macdonald IA, Wharrad HJ, Birmingham AT. Low plasma concentrations of adrenaline and physiological tremor in man. J Neurol Neurosurg Psychiatry 1986; 49:396–399.

9. Arnold JMO, McDevitt DG. Enhancement of physiological finger tremor by intravenous isoprenaline infusions in man: evaluation of its role in the assessment of β-adrenoceptor antagonists. Br J Clin Pharmacol 1984; 18:145–152.

10. Arnold JMO, O'Connor PC, Riddell JG, Harron DWG, Shanks RG, McDevitt DG. Effects of the β-adrenoceptor antagonist ICI 118,551 on exercise tachycardia and isoprenaline-induced β-adrenoceptor responses in man. Br J Clin Pharmacol 1985; 19:619–630.

11. Mansell PI, Fellows IW, Birmingham AT, Macdonald IA. Metabolic and cardiovascular effects of infusions of low doses of isoprenaline in man. Clin Sci 1988; 75: 285–291.

12. Watson JM, Richens A. The effects of salbutamol and terbutaline on physiological tremor, bronchial tone and heart rate. Br J Clin Pharmacol 1974; 1:223–227.

13. Basran G, Fentem PH, McGivern DV, Wharrad HJ. Clenbuterol-induced reduction in the tremor provoked by salbutamol. Br J Clin Pharmacol 1984; 18:283P.

14. Abila B, Wilson JF, Marshall RW, Richens A. The tremorolytic action of β-adrenoceptor blockers in essential, physiological and isoprenaline-induced tremor is mediated by β-adrenoceptors located in a deep peripheral compartment. Br J Clin Pharmacol 1985; 20:369–376.

15. Calzetti S, Findley LJ, Perucca E, Richens A. Controlled study of meloprolol and propranolol during prolonged administration in patients with essential tremor. J Neurol Neurosurg Psychiatry 1982; 45:893–897.

16. Wharrad HJ, Birmingham AT, Wilson CG, Williams EJ, Roland JM. Effect on finger tremor of withdrawal of long-term treatment with propranolol or atenolol. Br J Clin Pharmacol 1984; 18:317–324.

17. Ljung O. Treatment of essential tremor with metoprolol. N Engl J Med 1979; 301: 1005.

18. Larsen TO, Teräväinen H, Calne DB. Atenolol versus propranolol in essential tremor: a controlled quantitative study. Acta Neurol Scand 1982; 66:547–554.

19. Wharrad HJ, Patrick JM, Birmingham AT, Wilson CG. Effects of the cardioselective drugs, atenolol and betaxolol on normal finger tremor. Proc 9th Int Cong Pharmacol 1984; 938P.

19a. Woods PB, Robinson ML. An investigation of the comparative liposolubilities of β-adrenoceptor blocking agents. J Pharm Pharmacol 1981; 33:172–173.

20. Cruikshank JM, Neil-Dwyer G, Cameron MM, McAinsh J. β-Adrenoceptor-blocking agents and the blood–brain barrier. Clin Sci 1980; 59:453S–455S.

21. Cleeves L, Findley LJ. beta-Adrenoceptor mechanisms in essential tremor: a comparative single dose study of the effect of a non-selective and a β_2 selective adrenoceptor antagonist. J Neurol Neurosurg. Psychiatry 1984; 47:976–982.

22. Jefferson D, Wharrad HJ, Birmingham AT, Patrick JM. The comparative effects of ICI 118551 and propranolol on essential tremor. Br J Clin Pharmacol 1987; 24: 729–734.

23. McGuire EAH, Helderman JH, Tobin JD, Andres R, Bergman R. Effects of arterial versus venous sampling on glucose kinetics in man. J Appl Physiol 1976; 41:165–173.
24. Clutter WE, Bier DM, Shah SD, Cryer PE. Epinephrine plasma metabolic clearance rates and physiological thresholds for metabolic and hemodynamic actions in man. J Clin Invest 1980; 66:94–101.
25. Sjöstrom L, Schutz Y, Gudinchet F, Hegnell L, Pittet PG, Jéquier E. Epinephrine sensitivity with respect to metabolic rate and other variables in women. Am J Physiol 1983; 245:E431–E442.
26. Warren JB, O'Brien M, Dalton N, Turner CT. Sympathetic activity in benign familial tremor. Lancet 1984; 1:461–462.
27. Kilfeather SA, Massarella A, Gorgolewska G, Findley LJ, Ansell E, Turner P. Normal lymphocyte β-adrenoceptors in essential tremor and migraine and normal responsiveness to epoprostenol in migraine. Br J Clin Pharmacol 1984; 18:299P.
28. Heller SR, Macdonald IA, Herbert M, Tattersall RB. Influence of sympathetic nervous system on hypoglycaemic warning symptoms. Lancet 1987; 2:359–363.
29. Kerr D, Macdonald IA, Heller SR, Tattersall RB. A randomised, double-blind placebo controlled trial of the effects of metoprolol CR, atenolol and propranolol LA on the physiological responses to hypoglycemia in nondiabetic subjects. Br J Clin Pharmacol 1990; 29:685–694.
30. Growdon JH, Shahani BT, Young RR. The effect of alcohol on essential tremor. Neurology 1975; 25:259–262.
31. Kerr D, Macdonald IA, Heller SR, Tattersall RB. Alcohol causes hypoglycaemic unawareness in healthy volunteers and patients with type 1 (insulin-dependent) diabetes. Diabetologia 1990b; 33:216–221.
32. Wharrad HJ, Birmingham AT, Macdonald IA, Inch PJ, Mead JL. The influence of fasting and of caffeine intake on finger tremor. Eur J Clin Pharmacol 1985; 29:37–43.
33. Mansell PI, Macdonald IA, Fellows IW. 48-hr starvation enhances the thermogenic response to infused epinephrine. Am J Physiol 1990; 258:R87–R93.
34. Silverberg AB, Shah SD, Haymond MW, Cryer PE. Norepinephrine: hormone and neurotransmitter in man. Am J Physiol 1978; 234:E252–E256.
35. Izzo J. Cardiovascular hormonal effects of circulating norepinephrine. Hypertension 1983; 5:787–789.
36. Buck J, Haigh R, Macdonald IA, Birmingham AT. Effect of food intake on orthostatic tolerance and finger tremor in healthy young subjects. Proc Nutr Soc 1989; 48:134A.
37. Birmingham AT, Macdonald IA, Sainsbury R. Food intake, orthostatic tolerance and finger tremor in healthy elderly women. J Physiol 1988; 406:102P.
38. Schwartz RS, Jaeger LF, Silberstein S, Veith RC. Sympathetic nervous system activity and the thermic effect of feeding in man. Int J Obes 1987; 11:141–149.
39. Berne C, Fagius J, Niklasson F. Sympathetic response to oral carbohydrate administration. Evidence from microelectrode nerve recordings. J Clin Invest 1989; 84:1403–1409.
40. Hunt CC. The effect of sympathetic stimulation on mammalian muscle spindles. J Physiol 1960; 151:332–341.
41. Hodgson HJF, Marsden CD, Meadows JC. The effect of adrenaline on the response to muscle vibration in man. J Physiol 1969; 202:98P.

10

Positron Emission Tomography in Tremor Disorders

David J. Brooks
Hammersmith Hospital
London, England

I. INTRODUCTION

Tremor can be conveniently classified in terms of appearance as postural, resting, and kinetic or intention. *Essential tremor* (ET) is usually defined as a postural tremor not exacerbated by movement, in the absence of parkinsonian features or cerebellar ataxia (1). A low-amplitude rest component may be present in severe cases. The tremor frequency generally falls within the 4- to 8-Hz range. In spite of the high prevalence of ET, 12% of persons older than 70 years are affected (2), its etiology remains uncertain. Histopathological assessment of the nine cases reported to date has revealed only nonspecific changes (3–5). There are, however, some clues to the pathways involved in conducting essential tremor. Lesions of the contralateral thalamic nucleus ventralis intermedius (Vim), hemiparesis, and ipsilateral cerebellar stroke, all can abolish ET in humans (6–8). If monkeys with brainstem lesions involving the olivocerebellar–dentatorubral loop are given intravenous harmaline, they develop a 6- to 8-Hz postural tremor. Lamarre has reported that cells in the inferior olive that are firing at the tremor frequency can be identified in these lesioned primates (9). The foregoing findings are all compatible with ET being generated by olivocerebellar projections, and conducted by cerebellothalamocortical projections to the pyramidal tracts and spinal cord.

Peripheral factors are also important in determining essential tremor amplitude and frequency. Those β-adrenergic receptor blockers that are effective in reducing the amplitude of postural tremor all act on peripheral β_2-adrenergic receptors (10).

In addition, essential tremor frequency can be reset by large-amplitude external limb perturbations (11). Small-amplitude perturbations, however, are ineffective in resetting postural tremor, whereas passive rhythmic oscillations of outstretched fingers at near tremor frequencies cause beats to be set up, rather than entraining the tremor (12). These findings suggest that, although sensory feedback may be involved in modulating tremor frequency and amplitude, essential tremor is most likely to arise from a central generator. Having said that, patients with demyelinating peripheral neuropathies associated with IgM paraproteinemia can manifest postural tremors that are clinically indistinguishable from essential tremor (13). The frequency of such tremors correlates with nerve conduction velocity, and it has been postulated that such neuropathic tremors arise as a consequence of mismatch of afferent and efferent traffic in affected peripheral nerves, rather than from a central oscillator.

Parkinson's disease (PD) is characterized by a resting tremor in the 3- to 5-Hz range, but can also be associated with a 4- to 8-Hz postural tremor. This has led to some debate over the relation between PD and essential tremor. Between 3 and 19% of patients initially diagnosed as having ET are reported to become parkinsonian (14,15), and there is an increased incidence of tremor in relatives of PD patients (16). The primary pathology of PD involves degeneration of the dopaminergic cells in the substantia nigra compacta and ventral midbrain tegmentum. Pure lesions of the substantia nigra in primates do not result in a tremor (17). If the rubrospinal and dentatothalamic tracts are additionally lesioned, a typically parkinsonian 3- to 5-Hz tremor may result, although additional administration of harmaline is often necessary (18,19). Cells firing at rest tremor frequency have been identified in the contralateral ventrolateral thalamus and sensorimotor cortex of such lesioned primates, even when their limbs were deafferented or paralyzed with gallamine (20). Cooling of the contralateral sensorimotor cortex abolishes the 3- to 5-Hz tremor, but not the associated ventrolateral thalamic activity (9). This has led to the postulate that rest tremor is generated by disinhibited firing of a ventral thalamic generator and conducted by thalamocortical projections. Sectioning the pyramidal tracts of primates does not abolish 3- to 5-Hz tremor, suggesting that it may be conducted by extrapyramidal pathways (19).

Positron emission tomography (PET) provides a noninvasive means of studying regional cerebral blood flow (rCBF) and metabolism, and the integrity of neurotransmitter systems, in humans. Tracers labeled with short-lived positron-emitting isotopes, such as ^{15}O, ^{11}C, and ^{18}F (half-lives 2, 20, and 110 min, respectively) are administered, and their regional cerebral distribution quantitatively determined, The rCBF is usually measured by infusing $H_2^{15}O$, or asking subjects to inhale $C^{15}O_2$, and comparing levels of regional cerebral and arterial plasma ^{15}O activity. Measurement of rCBF changes while subjects perform motor tasks provides a sensitive means of defining which areas of the brain are focally activated by the paradigm (21). Stereotyped, repetitive arm movements result in increased blood flow in the contralateral sensorimotor cortex (SMC), the caudal lateral premotor cortex (PMC), and supplementary motor area (SMA) (22). Spontaneous free selection of the direction of limb movement results in additional activation of rostral PMC and SMA, and the dorsolateral prefrontal cortex (23,24).

The integrity of the terminals of the nigrostriatal dopaminergic system can be assessed with PET by measuring caudate and putamen 6[^{18}F]fluorodopa uptake. This L-dopa analogue is transported across the blood–brain barrier by the neutral amino acid carrier and taken up specifically by the striatum, where it is converted to ^{18}F-dopamine by aromatic acid decarboxylase (AADC). In patients with clinically diagnosed Parkinson's disease mean putamen ^{18}F-dopa uptake is reduced to 50% of normal levels, whereas caudate tracer uptake is relatively spared (25). Measurement of putamen ^{18}F-dopa uptake, therefore, provides a sensitive means of detecting the presence of abnormalities of the nigrostriatal dopaminergic system, and has been used to demonstrate subclinical nigral lesions in subjects exposed to the toxin 1-methyl-4-phenyl-1,2,3,6-tetrahydropyridine (MPTP) (26).

In this chapter, the use of PET for studying patterns of regional cerebral activation associated with different forms of tremor (essential, neuropathic, parkinsonian rest) measured as increases in rCBF, is presented. The relation between essential tremor (familial and sporadic), isolated rest tremor, and dysfunction of nigrostriatal dopaminergic projections (as evidenced by reduced striatal ^{18}F-dopa uptake) is also examined. The clinical relevance of possible predictors of underlying nigral disfunction in ET patients, such as the presence of reduced arm swing, and cogwheel rigidity, is also discussed.

II. POSITRON EMISSION TOMOGRAPHY ACTIVATION STUDIES

Dubinsky and Hallett were the first to study essential tremor patients with 2-deoxy-2-[^{18}F]fluoro-D-glucose ([18]FDG) PET (27). They have reported, in abstract, that the presence of postural tremor was associated with abnormally high medullary glucose metabolism, presumed to be arising from the inferior olive, and suggested that their findings provided evidence that essential tremor (ET) is associated with abnormal overactivity of olivocerebellar connections.

Colebatch et al. subsequently measured rCBF in four patients with essential tremor and compared their findings with those of four age-matched controls (28). None of the ET patients had a tremor at rest, and all had a postural tremor with their arms extended. The rCBF was determined by asking subjects to inhale $C^{15}O_2$ continuously for 2 min during PET scanning. Tremor patients were scanned under three separate conditions: at rest with the arms relaxed (no tremor), with the right arm extended (involuntary postural tremor), and at rest with the right wrist being passively flexed and extended at tremor frequency (passive oscillation). Controls were also scanned under three conditions: at rest, while holding the right arm extended without tremor (posture), and while mimicking a postural tremor at the right wrist (mimic). Subjects had two estimations of rCBF under each condition.

Scans were performed on an ECAT 931/08/12 scanner (CTI, Knoxville, Tennessee), with an intrinsic spatial resolution of $5.5 \times 5.5 \times 7.0$ mm at full-width–half-maximum. This tomograph produces 15 axial contiguous planes, with a total axial field of view of 10.5 cm. To include cerebellum and premotor areas in the field of view, the rings were tilted 15° back from the orbitomeatal line. Scans were transformed into standard stereotactic space, using anatomical landmarks, and rescaled to correspond to the atlas of Talairach and Tournoux. Statistical analysis was performed using pixel-by-pixel analysis of covariance over the different baseline and activation conditions for the two groups of subjects. This analysis normalizes rCBF images to the group global blood flow and removes the effects of changes in global blood flow caused by activation. Statistically significant focal changes in blood flow, assumed to be independent of global blood flow changes, can then be detected. Blood flow increases were measured at the peaks of sites of significant focal increases.

Figure 1 shows an axial tomographic map of the focal regions of significantly increased rCBF in association with postural tremor of the right arm for the group of four ET patients. Equivalent axial levels from the stereotactic atlas are shown on the right of the statistical maps for reference. Involuntary unilateral postural tremor was associated with significant contralateral sensorimotor cortex, bilateral premotor cortex, and bilateral cerebellar hemisphere activation. Passively imposed wrist oscillation in the ET group was associated with contralateral SMC and bilateral PMC activation, but no significant increase in cerebellar blood flow. When the control group voluntarily extended their right arms without tremor the contralateral SMC and SMA was activated, but not the cerebellum. Table 1 details the percentage focal rCBF increases that were associated with these various motor conditions for the tremor and control groups of subjects. Postural tremor can be considered as a combination of the voluntary act of posture with superimposition of an involuntary tremor. The cerebellar activation seen in association with involuntary postural tremor was not evident when normal subjects held one arm extended, nor did it occur as a consequence of proprioceptive input when the wrist was passively oscillated. It can be seen, therefore, that bilateral cerebellar activation was specifically associated with the presence of involuntary unilateral postural tremor.

The study by Colebatch et al. (28) has now been extended. Brooks et al. compared PET findings for 11 ET patients with those for 8 controls (29). With these greater numbers, it became apparent that, even at rest without tremor, ET patients had an abnormally globally raised mean cerebellar blood flow that was 12% higher than that of controls. Additionally, the presence of involuntary postural tremor was associated with significant contralateral striatal and thalamic, as well as global cerebellar, activation. Interestingly, when the control subjects mimicked a tremor,

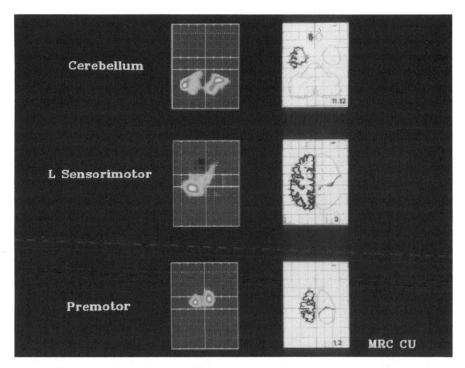

Figure 1 Axial tomographic maps showing focal regions of significantly increased mean rCBF associated with involuntary postural tremor of the right arm. Tremor leads to bilateral cerebellar and premotor cortex, and contralateral sensorimotor cortex activation.

Table 1 Significant Percentage rCBF Increases Associated with Postural Tremor, Voluntary Arm Extension, and Passive Wrist Oscillation

Action	Location[a]	Percentage rCBF increase
R arm extension (+ involuntary tremor)	L and R cerebellum	7.7, 6.9
	L SMC	13.6
	L and R PMC	6.7, 4.5
R arm extension (no tremor)	L SMC	9.1
	SMA	6.8
R passive wrist oscillation	L SMC	14.8
	L and R PMC	6.9, 5.4

[a]SMC, sensorimotor cortex; PMC, premotor cortex; SMA, supplementary motor area; R, right; L, left.

only significant ipsilateral, rather than bilateral, cerebellar activation was evident. This finding could potentially provide a means of distinguishing psychogenic from involuntary postural tremor. Liao et al. have also compared resting rCBF in ET and normal subjects (30). Similar to Brooks et al. (29), these workers found that mean resting cerebellar blood flow was bilaterally increased in ET, but also found raised resting thalamic activity.

Brooks et al. also studied seven patients with neuropathic 4- to 8-Hz postural tremor (NT) (29). All had a demyelinating peripheral neuropathy demonstrated with nerve conduction studies; in six cases this was associated with IgM paraproteinemia, and in the seventh case with chronic inflammatory demyelinating peripheral neuropathy (CIDP). All patients had impaired light-touch and pain sensation in a glove-and-stocking distribution, but none were deafferented. As with ET, the seven NT patients showed abnormally raised global mean levels of cerebellar blood flow at rest, without tremor, 10–15% higher than that of normal. Unilateral involuntary postural tremor was associated with additional bilateral cerebellar and contralateral thalamic and SMC activation. This finding is against the hypothesis that neuropathic tremor (NT) arises simply as a consequence of mismatch of afferent and efferent traffic in peripheral nerves and suggests that, like ET, NT is associated with abnormal overactivity of cerebellar connections.

Parker et al. have recently reported PET rCBF findings in seven patients with unilateral parkinsonian rest tremor resistant to levodopa (31). These patients had an electrode stereotactically placed in the contralateral ventral intermediate nucleus (Vim) of the thalamus. Electrical stimulation abolished the tremor and led to a global fall in cerebellar, and ipsilateral fall in SMC blood flow. These findings suggest that overactivity of cerebellar connections may underlie all forms of tremor, whether the tremor be essential, neuropathic, or parkinsonian in etiology.

III. TREMOR AND THE DOPAMINERGIC SYSTEM

We have studied 19 patients diagnosed as having essential tremor with ^{18}F-dopa PET scans. These patients were segregated into a group of 8 who had a clear family history of postural tremor, and a group of 11 with sporadic tremor. The ages of the familial tremor patients ranged from 39–74 years, and their tremor duration from 1–55 years. Tremor involved both arms in all eight subjects, and titubation was evident in five. Only one patient had leg tremor and this was low-amplitude. Four of the eight showed intermittent low-amplitude tremor seated in repose, and one had sustained cogwheel rigidity on synkinesis. One subject had reduced arm swing. Four of the eight had ethanol-, and three propranolol-responsive tremors.

The age range and tremor duration of the 11 patients with sporadic postural tremor were 28–77, and 2–60, years, respectively. Tremor involved both arms in 10, and the right arm in 1 subject. Five patients had leg, 3 had head, and 5 jaw tremor. Eight had intermittent low-amplitude rest tremor, and 5 had cogwheel rigidity on synkinesis. Six of the 11 had reduced arm swing. Two patients had alcohol- and 4 propranolol-responsive tremors.

We have also performed ^{18}F-dopa PET on ten patients with isolated predominant rest tremor; that is, with no evidence of sustained rigidity or akinesia. Their age range was 47–70 years, and their tremor duration 1–20 years, respectively. The tremor involved one arm in seven, both arms in two, one leg in five, and both legs in three subjects. Two patients had involvement of only one limb, and four had hemitremor. Nine of the ten also had a lower amplitude 4- to 8-Hz postural tremor of the affected limbs, and five had reduced arm swing. Only three out of the eight treated with levodopa showed a good response of their tremor to this agent.

Results of the ^{18}F-dopa PET scans for the three tremor groups were compared with those obtained for a group of 30 controls, aged 30–77 years, and for a group of 16 L-dopa responsive PD patients aged 38–76 years, who all had rest tremor, rigidity, and bradykinesia, and ranged from 1 to 4 on the Hoehn and Yahr disability scale. The ^{18}F-dopa scans were performed on an ECAT 931/08/12 scanner (CTI, Knoxville, Tennessee) with a reconstructed resolution of $5.5 \times 5.5 \times 7.0$ mm. Regions of interest (ROIs) were placed in a standard arrangement (25): one square region length, 8.2 mm, was placed over the head of the caudate, and three more were lined along the axis of the putamen, for each hemisphere in both normal subjects and patients. One circular region diameter, 32.8 mm, was placed over the occipital lobe of each hemisphere. This array of ROIs was defined on the integrated images of the two optimum contiguous 7-mm planes for each cerebral structure, and then superimposed on individual time frames. Averaged values for each structure (caudate, putamen, occiput) over two planes were then calculated from the individual hemispheric ROI data.

Following decay correction, regional time activity curves were plotted for ^{18}F-dopa. Specific striatal ^{18}F-dopa uptake was determined by using a modified multiple time graphic analysis (MTGA) approach with an occipital nonspecific tissue, rather than a plasma input function (32). This MTGA approach linearizes striatal ^{18}F uptake curves over 30–90 min of real time, and the gradients of the plots obtained using this approach can be considered as influx constants, K_i, which reflect the rate of striatal decarboxylation of ^{18}F-dopa and its storage as ^{18}F-dopamine and its metabolites.

Figure 2 shows the individual ^{18}F-dopa putamen influx constants for 30 normal subjects, 16 patients with L-dopa-responsive PD, and the groups of tremor patients. It can be seen that all eight patients with familial essential tremor had K_i values within the normal range. Only 1 of the 11 patients with sporadic postural tremor had a putamen K_i value within the parkinsonian range. This patient's tremor had been evident for 2 years, and a low-amplitude rest tremor, hypomimia, reduced arm swing, and cogwheel rigidity on synkinesis, were also present. He has subsequently become bradykinetic over the last 18 months.

Figure 3 shows PET scans of striatal ^{18}F-dopa uptake for a normal subject and a

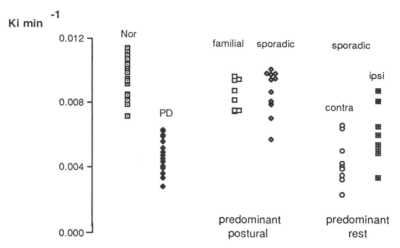

Figure 2   A column graph of mean putamen ^{18}F-dopa K_i values for the groups of tremor patients. Using t statistics, with Bonferroni's correction for multiple comparisons, only the rest tremor group show significantly reduced mean putamen ^{18}F-dopa uptake, being affected to a similar extent as the PD group.

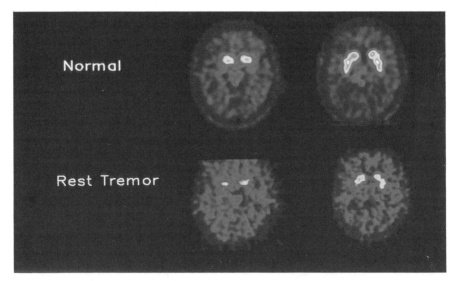

Figure 3   PET scans of striatal ^{18}F-dopa uptake for a normal subject and a patient with isolated rest tremor. It can be seen that putamen tracer uptake is severely reduced in the rest tremor subject, typical of PD.

patient with isolated rest tremor. It can be seen that putamen tracer uptake is severely reduced in the rest tremor subject. Figure 2 shows that in the ten patients with preponderant rest tremor, putamen ^{18}F-dopa K_i values contralateral to the more affected limbs were consistently below the normal range. Nine of ten contralateral, and eight out of ten ipsilateral, putamen K_i values fell in the parkinsonian range. Figure 4 is a column graph of mean putamen ^{18}F-dopa K_i values for the groups of tremor patients. From Bonferroni statistics, only the rest tremor group showed significantly reduced mean putamen ^{18}F-dopa uptake, being affected to an extent similar to the PD group.

Our findings argue against an association between essential tremor and Parkinson's disease. None of our eight patients with familial postural tremor, and only 1 of our 11 patients with sporadic postural tremor, showed reduced putamen ^{18}F-dopa uptake. Asymmetric tremor onset, the presence of low-amplitude tremor seated in repose, poor arm swing, and the presence of cogwheel rigidity on synkinesis, all were unreliable predictors of dysfunction of the nigrostriatal dopaminergic system. Only two subjects with postural tremor had poverty of facial expression, and one of these had abnormal putamen ^{18}F-dopa uptake.

All ten of our patients with predominant rest tremor showed abnormal ^{18}F-dopa uptake by one or both putamens. Nine of these subjects also had low-amplitude postural tremor, but only five had reduced arm swing, and only four had cogwheel rigidity on synkinesis. Interestingly, only four of these rest tremors were respon-

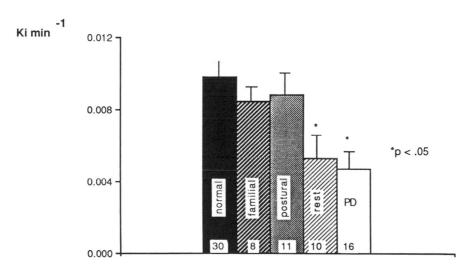

Figure 4 A diagram showing individual ^{18}F-dopa putamen influx constants for the 30 normal subjects, 16 patients with L-dopa responsive PD, and the groups of postural and rest tremor patients.

sive to levodopa. Currently we are unable to predict how many of these patients will develop a full parkinsonian syndrome with rigidity and akinesia. In eight of these patients, rest tremor had been present for only 1–5 years, but two patients had had tremor for 14 and 20 years, respectively, without evidence of bradykinesia. Our findings would support the concept of an entity of "tremulous parkinsonism," but its exact prognosis remains to be determined.

IV. CONCLUSIONS

In this chapter the ways in which PET can be used to demonstrate the abnormal patterns of cerebral activation associated with tremor, and how tremor relates to dysfunction of the nigrostriatal dopaminergic system, have been reviewed. Involuntary tremors, whether essential, neuropathic, or parkinsonian, appear to be associated with globally abnormal overactivity of the cerebellum. Isolated postural tremor is rarely associated with reduced putamen ^{18}F-dopa uptake, and soft signs of parkinsonism, such as reduced arm swing and cogwheel rigidity on synkinesis, are unreliable predictors of an underlying nigral disorder in patients with postural tremor. Isolated rest tremor appears to be consistently associated with nigral dysfunction. Currently, we are unable to predict how many patients with isolated rest tremor will go on to develop a full parkinsonian syndrome.

REFERENCES

1. Marsden CD. Origins of normal and pathological tremor. In: Movement Disorders: Tremor. Findley LJ, Capildeo R, eds. London: Macmillan, 1984:37–84.
2. Rautakorpi I, Takala J, Marttila RJ, Sievers K, Rinne UK. Essential tremor in a Finnish population. Acta Neurol Scand 1982; 66:58–67.
3. Herskovitz E, Blackwood W. Essential (familial, hereditary) tremor: a case report. J Neurol Neurosurg Psychiatry 1969; 32:509–511.
4. Larsen TA, Calne DB. Essential tremor. Clin Neuropharmacol 1983; 6:185–206.
5. Rajput AH, Rozdilsky B, Ang L, Rajput A. Clinicopathologic observations in essential tremor: report of six cases. Neurology 1991; 41:1422–1424.
6. Hirai T, Miyazaki M, Nakajima H, et al. The correlation between tremor characteristics and the volume of effective lesions in stereotaxic nucleus ventralis intermedius thalamotomy. Brain 1983; 106:1001–1018.
7. Young RR. Essential–familial tremor. In: Vinken PJ, Bruyn GW, Klawans HL, eds. Handbook of Clinical Neurology. Vol. 49. Amsterdam: Elsevier, 1986:565–581.
8. Dupuis MJM, Delwaide PJ, Boucquey D, et al. Homolateral disappearance of essential tremor after cerebellar stroke. Mov Disord 1989; 4:183–187.
9. Lamarre Y. Animal models of tremors. In: Findley LJ, Capildeo R, eds. Movement Disorders: Tremor. London: Macmillan, 1984:183–194.
10. Leigh PN, Jefferson D, Twomey A, Marsden CD. beta-Adrenoceptor mechanisms in essential tremor; a double-blind placebo-controlled trial of metoprolol, sotalol, and atenolol. J Neurol Neurosurg Psychiatry 1983; 46:710–715.

11. Lee RG, Stein RB. Resetting of tremor by mechanical perturbations: a comparison of essential tremor and parkinsonian tremor. Ann Neurol 1981; 10:523–531.

12. Marsden CD, Obeso J, Rothwell JC. Benign essential tremor is not a single entity. In: Yahr MD, ed. Current Concepts in Parkinson's Disease. Amsterdam: Excerpta Medica, 1983:31–46.

13. Smith IS, Kahn SN, Lacey BW, et al. Chronic demyelinating neuropathy associated with benign IgM paraproteinaemia. Brain 1983; 106:169–195.

14. Geraghty JJ, Jankovic J, Zetusky WJ. Association between essential tremor and Parkinson's disease. Ann Neurol 1985; 17:329–333.

15. Cleeves L, Findley LJ, Koller W. Lack of association between essential tremor and Parkinson's disease. Ann Neurol 1988; 24:23–26.

16. Lang AE, Kierans C, Blair RDG. Family history of tremor in Parkinson's disease compared with those of controls and patients with idiopathic dystonia. Adv Neurol 1987; 45:313–316.

17. Larochelle L, Bedard P, Poirier LJ, Sourkes TL. Correlative neuro-anatomical and neuropharmacological study of tremor and catatonia in the monkey. Neuropharmacology 1971; 10:273–288.

18. Poirier LJ, Sourkes TL, Bouvier G, Boucher R, Carabin S. Striatal amines, experimental tremor, and the effect of harmaline in the monkey. Brain 1966; 89:37–52.

19. Poirier LJ, Bouvier G, Bedard P, Boucher R, Larochelle L, Oliver A, Singh P. Essai sur les circuits neuronaux impliqués dans le tremblement postural et l'hypokinesie. Rev Neurol 1969; 120:15–40.

20. Lamarre Y, Joffroy AJ. Experimental tremor in monkey: activity of thalamic and precentral cortical neurons in the absence of peripheral feedback. Adv Neurol 1979; 24:109–122

21. Raichle ME. Circulatory and metabolic correlates of brain function in normal humans. In: Mountcastle VB, ed. Higher Functions of the Brain. Part 2. Handbook of Physiology Section 1, Vol 5. Bethesda: American Physiological Society 1987: 643–674.

22. Colebatch JG, Deiber MP, Passingham RE, Friston KJ, Frackowiak RSJ. Regional cerebral blood flow during voluntary arm and hand movements in human subjects. J Neurophysiol 1991; 65:1392–1401.

23. Deiber MP, Passingham RE, Colebatch JG, Friston KJ, Nixon PD, Frackowiak RSJ. Cortical areas and the selection of movement: a study with PET. Exp Brain Res 1991; 84:393–402.

24. Playford ED, Jenkins IH, Passingham RE, Nutt J, Frackowiak RSJ, Brooks DJ. Impaired mesial frontal and putamen activation in Parkinson's disease: a PET study. Ann Neurol 1992; 32:151–161.

25. Brooks DJ, Ibanez V, Sawle GV, et al. Differing patterns of striatal ^{18}F-dopa uptake in Parkinson's disease, multiple system atrophy, and progressive supranuclear palsy. Ann Neurol 1990; 28:647–655.

26. Calne DB, Langston WJ, Martin WRW, et al. Positron emission tomography after MPTP: observations relating to the cause of Parkinson's disease. Nature 1985; 317: 246–248.

27. Dubinsky R, Hallett M. Glucose hypermetabolism of the inferior olive in patients with essential tremor. Ann Neurol 1987; 22:118.

28. Colebatch JG, Findley LJ, Frackowiak RSJ, Marsden CD, Brooks DJ. Preliminary report: activation of the cerebellum in essential tremor. Lancet 1990; 336:1028–1030.

29. Brooks DJ, Jenkins IH, Baines P, Thompson PD, Findley LJ, Marsden CD. A comparison of the abnormal patterns of cerebral activation associated with neuropathic and essential tremor. Neurology 1992; 42(supp 3):423.

30. Liao K-K, Zeffiro T, Kertzman C, Hallett M. Regional cerebral blood flow abnormalities in essential tremor. Mov Dis 1992; 7(supp 1):46.

31. Parker F, Tzourio N, Blond S, Petit H, Mazoyer B. Evidence for a common network of brain structures involved in parkinsonian tremor and voluntary repetitive movement. Brain Res 1992; 584:11–17.

32. Brooks DJ, Salmon EP, Mathias CJ, et al. The relationship between locomotor disability, autonomic dysfunction, and the integrity of the striatal dopaminergic system in patients with multiple system atrophy, pure autonomic failure, and Parkinson's disease, studied with PET. Brain 1990; 113:1539–1552.

11

Analysis of Tremor Waveforms

David Buckwell and Michael A. Gresty
Institute of Neurology
National Hospital for Neurology and Neurosurgery
London, England

I. USES OF TREMOR WAVEFORM ANALYSIS

This chapter is concerned with the analysis of tremor waveforms. The first question that must be addressed is "what do we want from tremor waveform analysis?" There are several possibilities that include characteristics of the waveform, clues to possible mechanisms and to differential diagnosis, and methods of studying the relation between tremor and other phenomena, such as neurophysiological processes, and measurements, such as disability-rating scales.

First, tremor waveform analysis is aimed at establishing the physical trajectory characteristics of motion of the tremulous part of the body. This itself is a very complicated question and involves measurement of the amplitude of tremor and of the patterns of variation in amplitude; the frequency of the tremor and pattern variations therein; and the actual shape of the trajectory, whether it be a symmetric sine wave, as with much "essential tremor," or asymmetric, with distortions that, as we shall see, are characteristic of the resting tremor of Parkinson's disease.

Once we have achieved an adequate description of the physical characteristics of the tremor, and it is by no means evident that currently available techniques are capable of doing this, the next and more interesting question can be addressed, which is whether the results of our analysis of the tremor suggest the type of mechanism that may be responsible. Here an example may be given of what is meant by this possibility. If one, say, clamps a ruler to the edge of a bench so that it overhangs the edge and then taps the free end, the ruler will execute a series of oscillations that gradually die out. One can imagine the trajectory of the ruler's motion commencing with a step in the direction of the tap with a gradual return back to resting position superimposed on which will be sinusoidal oscillations. The equation of this type of motion can be written, by inspection, as the product of an exponential decay term and a sine wave. This type of equation is well known in physical systems and is referred to as a second-order differential equation. The exponential decay term of this equation describes the effect of the viscosity of the material from which the ruler is made on the motion. Its effect is generally to dampen down any movement. The sinusoidal term relates to the relation between the mass of the ruler and the elasticity of its material, and it is this relation that makes the ruler oscillate, much as a weight would bob up and down on the end of a piece of elastic. Thus, when we tap the end of the ruler, we stretch the elastic component of its material. This restores the position of the ruler, but its weight makes it overshoot that position and, in turn, causes a further elastic stretch that tends to restore the position, and so cycles of oscillation are set up. These cycles are subject to an overall dampening effect of the viscosity of the ruler so that they eventually die out. Thus, we see that recording the ruler's waveform motion allows us to write a mathematical description of its motion which, in turn, relates to physical entities that "explain" why the ruler is moving thus. The behavior of many simple mechanical, chemical, and electrical systems can be described by linear differential equations; consequently, if one can describe the behavior of any system with a linear differential equation, an important clue is obtained to the nature of the underlying mechanism. One should always have at the back of one's mind the notion that the system one is investigating is of indefinite complexity, and a particular phenomenon may be caused by an infinite number of possible mechanisms. However, in thankful evocation of the principle of parsimony, one is usually looking for a fairly obvious and simple one.

Even when dealing with fairly simple, and, in particular, second-order systems, the results of analysis can be equivocal. As an example highlighted later in this chapter, the task of distinguishing between the oscillation of a second-order system, subject to statistical variability in amplitude and frequency, and noise that is highly filtered so that it becomes of an almost "pure color," can present great difficulty. Their respective waveforms are similar, and the results of any analyses we have at our disposal for such waveforms can be similar.

Unfortunately, as soon as we move away from the realm of simple linear systems, the techniques of waveform analysis at our disposal rapidly lose potency. For more complex systems to which most, if not all tremors, almost certainly belong, there are no universally applicable techniques of waveform analysis that are powerful enough to identify the type of mechanism, or at least the describing equations, that are responsible for the waveform under study.

A third application of waveform analysis may be to distinguish between phenomena that are superficially similar. A prime example of this is afforded by the familiar clinical problem of distinguishing between essential tremor and tremor as an early manifestation of basal ganglia disease, when presented with a patient who has a postural tremor and minimal rigidity. We do not know if the postural tremor of Parkinson's disease has the same mechanism as essential tremor. They can look similar and their appearance on spectral analysis can be similar. However, if we possessed a technique of waveform analysis capable of reliably identifying systematic differences between known samples of the two types of tremor or, alternatively, of showing that they are ultimately indistinguishable, then one would be on the way to specifying underlying mechanisms and, possibly, of establishing an objective means of differential diagnosis.

The final use we may expect from techniques of waveform analysis of tremor concerns how tremor relates to other functions; on the one hand, to studies of underlying neurophysiological processes and, on the other hand, to questions of how tremor interacts with other movement and impairs and disables (1).

II. BASIC ASSUMPTIONS ON THE NATURE OF TREMOR

Before reviewing the techniques we have at our disposal for analyzing tremor waveforms, it may first be wise to consider our basic assumptions concerning the nature of tremor. Treatises on tremor usually commence with a definition along the lines of "tremor is a rhythmical oscillation of a part of the body . . ." (2,3). This definition is adequate in that encapsulates an essential ingredient on which most would agree, which is that tremulous movements appear to the human observer as having a certain periodicity that is relatively fixed and is not only apparently constant from second to second, but is also constant from hour to hour or day to day (4). Thus, an individual patient may be recognizably described as having a "fast, fine" postural tremor, whereas another would be described characteristically as having a "slow, coarse" tremor. The definition is inadequate in that many movements of the body are periodic, as in walking or running, breathing, or in the heart beat or as with voluntary movements such as writing and painting. One may say that surely it is self-evident that these movements are not tremulous and, yet, on closer investigation, it can be that, under certain circumstances, their respective mechanisms can display behavior that could be thought of as tremulous: for example, when the heart goes into fibrillation its motion is very much like the movement of a muscle in a tremulous limb. Indeed, the circumstances under which mechanisms of walking, heart beat, and so-forth may go wrong, give us insight into the possible nature of mechanisms underlying pathological tremor of the head, trunk, and limbs. However, we do not refer to the heart beat as tremor, and so limitations that, to some extent, may be arbitrary, are set upon the frequency range of phenomenon we are inclined to refer to as tremulous, and these are a lower cutoff at about 2 Hz and a higher cutoff at about 20 Hz, which is more or less the fusion rate of motor units (2,3). Within this frequency range, all phenomena we clinically refer to as tremor are distributed. At the lowest frequency, we have the tremor associated with truncal ataxia in multiple sclerosis and cerebellar disease at about 2–3.5 Hz. Between about 4 and 10 Hz, most of the essential tremors are distributed. The resting tremor of Parkinson's disease is in the region of 4–5.5 Hz, whereas the postural tremor of the hands may be 6–8 Hz. Enhanced physiological tremor is in the region of 8–13 Hz. Orthostatic tremor scores the highest frequency at about 16–18 Hz. Only the eye exhibits behavior that is exceptional to the tremors subsumed within this frequency band. Because of its unique muscular control and its inertial properties, tremor of the globe has been measured at frequencies ranging between about 2 Hz and in the region of 70 Hz (4). The higher frequencies of motion are referred to as ocular microtremor.

All our clinical experience informs us that, in a well-formed tremor of all these types, there is little variation in frequency under the same conditions of observation (5). For example, a distinct postural tremor of the hand in a patient with essential tremor will vary by only, say ±0.5 Hz. A tremor may shift frequency more significantly when the limb is undergoing a maneuver; thus, for example, an essential tremor of the hand that in posture is 4 Hz may shift up to 6 Hz when the hand grasps an object. This is a more complex matter and we do not know to what extent the action of grasping fundamentally changes the nature of the underlying tremor mechanism.

The only involuntary movements commonly referred to as a tremor that are not so easy to characterize with a single frequency and small-frequency deviation, are some tremors of the head which, although having an overall oscillatory appearance, are sufficiently irregular in amplitude and frequency to bring into question whether the term tremor is an appropriate label. Such movements may call into question the adequacy of our classification of involuntary movement disorders, and clearly, they may cross the boundaries between tremor and other phenomenon, such as dystonic tremors.

Because the constant feature of tremor is its frequency, much labor has been spent on characterizing various tremors in terms of their frequency and in attempting classification of tremors relative to frequency criteria. Frequency is probably of importance in terms of identifying the underlying mechanism of the tremor (6–11). For example, enhanced physiological tremor has a characteristic frequency that can be related to timing relations in the peripheral and spinal neuromuscular control of the limb. Similarly, "basal ganglia" and "rubral" type tremors may be attributable to rhythmic instability in thalamic neurons, causing repetitive discharges at a rate proportional to the tremor frequency. However, for many purposes, and particularly since frequency is so constant and identifiable, frequency is the least interesting or important aspect of the tremor. Factors provoking the suppression, enhancement, or release of the tremor; the absolute amplitude of tremor; and the impairment and disability that it may impart are, to both the clinician concerned with therapy and the patient concerned with his or her plight, more important measures of the tremulous movement than its frequency.

There is the considerable problem that amplitude fluctuations in tremor may follow highly complex patterns that are extremely difficult, or sometimes impossible, to analyze with the current state of knowledge of signal processing, and we will see that only for repetitive patterns of amplitude fluctuation, or amplitude fluctuations following a simple statistical distribution, are there adequate techniques for characterizing the amplitude variability. It is not surprising that characterization of tremor amplitude poses such difficulties, for whereas the frequency of the tremor may be determined by a fairly simple mechanism, for example, a local chemical instability at the level of a neuronal membrane, the ways this instability may be triggered, enhanced, or suppressed might be determined by the universe of physiological and external environmental factors. In other words, to understand tremor expression, one might have to understand the entire organism and its relation to the environment, and philosophical issues are raised over whether this could ever be achieved. The raising of quasiphilosophical issues, such as these, could be interpreted as overstressing the point; however, anyone who has taken recordings of the rest tremor of Parkinson's disease must have been impressed by the complex pattern of amplitude fluctuations it presents. Major fluctuations in amplitude occur that seem to be related to the "general state of arousal" of the subject. Other amplitude fluctuations seem to be determined by small adjustments in the precise attitude of the limb, whereas, within any short epoch of tremor, during which the condition of the subject and position of the limbs seem fairly constant, fluctuations in amplitude, occurring over a very different time scale of only a few seconds, may be seen that have no obvious correlation with any other observable features.

III. RECORDING TECHNIQUES

Before reviewing some of the techniques available for waveform analysis of tremor and the kind of results they can offer, it is opportune to consider the type of techniques we should be using to record tremor and the conditions under which the recordings should be made. Almost all movements of the above involve rotations about joints. The rotation should be transduced with an appropriate angular rate or by acceleration transducing; the trajectory of any part of the moving limb can be then reconstructed (on a computer) by summing the rotation about successive joints while taking the metrics of the individual segment lengths of forearm and finger phalanges and so-forth into account. The overall result would be something like an animated matchstick man model of body movement, similar to the animations with which we are familiar, or a structural dynamics model of an oil rig or airplane. Obviously, few practicing "tremorologists" actually do this form of analysis, partially because of its complexity, although appropriate systems are available from commercial companies, such as Solartron Shlumberger and

Hewlett Packard. In addition, it is extremely difficult to equip the body with a suitable assembly of transducers because of the size of current devices and their encumbrances of wiring. In practice, what is commonly done is to mount a single transducer, such as a linear accelerometer, on to the limb to record in the predominant plane of motion of the limb and to simplify the maneuver under which tremor is provoked. Although we may be forgiven for this simplification, the practice is hardly adequate to characterize tremor, because the complex reaching and grasping movements that are particularly provocative of tremor, for example, curling the fingers around and picking up a tea cup by the handle, involve extremely complicated movement trajectories, which we have hardly begun to investigate. This point is very important, as it is most frequently the interaction of the limb prone to tremor with the external environment in such acts as manipulation that is particularly provocative of tremor and that causes disability to the patient. There is a noticeable paucity of literature concerned with waveform analysis of tremor during such maneuvers; however, the exceptions are valuable source references (12–19).

A.   Which Recording Scenario to Use?

Almost all studies extant have examined simple resting or postural tremor. The exceptions quoted in the foregoing are notable. It is important and opportune that studies should be done to assess the particular features of interaction between the limb and the manipulandum that are particularly provocative of tremor and of the characteristics of the type of tremor provoked by manipulation. For example, picking up a cupful of tea will provoke disabling tremor in a subject prone to intention tremor; however, we know of no studies of what kind of tremor is provoked by this task. It is interesting that the particular physical characteristic of a cup of tea is that of an unstably balanced inertial load with relatively negligible viscous or elastic components. Accordingly, one may ask why an unstable load particularly provokes tremor, whereas weighting a limb with a stable load can suppress tremor. Is this because the motion of the load sets up certain conditions of sensory feedback that aggravate the tremulous process? In contrast, viscous dampening seems to suppress tremulous oscillations, and this feature is used in orthoses to assist violently tremulous patients in manipulating spoons for eating; the principle being to attach the limb to a jointed rod framework that follows the limb's motion and contains friction dampers at the joints so that the overall limb movement encounters viscous resistance. As with unstable inertial loading, elasticity exacerbates tremor. What happens to the tremor in a limb when these types of loading are encountered during a manipulation task is an open question for study, the answers of which will have implications for the nature of the tremogenic mechanism as well as for the factors that render patients disabled.

IV. ANALYSIS TECHNIQUES

A. Spectral Analysis

Because of the periodic nature of tremor, the preferred technique for condensing long time records of tremor waveform into a readily available single picture is spectral analysis (20). Several useful techniques for examining the relations between signals can be derived from spectra, which afford additional advantages (7). For reference, the results of spectral analysis on various types of tremor and the meaning of the shapes of the spectra resulting from analysis are shown in the Appendix. Here, we will restrict ourselves to some of the disadvantages in limitations of spectral analysis.

By a curious paradox, the spectrum that derives from spectral analysis of a time record of tremor is only interpretable with surety if one already has a fairly good idea of how the signal is composed in the first place. For example, if the frequency of the tremor varies with some statistical distribution about a certain central frequency, then the spectrum will show a peak at the central frequency with side bands above and below this peak, the shape of which is indicative of the statistical distribution of the frequency jitter. This frequency jitter could possibly be equally well observed by superimposing successively triggered cycles of tremor on the oscilloscope or by constructing a histogram of the instantaneous frequency, or the inverse, the period of the tremor. Similarly, fluctuations in tremor amplitude, which follow a recognizable distribution, can be identified either in the sidebands, on oscilloscope pictures, or in histograms of instantaneous amplitude. Likewise, if a tremor "spindles," that is waxes and wanes regularly in amplitude, the spectrum of the tremor will how a central peak with upper and lower sidebands separated from the main peak by the frequency of the spindling. For a 5-Hz tremor with amplitude fluctuations at cycles of 2 s, the spectrum will have a central peak at 5 Hz, with an upper sideband at 5.5 Hz, and a lower sideband at 4.5 Hz. The sidebands corresponding to the frequency of 0.5 Hz have a period of 2 s. Unfortunately, if the amplitude or frequency fluctuations of a tremor follow a complex pattern, then the structure of the sidebands will become uninterpretable and, eventually, if enough tremor spectra are averaged together, which is commonly the practice, they will merge into a statistical smear that may give the erroneous impression that amplitude and frequency fluctuations are statistically distributed, whereas, in fact, they may follow highly deterministic, but complicated patterns.

Looking on the brighter side of things, spectral analysis does retain the facility for being able to identify the presence of multiple stable frequencies within a complex signal. An accelerometer placed on the hand is quite sensitive enough to record not only the tremor of that limb, but also of any tremor passively transmitted from some other part of the body. The resulting raw signal may look rather irregular, but spectral analysis is capable of distinguishing therein separate tremor frequencies if they are present as a fairly constant feature through the recording, a task that would be impossible to perform by eye which, at best, can pick out only two concurrent frequencies within a signal and, even then, only in the absence of any significant noise level.

From the sensitivity of recording devices and the frequency-resolving power of spectral analysis derives an important technique for tremor analysis that is of value in determining the degree of relation between tremors in different parts of the body, or indeed between tremor and underlying neurophysiological recordings in the nervous system. This is the coherence (or coherency) function. The *coherence function* is the ratio of the product of the averaged power spectra of two signals to the average of the product of the individual power spectra from coincidental epochs of signal. At each frequency present in the spectra, the coherence may vary between a value of 0 and 1, depending on the degree to which the amplitudes of a particular frequency in the two spectra covary. If one amplitude increases or decreases and the other follows in a linear fashion, then the coherence value for this frequency will remain close to unity. As the amplitude of the frequency component in one spectrum varies independently of its amplitude in the other spectrum, the coherence will fall toward 0. If the spectral resolution is adequate and sufficient number of averages are taken, a high coherency value for a particular frequency indicates that the two signals at this frequency are highly related, and this is probably as close as we have to a test of causality, although it must be stressed that the direction of the causal relation is not indicated by the coherence function. Clearly, however, the application of this function has use in establishing the degree of relation between signals and of testing whether signals are truly related or have merely chance concurrence. Having said this, it is surprising that so few studies in the entire biomedical literature bother to establish a coherence relation between signals when studying the presumed input–output relations of a system.

B. Nonlinear Dynamic Analysis and Deterministic Versus Noisy Mechanisms

The interpretation of other forms of waveform analyses that can be applied to tremor, particularly of the newly appearing nonlinear analyses, which derive from so-called chaos theory, depend heavily on some prior intuitive understanding or guess about the nature of the process being studied and, at this stage, it is appropriate to try and make as clear a statement as possible about what sort of processes may contribute to tremor (21). For convenience, let us think of these as components that we may use in various combinations to construct a tremor. The first component we may use is an oscillator, which may be in the form of a simple second-order system, such as a feedback circuit on an analog computer, or a mechanical system, such as our ruler, or possibly some oscillatory instability in a neuronal membrane that approximates a sinusoidal process. In the absence of the application of external forces, the oscillations of these simple systems will vary in amplitude and frequency terms only at the statistical level of noise in the system. Thus, the second component we have to consider in building a model of tremor is to what extent noise or statistical variability is involved in the process. This may affect tremor frequency or tremor amplitude. The third type of block we may consider using in modeling tremor is a deterministic system that produces waveforms looking like sinusoidal oscillations, the amplitude or frequency of which may vary in an irregular or surprising manner and yet that overall maintains a certain identifiable characteristic. It is this type of process that is the subject of nonlinear dynamic analysis. The important characteristic is that the irregular or regular fluctuations in amplitude or frequency are determined by the equations of motion of the process and are not due to noise in the system. These are so-called chaotic processes. Despite their irregularities they maintain a general recognizable identity because of the presence of an attractor that maintains the process in an orbital pattern. When we recognize some similarity between the shape of the first couple of cycles of tremor we observe and the thousandth or hundred-thousandth cycles, we are really recognizing the characteristic of orbiting around the attractor of which examples are given in the Appendix.

Unfortunately, for practical purposes, making the distinction between noise in a signal and fluctuations because of an underlying nonlinear characteristic can be difficult, to say the least. To focus on this point a little more, consider the jitter in the timing of an action potential evoked from stimulating a neuron. The jitter could be due to noise in the underlying biochemical process, ultimately related to something like Brownian noise, or the statistical availability of transmitter substances; or, alternatively, could be due to the chaotic behavior of the underlying process. At this level, it is probably a bit of both, which makes the business of analysis even more difficult. However, at the level of whole-limb movement, noise may be not such an important factor. For example, the arm outstretched in the act of pointing can rotate through more than $180°$ from adduction to complete abduction. When held still to point at an object, the natural tremor of the hand, which could be considered as residual noise level, is perhaps of the order of $0.2°$. Therefore, the signal-to-noise level relative to the maximum possible amplitude of signal, is something like 1000:1; much less than the fluctuations one might expect in the timing jitter of an individual motor unit. Thus, on appearances, at the macroscopic level of behavior, noise in the nervous system is very well controlled.

The nature of noise in a biological system draws attention to a possible source of tremor that is notably missing from the literature of speculations on the nature of tremor mechanisms. As an alternative to tremor arising from an oscillatory process that is released (which may or may not have a nonlinear dynamical characteristic to render a noisy appearance), it is possible that tremor is generated through a massive release of noise in the system which becomes filtered into individual frequency bands.

In certain diseases, such as demyelination, one could easily envisage how disruption of normal signal processing in the nervous system gives rise to a pool of noise that channels through the motor system and is filtered into certain frequency bands by a combination of the filter properties of neuronal machinery through which signals pass, combined with mechanical filtering of efferent signals in "neuromuscular–sensory" motor loops. If the liberation and filtering of noise is not itself the immediate cause of tremor, the presence of noise can certainly be the cause of fluctuation in tremor characteristics. In direct contrast and as an example of the oscillator theory, consider the adrenergic enhancement of physiological tremor. The adrenergic enhancement improves the timing and efficiency of normal processes to the extent that they undergo cycles of self-activation. Think of this process in terms of a drug adjusting the parameters of an equation that describes some aspect of neuronal control of limb dynamics. The equations of motion are altered so that they describe an oscillation and, if the oscillation is irregular in certain ways, the equation is characteristic of a chaotic process. As with chaotic models of other physical systems, such as the atmosphere, very small adjustments to the terms of the equations of motion or small differences in initial conditions may lead to drastic changes in overall behavior. Our problem in analyzing tremor is that the appearances of narrow-bandwidth filtered noise and an oscillating chaotic process or a noisy linear oscillator are similar.

From clinical observation of tremor we may already derive an intuitive feel for what aspects of the tremulous process may be statistical in their variability and what may be chaotic. For example, some essential tremors maintain at fairly reliable frequencies and amplitudes over periods of several years. Their frequencies may change within or between recording sessions by only a fraction of a herz and their amplitudes may fluctuate in a random fashion, perhaps Gaussian, by 30%. It is quite easy to model the behavior of such tremors on an analog computer, using a noise source for frequency and amplitude modulation, and there is no reason why we should look to any more complicated model of this type of tremor. Such behavior is in marked contrast with that previously described for the resting tremor of Parkinson's disease, which may suddenly switch in or switch out, wax or wane in ways that are unfamiliar in terms of the statistical distributions we expect to encounter in biological processes. On the other hand, this type of behavior can be modeled by using fairly simple nonlinear equations, which persuades us, again through the principle of parsimony, to look to nonlinear dynamic analysis as a way of investigating these tremors. As an aside, this last point also raises the interesting question of just how deeply we should look into the nervous system to find an adequate explanation for the variability of tremor, for example, in Parkinson's disease. Often one has read, as earlier in this text, of referrals to high-level cognitive processes involving arousal and other more hypothetical psychological variables as an explanation for fluctuations in the tremor of Parkinson's disease and, indeed, of other motor features of the disorder. This may well be true, but it is interesting to consider that a very simple mechanism, perhaps a small group of neurons in the spinal cord or in the thalamus, could be responsible for abrupt and unpredictable fluctuations in behavior if the dynamics of their behavior are nonlinear. The only representation in a tremor of the "psychological state" of the individual may consist of a net energy input to these neuronal assemblies.

In the Appendix to this chapter we present the results of our own experience with applying currently available techniques of nonlinear dynamic analysis to tremor signals, together with comparative analyses of simulated signals of known composition. Because nonlinear analyses are so time-consuming, we have been unable to amass a comprehensive library of data on various types of tremor to see whether they show promise in characterizing the complexity and, therefore, possibly the type of process involved in tremor or of differentiating between different tremors as an aid to diagnosis. However, since the interpretation of the pictures that result from such types of analyses is to a large extent intuitive, the readers can make up their own minds from the "feel" they get from the examples given, as to whether they wish to pursue this avenue into the tangled pathways of tremor signals.

V. CONCLUSIONS

The dynamic analysis of the more simple rest tremor shows that the simulated tremor has an integral dimensionality, whereas the actual rest tremor has a fractional dimensionality characteristic of a nonlinear chaotic process. The simulated postural tremor still has an integer dimensionality, whereas the dynamic analysis of the actual postural tremor shows a trend to indefinitely increasing dimensionality characteristic of noise, with no clear indication of an asymptote to suggest a definite measurement of dimensionality.

Thus, on the one hand, the nonlinear analysis has told us that the rest tremor in the patient studied is a chaotic process and, therefore, different in nature from the simulation. However, it has failed to reveal more of the nature of the postural tremor signal relative to the extent to which linear or nonlinear oscillators and noise are involved in the tremor signal than was already known by inspection of the raw signal. This is a pertinent example of the inability of present analytic techniques to distinguish narrow band noise from nonlinear signal, which is so often the problem with the type of signals encountered in clinical neurology.

APPENDIX

Comparison of spectral analysis and nonlinear dynamic analysis on simulated and actual tremor waveforms (Figs. 1–4).

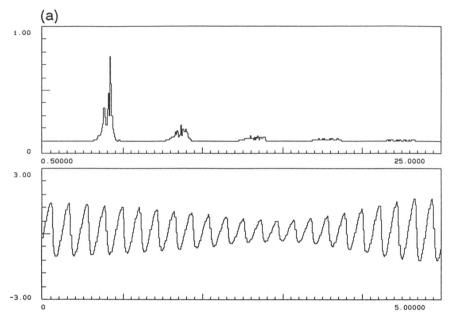

Figure 1 (a) Spectral analysis of the results of an analog computer simulation of an amplitude- and frequency-modulated, skewed sinusoidal signal made to resemble the typical appearance of the resting tremor of Parkinson's disease. This example illustrates all the features commonly seen in tremor spectra, but has the advantage that we know the constituent components beforehand and so can interpret the spectrum with confidence. The construction of this simulation commenced with a 5-Hz signal, which was skewed to generate asymmetry. The asymmetry is termed *harmonic distortion* and is shown by the harmonic components at ×2, ×3, ×4, and so-forth, of the fundamental frequency. The frequency was made to vary through a frequency multiplier to produce an approximately Gaussian jitter between limits of approx ±0.5 Hz. The amplitude of the signal was modulated by a noise source with similar Gaussian characteristics to vary between approximately 10 and 100% of full-signal strength. The combined amplitude and frequency modulation produces sidebands that are evident in the spreading out of the main peak of the spectrum (termed the *carrier frequency*). In this case, when frequency increased slightly through jitter, the amplitude was made to decrease, whereas when frequency decreased, the amplitude increased. This relation produces sidebands that are of greater magnitude at frequencies below the carrier. If the waveform amplitude was made to vary in proportion to frequency, the sidebands would be preponderantly at frequencies above the carrier. If frequency and amplitude modulation were independent, the sidebands would be equally distributed about the carrier and, by chance, there could be interaction between those due to frequency and those due to amplitude modulations. (b) Phase plane representation of the simulated rest tremor. This is a two-dimensional view of a three-dimensional trajectory. It is obtained by plotting the signal against itself (*x/y*-axes) lagged by a number of samples (five in this instance) and against itself again (*x/y/z*-axes) lagged by double this number of samples. The trajectory is a complex toroidal orbit around a single attractor. These trajectories can be constructed for any number of "embedding" dimensions (i.e., *x,y,z,p,q,r* . . .), although only three can be plotted in the phase plane. (c) Dynamic analysis of the simulated rest tremor. The analysis attempts to identify the value (integer or

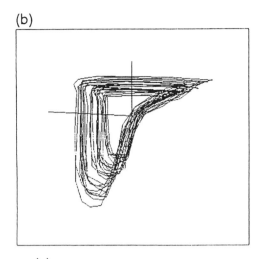

(c)

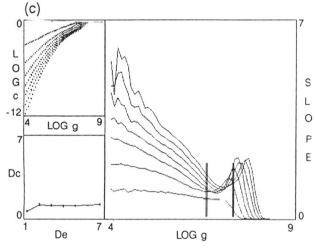

noninteger) of the correlation dimension (slope, Dc) of the time series. The correlation dimension is an indication of how completely the sample points of the signal fill space. Chaotic processes will have a noninteger dimensionality. Central to this method of analysis (22) is the scale length (g). Long scale lengths mask the signal fluctuations, and scale lengths that are too short are oversensitive to high-frequency noise in the signal. Thus, the scale length is appropriate to the frequency content of the signal. The factor g is determined experimentally to reveal a possible scaling region in the plot of the correlation dimension (slope and Dc) against scale lengths for various embedding dimensions. The scaling region is indicated by the parallel vertical bars. Each curve is the data analyzed for a different embedding dimension. For the analysis shown, seven dimensions were calculated that experimentally gave the most suitable scaling region. The correlation integral ($\log c$) is derived by computing the distances between all points in the time series and evaluating what fraction is less than a series of predetermined scale lengths. The plot of dimensionality against embedding dimensions shows an asymptote at a dimensionality of 0.95 showing a strong trend to an integer dimensionality of 1.0 and, therefore, not a chaotic process.

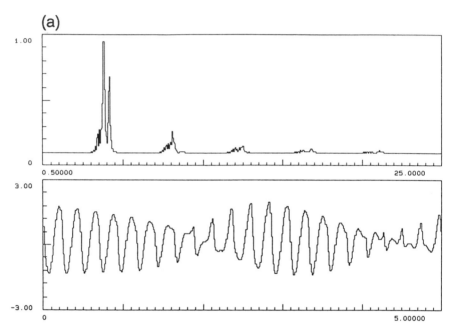

Figure 2 (a) Spectrum of an analog computer simulation of an amplitude- and frequency-modulated, skewed sinusoidal signal added to a nonskewed amplitude- and frequency-modulated signal made to resemble the appearance of complex postural tremor that is occasionally seen in Parkinson's disease. It has been suggested that such complex tremor is due to a combination of two independent tremors, represented here by the peaks occurring at 3.6 and 4.4 Hz. The harmonics are the distortion of the signal at 3.6 Hz. (b) Phase plane representation of the simulated postural tremor. (c) Dynamical analysis of the simulated postural tremor. The plot of dimensionality against embedding dimensions shows an asymptote at a dimensionality of 2.99, indicating an integer dimensionality and, therefore, not a chaotic process.

(b)

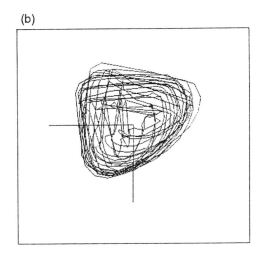

(c)

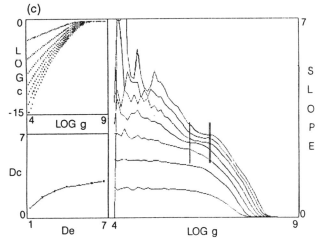

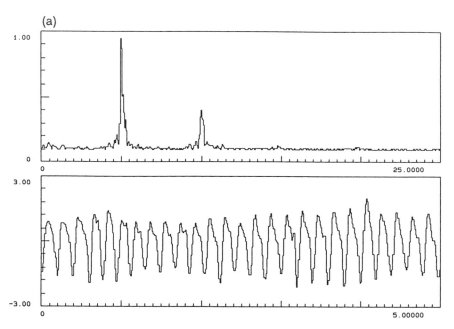

Figure 3   (a) Spectral analysis of typical rest tremor of the pronated outstretched hand in a
patient with Parkinson's disease. (b) Phase plane representation of the rest tremor. (c)
Dynamic analysis of the rest tremor. The plot of dimensionality against embedding
dimensions asymptotes as 1.76 with a 0 confidence interval, indicating a fractional
dimensionality and, therefore, possibly a chaotic process.

(b)

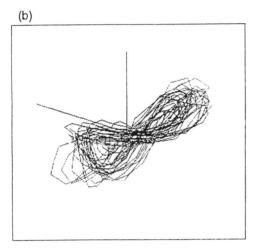

(c)

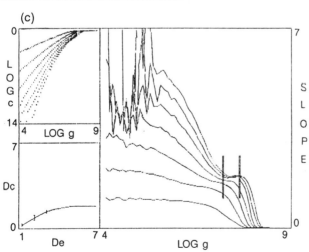

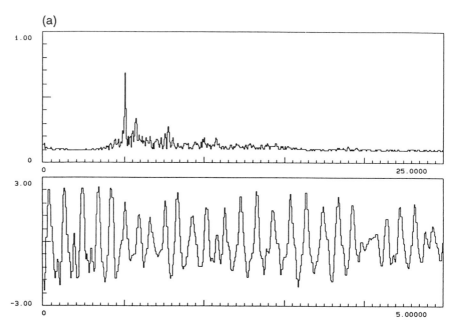

Figure 4   (a) Spectral analysis of complex postural tremor in the same patient whose rest tremor is shown in Figure 3. Note the presence of a dominant peak frequency at 5.0 Hz, with multiple upper sidebands between 5.3 and 11.0 Hz. (b) Phase plane representation of the postural tremor. (c) Dynamic analysis of the postural tremor. The plot of dimensionality against embedding dimension fails to show a trend to asymptote, indicating a process of high dimensionality suggestive of a chaotic process or a high noise content.

(b)

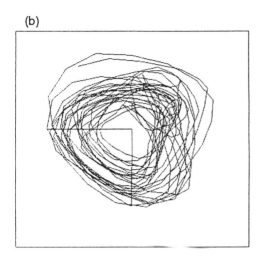

(c)

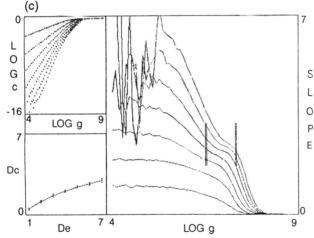

REFERENCES

1. Gath I, Yair E. Analysis of vocal tract parameters in parkinsonian speech. J Acoust Soc Am 1988; 84:1628–1634.
2. Fine EF, Soria ED, Paroski MW. Tremor studies in 1986 through 1989. Arch Neurol 1990; 47:337–340.
3. Gillespie MM. Tremor. J Neurosci Nurs 1991; 23:170–174.
4. Coakley D. Minute Eye Movement and Brainstem Function. Boca Raton: CRC Press Inc, 1983.

5. Hunker CJ, Abbs JH. Uniform frequency of parkinsonian resting tremor in the lips, jaw, tongue, and index finger. Mov Disord 1990; 5:71–77.

6. Ohye C, Shibazaki T, Hirai T, et al. A special role of the parvocellular red nucleus in lesion induced spontaneous tremor in monkeys. Behav Brain Res 1988; 28:241–243.

7. Lenz FA, Tasker RR, Kwan CH, et al. Single unit analysis of the human ventral thalamic nuclear group: correlation of thalamic "tremor cells" with the 3–6Hz component of parkinsonian tremor. J Neurosci 1988; 8:754–764.

8. Raeva SN. Unit activity of the human thalamus during voluntary movements. Stereotact Funct Neurosurg 1990; 54–55:154–158.

9. Jones MW, Tasker RR. The relationship of documented destruction of specific cell types to complications and effectiveness in thalamotomy for tremor in Parkinson's disease. Stereotact Funct Neurosurg 1990; 54–55:207–211.

10. Ohye C, Shibazaki T, Hirato M, Kawashima Y, Matsumura M. Strategy of selective Vim thalamotomy guided by microrecording. Stereotact Funct Neurosurg 1990; 54–55:186–191.

11. Raeva S, Lukashev A, Lashin A. Unit activity in human thalamic reticularis nucleus. I. Spontaneous activity. Electroencephalogr Clin Neurophysiol 1991; 79:133–140.

12. Lebedeva NN, Avakian GN, Sidorova OP. Visual motor co-ordination and its clinical significance. Zh Nevropatol Psikhiatr 1988; 88:19–22.

13. Hacisalihzade SS, Albani C, Mansour M. Measuring parkinsonian symptoms with a tracking device. Comput Methods Programs Biomed 1988; 27:257–268.

14. Sanes JN, Lewitt PA, Mauritz K-H. Visual and mechanical control of postural and kinetic tremor in cerebellar system disorders. J Neurol Neurosurg Psychiatry 1988; 51:934–943.

15. Cole JD, Philip HI, Sedgwick EM. The effect of fronto-parietal lesions on stability and tremor in the finger. J Neurol Neurosurg Psychiatry 1988; 51:1411–1419.

16. Cole JD, Philip HI, Sedgwick EM. Stability and tremor in the fingers associated with hemisphere and cerebellar tract lesions in man. J Neurol Neurosurg Psychiatry 1988; 51:1558–1568.

17. Elble RJ, Moody C, Higgins C. Primary writing tremor. A form of focal dystonia? Mov Disord 1990; 5:118–126.

18. Elble RJ, Sinha R, Higgins C. Quantification of tremor with a digitizing tablet. J Neurosci Methods 1990; 32:193–198.

19. Hore J, Wild B, Diener HC. Cerebellar dysmetria at the elbow, wrist and fingers. J Neurophysiol 1991; 65:563–571.

20. Gresty M, Buckwell D. Spectral analysis of tremor: understanding the results. J Neurol Neurosurg Psychiatry 1990; 53:976–981.

21. Deshmukh VD. A chain of suprasegmental neuro-oscillatory circuits: a human brain theory. Clin Electroencephalogr 1988; 19:7–13.

22. Grassberger P, Procaccia I. Measuring the strangeness of strange attractors. Physica 1983; 9D:189–208.

12

Is Essential Tremor Physiological?

Martin Lakie
University of Birmingham
Birmingham, England

I. INTRODUCTION

Tremor, defined as a rapid, involuntary rhythmic oscillation of a body segment, is ubiquitous; we all shake a little all of the time. We are not normally aware of this oscillation in our own bodies, and we cannot normally see it in the bodies of others, but it may come to our attention on occasion, as any apprehensive lecturer who has used a hand-held optical pointer in front of a critical audience will testify. similarly, musicians and others, faced with the stress of a public performance, may have recourse to drugs that reduce tremor.

Some persons have a tremor that is much larger; it may be readily observed by themselves and by others. It may cause them social embarrassment and interfere with their occupation. These people may seek medical advice and, in the absence of other symptoms, they will be told they have essential tremor. In some patients questioning will reveal that they have a family history of tremor. In the absence of any documented medical history, such hearsay evidence must be treated with some circumspection. With this caveat, 30–50% of cases may have a familial link. Nearly all the patients who suffer from this condition will already be aware that the symptoms are worsened by stress, and ameliorated to some degree by alcohol, although many report that the use of alcohol is associated with an unpleasant rebound. This probably materially decreases the risk of alcohol dependence. The incidence of the condition is difficult to estimate; in one United State study, there were 37 cases in a population of about 9000 people aged over 40 (1). Other studies have suggested a higher incidence, similar to that of Parkinson's disease.

It has been known for some time that there are probably two forms of the disease, which may be clinically rather easily confused (2). One form may represent little more than an enhanced physiological tremor, whereas, in the other form of essential tremor, the frequency is unusually low, and the movement very large. This "classic" form may involve abnormal movements of the neck or jaw.

As there are thought to be no other symptoms or diagnostic signs, essential tremor must be defined rather loosely as an abnormally large tremor. The question naturally arises of what exactly constitutes a normal (physiological) tremor. Are people with essential tremor simply representatives of one extreme of a whole range of normal tremors, or are they a separate subgroup of the population? The question is muddied by the occurrence of other pathological tremors and the associated difficulties of making a definite diagnosis of essential tremor. It has been said that tremor is easy to record, but difficult to interpret; there have been at least four recent studies of tremor in the population (3–6), but these have all been principally concerned with the effects of aging. A large-scale survey of tremor in the general population is described here; the results are compared with those from a small group of essential tremor patients.

The tremor of numerous subjects has been recorded and subjected to a comprehensive analysis. In making measurements of tremor, it has become customary to record movement of the fingers. There is, however, some ambiguity in the literature about what is meant by finger tremor. The contribution to the tremor of different parts of the body is sometimes uncertain, as the point of support of the upper limb is not always made clear. Here we have made two types of measurement. In both, tremor is recorded from the tip of the middle finger; the fingers are held horizontally and slightly abducted. When we record wrist tremor the hand is unsupported and the forearm rests on a padded support and is restrained by strapping, whereas when we record finger tremor the hand is additionally supported by a block shaped to fit the palmar surface and only the fingers are unsupported. In both situations, the resulting tremor would be classified as a modified postural type. On every occasion, tremor was recorded on both sides of the body at the same time.

II. SUBJECTS

A. Normal Subjects

Subjects are arbitrarily arbitrarily chosen from members of academic and medical staff of universities and hospitals, children from two schools, students, and members of various social and sporting clubs. We aimed only to preserve an approximate balance between the sexes. The subjects were not selected in any other sense; a consequence of this was that we had a larger number of subjects in the younger-aged groups (between 11 and 30). The distribution of numbers in each aged group is shown in Figure 1.

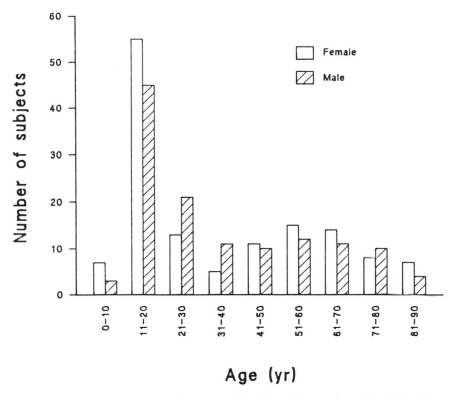

Figure 1 The age distribution of the normal subjects. Twenty-nine of the 245 subjects were left-handed; 118 were male.

This group is reasonably representative of the community. No form of medical screening was carried out; as many of the subjects who were investigated were active members of clubs, we assume that their general health was at least as good as the norm. In all, there were 245 persons in the survey.

B. Patients With Essential Tremor

Eleven patients with essential tremor were studied by the same method. These patients were chosen by a clinician on the basis of having well-established essential tremor. Their ages ranged from 21 to 81, and they had a history of tremor that ranged from 2 to 45 years. Nine were men, and five reported a family history (see Table 1 for details). All patients were asked to refrain from any tremor-related medication for 24 h before the investigation. This is a relatively small number of patients, but the main intention underlying the present study was not to investigate the condition itself, but to relate it to tremor levels prevailing in the general population. The investigation was carried out at Dundee Royal Infirmary; the permission of the hospital ethical committee was obtained.

III. METHODS

Tremor, in common with any other periodic oscillation, can be adequately described by decomposing the waveform into its frequency components and determining the size of each component. In principle, the size can be expressed in terms of amplitude, velocity, or acceleration. At resonance, all of these quantities are proportional to force, but in a nonresonant system, acceleration has the advantage that it most closely reflects the force generated by the muscles. It also emphasizes the higher-frequency components of the tremor. In all the investigations, the instrument used to record tremor was a solid-state strain-gauge accelerometer (ICS 3021) that was mounted on a light plastic plate attached to the middle finger by a Velcro strap. The whole device weighed less than 3 g and loaded the finger to a very small degree. Flying leads connected each transducer to an amplifier. Recordings were made simultaneously on both sides. The signals were amplified and low-pass filtered; the -3-dB point was 38 Hz. The resulting signals were digitized (CED 1401 interface) and stored on disk. Subsequently, Fourier analysis was used to extract three parameters: the peak frequency of the tremor, the size of the acceleration at the peak, and the mean acceleration level in each of nine bands of about 1.5-Hz width, ranging from 3.0 to 15.5 Hz. This latter procedure reduced the tremor on each side to nine numbers and expedited statistical analysis. To ensure that Fourier analysis produced a result that represented the entire recording period, the record was divided into 30 overlapping slices that were individually analyzed; the averaged result was then calculated and displayed. This meant that the effect of any minor external perturbation was minimized. In fact, analysis of serial samples of the signal revealed that there was little real variability throughout the recording period (Fig. 2).

The measurements were carried out in a variety of places, but care was taken to ensure that the rooms used were warm and quiet, and empty of persons other than the subject and the investigators. The procedure that was used was to ask the subject to extend the fingers of both hands, with the fingers slightly separated, using minimal force; 5 s later recording was started. The duration of recording period was 80 s. Two consecutive recordings were made of wrist and finger tremor; the first ones were discarded. Thus, the novelty of the situation could be largely discounted.

This method was compared with the tremorometric method used by Walsh et al. (see Chapter 5). We compared the results for finger and wrist tremor of 24 subjects, using both methods. In both cases the acceleration at the frequency peak was used as a measure of tremor. For finger tremor, the correlation coefficient was 0.67 for the broad-band tremorometer and 0.91 for the narrow-band instrument. For

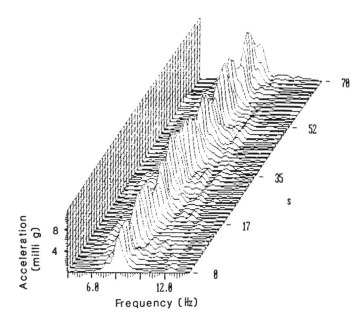

Figure 2 The frequency spectrum of a typical wrist tremor. Here, 50 overlapping segments of the record (lasting a total of 80 s) have been analyzed. There is some variation in acceleration, but very little variation in frequency. This is in good agreement with another study of hand tremor (10).

wrist tremor, the corresponding values were 0.61 and 0.84. The two methods, therefore, can be considered complementary; the tremorometer gave a fairly quick determination of the total tremor activity, and the computer analysis additionally permitted the calculation of the peak frequency and amplitude, and the construction of "average" tremor spectra. As the correlation coefficients were similar for wrist and finger tremor, either will provide a satisfactory measure of tremulousness.

Tremor is here expressed in "mg" where g is the acceleration due to gravity. One mg is essentially the same as one $cm\,s^{-1}\,s^{-1}$.

IV. RESULTS

A. The Composition of Normal Wrist Tremor

1. Frequency

Physiological tremor is often said to have a frequency peak between 8 and 12 Hz (7). From the present data, it appears that both these limits may be a little high.

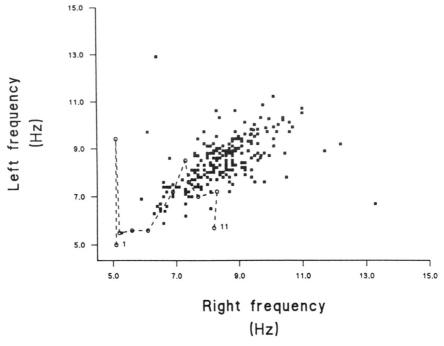

Figure 3 The peak frequency of tremor. Normal subjects (shown by squares) have frequencies that usually fall between 7 and 11 Hz and are broadly similar on both sides. There are exceptions (details in text). Patients with essential tremor are indicated by circles, the dotted line runs consecutively from patient 1 to 11.

Figure 3 shows the peak frequency of the tremor in left and right wrists; 216 of the subjects (88%) had a frequency between 7 and 11 Hz on both sides. This is in complete agreement with the values reported by Findley and Gresty (8). Every subject had a clearly defined peak.

Only seven subjects had a frequency greater than 11 Hz on either side. The significance of this is unknown. The frequencies on both sides were usually quite well matched (r value for left against right = 0.54), the obvious exceptions to this rule were elderly. There were 25 subjects who had a frequency of less than 7 Hz on either side; there was a striking relation with age. 10 of these 25 were older than 70, 8 were in their 60s, and 4 were in their 50s. Of the remaining 3, 1 was a man of 25 with a frequency of 6.7 on the right side, and the other 2 were girls of 12, 1 with a bilateral tremor at 6.3 Hz and the other with a left had 6.8-Hz tremor. These three are clearly exceptional; frequencies of less than 7 Hz are extremely rare in young subjects.

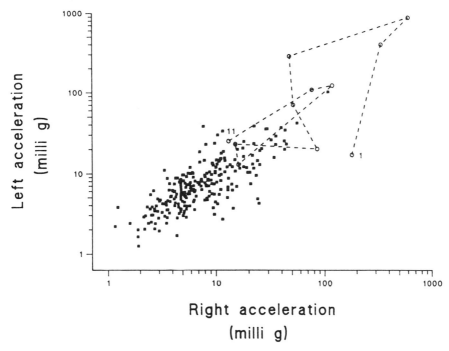

Figure 4 The peak acceleration of tremor. Normal subjects are indicated by squares. There is a large range (about 2 log units). There is little obvious difference between left and right wrists, but, as in Figure 3, considerable overlap with the normal subjects is obvious.

2. Tremor Level

It was obvious from an early stage that some normal individuals had much more tremor than others; the total range was about 100, or 2 log units (Fig. 4).

The same range was evident if the peak amplitudes or the total power of the spectrum was used as a measure. There was no obvious difference between left and right sides (r value of left against right = 0.83). Careful analysis of the pooled spectral data showed that, on average, persons had slightly more tremor on the right side (Fig. 5).

This difference was just significant in some of the bands. Surprisingly, this was also true of left-handed subjects (29 persons). The reason for this slight excess of tremor on the right side is unclear, but it may be that the ballistocardiogram is unexpectedly better transmitted to the right side of the body. Tremor contains a component that is related to the cardiac cycle (9), probably arising in part from transmitted thrust and in part from arterial pulsation. In some subjects tremor could be seen; the degree to which tremor is visible is probably dictated by the

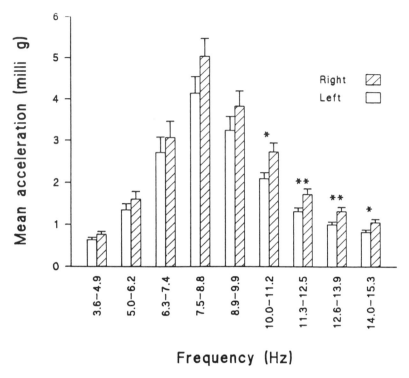

Figure 5 The right wrist was generally slightly more tremulous. The mean tremor levels in each of nine frequency bands have been calculated to produce an "average" tremor spectrum for each hand. The difference was significant in some bands (* $p < 0.05$, ** $p < 0.01$). The reason is not known. Curiously, left-handed subjects also had more tremor on the right side, and were also slightly, but significantly, less tremulous on both sides than right-handers.

amplitude of the oscillation, which is related to both acceleration and frequency. For subjects with a preponderant tremor rhythm at 10 Hz, movement is visible on close inspection at about 16 mg. At this frequency, the amplitude of displacement (using the formula for a sinusoidal oscillation, where f is frequency, x is displacement, and a is acceleration)

$$a = 4n^2 f^2 x$$

is about 40 μm. Lower-frequency tremors will be conspicuous at a lower acceleration level; an amplitude of 40 μm at 5 Hz corresponds to an acceleration of only 4 mg. For a given value of acceleration, tremor will be much more visible if it occurs at a low frequency. Forty-four of the normal subjects (18%) had tremor that was large enough to be readily visible.

Naturally, tremor amplitude in any one individual varies somewhat from day to day and from minute to minute; we made daily recordings of tremor in five subjects for 2 weeks; the maximum variation was a factor of 2.7. Thus, the intersubject variability is much greater than normal variation in any one subject. In a study of long-term variability of tremor, it has been shown that frequency is remarkably stable for periods up to 100 min (10). That study also revealed a variation in peak tremor power of about ninefold; this corresponds to a variation in peak acceleration of threefold. The agreement is close. Under unusual circumstances (e.g., emotional upsets), the variation may be greater than this; in recordings (unpublished) during which subjects are infused with epinephrine or insulin, we have observed increases in tremor greater than fivefold. We made no attempt to determine if there was a diurnal variation. One of the principal determinants of tremor level is limb temperature (11), and it would be very difficult to separate diurnal and temperature-related effects.

3. Age

There are several investigations suggesting that tremors become slower as persons age (3–6). There is also a belief that elderly persons shake more, but the evidence for this is less clear. Both of these claims were investigated. Figure 6 shows the peak frequency and peak amplitudes of tremor plotted against the age of the subjects.

The regression lines indicate that, on average, the oldest subjects have a peak frequency that is about 1 Hz less than the youngest, and also that, on average, they have about a doubling of acceleration at the peak. The combination of a decreased frequency and an increased acceleration will correspond to a considerably increased tremor amplitude (see foregoing). There is considerable scatter, and the coefficients of determinance (r^2) for frequency and acceleration are, on average, only 12 and 7%, respectively. Nonetheless, the effect seems to be real; the regression lines for left and right hands are practically identical. Close examination of Figure 6, and the use of a "best-fit" curve, suggest that the changes may not start until the fourth or fifth decade. There was no suggestion (see Ref. 3) that the frequency in children was slower than in young adults. There are two ways of interpreting these data. Either tremor generally slows and increases in size as persons age or, alternatively, some persons develop a large-amplitude, slow tremor rather abruptly, and the incidence of this condition increases with age. Without a longitudinal study it is impossible to say which of these hypotheses is correct. The wide range of acceleration levels and the asymmetric frequencies in older subjects may support the second theory; that is, the age-related development of an abnormal low-frequency, large-amplitude tremor in some subjects. The incidence of Parkinson's disease, for example, increases steeply with age, and the first sign of this is commonly a pathological tremor.

4. Sex

Analysis of an age-matched group of men and women revealed that the men generally had slightly more tremor than the women. The difference in acceleration, however, was not significant (Fig. 7).

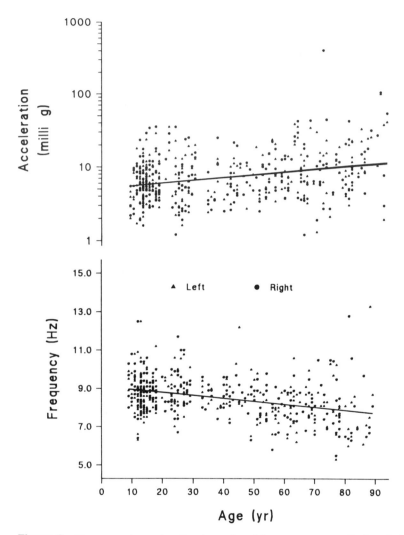

Figure 6 Tremor peak acceleration (upper) and frequency vs age. Left and right wrists are included. There is a tendency for tremor to slow and increase in size in older subjects. The regression lines are shown; they are virtually identical for left and right wrists. There is considerable scatter, particularly in size, this becomes even larger with older subjects.

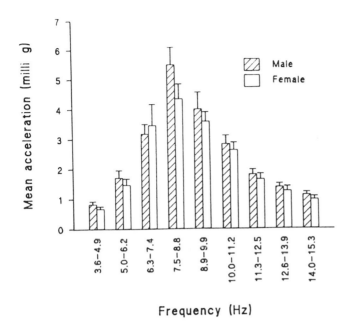

Figure 7 Mean tremor levels (as in Fig. 5) for men and women. The results include values from left and right wrists. Because of constraints of age-matching, these data were obtained from 126 age-matched subjects only. The men are generally slightly more tremulous than the women, for explanation see text.

The median peak frequencies for men and women were calculated. The men had a lower peak frequency (7.8 Hz as opposed to 8.6 Hz, $p < 0.01$). Both of these sex differences can probably be explained by the larger size of the male hand. The inertia of the larger hand and muscles is greater, and the resonant frequency is, consequently, less. As the length of the hand is greater, the resultant acceleration at the fingertip, where it is measured, is bigger. This is a consequence of employing a linear measure of an angular quantity. Thus, it appears that there is probably no fundamental difference in tremor in men and women. However, the amplitude of tremor in men will be generally larger than that in women, as the mean frequency is less.

B. Normal Finger Tremor

The results when finger tremor was recorded were qualitatively similar to those from the wrist. Thus there was the same general variability in amplitude and a tendency for amplitude to increase with age. Left and right tremor was again quite well matched in younger subjects. The frequency spectrum, however, was considerably different. The most significant finding was that the spectrum of pure finger tremor was usually bimodal, with one peak at 7–11 Hz and a second peak at 15–25 Hz (Fig. 8).

It was never certain which peak would be larger; sometimes consecutive recordings from a single subject would be different. Thus, there are two components in finger tremor of variable preponderance. There are different possible explanations for this. It may be that the higher-frequency peak is a harmonic of the first. Alternatively, the higher-frequency peak may be caused by a mechanical resonance. The resonant frequency of the relaxed finger when it is horizontally supported is about 12–18 Hz (12); when it is actively extended in a vertical plane, the resonant frequency will be higher (13). The high frequency may represent the mechanical resonance of the finger, and the lower frequency may represent the direct input of the motor units; many of which will be active at 7–11 Hz for these relatively trivial efforts. It is worth emphasizing that if tremor was recorded by a velocity-sensitive technique, the higher-frequency peak would have been reduced in size relative to the lower; and if a displacement-sensitive technique was used, the higher-frequency peak would have been almost invisible.

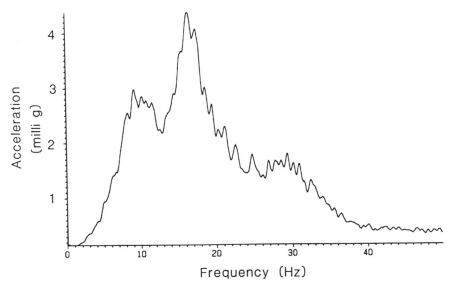

Figure 8 A typical spectrum of finger tremor. There are two peaks: one at 9 Hz probably represents the neural component and the one at 17.5 Hz is a mechanical resonance. In any individual spectrum, either peak may predominate. This is very different from the spectrum of wrist tremor (see Fig. 2).

Table 1 Patients With Essential Tremor[a]

Patient no.	Age (yr)	Sex	Family history	Duration (yr)	Left frequency (Hz)	Right frequency (Hz)	Left acceleration	Right acceleration (mg)
1	65	M	MAT	8	5.0	5.1	17	179
2	70	M	NO	45	9.4	5.1	398	332
3	34	F	NO	13	5.5	5.2	877	597
4	81	F	NO	14	5.6	5.6	283	47
5	62	M	NO	11	5.6	6.1	70	51
6	58	M	NO	2	7.2	6.9	20	85
7	46	M	MAT	30	8.5	7.3	23	15
8	57	M	PAT	10	7.6	7.4	13	16
9	21	M	MAT	19	7.0	7.7	122	117
10	29	M	MAT	3	7.2	8.3	108	76
11	62	M	NO	10	5.7	8.2	25	13

[a]Each patient has been indentified by a number (1–11) that is also used in Figures 3 and 4. Patients 6–10 inclusive have a tremor that is indistinguishable, on the basis of frequency or amplitude, from many of the normal subjects. They were also the patients most closely associated with a family history of tremor (MAT, maternal; PAT, paternal).

C. Patients With Essential Tremor

The peak frequencies and amplitudes of the 11 patients are summarized in Table 1. Their relation to the normal population can be seen at a glance, as these points have also been inserted in Figures 3 and 4. Five of the patients had tremor frequencies that fell within the normal range (7–11 Hz); their tremor amplitude, although large, considerably overlapped the range of the normal subjects. Their tremor apparently represents no more than an exaggerated physiological tremor; they represent one extreme of a distribution of tremor amplitudes. The remainder of the patients are different. Their tremor frequencies are unusually low, sometimes on both sides, but also commonly on only one side. Their peak accelerations are also high. This combination corresponds to a tremor with a very large amplitude. They do seem to represent a genuinely abnormal group. One interesting observation was that they did not show peaks in the frequency spectrum harmonically related to the main peak. The situation is very different in parkinsonian tremor, for which the peak frequency, although similar, is usually accompanied by harmonic overtones. It may be that the tremor of essential tremor patients is more sinusoidal in nature; a suggestion confirmed by inspection of the raw tremor traces.

V. DISCUSSION

A. Tremor Frequency

The frequency of physiological tremor falls in a fairly narrow band (7–11 Hz). We have previously suggested that one of the main determinants of the frequency is the resonant properties of the wrist, which are determined by the elasticity of the tissues (muscle and tendon) and the inertia of the moving parts (14). The shape of the spectrum for wrist tremor certainly suggests an underdampened resonant system. It is this relatively sharp tuning that justifies describing a single frequency peak and referring to a tremor rate. The "drive" to this resonant system is in the form of low-frequency impulses from the imperfectly fused contraction of motor units. There is, therefore, a component of the tremor spectrum that is determined by the mechanical properties of the limb, and a component that is determined by the firing rate of motoneurons. When these two frequencies coincide, the amplitude of the tremor will be very large (in engineering terms, a large magnification factor); if they are mismatched, the amplitude will be smaller. This is seen clearly in the finger tremor spectrum; the lower-frequency oscillation probably represents the neural input, and the higher-frequency the mechanical properties of the finger. The degree to which matching occurs may partly account for the considerable variation in tremor level in different individuals.

Tremor frequency was quite constant in each subject; it did not change significantly when several recording sessions were carried out. Indeed, with practice, it was often possible to identify individuals from the shape of their frequency spectrum. The frequency of physiological tremor is probably dictated by the basal rate of firing of the subject's motoneurons. In most subjects, there was a reasonable match between the frequencies of left and right tremor and, prima facie, one would expect this symmetry. In some cases, this matching broke down, sometimes spectacularly. It was noteworthy that the severe mismatches were confined to elderly subjects and to the essential tremor patients. Some of the normal subjects (and several of the essential tremor patients) had a tremor of one or both wrists that peaked at less than 7 Hz. It seems possible that some idiosyncratic properties of the wrist or hand may be responsible for slight departures from the norm. However, it is unlikely that this can explain the low frequencies (5–6 Hz) that were observed in several of the patients and in a few of the normal subjects. Nearly all the persons with low frequencies were elderly. It is possible that this decrease in frequency represents a natural slowing of the firing frequency of motoneurons with age. It is known that the twitch time in elderly muscle is often prolonged; motoneuron firing rate may be correspondingly decreased. Alternatively, a low-frequency tremor may be a sign of disease. As it is not known whether abnormal tremors develop progressively, it is now impossible to say whether low-frequency tremor is evidence of inchoate disease or a bizarre, but harmless, finding. However, in view of the age-related emergence of parkinsonism and other tremulous syndromes, really low frequencies, particularly when they are unilateral, may well be pathognomonic. This question is particularly pertinent for the two young subjects who had tremors that were not much over 6 Hz.

B. Tremor Level

The range of tremor levels that is seen in the general population is large; some persons are constitutionally much more tremulous than others. As tremors become larger, they also become slower. This progression is to be expected on purely energetic grounds; it requires four times as much energy to drive a tremor at 10 Hz than at 5 Hz. The reason for the variation is not known; it must reflect differences in the nervous system, or in the properties of the muscle or motor units themselves. The question of the "matching" of mechanical and neural properties (rate of motoneuron firing) has already been raised. Several other neural factors may be involved. The degree of synchronized motor unit activity may be different in different subjects. This may be a result of differences in the degree of inhibitory feedback in the spinal cord or at higher levels. Feedback from muscle afferents may play a role in certain conditions (15). It may be that low-frequency tremor represents an unusual degree of synchronized low-frequency motor unit activity; this would provide the combination of low-frequency activation and large-force pulsation that will cause a very large amplitude of oscillation. This would also account for the sinusoidal nature of the oscillation.

It is also possible that the variation in amplitude is a reflection of a difference in muscle properties. There are two possible explanations. The characteristics of motor units may vary subtly from subject to subject. A given rate of motor unit firing may produce a tetanic fusion if the motor unit is slow, whereas in subjects with faster motor units, a series of discrete twitches will result. The tremor level will be greater in the latter situation. Alternatively, the characteristics may be broadly similar, but the proportion of fast and slow motor units that are in use may vary from subject to subject. Evidence concerning this comes from experiments that alter the metabolism of the muscle. A brief period of ischemia causes a substantial decrease in tremor amplitude in normal subjects, as does lowering the temperature of the muscles involved. These procedures produce changes as a result of their direct effect on the muscle tissue. This can be shown by studying a "simulated" tremor that is produced by mild percutaneous electrical stimulation. The amplitude of this type tremor is subject to the same metabolically induced changes as real tremor (14). One explanation is that these maneuvers may slow the twitch properties of the motor units that are active and, thereby, produce a less "bumpy" input. An alternative view, which we favor, is that these procedures, by causing metabolic changes in muscle fibers that generate the tremor, may cause a shift in the relative contribution of different types of motor units. Thus, the contribution to the tension that is generated by large, fast motor units may be reduced, with a consequent diminution of tremor. It is arguable that some tremorogens (e.g., β-adrenergic agonists and thyroid hormone) may also act through a metabolic mechanism by causing a short- or long-term shift toward the recruitment of larger, faster motor units and the production of more tremor. Alterations in tremor level, consequently, would be a result of a shift in emphasis of fast and slow motor units.

C. Age

The age results confirm the belief that tremor peak frequency declines with age. A recent report (6) has suggested that there is no decline in modified postural tremor frequency, but the starting point for the study was at 65 years of age. There was no evidence that the frequency in children was much different from young adults. There was a tendency for tremor level to increase with age; close inspection of Figure 6 suggests that the level may actually be at its lowest in the middle years and slightly higher in children. This is similar to the results described by Birmingham et al. (5). The most striking finding was that there was very considerable variation between elderly individuals, and it was in older subjects that there were often differences between right and left hands.

D. Essential Tremor

It has been suggested that there are two types of essential tremor (2). This is supported by the results described here. One group of patients had tremors that fell within the normal frequency band, but that were rather large in acceleration. This appears to represent little more than an exaggerated physiological tremor. In patients with this form of tremor, both sides of the body appear to be more or less equally affected. There was considerable overlap with the normal subjects. Some 10% (25 people) of the normal subjects might have been classified as having this variety of essential tremor. Interestingly, at least in this small group of patients, this type of essential tremor showed the strongest familial link. [Note added in press: Since this chapter was written, an additional 14 essential tremor patients have been analyzed. In this group, there were four patients with a familial history of the condition who had a low-frequency tremor.] This suggests that the factor or factors that cause the increased amplitude may be an inherited characteristic. It also raises the intriguing possibility that there may be an inherited low-tremor syndrome. Most of the very tremulous normal subjects, when questioned, were aware that they had a large tremor, and many of these stated that it was a tendency that "ran in the family." Only one had sought medical attention. The clear implication is that this tremulous state is quite common and consistently under-reported. If the familial link can be confirmed, this condition might best be described as benign familial tremor.

The other patients who had low-frequency tremors, appear to form a separate subgroup. The frequency is distinctly lower than normal, and the acceleration (or force) is very large. These factors combine to produce an impressive oscillation. The abnormal tremor is often confined to one side. The disease creates the impression of a neurological problem, and it is difficult to see what could otherwise produce such a profound slowing and enlargement of the tremor. In a sense, the motion is more akin to a disordered movement, than to a tremor, as it represents about the maximum rate at which the wrist can be voluntarily flapped. Motoneurons cannot normally be persuaded to fire at frequencies less than their primary range (about 7–30 Hz); the reason is uncertain. Perhaps in these patients the basal rate of firing is unusually low. There is now evidence to implicate olivo-cerebellar or thalamocortical mechanisms (16,17) in some cases of essential tremor. However, it seems clear that if there is a connection between olivocerebellar oscillations and large-amplitude tremor (18), then, at least in humans, the rate of any central oscillator should be nearer to 5 than to 10 Hz. In the patients described here, with one exception, the disease had no familial link. The implication is that this form of the disease is mainly sporadic; this would be worth further investigation. It is doubtful that many of these patients would consider the condition benign. Thus, until a causative lesion is firmly identified, it seems that essential tremor is an entirely appropriate description.

VI. CONCLUSION

We can now address the question posed by the title. Benign familial tremor (peak frequency > 7 Hz) appears to be indistinguishable from the tremor that is found in quite a large proportion of the sample population; Therefore, it is by definition, physiological. Low-frequency essential tremor is more distinct. There was a small overlap with some (mainly older) subjects in the sample population, but it is quite possible that these apparently normal individuals actually had a pathological tremor. Tremor frequencies slower than 6 Hz are probably always unphysiological, as is a marked difference in frequency between left and right sides.

ACKNOWLEDGMENTS

It is a pleasure to thank the Wellcome Trust for support, Mr. L. A. Arblaster who provided invaluable assistance with the collection and analysis of the data, Dr. R. C. Roberts (Consultant Neurologist, Dundee Royal Infirmary) who selected the patients, and the patients and subjects themselves.

REFERENCES

1. Haerer AF, Anderson DW, Schoenberg BS. Prevalence of essential tremor. Results from the Copiah County study. Arch Neurol 1982; 39:750–751.
2. Marsden CD. Origins of normal and pathological tremor. In: Findley LJ, Caplideo R, eds. Movement Disorders: Tremor. London: Macmillan Press, 1984:37–84.
3. Marshall J. The effect of ageing on physiological tremor. J Neurol Neurosurg Psychiatry 1961; 24:14–17.
4. Marsden CD, Meadows JC, Lange GW, Watson RS. Variations in human physiological finger tremor, with particular reference to changes with age. Electroencephalogr Clin Neurophysiol 1969; 27:169–178.
5. Birmingham AT, Wharrad HJ, Williams EJ. The variation of finger tremor with age in man. J Neurol Neurosurg Psychiatry 1985; 48:788–798.
6. Kelly JF, Taggart HMcA, McCullagh. Physiological tremor in an elderly population. In: Bartko D, Gerstenbrand F, Turcani P, eds. Neurology in Europe. London: John Libbey & Co, 1989:541–545.
7. Lippold OCJ. Oscillation in the stretch reflex arc and the origin of the rhythmical 8–12 c/s component of physiological tremor. J Physiol 1970; 206:359–382.
8. Findley LJ, Gresty MA. Tremor. In: Harrison MJG, ed. Contemporary Neurology. London: Butterworths, 1984:168–182.
9. Van Buskirk C, Fink RA. Physiological tremor. An experimental study. Neurology 1962; 12:361–370.
10. Hefter H, Homberg V, Reiners K, Freund HJ. Stability of frequency during long term recordings of hand tremor. Electroencephalogr Clin Neurophysiol 1987; 67:439–446.
11. Arblaster LA, Elton RA, Lakie M, Walsh EG, Wright GW. Human physiological tremor—a relationship with limb temperature. J Physiol 1990; 423:71P.
12. Lakie M, Robson LG. Thixotropic changes in human muscle stiffness and the effects of fatigue. Q J Exp Physiol 1988; 73:487–500.
13. Randall JE, Stiles RN. Power spectral analysis of finger acceleration tremor. J Appl Physiol 1964; 19:357–360.

14. Lakie M, Walsh EG, Wright GW. Passive mechanical properties of the wrist and physiological tremor. J Neurol Neurosurg Psychiatry 1986; 49:660–676.
15. Hagbarth K-E, Young RR. Participation of the stretch reflex in human physiological tremor. Brain 1979; 102:509–526.
16. Lamarre Y. Animal models of physiological, essential and parkinsonian-like tremors. In: Findley LJ, Caplideo R, eds. Movement Disorders: Tremor. London: Macmillan Press, 1984:183–194.
17. Colebatch JG, Findley LJ, Frackowiak RSJ, Marsden CD, Brooks DJ. Preliminary report: activation of the cerebellum in essential tremor. Lancet 1990; 336:1028–1030.
18. Llinás R. Rebound excitation as the physiological basis for tremor: a biophysical study of the oscillatory properties of mammalian central neurons in vitro. In: Findley LJ, Caplideo R, eds. Movement Disorders: Tremor. London: Macmillan Press, 1984: 165–182.

13

Pathophysiology of Essential Tremor

J. C. Rothwell
Institute of Neurology
National Hospital for Neurology and Neurosurgery
London, England

I. INTRODUCTION

There are many theories about the possible role that peripheral and central mechanisms play in the genesis of tremor. These have been discussed in some detail in Chapter 5 in this handbook. However, from the physiological point of view, the crux of the matter is whether normal, physiological mechanisms have become disordered in patients with essential tremor. Presumably, if we could identify physiological abnormalities, then this might help us understand more clearly how tremor is generated. This chapter summarizes the neurophysiological studies that have been carried out in patients with essential tremor. Despite the prevalence of this condition, there are relatively few pathophysiological results available. Those that are can be grouped together under the following headings.

1. Central and peripheral nerve conduction velocities
2. Single motor unit-firing behavior
3. Stretch reflexes
4. Electrically elicited reflexes
5. Reciprocal inhibition

II. PERIPHERAL NERVE AND CENTRAL MOTOR CONDUCTION STUDIES

By definition, peripheral nerve conduction velocities, both in motor and sensory nerves are normal in patients with essential tremor. Thompson et al. have also reported that central motor conduction times in the pathways from motor cortex to spinal cord lie within the normal range (1).

III. SURFACE AND SINGLE UNIT ELECTROMYOGRAPHY STUDIES

The primary abnormality of essential tremor, as compared with normal physiological tremor is that there is segmentation of the electromyogram (EMG) during tonic muscle contraction. Bursts of activity are separated by a relative silence, occurring at the frequency of the tremor. The bursts of activity may be synchronous in antagonist muscles, or may alternate between them. Muscle groups that are usually studied are the flexors and extensors of the wrist, or the flexors and extensors of the elbow. Shahani and Young emphasized that, in their experience, there tended to be synchronized bursts of activity in antagonist muscles in patients with essential tremor (2). This feature distinguished the tremor from that of patients with Parkinson's disease. However, it is now clear that the presence or absence of synchronous bursts varies from patient to patient, from task to task, and from minute to minute. Synchronization between antagonists tends to be more prominent during horizontal extension of the arm. Other actions or postures may be accompanied by alternating activity. Patients with large-amplitude (and usually slow) tremors almost invariably have an alternative pattern of EMG activity between antagonist muscles.

Despite the variation from patient to patient, there may be some usefulness in distinguishing between preponderantly alternating and preponderantly synchronous tremors. Sabra and Hallett (3) and Deuschl et al. (4) found that patients with preponderantly synchronous tremor are more responsive to propranolol; patients with alternating tremor were more responsive to primidone (see Chapter 14).

The bursts of EMG activity seen in the surface EMG are not caused by synchronization of motor unit firing at the tremor frequency. Single motor unit studies show that within a tremor burst, individual units may fire twice or more at high frequency (5). Thus, tremor is produced by modulation of the firing frequency of the population of motor units.

Although each cycle of tremor is produced by a broad grouping of motor unit discharge, there is a tendency for synchronization of the discharge between individual motor units over a much shorter time interval. Cross-correlation histograms of the firing pattern of pairs of single units shows an increased tendency for the units to fire at approximately the same time, with cross-correlation peaks of up to 25 ms or so in duration. The interpretation of cross-correlation peaks between single motor units depends on the width of the peak. If the peak is narrow (up to about 15 ms), this suggests that the two motoneurons being studied receive synaptic input from a common source. If the cross-correlation peak is longer in duration, then the suggestion is that interneurons that project onto the two motoneurons under study receive input from a common source.

Is the synchrony between motor unit firing during bursts of essential tremor normal or pathological? Work by Logigian et al. (6) suggests that it is normal. They examined a group of normal subjects who were instructed to imitate tremor by rapid phasic voluntary flexion–extension movements at the wrist. Synchronization between pairs of motor units in the wrist extensor muscles was increased considerably during rapid wrist movements, compared with normal isotonic extension of the wrist. They suggest that the increased synchrony was caused by near maximal synaptic drive from phasically active voluntary supraspinal neurons as well as from muscle spindle afferents activated by the contraction. If the same is true in essential tremor, then short-term synchrony is a natural consequence of the bursting EMG pattern that is seen in surface recordings.

One peculiarity about the motor unit studies in patients with essential tremor, is that during a burst of tremor, the normal pattern of motor unit recruitment is disrupted This contrasts with the situation in patients with Parkinson's disease, in which motor units are recruited in their usual order during each burst of tremor (7).

IV. STRETCH REFLEX STUDIES

In view of the possibility that tremor could be caused by oscillation in a stretch reflex feedback circuit (see Chapter 5), there have been several studies of the response of muscles to stretch in essential tremor. All of these studies have used rapid, forcible extension of the wrist or thumb, delivered by a torque motor. Clinically, tendon jerks are normal in patients with essential tremor, so that most studies have concentrated on the long-latency components of the response to muscle stretch, which have a latency approximately twice that of the tendon jerk. In the human arm, two mechanisms probably contribute to this part of the stretch reflex response. The first mechanism, described by Marsden and associates (8) proposes that there is a transcortical reflex pathway involving rapid conduction from fast-conducting group Ia afferents to the sensorimotor cortex and back to the spinal cord. This mechanism is probably preponderant in intrinsic muscles of the hand and in those muscles in the forearm that act directly on the digits. The second mechanism, suggested by Matthews (9), is that stretch excites muscle spindle secondary endings, which, through slow-conducting group II afferents, produce late muscle reflexes by a totally spinal mechanism. This mechanism is probably important in more proximal muscles (for a discussion see, e.g., Ref. 10).

Marsden et al. examined the stretch reflex in the long flexor of the thumb, using ramp displacements of the interphalangeal joint at two different speeds (11). Elble et al. examined reflexes produced by 50-ms torque disturbances applied to the wrist (12). Both studies found that the latency and size of the long-latency component of the reflex was the same in patients with tremor as in normal subjects.

In addition, Marsden et al. said that the duration of the long-latency response was the same as normal (11), whereas Elble et al. confirmed that the short-latency (tendon jerk) component of the response was also normal (12). Thus, in some respects, the findings were disappointing, since if abnormalities of the timing or size of the stretch reflex responses had occurred, then obviously, they could have contributed to tremor.

Although the initial, reflex response to stretch is normal in tremor, the later parts of the response may be changed. Rothwell et al. asked subjects to hold their wrists flexed to about 160° against a small load offered by a torque motor (13). Every 4–5 s, the load on the wrist was increased by a factor of 2, 4, or 6 for a period of 800 ms. Stretches of this kind extend the wrist by 10°–40°. The initial stretch is followed by a dampened oscillation, which decays within a few cycles.

In patients with essential tremor, if the same stretch was given when there were no bursts of tremulous activity in the EMG, large-amplitude oscillations of the wrist occurred about the new extended position, which decayed only very slowly. This is shown for two subjects with essential tremor of different frequencies in Figure 1. On the time scale in this figure, the short- and long-latency components of the stretch reflex EMG response merged together into a single component, labeled B1. The size of this component was within the normal range in both patients. In control subjects without tremor, the long-latency stretch reflex often is followed by a period of relative silence that is terminated by a small, late burst of EMG. In patients with essential tremor, this burst was large (see B2 in Fig. 1) and could be equal in size to the long-latency reflex stretch itself. Moreover, the latency of the burst was longer than normal and was inversely related to the frequency of the patient's tremor. Thus, the abnormality in the response of the wrist flexor muscles to stretch lies not in the usual short- or long-latency stretch reflexes, but in the later component of the muscle activity.

Unfortunately, little is known about the mechanism of these later parts of the response to stretch (see B2 in Fig. 1), even in normal subjects. They lie within the limits of voluntary reaction time, yet under certain conditions, they may be influenced by nonvoluntary processes. For example, in the long flexor of the thumb, the size of a voluntary response made during this period can be adjusted automatically to the size of the preceding stretch reflex. The reflex varies considerably in size from trial to trial; when it is large, the voluntary burst of activity is small and vice versa. The net result is that the final end position of the thumb is constant, although different trajectories have been followed to get there (14). It is possible that the abnormal responses of patients with essential tremor reflect loss of this subtle mechanism that relates reflex to early voluntary effects.

Hore and Vilis have examined late responses to muscle stretch in some detail in the monkey (15). These authors gave short duration (40-ms) pulse stretches to the elbow of trained monkeys. The stretch generated a short- and long-latency stretch reflex in the biceps muscle, which produced force to flex the elbow against the

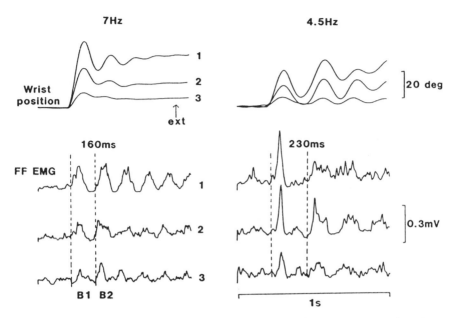

Figure 1 Average (of 24 trials) position (upper) and rectified EMG records from flexor muscles in the forearm (FF) to unpredictable wrist extension produced by a torque motor. Subjects maintained their wrist in a constant position against a small load while the flexor muscles were stretched by increasing the load randomly by a factor of 2, 4, or 6 (traces 3, 2, 1, respectively) for a period of 800 ms, starting 200 ms after onset of the recording sweep. Stretches were given only when there were no bursts of tremulous activity in the ongoing EMG. The EMG response in both subjects consists of a stretch reflex burst (labeled B1, with onset latency of approximately 50 ms after stretch), followed by a relative silence and further EMG bursts (B2, etc.). The patient on the left had a usual tremor frequency of 7 Hz, and the patient on the right a frequency of 4.5 Hz. The intervals between the onset of B1 and B2 EMG bursts were 160 ms and 230 ms, respectively for all three sizes of stretch.

increased load. However, since the load was removed after only 40 ms, much of the reflex force was unnecessary, and would, if unrestrained, drive the elbow past its initial starting position. Under conditions in which the monkey was expecting a pulse stretch, this stretch reflex activity was opposed by a burst in the antagonist (triceps) muscle, which started some 20 ms later than the stretch reflex in biceps. This activity stabilized the elbow at the initial position with minimal oscillation.

Hore and Vilis argued that, since the antagonist activity began before any stretch of that muscle, it must be part of a predictive response of the central nervous system (CNS) to the initial disturbance (15). If the monkey had been trained to expect a prolonged, step-torque increment, rather than a pulse, then the antagonist activity was no longer present. Indeed, a second burst of activity in the agonist muscle occurred, which was necessary to help restore the elbow to its initial position against the continuing load.

The timing of these later bursts of predictive activity (which may be in the agonist or the antagonist muscle) is regulated by the cerebellum. Cooling the dentate nucleus during regular pulse disturbances delayed the onset of activity in the antagonist muscle. Under these conditions, stretch produced unstable oscillation of the arm, because the antagonist activity was no longer timed correctly to compensate for the initial stretch reflex in the agonist. Indeed, Hore and Vilis argued that any antagonist activity that they saw was now driven by the muscle stretch reflexes, and that the oscillation was due to natural reverberation in the stretch reflex pathway, which under normal circumstances was prevented by predictive activity generated by the cerebellum (15). Such behavior is very reminiscent of that of the patients with essential tremor, and provides further evidence of a link between essential tremor and the cerebellum.

V. STUDIES OF ELECTRICALLY ELICITED REFLEXES

Only one other reflex pathway has been investigated in patients with essential tremor. This is described in detail in the Chapter 14. These authors have recorded the EMG from the abductor pollicis brevis muscle during voluntary contraction after motor threshold stimuli to the median nerve at the wrist. This electrical stimulus evokes reflex modulation of the tonic EMG, which has up to three different components. The precise relation of these components to the conventionally elicited stretch reflex is unknown. However, the presence or absence of the long-latency reflex 1 (LLR I) component correlates remarkably well with the response of the patient to treatment with propranolol or primidone.

VI. RECIPROCAL INHIBITION

It is now possible to investigate the function of many spinal cord circuits using modifications of H-reflex techniques. Such studies include the Renshaw circuit, Ib inhibitory circuits, Ia inhibitory interneurons, presynaptic inhibition, and propriospinal neurons. There are no published reports of investigations on any of these pathways in patients with essential tremor. However, in our laboratory we have preliminary data that indicate that the reciprocal Ia inhibitory pathway and the presynaptic inhibitory pathway between extensor muscle afferents and the flexor monosynaptic reflex is intact (at least at rest) in essential tremor.

The essence of the principle of reciprocal inhibition is that, during contraction of one group of muscles, there is active inhibition of their antagonists. One method that the CNS uses to achieve this is as follows. Tonic voluntary contraction of an agonist muscle is accompanied by an increase in discharge from the muscle spindles. The increased discharge in Ia afferent fibers activates Ia inhibitory interneurons in the spinal cord which, in turn, inhibit the α-motoneurons of the antagonist muscles. This is known as spinal disynaptic inhibition. In addition, the agonist Ia input appears to produce presynaptic inhibition of the terminals of Ia afferents from the antagonist muscle. Thus, if the antagonist muscle is stretched by the agonist contraction, then the antagonist stretch reflex (which may interfere with the progress of the movement) will be inhibited by two mechanisms: postsynaptic inhibition of α-motoneurons, and presynaptic inhibition of Ia afferents.

We have tested this system in the forearm of normal humans by giving single electric-conditioning stimuli at low intensity to the radial nerve in the spinal groove, and recording the effect on H-reflexes elicited in the flexor muscles of the forearm. A single radial nerve stimulus inhibits the H-reflex in forearm flexor muscles with a prolonged time course, such as that illustrated in Figure 2. The initial, short duration inhibition of the H-reflex is due to activity in the disynaptic

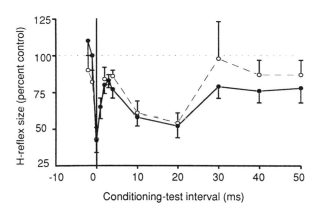

Figure 2 Time course of reciprocal inhibition between extensor and flexor muscles of the human forearm in a group of eight normal subjects (●) and eight patients with essential tremor (○). Motor threshold electrical-conditioning stimuli were given to the radial nerve in the spiral groove at $t = 0$ ms. H-reflexes were elicited in the forearm flexor muscles by stimulation of the median nerve in the cubital fossa at different times before (negative times) or after (positive timings). The size of the H-reflex was expressed as a percentage of the size of control H-reflexes elicited by median nerve stimulation given alone. The whole experiment was conducted with the subjects totally relaxed. The initial phase of inhibition can be seen with conditioning-test intervals of -1 to $+2$ ms. It is probably produced by activity in the spinal disynaptic Ia inhibitory pathway. The later inhibition at conditioning-test intervals of 10 and 20 ms is probably due to presynaptic inhibition of flexor Ia afferent fibers. Points are mean ± 1 standard error.

Ia inhibitory interneuron pathway. The later, longer-lasting period of inhibition is due to presynaptic inhibition of Ia afferents; this time course of inhibition is abnormal in patients with dystonia. Preliminary studies on eight patients with essential tremor show that these two phases of reciprocal inhibition are completely normal in this condition. We conclude that there is no disorder of reciprocal inhibitory pathways in the resting forearm muscles in patients with essential tremor.

VII. CONCLUSION

Most systems that have been studied using conventional electrophysiological techniques have been normal in patients with essential tremor. The only abnormality that has been described is the inappropriately large and late EMG burst that follows the conventional stretch reflex. In normal persons, this activity is thought to be a response triggered by the initial stretch, which prevents oscillation occurring in the limb after completion of the phasic stretch reflex response itself. Experiments in monkeys suggest that this predictive activity is under the control of the cerebellum. If a similar system is responsible for the abnormality in essential tremor, then this is further evidence to implicate cerebellar dysfunction in the genesis of the patient's tremor.

ACKNOWLEDGMENT

I should like to thank Dr. P. D. Thompson, Dr. B. L. Day, and Professor C. D. Marsden for much valuable discussion during the course of the work reported here. The data in Figures 1 and 2 was collected in collaboration with Drs. T. Kachi and K. Nakashima.

REFERENCES

1. Thompson PD, Dick JPR, Day BL, et al. Electrophysiology of the cortico-motoneurone pathways in patients with movement disorders. Mov Disord 1986; 1: 14–23.
2. Shahani BT, Young RR. Physiological and pharmacological aids in the differential diagnosis of tremor. J Neurol Neurosurg Psychiatry 1976; 39:772–783.
3. Sabra AF, Hallett M. Action tremor with alternating activity in antagonist muscles. Neurology 1984; 34:151–156.
4. Deuschl G, Lucking CH, Schenck E. Essential tremor: electrophysiological and pharmacological evidence for a subdivision. J Neurol Neurosurg Psychiatry 1987; 50:1435–1441.
5. Young RR, Shahani BT. Analysis of single motor unit discharge patterns in different types of tremor. In: Cobb WA, Duijin H, eds. Contemporary Clinical Neurophysiology. Amsterdam: Elsevier, 527–528.

6. Logigian EL, et al. Motor unit synchronisation in physiologic, enhanced physiologic and voluntary tremor in man. Ann Neurol 1988; 23:242–250.
7. Young RR. Pathophysiology and pharmacology of tremor. In: Shahani BT, ed. Electromyography in CNS Disorders: Central EMG. London: Butterworth, 143–159.
8. Marsden CD, Merton PA, Morton HB. Stretch reflex activity and servo-action in a variety of human muscles. J Physiol 1976; 259:531–560.
9. Matthews PBC. Evidence from the use of vibration that the human long latency stretch reflex depends on spindles secondary endings. J Physiol 1984; 348:383–415.
10. Thilmann AF, Schwarz M, Topper R, Fellows SJ, Noth J. Different mechanisms underlie the long latency stretch reflex response of active human muscle at different joints. J Physiol 1991; 444:631–643.
11. Marsden CD, Obeso JA, Rothwell JC. Benign essential tremor is not a single entity. Yahr MD, ed. Current Concepts in Parkinsons Disease. Amsterdam: Excerpta Medica, 1983:31–46.
12. Elble RJ, Higgins C, Moody CJ. Stretch reflex oscillations and essential tremor. J Neurol Neurosurg Psychiatry 1987; 50;691–698.
13. Rothwell JC, Kachi T, Thompson PD, Day BL, Marsden CD. Physiological investigations of parkinsonian rest tremor and benign essential tremor. In: Benecke R, Conrad B, Marsden CD, eds. Motor Disturbances 1. London: Academic Press, 1–17.
14. Rothwell JC, Traub MM, Marsden CD. Automatic and "voluntary" responses compensating for disturbances of human thumb movements. Brain Res 1982; 248: 33–41.
15. Hore J, Vilis T. A cerebellar-dependent efference copy mechanism for generating appropriate muscle responses to limb perturbations. In: Bloedel JR, Dichgans J, Precht W, eds. Cerebellar Functions. Berlin: Springer Verlag, 1984:24–35.

14

Physiological Classification of Essential Tremor

G. Deuschl, R. Zimmermann, H. Genger, and C. H. Lücking
University of Freiburg
Freiburg, Germany

I. INTRODUCTION

From a clinical point of view, essential tremor (ET) is usually considered to be a uniform disease characterized by the occurrence of a long-standing mono-symptomatic postural and action tremor, mainly bilaterally, with involvement of the arms, hand, and often the head (1–3). Nevertheless, the occurrence of postural tremors is found in a variety of neurological conditions, which has been recognized for a long time (for review see Ref. 1). An important attempt toward a clinical classification covering all these conditions was the classification of Marsden et al. (4) (Table 1).

Because of the need for careful studies of comparable patient populations, a very recent attempt has been made to classify the predominant postural tremors including ET on the basis of criteria separating *definite*, *probable*, and *possible* essential tremor (Tremor Investigation Group; TRIG; see Chapter 1) (Table 2). These clinical criteria are straightforward, useful, and necessary for the needs of clinical analysis, everyday practice, and treatment of these diseases. Nevertheless, it can be expected that future analysis will be able to better characterize, especially, some of the tremors presently summarized under the term of possible ET. Physiological and pharmacological differences have been demonstrated even among patients of the group with definite or probable ET, which may turn out to be meaningful and which, in the future, could help understand pathophysiological principles of ET. The present contribution will briefly summarize these attempts toward a physiological classification of ET.

Table 1 Clinical Classifications of Tremor

Type 1	Benign exaggerated physiological tremor, 8–12 Hz
Type 2	Benign pathological essential type, 5–7 Hz; frequently familial and responds to propranolol
Type 3	Severe pathological essential tremor, 4–7 Hz; frequently sporadic and non-responsive to therapy
Type 4	Symptomatic essential tremor, associated with other neurological conditions, such as dystonia and neuropathy

Source: Ref. 4.

II. METHODS

A. Tremor Recording

Tremor was recorded in all patients and controls according to a standardized protocol: They were seated in a comfortable chair and the forearm was fixed in a horizontal position. The hand could freely move in the vertical direction. The accelerometers (weight 8 g) were fixed 9 cm distal to the ulnar styloid process, exactly over the middle phalanx. Their signal was linear between 0.3 and 100 Hz. It was digitized at a rate of 300 Hz and stored on a personal computer. Further processing included fast-Fourier analysis of time-series of 6.8 s. The five spectra that were obtained were averaged, and the resulting spectrum thereby represents a 34-s period. From these power spectra, the maximum amplitude and the corre-

Table 2 Separation of ET Based on Clinical Criteria (TRIG)

Inclusion criteria for *definite essential tremor*
  1. Visible bilateral postural or action tremor of hands/forearms.
  2. A duration of more than 5 years.
  3. Other body parts may be involved, asymmetry may occur.
  4. Amplitude and disability is not critical for the definition.
Inclusion criteria for *probable essential tremor*: criteria 1–4 are present, except that
  1. Tremor may be confined to one body part other than hands.
  2. Duration has to be longer than 3 years.
Inclusion criteria for *"possible" essential tremor*:
The inclusion criteria for definite or probable ET, but additional features are allowed, such as

Type 1	Other recognizable neurological disorders (parkinsonism, dystonia, myoclonus, etc.)
Type 2	Monosynaptic and isolated tremors (task-specific tremors, primary orthostatic tremor, etc.)

Source: See Chapter 1.

sponding peak frequency were determined and are reported here. Statistical analysis included X^2 and t-tests as well as Mann–Whitney tests.

B. Long-Latency Reflexes

The method has been described in detail elsewhere. Briefly the subjects were asked to slightly contract the thenar, usually by leaning the thumb against the fifth finger. The electromyogram (EMG) was recorded from the abductor pollicis brevis with surface electrodes. The median nerve was stimulated at the wrist with stimuli just subthreshold for motor fibers, with rectangular pulses of 200-ms duration.

The EMG was filtered (1.5–1000 Hz), fullwave rectified, and averaged (256 sweeps). Reflex latencies were determined as onset latencies, and amplitudes were normalized to the baseline. The absolute amplitude measured as a difference of the peak and onset amplitude on the reflex was normalized to the baseline, measured at the first 20 ms. The normal values are reported elsewhere (5) and for the H-reflex are 24–32 ms; for the long-latency reflex (LLR) I, 38–45 ms; and for the LLR II, 44–57 ms. The relative amplitudes for the H-reflex are 0.5–5; for the LLR I, 0.1–1; for the LLR II, 0.3–2.3.

C. Subjects and Patients

The data reported here are based on 58 patients with essential tremor, 112 patients with Parkinson's disease (PD), and 85 normal subjects, who were used as controls.

III. PHYSIOLOGICAL CRITERIA CHARACTERIZING TREMOR

The physical properties of tremor can be described by frequency, amplitude, and waveform. Hence, the first attempt toward a physiological classification of tremor will use these criteria. Another feature characterizing a tremor is its pattern of EMG activity in antagonistic muscles. In addition to these aspects directly related to the tremor, additional features have been described for which the relation to the origin of tremor is not yet settled. Testing of reflexes and back-averaging of electroencephalographic (EEG) activity, using the tremor bursts as a trigger, belong to these features.

A. Frequency and Amplitude Characteristics of Pathological Tremors

The frequency of essential tremor has been found to have a bimodal distribution, with peaks at 6 and 10 Hz, respectively (6). Figure 1 shows our data, with the distribution of the tremor frequencies of 58 patients with essential tremor. It is evident that we cannot confirm a bimodal distribution of the tremor frequencies in this condition. Thus, in agreement with the observations of Elble (7), the tremor frequency does not allow a subdivision of ET.

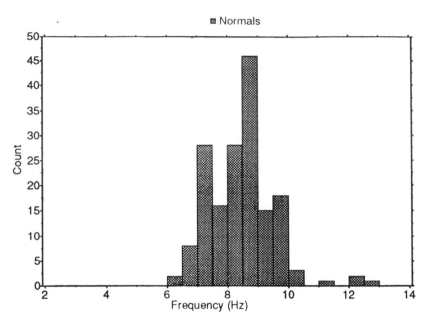

Figure 1 Distribution of the tremor frequencies in ET, Parkinson's disease, and physiological tremor.

The second question is whether the frequency of tremor may help separate ET from other pathological tremors. For this purpose the bilateral tremor frequencies of 128 patients with Parkinson's disease (PD) and 85 normal subjects with physiological tremor were included in the analysis. The mean frequencies are different in these three conditions, with 6.6 Hz $\pm$ 1.2 (mean $\pm$ SD) for essential tremor, 6.0 Hz $\pm$ 1.2 for tremor in Parkinson's disease, and 8.5 Hz $\pm$ 1.1 in physiological tremor. However, there is a considerable overlap of the frequencies in these tremors, as shown in Figure 1. As a rule of thumb, it is possible to make a differential diagnosis on the basis of tremor frequencies only at the extremes of the frequency spectrum. Below 4.6 Hz, we could find only patients with Parkinson's disease. Above 9 Hz we found only patients with postural tremor in Parkinson's disease and physiological as well as enhanced physiological tremor. Thus we conclude that tremor frequency is a poor indicator for the differential diagnosis of pathological tremors.

The amplitude of tremor is highly variable among different patients and even in a single patient over time. Therefore, it is unlikely to be of significant value in the differential diagnosis of tremor. Figure 2 shows the distribution of these amplitudes for essential tremor. It is clear that there is no evidence for a bimodal distribution and, therefore, no evidence for a subdivision into different subgroups

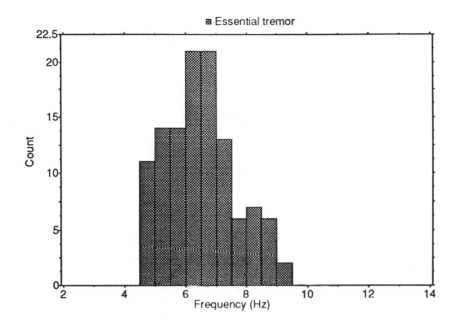

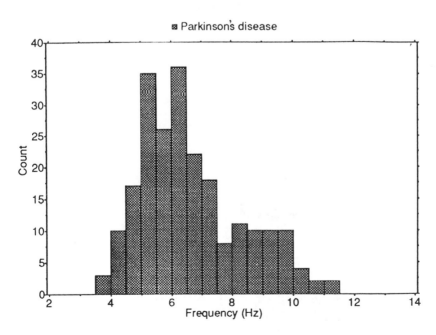

of essential tremor. The tremor amplitudes of ET differ clearly from those of other tremors. In our subjects, the mean amplitude of physiological tremor is 3.2 ± 2.3 mg (milligravity), the mean amplitude of ET is 111.2 ± 260 mg, and the mean amplitude of tremor in Parkinson's disease is 180 ± 377 mg. This feature does not allow separation of the various etiologies of tremor.

B. Waveform Characteristics of Tremor

The waveform of tremor measured with monoaxial accelerometry is another aspect characterizing tremors. Advanced mathematical methods of time series analysis can be applied to these data (19). It was found that characteristics of symmetry of the tremor curves bear some diagnostic significance. Without going too much into the details of mathematical analysis, this is exemplified in Fig. 3. Tremor curves of a normal subject, a patient with ET and a patient with parkinsonian tremor are displayed on the left side of the figure. On the right side the same curves are shown but with the time scale reversed. It is clear, that the curves look similar for normals and patients with ET but not for the patient with Parkinson's disease. This difference is due to the asymmetry of the curve. Different mathematical methods can be applied to quantify this feature of the curves (19). We found, that the separation based on this criterion is poor between normal subjects and patients with ET but valuable to separate patients with Parkinson's disease from these two conditions (5). Hitherto, our ongoing studies suggest that no subdivision among patients with essential tremor can be detected with this approach.

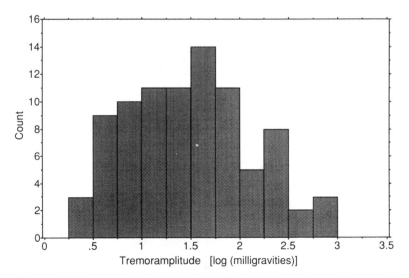

Figure 2 Tremor amplitudes in log (milligravity) in patients with essential tremor. A unimodal distribution was found.

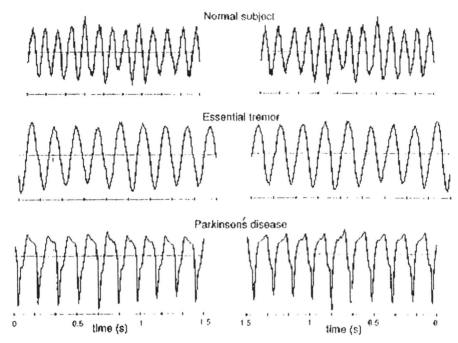

Figure 3 Normalized waveforms measured with accelerometers of a normal subject, a patient with ET and a patient with Parkinsonian tremor. These time series are displayed on the left side in original time order and on the left side in time reversed order. These curves look similar for normals and patients with ET but not for patients with Parkinson's disease. These differences can be exactly quantified with mathematical time series analysis, for example the invariance to time series reversal. (From Ref. 20.)

C. Electromyographic Pattern of Essential Tremor

Shahani and Young (8) emphasized that various patterns of EMG activity do occur in essential tremor. They have found synchronous activation of antagonists as well as reciprocal alternating activity. Moreover, tremulous activity of the agonist of the movement alone does occur (9,10). It has been observed that in a single patient synchronous and reciprocal alternating tremor bursts occasionally can occur (7) (Fig. 4). Although these features have been described by different investigators, it is not yet possible to define consistent differences on the basis of the EMG alone. On the other hand, the myographic pattern has been found to correlate with clinical and physiological aspects. Patients with reciprocal alternating patterns of EMG activity mostly had only a poor response to propranolol treatment (9). We have investigated the activation pattern as one criterion for the separation of tremors. We could confirm that reciprocal, alternating patterns occur more often in patients with abnormal hand muscle reflexes and poor response to propranolol treatment (10). However, prospective studies of these correlations are still lacking.

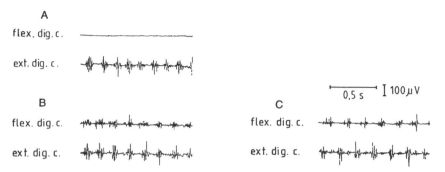

Figure 4 Patterns of electromyographic activity during forearm pronation in patients with tremor. The EMG activity of forearm flexors and extensors is shown with tremor bursts in the antigravity muscle alone and with synchronous or reciprocal alternating patterns.

We conclude that it is not yet possible to classify different forms of ET on the basis of the phase relations of antagonistic muscles alone, although a relation between the activation pattern in antagonistic muscles and pharmacological responsiveness has been described. Further investigations are mandatory.

D. Stretch Reflex Studies

Several reflex studies of tremor disorders have been conducted. The background of these studies is that insights about the underlying oscillator are expected: The easier it is to reset the tremor rhythm by external perturbations or electrical stimuli, the more this indicates that the oscillator underlying this tremor is likely to be stable or autonomous. Lee and Stein have investigated the resetting characteristics of patients with ET and tremor in PD (11). They demonstrated a higher probability for resetting the tremor rhythm in their patients with ET than for those with PD. Any subdivision of the patients with ET based on this criterion was not observed. More recent studies have shown that resetting the tremor rhythm depends on the frequency and amplitude of these tremors, rather than on the etiology of the tremor (ET or PD). Higher-amplitude tremors need a higher strength of perturbation (12). Accordingly, the resetting characteristics of the tremor in the different patients seemed to be ranked on a continuum, rather than ranked by different groups. Hence, it has been questioned if this pathophysiological aspect can be used as a differential diagnostic criterion of ET.

E. Electrically Elicited Hand Muscle Reflexes

Another test is the investigation of electrically elicited long-latency reflexes. This kind of test is not necessarily related to the resetting characteristics of tremor, as the tremor rhythm itself is not observed in this test, but the averaged EMG response of the thenar muscles to weak electrical stimuli applied to the median nerve is. However, it is not excluded that eventually existing abnormal reflexes detected by this method might contribute to the tremor. The normal reflex pattern consists of an Hoffmann reflex (HR) at about 29 ms and an long-latency reflex at 50 ms (LLR II) (Fig. 5). In normal subjects, an occasional small earlier LLR (LLR I) occurs at about 40 ms, with a small amplitude not exceeding the baseline amplitude. This LLR I is enhanced (larger amplitude than the baseline) in about one-third of the patients with ET (Fig. 6). Although ongoing investigations have shown that this abnormality is not restricted to ET (5), it has been observed in other extrapyramidal disorders; this finding could be confirmed in our more recent patients.

In our first report (10), we summarized 45 patients. The two groups, termed A and B, could be separated by means of the following criteria:

	Type A	Type B
Frequencies of tremor (Hz)	6–12	5.5–8
Long-latency reflexes	Normal	Enhanced LLR I
EMG pattern	Mostly synchronous	Mostly reciprocal alternating
Therapeutic results	Mostly responsive to propranolol	No response to propranolol

Meanwhile, we have followed 58 additional patients with reflex testing and with measuring the tremor frequencies and amplitudes based on an objective quantification (see methods). The patients were prospectively classified on the basis of LLR alone. The mean frequencies were 7.1 ± 1.2 Hz for the patients with ET type A ($n=30$ patients) and 6.23 ± 1.1 Hz for the patients with ET type B ($n = 28$ patients). The mean amplitudes were 60.6 ± 79.4 mg for the patients with ET type A and 149 ± 245 mg for the patients with tremor type B. Figure 7 displays the

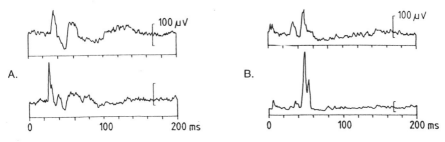

Figure 5 Long-latency reflexes of thenar muscles following median nerve stimulation: (A) The normal patterns with the Hoffmann reflex and the LLR II in the upper trace and a small LLR I in the lower trace. (B) The reflexes of patients with ET displaying an abnormally enlarged LLR I.

Type A   Type B

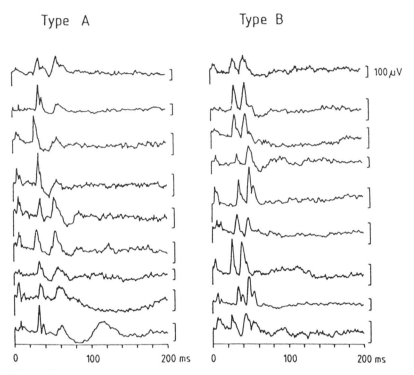

Figure 6 Long-latency reflexes of patients with ET showing normal (type A) or abnormal patters (type B). (From Ref. 10.)

amplitudes and frequencies of these two tremor types as percentage plots. The difference of the tremor frequencies was significant ($p < 0.01$, Mann–Whitney), but not the difference of the tremor amplitudes ($p > 0.5$). Somatosensory-evoked potentials were measured in ten of the patients with ET type B, and they did not show any abnormalities. Patients from the two groups were clinically indistinguishable. Analysis of the clinical data showed that the patients with type B tremor were significantly older and had a significant preponderance of women. Unfortunately, a follow-up of these patients concerning their response to pharmacotherapy could not be achieved.

Meanwhile, recent studies provide additional evidence for the occurrence of abnormal reflexes in patients presenting with the clinical picture of ET (13). These patients showed tremor, mainly during action, for more than 5 years. Additional signs were occasional grand mal seizures. One of the patients had a family history of action tremor. On physiological analysis the patients presented with a high-frequency, approximately 9-Hz, tremor showing an inconsistent, sometimes synchronous sometimes asynchronous, pattern (Fig. 8). These patients have to be

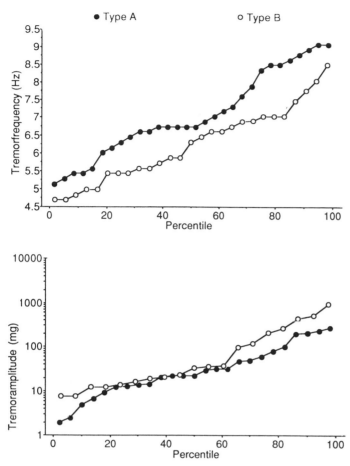

Figure 7 Percentage display of tremor amplitudes and tremor frequencies in patients with essential tremor type A and B.

discussed in the present context, as they had a reflex myoclonus of the thenar muscles to electrical stimulation of the median nerve. The latency of this reflex myoclonus was 43 ms. Although the HR latency was not reported, it is most likely, according to our own observations (5), that this reflex corresponded to the LLR I in these patients. Moreover, the authors could demonstrate, by means of jerk-locked averaging of the EEG and using the tremor bursts as a trigger, that both patients had a cortical positive–negative EEG discharge preceding the tremor bursts. Similar cortical equivalents have been observed in cortical myoclonus (14,15). Moreover, the resetting of the tremor rhythm following median nerve and cortical magnetic stimulation has been studied showing that only cortical stimulation

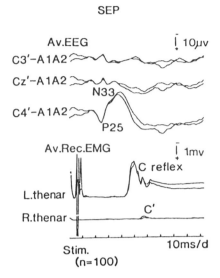

Figure 8 Somatosensory-evoked potential (SEP) and reflex myoclonus in a patient with cortical tremor. The SEP-amplitudes are normal and the latency of the C-reflex corresponds to the LLR I. (From Ref. 13.)

could reset the tremor frequency (Toro et al. 1993). The name "cortical tremor" has been proposed for this condition. Future experience will show if these studies provide evidence for a reliable pathophysiological classification.

IV. CONCLUSIONS

A physiological classification in essential tremor would be helpful, as we do not have an etiological approach to this disease. However, a physiological classification can be based only on proved pathophysiological mechanisms. The pathophysiological basis of tremor is still a matter of debate and has been extensively reviewed in other chapters of this volume. In essential tremor, there seems to be a general agreement that it is due to a central generator, rather than to a pure stretch reflex mechanism. This conclusion is based mainly on the observation, that loading of the trembling limb does alter the frequency of physiological, but not that of essential tremor or other so-called "central" tremors (7,16,17). Even this does not unequivocally exclude the involvement of reflex mechanisms (3).

Beyond this general statement about its central origin, which does not even separate essential tremor from other central tremors, there is only preliminary evidence for a classification of essential tremor on a physiological basis. We and others have shown that the physical properties of the movement disorder do not allow any subclassification. Neither the tremor amplitude nor the tremor frequency shows a clear-cut bi- or multimodal distribution. The EMG pattern seen in antagonistic muscles shows differences, but there is still an ongoing discussion about whether this pattern is stable and, therefore, reliable enough to allow a subdivision. Further investigations of the phase relations in tremor are mandatory. Evidence has been provided that stretch reflex studies show different resetting characteristics in various forms of tremor and could separate ET and the tremor of Parkinson's disease (11). However, recent studies have explained that these differences are gradual and depend mainly on the amplitude of tremor (12).

Nevertheless, there is ample evidence that different pathophysiological mechanisms may be active in ET:

1. The patients with ET differ in their clinical presentation. Some have a pronounced action tremor, so-called kinetic predominant tremor, whereas posture tremor amplitudes are small (18). Otherwise, the predominant activation of ET is seen in postural tasks.
2. Different patients may respond differently to pharmacological treatment with propranolol or primidone. Other respond only to clonazepam and present with the clinical picture of action tremor (18).
3. Different hand muscle reflexes to electrical median nerve stimulation can be found in patients with ET. Most patients have a normal pattern, but a smaller number have abnormal reflexes with an enhanced LLR I. The latter finding is possibly due to abnormal cortical excitability. Moreover, patients have recently been identified who have a cortical spike potential time-locked to the tremor bursts, possibly indicating a cortical origin or at least transmission of the rhythmic activity through the cortex in this condition. Hence, these patients share the physiological aspects of tremor and of cortical myoclonus. One, therefore, may speculate, whether cortical involvement differs among different forms of ET, and the patients with cortical tremor could represent one extreme of a mechanism that is more widespread and can already be demonstrated with our technique of LLR testing at an early stage.

Thus, we conclude that there are findings indicating possible different involvement of central pathways in ET as an indicator for different underlying pathophysiological mechanisms. Nevertheless, these findings do not justify subdivision of ET on the basis of clear-cut pathophysiological differences. The matter still remains experimental and open for future research.

REFERENCES

1. Findley LJ, Capildeo R, eds. Movement Disorders: Tremor. London: Macmillan Press, 1984.

2. Findley LJ, Koller WC. Essential tremor: a review. Neurology 1987; 37:1194–1197.
3. Elble RJ, Koller WC. Tremor. Baltimore: Johns Hopkins University Press, 1990.
4. Marsden CD, Obeso JA, Rothwell JC. Benign essential tremor is not a single entity. In: Yahr MD, ed. Current Concepts in Parkinson's Disease. Amsterdam: Excerpta Medica, 1983:31–46.
5. Deuschl G, Lucking CH. Physiology and clinical applications of hand muscle reflexes. Electroencephalogr Clin Neurophysiol 1990; 41(suppl):84–101.
6. Marshall J. Observations on essential tremor. J Neurol Neurosurg Psychiatry 1962; 22:122–125.
7. Elble RJ. Physiologic and essential tremor. Neurology 1986; 36:225–231.
8. Shahani BT, Young RR. Physiological and pharmacological aids in the differential diagnosis of tremor. J Neurol Neurosurg Psychiatry 1976; 39:772–783.
9. Sabra AF, Hallett M. Action tremor with alternating activity in antagonist muscles. Neurology 1984; 34:151–156.
10. Deuschl G, Lucking CH, Schenck E. Essential tremor: electrophysiological and pharmacological evidence for a subdivision. J Neurol Neurosurg Psychiatry 1987; 50:1435–1441.
11. Lee RG, Stein RB. Resetting of tremor by mechanical perturbations: a comparison of essential tremor and parkinsonian tremor. Ann Neurol 1981; 10:523–531.
12. Britton TC, Thompson PD, Cleeves L, et al. Phase resetting of postural tremor with mechanical stretches, peripheral nerve stimuli and magnetic brain stimulation. Mov Disord 1990; 5(suppl):32.
13. Ikeda A, Kakigi R, Funai N, Neshige R, Kuroda Y, Shibasaki H. Corticol tremor: a variant of cortical reflex myoclonus. Neurology 1990; 40:1561–1565.
14. Hallett M, Chadwick D, Marsden CD. Cortical reflex myoclonus. Neurology 1979; 29:1107–1125.
15. Deuschl G, Schenck E, Lucking CH, Ebner A. Corticol reflex myoclonus and its relation to normal long latency reflexes. In: Motor Disturbances. Benecke IR, Conrad B, Marsden CD, eds. London: Academic Press, 1987:305–319.
16. Stiles RN, Pozos RS. A mechanical reflex oscillator hypothesis for parkinsonian hand tremor. Ann Appl Physiol 1976; 40:950–998.
17. Homberg V, Hefter H, Reiners K, Freund HJ. Differential effects of changes in mechanical limb properties on physiological and pathological tremor. J Neurol Neurosurg Psychiatry 1987; 50:568–579.
18. Biary N, Koller WC. Kinetic predominant essential tremor: successful treatment with clonazepam. Neurology 1987; 37:471–474.
19. Gantert C, Timmer J, Honerkamp J. Analysing the dynamics of hand tremor time series. Biol Cybern 1992; 66:479–484.
20. Deuschl G, Timmer J, Genger H, Gantert C, Lücking CH, Honerkamp J. Frequency, amplitude and waveform characteristics of physiologic and pathologic tremors. In: Przuntek H, ed. Quantitative methods and assessment in extrapyramidal movement disorders. Exp Brain Research Series. Heidelberg: Springer, 1993 (in press).

15

Stereotaxis in the Management of Tremor: Physiological Basis and Current Practice

Albrecht Struppler
Klinikum rechts der Isar
Munich, Germany

I. INTRODUCTION

In the last two decades, the demand for stereotactic treatment of symptomatic tremor was decreasing owing to progress in drug therapy. Recently, however, the number of stereotactic procedures has increased throughout the world (1,2). We can confirm this trend and report an increase of 60% stereotactic procedures in the last 5 years.

The most obvious reasons are due to our increasing knowledge about the problems and limits in modern pharmacotherapy, especially that of tremor. In addition, there has been progress in technology. This includes the development of neuroimaging techniques, such as computed cranial tomography and magnetic resonance imaging (CCT and MRI). Computer-assisted techniques give us the chance to correlate physiological data with anatomical brain landmarks in the operating room during procedures. Furthermore, development of the use of microelectrodes for stimulation and recording, and the advances in computed electronic signal processing, have added to the effectiveness of stereotactic treatment.

In our experience, stereotactic treatment of different types of tremor should be considered if the effect of tremorlytic drugs are insufficient or their side effects are too intrusive. Furthermore, stereotaxis should be considered if the tremor is a

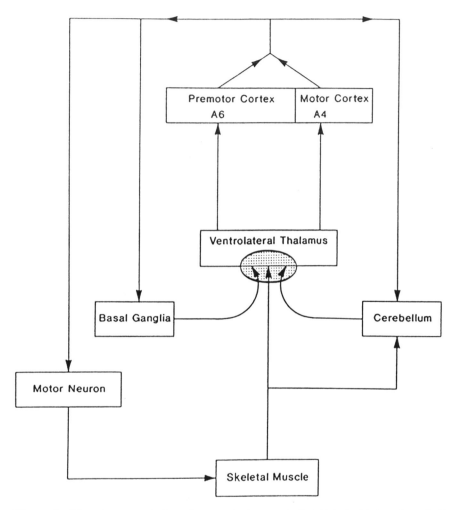

Figure 1   The scheme symbolizes the proposed concepts that disturbed interaction of all three inputs on the VL level lead to tremor, and the maintenance of all kinds of pathological tremor needs the integrity of a feedback loop originating in the skeletal muscle.

dominant symptom and is causing severe handicap in an individual patient's everyday life.

For satisfactory stereotactic treatment of pathological tremor one should be able:

1.   To abolish all kinds of pathological tremor
2.   To produce permanent results without recurrence

3. To ascertain that the lesions are small to avoid side effects as much as possible

To solve the problem of tremor by stereotaxis, one needs the best target point, which is based on a detailed functional anatomy (Fig. 1).

The development of the target point for treatment of pathological tremor ranges from lesions within the medial pallidum, to interruption within the pallidothalamic afferents. Lesions in this area could alleviate not only rigidity, but to some degree, parkinsonian tremor; however, they have to be quite large and can produce side effects. Therefore, combined lesions within the medial pallidum as well as in the ventrolateral (VL) and subthalamic area were used (3). Hassler showed that "the best effect on tremor will be gained by coagulation of the posterior portion of the oral ventral nucleus of thalamus (Vop; posterior basal part of VL)." Meanwhile there is general agreement, that all kinds of pathological tremor can be abolished by stereotactic lesions within the nucleus ventralis intermedius (*Vim*) or the corresponding area subthalamica, independent of tremor origin (reviewed in Ref. 4).

The optimal target point (i.e., the area in which the smallest lesions abolish pathological tremor) lies just rostral to the ventrocaudal (VC) nuclear representation of the lips or manual digits at or a little above the intercommissural (ACPC) line in the Vim or adjacent oralis posterior (Vop) of the thalamus (4,5).

II. PHYSIOLOGICAL BASIS

Stereotactic procedures for treatment of pathological tremor provide the unique chance to investigate sensory motor systems in alert humans. In addition, such physiological investigations may serve to improve functional neurosurgery.

My concept concerning the *physiology* is based on electrophysiological investigations during the intervention and on clinical observations, as well as on motor control studies in various stages following the lesion.

I will *concentrate* my interpretation of the physiological basis on our target point only. Furthermore, my own experiences in tremor treatment (376 interventions) are restricted to this area.

What are the characteristics of the movement-related zone within the target area?

A. Functional Anatomy

Histochemical and electrophysiological studies have recently shown (6) that the ventral nuclei both in human and monkeys can be divided into four pathways relaying pallidal, substantia nigral, cerebellar, and lemniscal information separately to the cerebral cortex (Fig. 2). In contrast with earlier investigations, there is no convergence within the VL. At least the first three pathways reveal separate relays to cortical territories defined as somatic sensory, motor, and premotor. Even

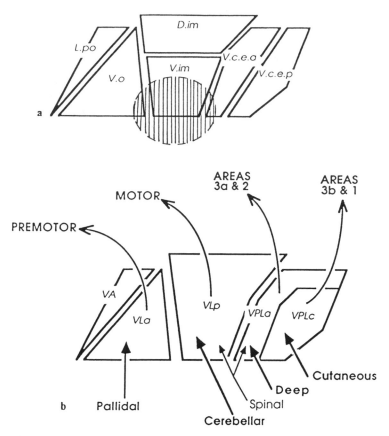

Figure 2 The scheme of (a) Hassler compared with that of (b) Hirai and Jones to which the input connections of the equivalent nuclei are added, as derived from experimental studies in monkeys (see text). (a) Schematic sagittal views of the major subdivisions of the human ventral thalamic nuclei, as made by Hassler. The circled area represents the general target of stereotactic thalamotomies for the relief of certain forms of spontaneous movement. (Modified from Ref. 6.)

within these three afferent systems, separate modality or otherwise specific parallel pathways exist. In the lemniscal path, the deep and cutaneous paths of the lateral segment of the ventoposterior (VPL) nucleus are clearly separate and relay separately to different cortical subfields of the somatic sensory cortex (7).

We may assume, therefore, that integration between these parallel afferent systems will be brought about by the corticocortical or corticosubcortical mechanisms. It seems unlikely that this can occur at the level of the ventral thalamic nuclei. Friedman and Jones (8) have also indicated from single-unit recording that the VPL should be divided into an anterodorsal shell, in which neurons responded only to stimulation of deep (muscle and joint) receptors and a central core in which neurons responded only to stimulation of cutaneous receptors. Furthermore, neurons in the anterodorsal shell project only to areas 3a or 2, whereas those in the central core project only to areas 3b and 1. Maendly et al. have shown that the anterior part of the shell of VPL is the principal input zone of group I muscle afferents (9). In the posterior VL (VLp), dentate, interpossital, and fastigial fibers terminate in separate, elongated regions that might also represent parallel pathways, whereby each of these deep cerebellar nuclei gains access to separate foci in the cerebral cortex (10).

The spinothalamic pathway seems to represent an *exception* to the theme of separate relays in the ventral nuclei of the monkey thalamus. Fibers in this pathway clearly terminate in VLp as well as VPL. It seems likely that the spinothalamic path through VLp is an essential route, whereby cutaneous and deep inputs could gain access to motor cortical neurons (7).

Coordinate date and the clear proximity of a cutaneous relay nucleus make it clear that most of such units have been recorded in the ventral part of VLp (Hassler's Vim) or in VPLa (Hassler's Vcae), but not in the anterior (VLa). The evidence that the region equivalent to the VPLa in monkeys is not only a deep relay, but specifically a group I afferent relay, supports our concept that, in the target area, muscle afferents are represented in a high density.

Tactile cells are located mostly posterior in the human nucleus ventralis caudalis. Cells responding to pressure, joint, and muscle movements are represented successively more rostrally in the nucleus (18). Cells responding to joint and muscle movement are located mainly in the Vim (19). These findings were recently extended by detailed studies, combining both microrecording and microstimulation techniques (4,13,15). Lenz et al. (13) could show that, in humans,

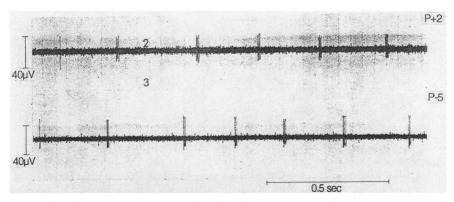

Figure 3 Rhythmic activity 2 mm above (Vop) and 5 mm below (radiatio prelemniscalis) the intercommissural plane, corresponding to the tremor cycle. (From Ref. 46.)

cutaneous and deep modalities are segregated according to Jones and Friedman's findings in monkeys, showing the same functional organization (20). Cells responding to deep stimulation could be classified into those responding to joint movement (63%), deep pressure (15%), or both (22%).

Repetitive electrical stimulation at the target point below the threshold for direct activation of the descending motor pathways augments the ongoing tonic activity associated with tremor and rigidity (Fig. 4). Such an increase of an ongoing electromyographic (EMG) activity could be evoked through the alpha or gamma system.

Microrecordings from Ia afferents (MNG) originating in a hand flexor muscle showed that the activity of a muscle spindle to stretch could be augmented by repetitive subthreshold stimulation at the target point (Fig. 5). These findings provide evidence that, at the target point, fibers are facilitating muscle tone, at least when the gamma system is involved.

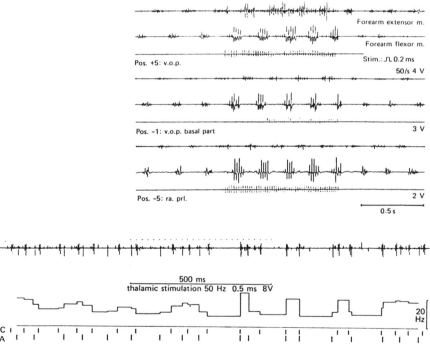

Figure 4 Recording of resting tremor activity in antagonistic muscle groups before, during, and after stimulation in the thalamus and subthalamus. Note that the spontaneous tremor activity can be facilitated by subthreshold stimuli within VOP and the radiatio prelemniscalis. (From Ref. 21.)

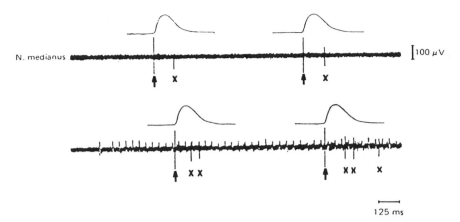

N. medianus

100 µV

X   X

X X   X X   X

125 ms

Figure 5 Effect of thalamic stimulation on muscle spindle discharges elicited by electrically induced twitch contraction. (Upper trace) Electrically evoked twitch contraction activity of one muscle spindle from a flexor muscle of the hand, firing during relaxation. (Lower trace) The activity is increased during subthreshold repetitive stimulation at the target point. Arrows indicate electrical stimulus artifact. (From Ref. 47.)

There is general agreement that repetitive stimulation with low frequencies and intensities at the Vim area usually facilitates tonic innervation. This can be shown in the relaxed state, as well as during automatic or intentional movements (5,22).

On the basis of anatomical studies we can conclude

1. The representation of the deep proprioceptive afferents, especially in the shell region of the VPLa, projecting to area 3a, is in accordance with our findings concerning muscle spindle recordings, sensation in deep tissue during stimulation, and superficial sensations, when touching the VPLc.

2. If *cerebellar* afferents, conducting processed information from the deep nuclei to the cortex, are involved in the lesion, they could contribute to only the control of muscle tone, in my experience. At least, I have never observed other cerebellar symptoms following my lesions (see p. 220). There are as yet no clear data from animal experiments that could be compared with the small stereotactic lesions in tremor patients.

3. In view of the *lack* of *convergence* in VL, let us assume that a deficiency in lemniscal and cerebellar information could be effective through a corticobasal ganglia–thalamocortical motor circuit (see p. 223). If we interrupt both systems, even with a small lesion, it would be interesting to analyze the interaction between reduced spinothalamic afferents and the feed-foreword function of the cerebellum.

The anatomical location must be confirmed by some physiological data, which can be obtained during the operation:

B. Electrophysiological Investigations During Intervention to Identify the Relevant Sensorimotor Systems in the Target Area

According to multi- and single-unit recordings from the human thalamus and area subthalamica, there is clear evidence that, in the target area, movement-responsive neurons are represented (11–17), as demonstrated in Fig. 3.

The same repetitive stimulation at the target point elicits the sensations projected to the corresponding somatic sensory area. These sensations are mostly interpreted as originating from deep structures, described sometimes as "strange" feelings, sometimes as tension. When the stimulation electrode moves ventro-caudally to the VC nucleus, the patients feel superficial sensations, especially in the fingers (see p. 227).

Evoked potentials recordings following electrical peripheral nerve stimulation give us information concerning the afferent pathway between the periphery and the target area. Evoked potentials of short-onset latency could be recorded within the target area following stimulation of contralateral mixed peripheral nerves. In contrast, no significant evoked potentials were recorded in the same area following electrical stimulation of skin afferents (Fig. 6).

Multielectrode recordings in the area of the calculated target point let us recognize the phase reversal from subthalamic to thalamic nuclear border region, indicating the generator was located here in this afferent system.

Recordings of evoked potentials following peripheral electrical stimulation of the peripheral nerve show single positive or positive–negative phasic configura-tions (Fig. 7). The first positive peak latency is between 12 and 20 ms in Vc evoked by median nerve stimulation (11,14,25–27). Goto et al. recorded a positive-phase latency of 13 ms and a negative of 16 ms after electric stimulation of the ulnar nerve at the elbow (25), which was thought to be due to muscle I fiber activation in Vim. Larson and Sances reported the peak latency in Vims as 13 ms (27), and Ohye and Narabayashi as 12–15 ms (14). Yamashiro et al. (28), using intra-thalamic single-unit recordings and somatic-evoked potentials (Th-SEP) that were evoked by percutaneous electrical median nerve stimulation and intrathalamic microstimulation, showed that the format of Th-SEP varied in anteroposterior, mediolateral, and dorsoventral direction in the ventrocaudal nucleus (Vc). The positive response peak latency was shortest from the caudal part of Vc and long-est in the anterior part of Vc, according to our findings.

On the basis of the experiments during these procedures, we suggest that, in the target area, a fiber system is densely represented that is involved in skeletal muscle tone, probably through the gamma-loop system.

1 + 3   Stimulation of med. nerve at the wrist

2 + 4   Stimulation of skin afferents (fingers)

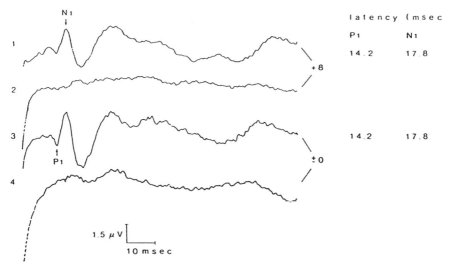

Figure 6 In contrast with stimulation of mixed nerves, stimulation of skin afferents evokes no significant potential within the target region. For the anatomical localizations see Figure 7a. ±0 and −3 symbolize the depth according to the stereotaxic system. (From Ref. 23.)

C. Postoperative Clinical and Neurophysiological Investigations of Motor Control

Following a lesion in the optimal target point, the tremor is replaced by a tonic activity during slight isometric contraction (Fig. 8). The previous tremor cycles no longer occur.

In addition to the abolition of tremor, the following clinical symptoms were observed:

1. Resistance to passive limb displacement in the relaxed state (rigidity) was reduced, there was no more spontaneous muscle activity. Reinforcement (Jendrassik's maneuver or mental drive) no longer evoked tremor or rigidity.
2. Normal maximal voluntary force in proximal as well as in distal muscles, rapid movements, and phasic stretch reflexes remained unchanged; rapid movements were mostly more synchronized.

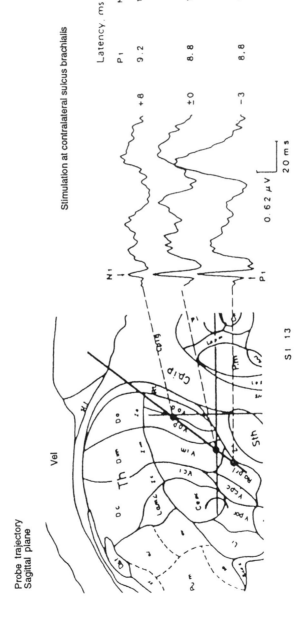

Figure 7 (a) Evoked potentials following mixed nerve stimulation in reference to the stereotactic atlas of Schaltenbrand and Wahren (plane sagittal lateral 13). The evoked potentials initially are triphasic. The latencies of the first positivity (PI) and the first negativity (NI) show a slight decrease with depth (9.2 to 8.8 ms, 12.4 to 12.0 ms, respectively), whereas the amplitudes show a slight increase. The probe passes ventralis oralis posterior (Vop), ventralis intermedius (Vim) on the way to the subthalamus (radiatio prelemniscalis; ra prl). The target point is located in the Vim and Vim radiatio prelemniscalis border region (depth 0 to −3).

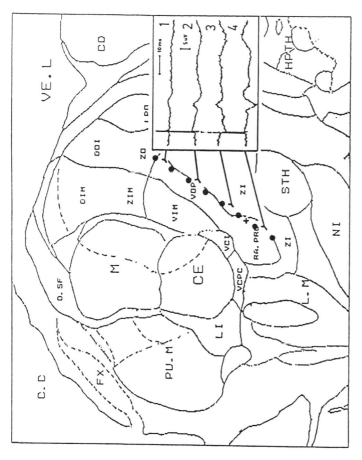

Figure 7 (b) Evoked potentials following contralateral median nerve stimulation recorded within the thalamic area by a multipole electrode. Phase reversal occurred between trace 3 and trace 4 that was related to the thalamic–subthalamic border (+). Active areas of the multielectrode (●) were related to Schaltenbrand and Wahren's sagittal atlas plane 10.5. (From Refs. (a) 23; (b) 24.)

Isometric contraction (10 N) before (a) and after (b) subthalamotomy

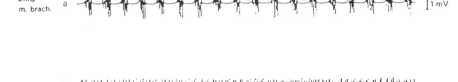

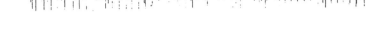

250 ms

Figure 8   Isometric contraction (10 N) before (a) and after (b) subthalamotomy.

3.   There was a slight postural hypotonia, especially in the lower extremity, which is more tonically innervated. Following sudden perturbation of an isometrically contracted muscle, the displacement and the overshoot were enhanced (Fig. 9).

4.   There was no deficiency in coordination, as in ataxia, dysdiadochokinesia, and dysmetria, and no lack in initiation of movement. The so-called epicritic sensitivity, such as perception of touch, joint movement, and position sense, remained unchanged. However, there was a deficiency in the estimation of force during isometric contraction tasks.

Two postoperative symptoms are especially important and need more detailed analysis. These are the deficiencies in sudden load compensation and in estimation of force. Both are probably due to an interruption in a feedback system controlling adequate muscle stiffness.

This clinical phenomenon is demonstrated in a clinical example for controlled load compensation of the deltoid muscle (see Fig. 9).

If the patient was asked to hold both arms horizontally, he or she showed a deficiency in control of appropriate tone or stiffness to maintain position. These phenomena seem to be correlated with the abolition of tremor. If these symptoms are not produced by the lesions, the tremor will recur.

The tremor remained abolished in approximately 80% of patients. The deficiency in rapid load compensation was usually clinically compensated after a few weeks or months. Neurophysiological studies however allow us to examine the remaining deficiencies (30). Modern neurophysiological NI methods give one the chance to correlate structure and function, even after years, and to follow-up the compensation of this open-loop condition.

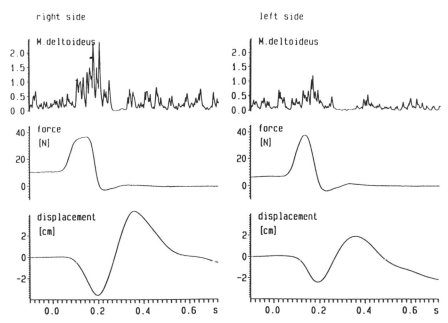

Figure 9 On the hypotonic side (right) there is a longer elongation and overshoot as well as a larger reflex component of the EMG. Under this nonstandardized condition the applied force on both sides is not identical. However, in this example the force on the right hypotonic side is at least no greater on the left side and cannot be the cause of the difference in the two sides. Therefore, we assume that the overshoot is at least partly caused by this enlarged EMG in the agonistic muscle. (From Ref. 29.)

To obtain more insight into the changed motor control, we investigated the mechanics and the EMG in forearm and finger flexor muscles during stretch and unloading under isometric contraction, and the rapid movements as well as the firing rate of motor units near the recruitment level. Given our investigations so far, we assume that, under this open-loop condition, the mode of innervation during tonic activity is changed, with a shift in the population of active motor units from a preponderantly static to a more phasic type (31).

D. How Could the Alleviation of Tremor by Vim Lesions be Interpreted on the Basis of the Concept of a Disinhibition of the Subthalamic Nucleus in Parkinson's Syndrome?

In 1-methyl-4-phenyl-1,2,3,6-tetrahydropyridine (MPTP)-treated monkeys showing parkinsonianlike symptoms, the subthalamic nucleus (STN) is abnormally overactive. Therefore, it was concluded that the STN is essential for the pathophysiology of parkinsonism. This concept is based on a shift in the balance between activity in two parallel pathways: a direct one from the cortex through putamen to the SNr, and an indirect one through GPe and STN, resulting in an alteration in GPe–SNr output, which may account for the hypo- and hyperkinetic features in basal ganglia disorders. Parkinsonism, as a hypokinetic–hypertonic syndrome plus tremor, results in large part from increased thalamic inhibition by the excessive excitatory drive from the STN to the output nuclei of the basal ganglia, the GPi and SNr (32).

Obviously, the interruption of the subthalamopallidal pathway by inactivation of the STN could ameliorate motor disturbances such as Parkinsonian tremor (33,34).

This concept of a parallel processing of basal ganglia information sheds new light on the treatment of tremor by Vim lesion.

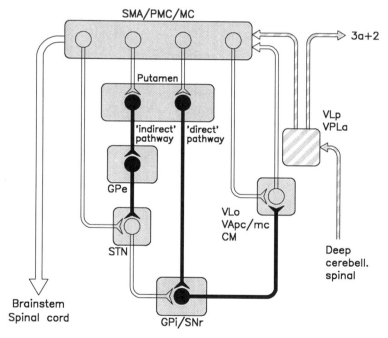

Figure 10   The two-pathway concept of parkinsonism. Inhibitory neurons are filled symbols, excitatory neurons are open symbols. Abbreviations: CM, centromedian nucleus; GPe, external segment of globus pallidus; GPi, internal segment of globus pallidus; SNr, substantia nigra pars recitulata; STN, subthalamic nucleus; VAmc, nucleus ventralis anterior pars magnocellularis; VApc, nucleus ventralis anterior pars parvocellularis; VLo, nuclcus ventralis lateralis pars oralis. In addition, the hatched VLp and VPLa (6) represent the Vim (5). (Modified from Ref. 35.)

The imbalance in these proposed loops could be modified by Vim lesions directly or indirectly. Could the Vim lesion additionally interrupt pallido- or nigrothalamic afferents? Considering the representation of these afferent systems on the target point, this seems to be unlikely (see Ref. 7). The Vim lesion could diminish the disinhibition of the STN system by involving the STN system in the Vim lesion to some degree. This is also unlikely because of the anatomy and the size of lesions. Therefore, it seems most likely that the shift in the balance can be produced by the lesion at the Vim level, itself. Accordingly, we could assume that the lesion at the Vim level can elicit a shift in the balance by a separate and indirect route.

This leads to the following hypotheses: Rigidity, caused by increased inhibitory pallidothalamic drive and independent of pathological tremor, can be abolished separately by lesions in the pallidum internum. Tremor, however, can be abolished by lesions within the Vim area by modifying the balance caused by a change in motor control on the level of the basal ganglia, thalamic, and cortical circuits. This independently and simultaneously abolishes rigidity, as according to our experience, Vim lesion alleviates both tremor and rigidity. This may be illustrated in Figure 10, in which the concept of the tremor treatment by Vim lesion is symbolized in the diagram of Alexander and Crutcher (35).

III. STEREOTAXIC MANAGEMENT OF TREMOR

A. The Localization of the Target Point

To determinate the target point, we have two methodological approaches:

1. On the basis of *neuroimaging* methods of ventriculography (VG) and CT, the position of the target point is calculated by reference to the imaged structures.
2. The definite position of the target point relative to the function is determined by *physiological tests*, such as recording and stimulation. Even the best neuroimaging facilities will not replace these tests in the future because of interindividual anatomical variations (Fig. 11).

1. Coordinates

Coordinates from the individual *brain* are commonly transferred to the *atlas*, proportional to the Ca–Cp distances of the individual brain and the atlas. So far, positive ventriculography is the most accurate method to identify Ca and Cp in the human brain and should not be avoided. However, the lateral distances of the Vim, mostly those of the upper extremity neurons from the midline of the third ventricle vary remarkably, depending on width of the third ventricle (36). Therefore, a further method was developed that included the individual lateral extension of the target area, using CT scans.

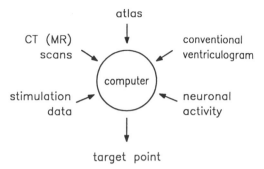

Figure 11 Neuroimaging, electrophysiological, and morphological parameters to determine the target point.

To optimize target point evaluation *mathematical transformation modes* must be defined to allow comparison of individual brains. The bicommissural axis (Ac–Pc line), in the ventriculogram lets us determine a coordinate system of the thalamus and its adjacent structures. In reference to this axis a localization system may permit the comparison of different individual brains by proportional standardization on the basis of the CT scan (37).

Our procedure includes, neuroradiological examination by VG and CT to reconstruct the bicommissural axis in vivo. Digital images of CT scans are created in parallel with the bicommissural axis by linear gray tone interpolations. The individual outlines of the thalamus are constructed from these images.

Given these data, a "mean" of the thalamus and its adjacent structures is computed. This calculated model structure of the thalamus serves as a reference for individual target points. A statistical analysis is performed to evaluate the relation between individual lesion sides and geometric parameters of the mean thalamus. Finally, the geometrical parameters are used to match individual brains with Schaltenbrand and Wahren's stereotactic atlas (Fig. 12).

The transfer of the borders of anatomical regions or sets of coordinates from one model taken as standard (the atlas) to the individual brains of actual patients to calculate "nonvisible" targets in a three-dimensional stereotactic atlas has been done (38–40).

Recently, MRI has been used, since the target area can be demonstrated with more definition. However, when using MRI for accurate spatial information—critical for effective stereotaxy—a homogeneous static field and linear gradients are necessary (41). Correction of spatial distortion by inhomogeneities and nonlinearities may provide an opportunity in the future to use MRI instead of CT, with the same accuracy (42).

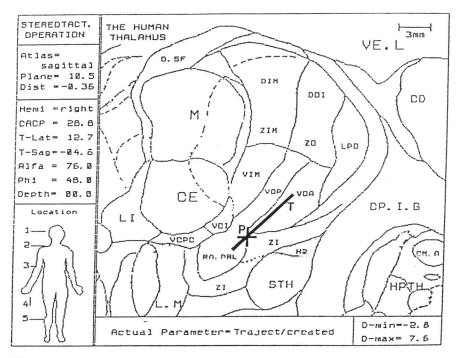

Figure 12 Computer graphic multidisplay. Correlation of a trajectory (T) and the tip (+) of the electrode at position P and Schaltenbrand and Wahren's sagittal atlas plane 10.5. The patient was operated on for the left side, the AC–PC distance was 28.8 mm, the target laterality relative to the midventricular plane was 12.7 mm, the target was 4.6 mm behind the half of AC and PC. The tilt angles of the electrode in the spherical frame coordinate system were α = 76 and φ = 48. The tip of the electrode matched the target coordinates (depth = 0.0). (From Ref. 24.)

The definitive position of the target point relative to the *function* is monitored by physiological tests, such as recording and stimulation.

2. Recording

Recording the spontaneous activity of a neuronal cell, and the fiber activity along the probe trajectory, determines the entrance to the VL (Fig. 13) (nucleus reticularis) and the subthalamic border. The audiovisual monitoring of neuronal noise is a very useful method to recognize the location and extent of various subcortical structures along a trajectory and, furthermore, to understand the extent of individual and anatomical variation. Frequency power spectrum analysis is a new approach to characterize neuronal noise (43). It is suggested that characteristics of neural noise are primarily determined by cytoarchitecture and

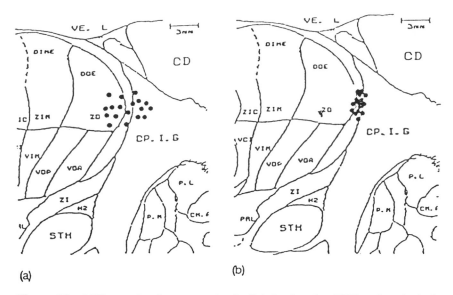

Figure 13 (a)The results of a computation for Schaltenbrand and Wahren's sagittal atlas, plane 12. (b) The CT-based transformation gives a better correlation between electrophysiological registered thalamus borders and the corresponding atlas borders. (For details see text.)

physiology, possibly secondarily modified by the underlying pathology and functional state, such as in multiple sclerosis (MS) demyelination. For use in the operating room, a three-dimensional display of frequency power spectrum along the trajectory may be a helpful guide for exploring neuronal cell and fiber systems. Sites of noise changing, determined using our compound transformation, are compared with the atlas thalamus borders (37). Figure 13a shows the result of that computation for Schaltenbrand and Wahren's sagittal atlas plane 12.0. In contrast with the AC–PC transformation, the CT-based transformation gives a better correlation between electrophysiologically registered thalamus borders within the patient's brain and the corresponding atlas borders (see Fig. 13b).

Recording evoked potentials following peripheral stimulation give us important information about the representation of afferent systems in the target area. This method is time-consuming, but useful for elaborating functional anatomy close to the target area.

3. Electrical Stimulation

Repetitive electrical stimulation in the target area is an essential test and cannot be missed. The observation of *motor responses* show, if the probe is localized within facilitatory systems for muscle tone and which part of muscle groups can be activated while advancing the trajectory.

In analogy, the described *sensations* of the patient let us differentiate whether the probe is localized in the lemniscal somatosensory afferents responsible for superficial sensations, such as touch; or in a sensory system, conducting signals of so-called deep tissue, such as muscle or joint. Videomonitoring gives the chance to correlate motor effects of stimulated structures with postoperative evaluations.

B. The Lesion: Preoperative Control of Electrode Position: Control of Lesion Effect

Preoperatively, it is necessary, for ethical reasons, to control the position of the coagulation electrode by neuroimaging—even when the evaluation had been perfect. Postoperatively, the size of the lesion should be controlled in various stages by neuroimaging. This now gives us the chance to correlate structure and function (Fig. 14).

1. What Could be Improved in the Future?

According to our experience, two technical developments could be helpful: An optimal method to perform a reversible block could offer the chance to predict the lesion effect—at least for the acute stage. In addition, the size of the conventional thermocoagulation depends on the individual properties of the brain tissue. Therefore, we are not able to predict sufficiently accurately the final lesion. One may expect that laser techniques will be adapted to stereoencephalotomy.

C. Lesion Versus "Deep Brain Stimulation"

The observation that repetitive stimulation, with a frequency of 100 Hz or more, at the target point can inhibit tremor activity has encouraged the development of the deep brain stimulation (DBS) method, with long term implanted electrodes for the treatment of movement disorders, such as dystonia, spasmodic torticollis, and spasticity, by constant stimulation. Sites include the VL, pulvinar and dentate nucleus (44). Recently, Benabid and co-workers (45) described the suppression of tremor by long-term stimulation of the Vim in tremor patients older than 65 years, in whom a second operation contralateral to a previous thalamotomy was necessary. It was thought that the risk of a coagulation would be greater than an implantation of a long-term intrathalamic stimulation electrode.

This raises some important considerations in comparing Vim lesions with the long-term stimulation method. The lesion usually needs only a single intervention, the tremor is in 90% permanently alleviated or abolished, and the side effects have been reduced with the newer techniques. Long-term stimulation requires a permanent stimulation electrode in the brain for the rest of the patient's life. Although the stimulation can be reduced or stopped, when side effects, such as paresthesias, are

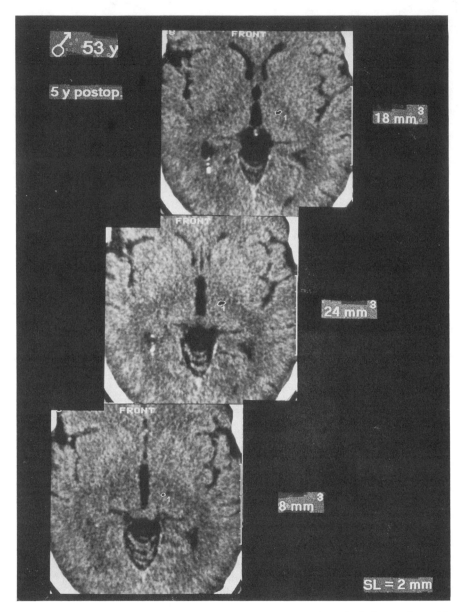

Figure 14 An example of a stereotactic lesion 5 years postoperatively in a patient with parkinsonian tremor (2-mm slides; MRI).

elicited, the tremor then recurs, as a rebound effect. Furthermore, one should keep in mind, that the physiological basis is unknown. Therefore, the indication for this stimulation technique must be very strict, especially if the tissue at the target point is altered (e.g., in demyelinating disease).

IV. CONCLUSION

What can we conclude from our findings and from the literature concerning the treatment of tremor by stereotactic lesions? All kinds of pathological tremor can be alleviated or even abolished by small lesions in a small area (Vim and area subthalamica), independently of the types of tremor (e.g., resting, postural, action, or intention) or of its origin (e.g., cerebellar, mesencephalic, or basal ganglia systems).

Therefore, one can assume that the pathological tremor is due to an imbalance between facilitatory and inhibitory afferents to the VL, controlling the postural component of motor performance. Even when there are pacemaker cells (so-called tremor cells), the cells can produce tremor only with a higher level of excitability. The main task to alleviate tremor is to reduce this imbalance by lowering facilitatory inputs. According to our findings, we assume that interruption of afferents controlling muscle tension—not only for automatic, but also for cortically controlled intentional movements—produces alleviation of tremor by changing motor control at the level of basal ganglia–thalamocortical circuits.

The fact that all kinds of pathological tremor can be abolished by lesions in one place supports the idea that the origin of tremor depends mainly on the state of excitability of different systems, rather than from the presence of some pacemaker in different areas. It does not mean that all kinds of tremor have the same origin. The manifestation of tremor is dependent on different types of motor performances. The more information we have about the pathophysiology of different types of tremor, the more individualized (specific) the target points can become.

REFERENCES

1. Gildenberg PL. Whatever happened to stereotactic surgery? Neurosurgery 1987; 20: 983–987.
2. Siegfried J, Rea GL. Thalamotomy for Parkinson's disease. In: Lunsford D, ed. Modern Stereotactic Neurosurgery. Boston: Martinus Nijhoff, 1988:333–340.
3. Laitinen LV. Brain targets in surgery for Parkinson's disease: results of a survey of neurosurgeons. J Neurosurg 1985; 62:349–351.
4. Tasker RR, Lenz FA, Dostrovksy JO, Yamashiro K, Chodakiewitz J, Albe-Fessard DG. The physiological basis of VIM thalamotomy for involuntary movement disorders: In: Struppler A, Weindl A, eds. Clinical Aspects of Sensory Motor Integration. Berlin: Springer-Verlag, 1987.

5. Hassler R, Riechert T, Mundinger F, Umbach W, Ganglberger A. Physiological observations in stereotaxic operations in extrapyramidal motor disturbances. Brain 1960; 83:337–350.

6. Jones EG. Correlation and revised nomenclature of ventral nuclei in the thalamus of human and monkey. Proceedings of the 10th Meeting of the World Society for Stereotactic and Functional Neurosurgery, Maebashi, Japan. Stereotact Funct Neurosurg 1990; 54–55:1–20.

7. Jones EG. Afferent pathways for short latency sensory input to primate motor cortex. In: Motor Mechanisms in Health and Disease. New York: Raven Press, 1983: 111–121.

8. Friedman DP, Jones EG. Thalamic input to areas 3a and 2 in monkeys. J Neurophysiol 1981; 45:59–85.

9. Maendly R, Ruegg DG, Wiesendanger M, Wiesendanger R, Lagowsky J, Hess B. Thalamic relay for group 1 muscle afferents of forelimb nerves in the monkey. J Neurophysiol 1981; 46:901–917.

10. Asanuma C, Thach WT, Jones EG. Cytoarchitectonic delineation of the ventral lateral thalamic region in monkeys. Brain Res Rev 1983; 5:219–235.

11. Albe-Fessard D, Guiot G, Hardy J. Electrophysiological localization and identification of subcortical structures in man by recording spontaneous and evoked activities. Encephalogr Clin Neurophysiol 1963; 15:1052–1053.

12. Jasper HH, Bertrand G. Thalamic units involved in somatic sensation and voluntary and involuntary movements in man. In: Purpura DP, Yahr MD, eds. The Thalamus. New York: Columbia University Press, 1966:365–390.

13. Lenz FA, Tasker RR, Kwan KC, et al. Single unit analysis of the human ventral thalamic nuclear group: correlation of thalamic "tremor" cells with the 3–6 Hz component of parkinsonian tremor. J Neurosci 1988; 8:754–764.

14. Ohye C, Narabayashi H. Physiological study of presumed ventralis intermedius neurons in the human thalamus. J Neurosurg 1979; 50:290–297.

15. Ohye C, Shibazaki T, Hirai T, Wada H, Hirato M, Kawashima Y. Further physiological observations on the ventralis intermedius neurons in the human thalamus. J Neurophysiol 1989; 61:488–500.

16. Lücking HG, Struppler A, Erbel F, Reiss W. Stereotactic recording from human subthalamic structures. In: Somjen Neurophysiology Studies in Man. Amsterdam: Excerpta Medica, 1972:95–99.

17. Struppler A, Lücking CH, Erbel F. Neurophysiological findings during stereotactic operation in thalamus and subthalamus. Confin Neurol 1972; 34:70–73.

18. Bertrand G, Jasper H, Wong A. Microelectrode recording during stereotactic surgery. Clin Neurosurg 1969; 16:328–355.

19. Hardy TL, Bertrand G, Thompson CJ. Position and organization of thalamic cellular activity during diencephalic recording: II: joint and muscle evoked activity. Appl Neurophysiol 1980; 43:28–36.

20. Jones EG, Friedman DP. Projection pattern of functional components of thalamic centrobasal complex on monkey somatosensory cortex. J Neurophysiol 1982; 48: 521–544.

21. Struppler A. Contribution of electromyography to stereotaxy. In: Schaltenbrand G,

Earl Walker A, eds. Stereotaxy of the Human Brain. New York: Thieme-Verlag, 1982: 436–448.

22. Narabayashi H. Muscle tone conducting system and tremor concerned structures. In: Third Symposium on Parkinson's disease. Edinburgh: E&S Livingstone, 1968: 246–251.

23. Birk P, Riescher H, Struppler A, Keidel M. Somatosensory evoked potentials in the ventrolateral thalamus. Appl Neurophysiol 1986; 49:327–335.

24. Struppler A, Lipinski HG. Computer processing and anatomical correlation of somatosensory evoked potentials in VL thalamus. In: Kelly PJ, Kall BA, eds. Computers in Stereotactic Neurosurgery. Cambridge, MA: Blackwell Scientific Publ, 1991.

25. Goto A, Kosaka K, Kubota K, Nakamura R, Narabayashi H. Thalamic potentials from muscle afferents in the human. Arch Neurol 1968; 19:302–309.

26. Hankinson J, McComas AJ, Upton ARM, Wilson P. Properties of somatosensory cells in the human thalamus. J Physiol 1971; 216:23–24.

27. Larson SJ, Sances A. Averaged evoked potentials in stereotaxic surgery. J. Neurosurg 1968; 28:227–232.

28. Yamashiro K, Tasker RR, Iwayama K, et al. Evoked potentials from the human thalamus: correlation with microstimulation and single unit recording. Stereotact Funct Neurosurg 1989; 52:127–135.

29. Struppler A, Gurfinkel V, Mathis J. Hypotonia of central origin and motor performance [abstr] in: Proceedings International Society Pathophysiology I, Moscow, 1991: Sect 1.

30. Keidel M, Klein W, Struppler A. Stretch reflex modification by subthalomotomy: a follow up study in parkinsonian patients. J Psychophysiol 1990; 4:103–114.

31. Struppler A, Plant T, Jahnke MT, Riescher H. Stereoencephalotomy and control of skeletal muscle tone. Stereotact Funct Neurosurg 1990; 54–55:136–139.

32. DeLong Mahlon R. Primate models of movement disorders of basal ganglia origin. TINS 1990; 13:281–285.

33. Bergmann H, Wichmann T, DeLong MR. Amelioration of parkinsonian symptoms by inactivation of the subthalamic nucleus (STN) in MPTP treated monkeys. [abstr] Mov Disord 1990; 5:79, No 284.

34. Brotchie JM, Mitchell IJ, Sambrook MA, Crossman AR. Alleviation of parkinsonism by antagonism of excitatory amino acid transmission in the medial segment of the globus pallidus in rat and primates. Mov Disord 1991; 6:133–138.

35. Alexander GE, Crutcher MD. Functional architecture of basal ganglia circuits: neural substrates of parallel processing. TINS 1990; 13:266–271.

36. Maeda T. Lateral coordinates for nucleus ventralis intermedius target for tremor alleviation. Stereotact Funct Neurosurg 1989; 52:191–199.

37. Lipinski HG, Struppler A. New trends in computer graphics and computer vision to assist functional neurosurgery. Stereotact Funct Neurosurg 1989; 52:234–241.

38. Cerchiari U, Del Panno G, Giorgi C, Garibotto G. 3-D correlation technique for anatomical volumes in functional stereotactic neurosurgery. In: Proceedings of 2nd International Workshop on Time Varying Image Processing and Moving Object Recognition. Florence, September 1986.

39. Tasker RR, Hayrylyshyn P, Organ LW. Computerized graphic display of physiological data collected during human stereotactic surgery. Appl Neurophysiol 1978; 41: 182–187.

40. Thompson CT, Hardy T, Bertrand G. A system for anatomical and functional mapping of the human thalamus. Comput Biomed Res 1977; 10:9–24.

41. Villemure JG, Marchand E, Peters T, et al. Magnetic resonance imaging stereotaxy: recognition and utilization on the commissures. Appl Neurophysiol 1987; 50:57–62.

42. Schad L, Lott S, Schmitt F, Sturm V, Lorenz WJ. Correction of spatial distortion in MR imaging: a prerequisite for accurate stereotaxy. J Comput Assist Tomogr 1987; 11:499–505.

43. Yoshida M. Electrophysiological characterization of human subcortical structures by frequency spectrum analysis of neural noise (field potential) obtained during stereotactic surgery. Proceedings of the Microelectrode Meeting, Evian-les-Bains, France, September 1987. Stereotact Funct Neurosurg 1989; 52:157–163.

44. Mundinger F. Neue stereotaktisch-funktionelle Behandlungsmethode des Torticollis spasmodicus mit Hirnstimulatoren. Med Klinik 1977; 72:1982–1986.

45. Benabid AL, Pollak P, Gervason C, et al. Long term suppression of tremor by chronic stimulation of the ventral intermediate thalamic nucleus. Lancet 1991; 337:403–406.

16

Pathological and Neurochemical Basis of Essential Tremor

Ali H. Rajput
University of Saskatchewan
Saskatoon, Saskatchewan, Canada

I. INTRODUCTION

Essential tremor (ET) has been recognized for more than 100 years and is the most common variety of pathological tremor in humans (1). In spite of remarkably higher prevalence of ET compared with Parkinson's disease (PD) reported in several epidemiological surveys of these two disorders conducted in the same communities (2–7), and that histological and biochemical studies have had a major impact on the understanding of PD, similar studies in ET have been minimal (1).

In this chapter I will review the literature pertinent to the pathological and neurochemical observations in essential tremor.

Only eight autopsies have been reported previously (1), and we have added six more cases (8). In this review, I will also consider the two more recently studied cases, thus bringing the total reported cases of ET pathology in the literature to 16.

II. REASONS FOR THE SCARCITY OF LITERATURE ON ESSENTIAL TREMOR

There are several reasons for the limited scientific literature on this subject. In most ET patients during the early stage and in some patients throughout life, there is no major psychological or functional disability, and the life expectancy in these patients is normal (2). Therefore, the term benign essential tremor has been frequently used to describe this disorder. In several cases ET is dominantly inherited, and the family is well aware of the presence of tremor in more than one generation. Most families are also aware of the lack of specific therapy. The families of the deceased persons, therefore, have limited interest in autopsy studies. The pathological studies have not yet identified any characteristic abnormality; hence, some autopsy reports could have been rejected for publication. Another handicap is the lack of a suitable animal model that would permit in-depth scientific studies.

III. SUSPECTED SITE OF PATHOLOGY

When harmaline is administered to a monkey that has a lesion in the olivodentato-rubral system, the animal develops tremor that has some characteristics of ET (9). In one ET patient, improvement in tremor on the ipsilateral side following cerebellar infarction (10) has been reported. A recent study by Colebatch et al. (11) noted increased cerebellar blood flow in ET patients compared with normal controls. Lee, in his review of ET, concluded that the most likely site of lesion in this disorder is in the rubroolivocerebellar loop (12). All of the foregoing indicate that the possible site of pathology in ET is in the cerebellum or the brainstem loop, connecting the cerebellum with the inferior olive and the red nucleus.

IV. POSSIBLE ASSOCIATION BETWEEN ESSENTIAL TREMOR AND PARKINSON'S DISEASE

Typical ET cases are easily distinguishable from classic PD patients. However, some ET patients during the later stage may develop clinical features of PD—resting tremor (RT) and cogwheeling with minor increase in tone—thus making the distinction from PD difficult. The most common misdiagnosis in ET patients is PD (1) and, in our experience, the most common misdiagnosis in PD is ET.

An epidemiological (13) and a large clinical study (14) each reported a remarkably higher prevalence of PD among the ET cases than expected in the general population. The high coprevalence of the two disorders may indicate that ET patients are predisposed to PD. Alternatively, ET could represent an unusual and slowly progressive form of PD in which the other parkinsonian manifestations emerge late in the course of illness. Since the pathological characteristics in PD (15) are well known, the histological studies focusing on the substantia nigra (SN) and presence of Lewy body (LB) inclusions will help understand the coprevalence of ET and PD. Lewy body inclusions were first described in 1912, but the pathological changes in the SN were not linked with parkinsonism until 1919 (16).

The ET autopsy reports before 1919, therefore, will not be useful in understanding the relation between ET and PD.

V. PATHOLOGICAL FINDINGS

Table 1 is a summary of the 14 known ET autopsies since 1919, including our 8 cases. The two ET autopsy cases before 1919 had brief pathological description and are not included in the summary table.

The 14 patients who had pathological studies will be reviewed in an attempt to identify characteristic anatomical and histological lesion(s).

It is not possible to identify all the areas of brain that were histologically examined in the six cases reported by other workers. In each of our eight patients (cases 7–14), the histological examination included the neocortex and adjacent white matter, basal ganglia, hippocampi, brainstem, and cerebellum. Included was examination of substantia nigra, red nucleus, superior cerebellar peduncle, locus coeruleus, and inferior olives. Hematoxylin and eosin (H&E) staining was done on all sections and special stains were performed only when deemed necessary for the diagnostic accuracy. We did not conduct a formal cell count at any of the sites (8).

Systemic atherosclerosis was noted in 9 of the 14 and cerebral atherosclerosis or arteriosclerosis, with or without cerebral ischemia, was detected in 8 of the 14 cases.

The most common anatomical site of brain abnormality was reported in the basal ganglia—striatum and globus pallidus. The abnormalities in these regions fall into two categories: ischemic changes, and selective neuronal loss.

Evidence of old or recent ischemia in the striatum or the globus pallidus was found in 6 of the 14 cases (see Table 1). Hassler (17) noted ischemic changes in the putamen and the caudate in one case (No. 2). Mylle and van Bogaert (18) reported ischemic changes in the caudate, putamen, and the globus pallidus in their patient (No. 4), and Herskovits and Blackwood (19) detected areas of softening in the putamen in one case (No. 5). We have observed ischemic basal ganglia abnormality in (2) cases (7 and 11).

Selective basal ganglia neuronal loss is reported by Hassler (17) and by Mylle and van Bogaert (20). Hassler noted reduction in the *small* cells in the striatum in two cases (17), whereas Mylle and van Bogaert (20) noted loss of *large* cells in the striatum and the pallidum in one patient (No. 3). These cases of Hassler and of Mylle and van Bogaert were all men, and all had a family history of ET (17,20).

Cerebellar Purkinje loss is reported in 4 of the 14 cases, and dentate nucleus abnormality in 1 case (20). Inferior olive atrophy has been reported in only 1 (4) and gliosis of the superior cerebellar peduncle in 1 case (3).

There is no abnormality reported in the red nucleus or the locus coeruleus and

Table 1 Summary of the 14 Known Essential Tremor Atopsies Since 1919

Author (ref.) yr, c no.	Sex/age at death	Familial or sporadic	Age at onset	Site of tremor	Other pertinent clinical information	Gross and microscopic findings
1. Hassler (17) 1939	Male 71 yr	Familial	45 yr	Hands, head	History of alcoholism	Grossly normal brain microscopically—reduced number of small neurons in the striatum
2. Hassler (17) 1939	Male 80 yr	Familial	Unknown	Hands	Choreoathetoid movements of the feet	Advanced and diffuse cerebral arteriosclerosis; reduced number of small nerve cells in the striatum; small areas of softening in the putamen and caudate; rarefaction of the cerebellar Purkinje cells and laminar atrophy
3. Mylle and van Bogaert (18) 1940	Male 61 yr	Familial	When in his 40s	Arms and head	Family history of psychopathy; patient suffered stroke which resulted in improvement of tremor on the paralyzed side. Patient was in psychiatric hospital at time of death.	Grossly right internal capsule infarction; gliosis of the superior cerebellar peduncles, cerebellar white matter, globus pallidus, and the dentate nuclei; loss of cerebellar Purkinje cells and of large nerve cells in the striatum and the pallidum
4. Mylle and van Bogaert (18) 1940	Female 72 yr	Sporadic	At aged 16 yr	Head, hands	Patient had psychiatric illness and was confined to psychiatric hospital when in her 50s.	Small areas of softening and status cribrosus in caudate and putamen; atrophy and gliosis of the globus pallidus and atrophy of the inferior olive; cerebellar Purkinje cell loss

	Sex/Age	Type	Onset	Tremor	Clinical/cause of death	Pathology
5. Herskovits and Blackwood (19) 1969	Male 68 yr	Familial	Onset in early 40s	Hands, voice, tongue, chin; resting tremor in hands	Death attributed to myocardial infarction	Moderate cerebral atherosclerosis; old right occipital infarct; numerous small hemorrhagic softenings in the putamen
6. Lapresle et al. (41) 1974	Female 74 yr	Sporadic	68 yr	Hands, voice, jaw, tongue	Died of pneumonia	Cerebral atherosclerosis; histologically no abnormalities; no Lewy body inclusions; normal substantia nigra and red nucleus
7. Rajput et al. (8) 1991	Female 78 yr	Familial	Childhood	Hands, head, jaw; resting tremor at ankle	Cerebral ischemia, myocardial infarction and nonprogressive Parkinson's syndrome beginning at aged 60 yr	Left half brain examined histologically; ischemic changes left hippocampus and in the occipital regions of the cortex; status lacunaris and status cribrosus in the globus pallidus and the putamen (right half of brain neurochemical analysis)
8. Rajput et al. (8) 1991	Male 58 yr	Sporadic	Childhood	Upper limbs, head	Had severe anxiety and drug-induced parkinsonism; attempted suicide three times; severe coronary artery disease; died after aortocoronary bypass	Severe generalized atherosclerosis; brain grossly and microscopically normal
9. Rajput et al. (8) 1991	Male 69 yr	Familial	51 yr	Upper limbs, head	Hypertension and leukemia	Brain grossly and microscopically normal

Table 1 Continued

Author (ref.) yr, c no.	Sex/age at death	Familial or sporadic	Age at onset	Site of tremor	Other pertinent clinical information	Gross and microscopic findings
10. Rajput et al. (8) 1991	Male 56 yr	Familial	Childhood	Hands	Hypertension, alcoholism; systemic atherosclerosis; died of presumed cardiac dysrhythmia	Brain grossly and microscopically normal
11. Rajput et al. (8) 1991	Female 83 yr	Sporadic	25 yr	Head, hands	Abdominal aortic aneurysm rupture resulted in death	Multiple lacunes and foci of perivascular atrophy in basal ganglia
12. Rajput et al. (8) 1991	Male 85 yr	Familial	68 yr	Hands, head, voice	Myocardial infarction, atrial fibrillation and leukemia	Brain normal grossly and microscopically
13. Rajput (unpublished)	Female 62 yr	Familial	30 yr	Upper limbs	Depression; chronic bronchitis; hypertension; drug-induced parkinsonism; died of neuroleptic malignant syndrome	Generalized atherosclerosis; microscopic foci of hemmorhage in the right occipital hypothalamus, and medial thalamus; midbrain, pons, medulla, cerebellum, substantia nigra, locus, coeruleus normal; no Lewy body inclusions
14. Rajput (unpublished)	Male 67 yr	Familial	61 yr	Upper limbs	Angina pectoris; depression; paranoia; given phenothiazines and ECT; drug-induced parkinsonism; myocardial infarction resulting in death	Generalized atherosclerosis; cerebral atherosclerosis; myocardial infarction (recent); brain grossly and histologically normal; no Lewy body inclusions

the SN has been reported normal for age (21) in all ET cases. None of the 14 cases revealed LB inclusions in the SN or at any other site.

VI. LABORATORY INVESTIGATIONS IN ESSENTIAL TREMOR PATIENTS

There are very few studies aimed at identifying biological markers in ET. Results of routine laboratory investigations of the blood, urine, and cerebrospinal fluid (CSF) are normal (1). Barbeau and co-workers noted that hyperthyroidism "appeared" to be more frequent in ET and in "essential tremor-related parkinsonism" kindreds (22,23). There are no other studies to substantiate that (1). Other laboratory investigations, such as electroencephalogram, pneumoencephalogram, and so forth, are nonspecific and unrewarding for localizing the site of the disorder in ET (1).

Colebatch et al. (11) conducted cerebral blood flow studies with positron emission tomography (PET) while the subjects held the arms outstretched against gravity. These studies revealed an increased cerebellar blood flow in the four ET patients compared to the normal controls.

Williams et al. compared tetrahydrobiopterin (a hydroxylase cofactor) levels in the cerebrospinal fluid of ten ET patients and normal controls (24). Lower levels of tetrahydrobiopterins in the ET were noted. This observation, however, was not specific for ET, as lower levels were also noted in Parkinson's disease, progressive supranuclear palsy, Alzheimer's disease, and Huntington's disease patients.

Stibler and Kjellin studied CSF proteins with isoelectric focusing and electrophoresis in 16 ET patients (25). They detected abnormal CSF proteins in 94% of the ET cases, but similar abnormalities were also noted in the cases with cerebellar dysfunction consequence to chronic alcoholism.

Barkhatova and Ivanova-Smolenskaia studied catecholamine metabolic indices in 40 ET patients (26). Urinary catecholamine (especially the norepinephrine) excretion was considerably reduced in the ET patients, but the urinary level of the catecholamine precursor dihydroxyphenylalanine (DOPA) was normal. The urinary excretion of vanillylmandelic acid, the major metabolite of epinephrine and norepinephrine tended to be low. Blood catecholamines levels, on the other hand, were normal in ET (26). They concluded that the general catecholamine pool in the body in ET patients is reduced (26).

Pharmacological effects of different drugs is another method for identifying biological markers in ET. Alcohol intake may temporarily relieve tremor in 60–80% of ET (1). The widely used, and perhaps the most effective, drug for the ET today is the β-adrenergic blocking agent propranolol. Neither alcohol nor propranolol, however, has specific tremorlytic effect on ET. Action tremor caused by other illnesses, including Parkinson's disease, also may improve with these agents (27).

There is no literature report on the neurochemical analysis of an ET brain. We

Table 2 Concentrations of Dopamine in Autopsied Human
Brain: Controls vs Essential Tremor[a]

Brain region	Controls $N = 8$	Essential tremor $N - 1$	Percentage of controls
Caudate head			
Rostral	2.94 ± 0.47	1.51	−49
Intermediate	4.03 ± 0.64	1.68	−51
Caudal	3.63 ± 0.45	0.45	−88
Putamen			
Rostral	5.33 ± 0.77	1.80	−66
Intermediate	4.73 ± 0.52	1.81	−62
Caudal	5.47 ± 0.90	2.52	−54

[a]Values (ng/mg tissue) represent mean ± SE of eight controls and one
patient with essential tremor (case 7).

have conducted a preliminary study in one-half of the brain in one patient (No. 7).
Table 2 shows dopamine levels in different striatal regions in this patient compared
with age-matched control brains (28).

VII. DISCUSSION

From the monkey experiments (9), cerebellar infarction resulting in ipsilateral ET
improvement in one case (10), and PET scanning studies (11), the cerebellum or
olivocerebellorubral loop have been considered as the most likely site of abnormality in ET.

Routine histological studies of the cerebellum have revealed Purkinje cell
loss in only 4 of the 14 autopsies. Each of these patients had history of electrocon-
vulsive therapy or cerebral hypoxia, which probably accounted for the cell loss. In
one of these cases, dentate nucleus cell loss was noted. In the same patient superior
cerebellar peduncle ischemic changes were observed. On the other hand, the
cerebellar histological structure was normal in 10 of the 14 autopsies. Therefore,
the cerebellar abnormalities reported in the literature to date cannot be the basis of
ET. Inferior olive abnormality (most likely due to ischemia) was noted in one
patient (No. 4); however, none of the patients had pathological changes in the red
nucleus.

The absence of consistent histological abnormality in the olivocerebellorubral
system on routine microscopic examination, does not rule out the possibility that
an, as yet unidentified, abnormality in these regions exists. Careful studies using
advanced staining techniques, including immunohistochemistry and electron
microscopy, may provide valuable information in the future.

The most common site of the abnormality reported in the 14 ET autopsies is in the basal ganglia. Seven of the 14 (50%) cases had basal ganglia abnormality. In 6 of the 14 cases, ischemic basal ganglia changes—status lacunaris or status cribrosus were noted. Status cribrosus, however, is common in the elderly and may or may not be associated with neurological abnormalities. These abnormalities, therefore, cannot constitute the basis of ET.

Selective basal ganglia cell loss was noted by Hassler (17) and by Mylle and van Bogaert (20). One case of Hassler (No. 2) and the case reported by Mylle and van Bogaert (No. 3), who had selective cell loss, also had evidence of basal ganglia ischemia. In view of the contradictory observations on the morphology of the vulnerable cell type and the lack of similar observation by other workers, specific cell loss in the striatum is not the pathological basis of ET.

No striatal or pallidal abnormality was detected in the remaining half of the patients, indicating that the reported basal ganglia abnormality is not related to the production of ET.

Resting tremor is a well-known and almost a constant feature in Parkinson's disease (29), and cogwheel rigidity is another characteristic feature of PD. Both these may also be seen in some advanced essential tremor patients. Therefore, the clinical distinction between ET and PD is sometimes difficult (28,30–32).

Some studies indicate an extraordinarily higher (24–35 times) prevalence of PD in the ET patients than in the general population (13,14). If those observations were accurate, there are at least two possible explanations: ET is an unusual and slowly evolving variant of PD, or ET patients are excessively predisposed to PD. Since the disorder of PD is characteristic and easily recognizable (15), these hypotheses can be tested using the analysis of the current autopsy literature.

Lewy body inclusions that are considered the hallmark of PD (33) are detected in 3.8–12.8% of the brains of neurologically normal (but presumed presymptomatic PD) elderly general population (33,34). If the ET cases had 24 times higher than expected coprevalence of PD (14), 91% (3.8% × 24) or more ET cases would manifest LB inclusions. None of the 14 ET autopsies reported since 1919 had LB inclusions. Additionally, no SN neuronal loss out of keeping with the age of the patient was noted (21). Even if the prevalence of PD in ET were twice that of the general population, we would expect that 1 of the 14 autopsy cases would have LB inclusions. The normal SN cell complement and the absence of LB inclusions in the reported literature are, therefore, strong indications that ET is neither an unusual variant of PD, nor represents an extraordinary risk for PD. Similar conclusions have also been made in some clinical studies (2,35,36).

Parkinson's syndrome (PS) is a clinical entity resulting from a variety of causes (37). In three (Nos. 7, 13, and 14) of our eight ET patients, a second diagnosis of PS was made. In case 7, the PS was attributed to status cribrosus and lacunaris in the basal ganglia, and in the other two patients, the PS was consequent to neuroleptic agents.

Reduced striatal dopamine (DA) (38) levels and substantia nigra neuronal loss (21) are consequent to normal aging. It is possible that the normal age-related striatal DA loss modifies the tremor pattern in some ET cases, resulting in RT, and leads to mild cogwheel rigidity. For the same reason, the elderly ET patients may be predisposed to drug-induced parkinsonism (39).

Biochemical analysis of the ET brain is limited to only one patient who also had mild parkinsonism. On the basis of recently reported subregional pattern of DA loss in the caudate and putamen of Parkinson's disease patients (40), studies of DA levels in the striatum of this patient were conducted. The pattern in PD is characterized by specific rostral–caudal and dorsal–ventral gradients. Analysis of the subregional pattern of the dopamine loss in the striatum of our ET patient revealed a different pattern from that observed in PD (40). In PD patients, the putamen is affected much more than the caudate by the dopamine loss, whereas in this ET case, it was the caudal portion of the head of the caudate that suffered the most severe dopamine loss (see Table 2). The subregional pattern of striatal DA loss suggests that this ET patient was not afflicted with idiopathic Parkinson's disease (28). The significance of these DA findings to ET, however, remain to be elucidated.

VIII. SUMMARY

There is no known anatomical site or histological abnormality characteristic of ET. Careful analysis of pathological studies indicates that the risk of PD among the ET cases is comparable with that in the general population. From animal experiments, clinical observations, and PET-scanning studies, there is strong indication that the cerebellum or its brainstem connections are critical in the production of ET. Future studies using more advanced histological techniques and chemical analyses of the brain are necessary to identify the site and the nature of lesion(s) in ET.

REFERENCES

1. Larsen TA, Calne DB. Essential tremor. Clin Neuropharmacol 1983; 6:185–206.
2. Rajput AH, Offord KP, Beard CM, Kurland LT. Essential tremor in Rochester, Minnesota: a 45-year study. J Neurol Neurosurg Psychiatry 1984; 47:466–470.
3. Rajput AH, Offord KP, Beard CM, Kurland LT. Epidemiology of parkinsonism: incidence, classification, and mortality. Ann Neurol 1984; 16:278–282.
4. Rautakorpi I, Takala J, Marttila RJ, Sievers K, Rinne UK. Essential tremor in a Finnish population. Acta Neurol Scand 1982; 66:58–67.
5. Marttila RJ, Rinne UK. Epidemiology of Parkinson's disease in Finland. Acta Neurol Scand 1976; 53:81–102.
6. Haerer AF, Anderson DW, Schoenberg BS. Prevalence of essential tremor: results from the Copiah County study. Arch Neurol 1982; 39:750–751.

7. Schoenberg BS, Anderson DW, Haerer AF. Prevalence of Parkinson's disease in the biracial population of Copiah County, Mississippi. Neurology 1985; 35:841–845.

8. Rajput AH, Rozdilsky B, Ang L, Rajput A. Clinicopathological observations in essential tremor. Report of 6 cases. Neurology 1991; 41:1422–1424.

9. Lamarre Y, Animal models of physiological, essential and parkinsonian-like tremors. In: Findley LJ, Capildeo R, eds. Movement Disorders: Tremor. London: Macmillan Press, 1984:183–194.

10. Dupuis MJM, Delwaide PJ, Boucquey D, Gonsette RE. Homolateral disappearance of essential tremor after cerebellar stroke. Mov Disord 1989; 4:183–187.

11. Colebatch JG, Findley LJ, Frackowiak RSJ, Marsden CD, Brooks DJ. Preliminary report: activation of the cerebellum in essential tremor. Lancet 1990; 336:1028–1030.

12. Lee RG. The pathophysiology of essential tremor. In: Marsden CD, Fahn S, eds. Movement Disorders 2. London: Butterworths & Co, 1987:423–437.

13. Hornabrook RW, Nagurney JT. Essential tremor in Papua, New Guinea. Brain 1976; 99:659–672.

14. Geraghty JJ, Jankovic J, Zetusky WJ. Association between essential tremor and Parkinson's disease. Ann Neurol 1985; 17:329–333.

15. Duvoisin R, Golbe LI. Toward a definition of Parkinson's disease. Neurology 1989; 39:746.

16. Alvord EC Jr, Forno LS. Pathology. In: Koller WC, ed. Handbook of Parkinson's Disease. New York: Marcel Dekker, 1987:209–236.

17. Hassler R. Zur pathologischen anatomie des senilen und des parkinsonistischen tremor. J Psychol Neurol 1939; 49:193–230.

18. Mylle G, van Bogaert L. Du tremblement essential non familial. Monatsschr Psychiatr Neurol 1948; 115:80–90.

19. Herskovits E, Blackwood W. Essential (familial, hereditary) tremor: a case report. J Neurol Neurosurg Psychiatry 1969; 32:509–511.

20. Mylle G, van Bogaert L. Etudes anatomo-cliniques de syndromes hypercinetiques complexes. Monatsschr Psychiat Neurol 1940; 103:28–43.

21. Thiessen B, Rajput AH, Laverty W, Desai HB. Age, environments and the number of substantia nigra neurons. In: Streifler MB, Korczyn AD, Melamed E, Youdim MBH, eds. Advances in Neurology. New York: Raven Press, 1990:201–206.

22. Barbeau A, Pourcher E. New data on the genetics of parkinson's disease. Can J Neurol Sci 1982; 9:53–60.

23. Roy M, Boyer L, Barbeau A. A prospective study of 50 cases of familial Parkinson's disease. Can J Neurol Sci 1983; 10:37–42.

24. Williams AC, Levine RA, Chase TN, Lovenberg W, Calne DB. CSF hydroxylase cofactor levels in some neurological diseases. J Neurol Neurosurg Psychiatry 1980; 43:735–738.

25. Stibler H, Kjellin KG. Isoelectric focusing and electrophoresis of the CSF proteins in tremor of different origins. J Neurol Sci 1976; 30:269–285.

26. Barkhatova VP, Ivanova-Smolenskaia IA. Catecholamine metabolism in essential tremor. Zh Nevropatol Psikhiatr 1990; 90(3):10–14.

27. Rajput AH, Jamieson H, Hirsch S, Quraishi A. Relative Efficacy of alcohol and propranolol in action tremor. Can J Neurol Sci 1975; 2:31–35.

28. Rajput AH, Rozdilsky B, Kish S, Hornykiewicz O. Parkinson's disease association with essential tremor [abstr]. Mov Disord 1990; 5(suppl 1):14.
29. Rajput AH, Rozdilsky B, Ang L. Occurrence of resting tremor in Parkinson's disease. Neurology 1991; 41:1298–1299.
30. Findley LJ, Gresty MA, Halmagyi GM. Tremor and cogwheel phenomena and clonus in Parkinson's disease. J Neurol Neurosurg Psychiatry 1981; 44:534–546.
31. Salisachs P, Findley LJ. Problems in the differential diagnosis of essential tremor. In: Findley LJ, Capildeo R, eds. Movement Disorders: Tremor. London: Macmillan Press, 1984:219–224.
32. Marsden CD. Origins of Normal and Pathological Tremor. In: Findley LJ, Capildeo R, eds. Movement Disorders: Tremor. London: Macmillan Press, 1984:37–84.
33. Gibb WRG, Lees AJ. The relevance of the Lewy body to the pathogenesis of idiopathic Parkinson's disease. J Neurol Neurosurg Psychiatry 1988; 51:745–752.
34. Gibb WR. Idiopathic Parkinson's disease and the Lewy body disorders. Neuropathol Appl Neurobiol 1986; 12:223–234.
35. Cleeves L, Findley LJ, Koller W. Lack of association between essential tremor and Parkinson's disease. Ann Neurol 1988; 24:23–26.
36. Marttila RJ, Rautakorpi I, Rinne UK. The relation of essential tremor to Parkinson's disease. J Neurol Neurosurg Psychiatry 1984; 47:734–735.
37. Jellinger K. The pathology of parkinsonism. In: Marsden CD, Fahn S, eds. Movement Disorders 2. London: Butterworths & Co, 1987:124–165.
38. Martin WRW, Palmer MR, Patlak CS, Calne DB. Nigrostriatal function in humans studied with positron emission tomography. Ann Neurol 1989; 26:535–542.
39. Rajput AH, Rozdilsky B, Hornykiewicz O, Shannak K, Lee T. Reversible drug-induced parkinsonism. Clinicopathologic study of two cases. Arch Neurol 1982; 39:644–646.
40. Kish SJ, Shannak K, Hornykiewicz O. Uneven pattern of dopamine loss in the striatum of patients with idiopathic Parkinson's disease. N Engl J Med 1988; 318:876–880.
41. Lapresle J, Rondot P, Said G. Tremblement idiopathique de repos, d'attitude et d'action: etude anatomo-clinique d'une observation. Rev Neurol Paris 1974; 130:343–348.

17

Essential Tremor and Other Movement Disorders

Joseph Jankovic
Baylor College of Medicine
Houston, Texas

I. INTRODUCTION

Two or more movement disorders may coexist in a patient because they are pathogenically linked or because of a chance occurrence. The study of such associations may provide insights into the pathogenesis of the various disorders. Essential tremor (ET) is the most common movement disorder and, therefore, its association with other disorders may be purely coincidental (1–3). This is particularly true if ET is defined as a monosymptomatic illness. In this case, ET-like postural tremor associated with other diseases must be considered some other clinical entity. Alternatively, it is possible that postural tremor associated with some other disorders indeed represents ET; hence, the coexistence of the two disorders may be pathophysiologically important. Postural ET-like tremor is frequently seen in patients with Parkinson's disease (PD), dystonia, and hereditary peripheral neuropathy. This review will focus on the relations between these three disorders and postural tremor which, for the purposes of this review, will be termed ET. Our understanding of these relations will immensely improve, once disease-specific biological markers are identified. However, until then, a thoughtful examination of these relations may improve the understanding of not only ET, but also of the associated diseases.

II. ESSENTIAL TREMOR AND PARKINSON'S DISEASE

Whether ET and PD are pathogenically related has been debated since 1817, when
James Parkinson first attempted to differentiate paralysis agitans from senile
(essential) tremor (4). One of the chief reasons for the controversy is that the
diagnostic criteria for either ET or PD have not been well defined. Furthermore,
the two disorders share common clinical features. Parkinson's disease and ET may
be difficult to differentiate clinically when a prominent postural tremor is the
dominant manifestation and PD symptoms are relatively mild, and when resting
tremor, cogwheeling, reduced arm swing, and bradykinesia are present in patients
with typical ET. Since ET is difficult to diagnose in patients with PD, certain
criteria must be established before the diagnosis of ET–PD combination can be
accepted. We insist on the presence of clinically evident postural tremor for at least
5 years *before* the onset of PD symptoms, represented by at least three of the four
cardinal features: resting tremor, rigidity, bradykinesia, and postural instability.
These criteria, however, cannot be validated until a disease-specific biological
marker is identified. Without it, the question whether parkinsonian features in ET
represent one end of the spectrum of ET, or whether they are a manifestation of
coexisting PD, will be difficult to answer with any degree of certainty. Alternatively, bradykinesia, rigidity, rest tremor, postural instability, and other parkinsonian findings in ET patients may be due to a disorder other than PD. Since the
diagnosis of PD cannot be confirmed without an autopsy, the term *parkinsonism*
(P), rather than PD, may be more appropriate. This implies that the parkinsonian
features associated with another movement disorder are either due to PD or to
some other parkinsonian disorder.

Evidence for an association between ET and P has been provided by some (5–
11), but not all (12,13), studies. In a population study, Hornabrook and Nagurney
found the risk of PD to be 35 times higher in patients with ET than in the control
population (10). We found 25 patients with P among 130 with ET (5). Although our
study was based on a selected population of patients referred to our movement
disorders clinic, the 18.5% prevalence of PD among these ET patients seemed
much higher than the expected 0.35% prevalence estimated from a door-to-door
survey of a general population (14). In another study of 350 ET patients, 71
(20.2%) had associated P (6). The following diagnostic criteria for ET were
required: (1) intermittent or constant tremor of hand, head, or voice present for at
least 1 year; (2) tremor must be predominantly postural; and (3) absence of other
diseases, toxins, or drugs that can cause tremor. Positive family history and
attenuation of tremor with alcohol, propranolol, or primidone supported, but were
not required for, the diagnosis of ET. The distribution of age at onset of tremor
showed a bimodal distribution with peaks at second and sixth decades for both
groups of patients: ET with P and ET without P. Although most patients in both
groups had tremor of head and hand, those with ET–P combination had more

tremor in their legs compared with the group of patients with ET alone (21.1% vs 11.1%, $p < 0.05$) (Table 1). Furthermore, patients with ET alone were more likely to have dystonia than patients with ET–P ($p < 0.001$). There were no significant differences in sex ratio, age at onset, family history, or response to treatment.

In contrast with ours and some other studies suggesting possible link between ET and PD (5–11), Cleeves et al. (12) concluded that the two disorders were unrelated. They studied 237 patients with ET, 100 PD patients, and 100 normal control subjects, and found mild extrapyramidal signs, such as reduced arm swing, abnormal posture, bradykinesia, and masked facies in 4.5% of their ET patients. These parkinsonian signs were attributed by the authors to normal aging, which may possibly explain the relatively low prevalence of P among their ET patients. In our patients with the ET–PD combination, the parkinsonian symptoms were more disabling than the ET symptoms and were the reasons for referral to the movement disorder clinic. It must be emphasized, however, that the methods used in ours and other clinical studies have significant limitations. For example, because ET must be present before the onset of PD symptoms, the diagnosis of preexisting ET may be difficult to make in a patient who is chiefly troubled by PD. Many patients with ET are not disabled by their postural (ET) tremor before the onset of their PD symptoms and, therefore, the history of preexisting tremor in patients with PD may not be volunteered by the patient or spouse, and the presence of tremor is often difficult to verify without an examination. Furthermore, it is not

Table 1 ET Versus ET–P

Variable	ET without parkinsonism $N = 279$	ET with parkinsonism $N = 71$	p
Male (%)	49.0	57.9	NS
Age at onset	40.2 ± 22.1	38.5 ± 21.0	NS
Anatomical (%)			
Hand	88.5	94.3	NS
Head	41.9	36.6	NS
Voice	19.0	11.1	NS
Leg	11.8	21.1	<0.05
Associated (%)			
Dystonia	53.2	21.1	<0.001
Family history	63.0	59.1	NS
Effectiveness (%)			
Alcohol	65.0 (76/117)	74.0 (21/27)	NS
Propranolol	64.3 (18/28)	100.0 (4/4)	NS
Primidone	75.0 (12/16)	50.0 (1/2)	NS

uncommon for patients with ET to wrongly attribute their tremor, and the tremor in their relatives, to a natural consequence of aging, anxiety, alcoholism, and other reasons. By paying careful attention to these potential pitfalls, we found 8.5% prevalence of ET among our 1288 PD patients, nearly three times greater that the 3% prevalence noted in the 100 PD patients studied by Cleeves et al. (12). In the last 10 years we have prospectively collected data on 504 patients with ET, 110 (21.8%) of whom later developed parkinsonian symptoms. This figure is nearly identical with the estimated prevalence (18.5 and 20.2%) of P among ET patients based on an analysis of retrospective data (5,6). Since we did not include patients in whom postural tremor developed *after* the onset of parkinsonian symptoms and, thus, excluded those who may have developed ET later in life (after onset of PD), our estimated prevalence rates of ET–P may be actually falsely low.

Another evidence in support of an etiological link between PD and ET is the relatively high frequency of familial tremor among patients with PD. Barbeau and Pourcher (7) found that 17 of 67 patients with young-onset PD (onset of symptoms before aged 40) had familial history of ET. They suggested that these patients had increased genetic susceptibility to PD. In another study of 50 families of patients with young-onset PD, Roy et al. (8) found relatively high prevalence of ET in family members, and the authors classified 34 of these 50 families as "essential tremor-related parkinsonism." Cleeves et al. found that 15% of PD patients had family history of tremor, compared with only 6% of the control population (12). This difference, however, failed to reach statistical significance, probably partly because of a small sample size. Among 159 PD patients studied by Lang et al. (11), there were 17% with family history of tremor compared with 5.6% of controls ($p < 0.01$). We found that 21% of our patients with PD had at least one first-degree relative with tremor. It is doubtful that the high frequency of tremor among family members of PD patients can be explained by a selection bias, since only 11% of carefully studied normal controls, spouses of patients referred to our clinic, had tremor among first-degree relatives (14a). Similarly, only 11% of our 99 patients with progressive supranuclear palsy (PSP), a nongenetic neurodegenerative disorder, had family history of tremor. Further analysis showed that among 1874 parents and siblings of patients with PD, there were 96 (5.1%) with tremor; tremor was present in 152 of 650 (23.4%) relations of patients with ET and 91 of 439 (20.7%) relatives of patients with ET–P. In contrast, only 12 of 462 (2.6%) relations of patients with PSP and 10 of 448 (2.2%) of relations of normal controls had tremor. We also found that parents with tremor lived nearly 10 years longer than those without tremor, confirming earlier anecdotal evidence that familial tremor confers some antiaging influence.

The controversy about a relation between PD and ET will be resolved when a diagnostic marker for either or both diseases is found. Until then, some clues may be provided by in vivo studies using positron emission tomography (PET) and by postmortem studies of brains. Brooks et al. found that the mean influx constant for striatal ^{18}F-dopa uptake was lower in eight patients with postural familial tremor (four also had rest tremor) compared with normal age-matched controls, but this difference did not reach statistical significance (15). However, two of ten patients with sporadic and predominantly postural tremor had subnormal putamen ^{18}F-dopa uptake, and both had subsequently developed parkinsonism. Although the authors concluded that the PET studies failed to provide evidence of nigral abnormality in patients with familial postural tremor and that the presence of cogwheeling and reduced arm swing were not useful predictors of nigral disfunction, long-term follow-up is needed to explain why some patients with familial postural tremor have ^{18}F-dopa uptake in a low range. Re-analysis of the data suggest that the 13% reduction in ^{18}F-dopa uptake may indeed be significant (15a). In a postmortem study of nine brains of patients clinically diagnosed as ET, three of whom had parkinsonian symptoms, Rajput et al. (16) found over a 50% reduction in dopamine in all regions of the basal ganglia in one patient. This was attributed to a combination of status cribrosus and age-related decline in striatal dopamine. In the other two patients, the clinically evident parkinsonism was attributed to neuroleptic drugs, and the authors proposed that ET patients were predisposed to neuroleptic-induced parkinsonism. Although Lewy bodies were not found in these brains, it is possible that nigral abnormality may be more evident in more advanced ET–P combination. The contention that ET patients are particularly susceptible to develop neuroleptic-induced parkinsonism has been supported by recent studies of Gimenez-Roldan and Mateo (17). In 24 of their patients with cinnarizine-induced P, they found 56% with at least one family member having tremor. This contrasted with 17% frequency of familial tremor among 124 patients with PD and only 6% in nonneurological controls. Genetic predisposition, as a potential risk factor for drug-induced movement disorders, is of growing interest. In one study of 16 patients with metoclopramide-induced movement disorders, we found a family history of movement disorders, particularly ET, in a third of all subjects (18).

Although current theories about the etiology of PD seem to favor "environmental" over "genetic" hypotheses, the confirmation of a pathogenetic link between ET and PD may add to the importance of genetic factors in the pathogenesis of at least some forms of PD. The "tremor-dominant" form of PD, for example, appears to be more likely associated with family history of tremor than the "postural instability–gait difficulty" form (19). It is possible that the tremor-dominant PD is more related to ET than the other forms. Additional indirect evidence in support of the hypothesis that PD and ET may be pathogenically related is the observation the certain disorders, such as orthostatic tremor (20) and dystonia (21–25) may occur in both disorders.

III. ESSENTIAL TREMOR AND DYSTONIA

The frequency coexistence of tremor and dystonia, although recognized by clinicians, is also a controversial subject. Baxter and Lal (22) found that 12 of 100 patients with ET had dystonic symptoms. Some patients with postural hand tremor also have dystonic writer's cramp, a form of task-specific focal dystonia (26–30). In a study of 28 patients with task-specific movement disorders, 10 had a combination of focal tremor and dystonia (27). Ravits et al. (28) reported four patients with primary writing tremor and suggested this task-specific tremor was a variant of dystonia. Marsden and Sheehy (30) proposed that patients who presented with primary writing tremor had a variant of ET or a tremulous form of dystonia.

Essential tremor is often defined as a monosymptomatic disorder, but this definition may be too restrictive, and the presence of related disorders should not exclude the diagnosis of ET. For example, ET is often associated with dystonia, and dystonic patients often have postural tremor, clinically similar to ET. In a detailed analysis of 350 patients with ET, we found 165 (47.1%) with coexistent dystonia (6). Cervical dystonia (26.8%) was most common, followed by writer's cramp (13.7%), blepharospasm (7.4%), and laryngeal dystonia (4%) (Table 2). Both groups, ET without dystonia and ET with dystonia (ET–D), showed a bimodal distribution of age at onset, with peaks at second and sixth decades. There were more females in ET–D group (58.5%) then in ET group (43.3%), and P was more likely to develop in ET patients without dystonia than in those with dystonia ($p < 0.001$). There was no difference between these two groups in the anatomical distribution of tremor, family history, or response to alcohol, propranolol, and primidone (Table 3). Again, it is important to emphasize that this study is based on a group of selected patients referred to a specialty clinic. Patients with more severe symptoms of ET and those with associated neurological conditions may be more likely to be referred to a movement disorders clinic. Although the results of this study should not be extrapolated to the ET population in general, the findings are applicable to a patient population seen in specialized clinics and may provide evidence that ET and dystonia are pathogenically related.

Table 2 Distribution of Dystonia in ET Patients

$N = 350$		
Dystonia	165	(47.1%)
Cervical	94	(26.8%)
Writer's cramp	48	(13.7%)
Blepharospasm	26	(7.4%)
Laryngeal spasm	14	(4.0%)
Cranial–cervical	9	(2.5%)
Others	21	(6.0%)

Table 3 ET Versus ET–D

Variable	ET without dystonia N = 185	ET with dystonia N = 165	p
Male (%)	56.7	41.5	<0.05
Age at onset (yr)	42.5 ± 21.81	36.6 ± 21.4	NS
Anatomical (%)			
Hand	92.4	86.7	NS
Head	37.3	44.8	NS
Voice	16.7	18.1	NS
Leg	7.0	9.7	NS
Associated (%)			
Parkinsonism	30.2	9.1	<0.001
Family history	61.6	63.6	NS
Effectiveness (%)			
Alcohol	60.8 (45/74)	72.8 (51/70)	NS
Propranolol	73.7 (14/19)	62.5 (8/13)	NS
Primidone	71.4 (10/14)	75.0 (3/4)	NS

Although tremor is frequently found in patients with dystonia, it is not always clear whether the oscillatory movement is a form of dystonia; hence, a dystonic tremor, or whether it represents coexistent ET. Couch noted that 26 of 30 patients with idiopathic spasmodic torticollis had evidence of ET (21). In a study of 100 patients with cranial–cervical dystonia (31), a third were found to have postural tremor, phenomenologically similar to ET. In a separate study involving 300 patients with cervical dystonia, we found head–neck tremor in 60%, and 32% had postural tremor in other body parts (32). We defined dystonic tremor of the head–neck region as a tremor that increased in amplitude as the patient resisted the force of the primary contracting muscles; ET of the head–neck region was presumably independent of the head position. This separation, however, was not always possible and, in some patients, dystonic tremor may have been superimposed on or coexisted with ET in the same body part. Some investigators argue that the postural tremor seen in patients with dystonia has different clinical characteristics, such as an irregularity and a broader range of frequencies, asymmetry, and the presence of associated myoclonus, which distinguish this tremor from ET (33). Three separate large series of cervical dystonia found that 21 to 27% of all such patients have postural hand tremor that is phenomenologically similar to ET (32,32a,32b). This frequency is much higher than that found in one recent study in which only 8 of 193 (4.1%) patients with cervical dystonia were considered to have ET (32c). The implication from these and other studies (34) is that postural tremor, phenomenologically identical with ET, may precede or be the sole manifestation of dystonia. Our own studies suggest that postural hand tremor, frequently noted in patients with dystonia, even when distant from the site of tremor (e.g., hand tremor in patients with cranial–cervical dystonia), cannot be clinically differentiated from typical ET. The lack of demographic and other differences between ET and ET–P group and between ET and ET–D group (see Tables 1 and 3) supports the notion that ET is a single disease entity and that ET–D and ET–P combinations represent a spectrum of the same disease, namely, ET (6). This dilemma will be relatively easy to resolve once an ET-specific genetic marker is identified. The application of ET- and dystonia-specific genetic markers in large kindreds with dystonia and postural tremor (35), may elucidate the mechanism of this association. The exclusion of the DYTI locus on chromosome 9q32–34 in families with ET suggests that dystonia and ET are not genetically linked or that a mutation other than DYTI is responsible for the frequent association of dystonia and ET (35a,35b). Another possibility is that postural tremor and dystonia are linked pathophysiologically, rather than genetically.

IV.   ESSENTIAL TREMOR AND HEREDITARY PERIPHERAL NEUROPATHY

The coexistence of hereditary motor–sensory neuropathy (HMSN) and ET has been previously recognized, but the nature of this association is still not understood (36–42). We studied four unrelated patients with the combination of HMSN, ET, P, and blepharospasm (Table 4). The occurrence of these disorders in the probands and in some of their relatives suggests that a genetic linkage exists between HMSN and these movement disorders. Clinical, neurophysiological and genetic characterization of such families may provide insight into the etiology of these progressive neurological disorders.

Table 4   Coexistence of HMSN with ET

Pt/sex/ age	HMSN			ET (age at onset)	Bleph (age at onset)	Parkinsonism (age at onset)
	Age at onset	NCV[a]				
		Per	Med			
1/M/64	9	15	0	54	53	60
2/M/78	8	30	42	53	75	76
3/M/50	<1	32	43	23	47	44
4/M/79				20	69	69

[a]NCV, nerve conduction velocity; Per, peroneal nerve; Med, median nerve; Bleph, blepharospasm.

Patient 1. The proband of this large family was a 64-year-old man who had had progressive weakness in his feet and hands since aged 9. He was able to walk independently until aged 52, when he began to fall and needed a cane. He also noted weakness in his hands, and a year later he had involuntary squinting of his eyes. Because of progressive blepharospasm, which prevented him from driving and practically rendered him blind, he had bilateral facial nerve resection at aged 58. This partially controlled his blepharospasm, but the procedure was complicated by residual left facial weakness. He also noted bilateral action and postural hand tremor, which increased in amplitude and interfered with writing, feeding, and other activities of daily living. At aged 60, he noted progressive slowness and postural instability and, on examination, he had marked hypomimia and left facial weakness; marked atrophy of small muscles of both hands, with clawlike deformities; and atrophy of distal forearm muscles (Fig. 1). There was also marked atrophy of the anterior compartment of both legs, with high foot arches and hammertoe deformities (Fig. 2). The peripheral nerves did not seem hypertrophied on palpation. A marked 4- to 5-Hz supination–pronation tremor was present in both hands at rest; a high amplitude flexion–extension tremor occurred when arms were outstretched in front of his body and when he held them in a "wing-beating" position. The tremor was also present on finger-to-nose test, but

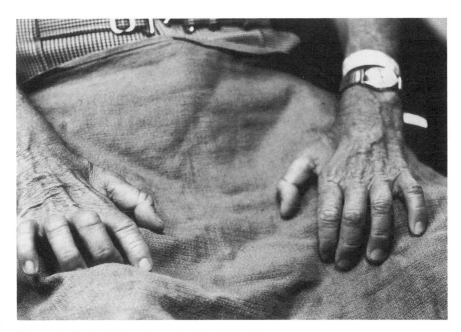

Figure 1 Patient 1 showing marked hand atrophy.

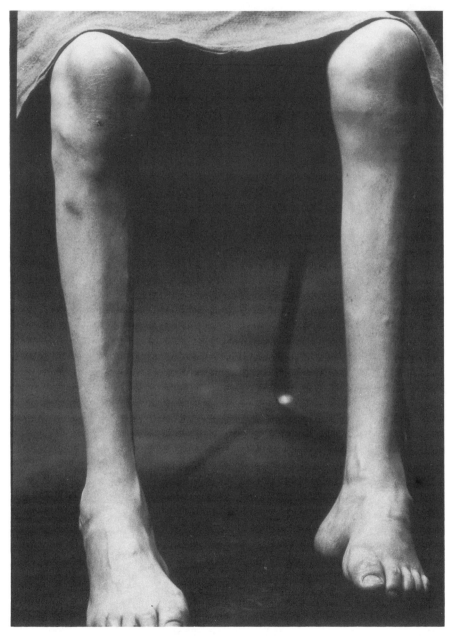

Figure 2 Patient 1 showing marked distal leg atrophy and high arches.

there was no dysdiadochokinesia. He had moderate cogwheel rigidity and body bradykinesia, and marked weakness in both hands and distal legs. The tendon reflexes were absent, and the plantar response was flexor. Vibratory and position sense were absent in both hands and feet, and there was a moderate impairment of light-touch and pain in the same glove–stocking distribution. His gait was high-steppage and unsteady, and he needed assistance with ambulation.

The blood and cerebrospinal fluid (CSF) studies, electroencephalogram (EEG), and computed tomography (CT) scan of the head were normal. Nerve conduction velocities (NCV) were slow, and electromyography (EMG) showed denervation (see Table 4). Because of gastrointestinal side effects he could not tolerate levodopa; a combination of primidone and amantadine provided modest improvement in his tremor.

All four daughters of the proband had atrophy and weakness in the distal muscles of the upper and lower limbs, hammertoes, and pes cavus, one also has postural tremor and blepharospasm. The family pedigree indicates autosomal dominant inheritance of the peripheral neuropathy.

Patient 2. This was a 78-year-old man who has had painful cramps in his legs since aged 8. At aged 53 he noted postural tremor in both hands, and 22 years later, he had resting tremor in both hands, shuffling gait, and slowness in activities of daily living. He also had involuntary eye closure, and examination revealed bilateral blepharospasm. There was a 4- to 5-Hz supinating–pronating tremor in both hands, right more than left, and an 8- to 9-Hz postural flexion–extension tremor. He had moderate cogwheel rigidity, bradykinesia, and typical parkinsonian gait. The tendon reflexes were diminished, and ankle jerks were absent; the plantar response was flexor. Distal glove–stocking sensory impairment was present in both hands and feet. His feet showed abnormally high arches and hammertoes. All laboratory studies, including brain CT were normal, except for slow NCVs (see Table 4). He had moderate improvement in his tremor with combination of levodopa, atenolol, and ethopropazine.

His father had hammertoes and died at aged 45 of "postencephalitic" parkinsonism. His father's sister and the patient's son had postural hand tremor.

Patient 3. This was a 50-year-old man with lifelong pes cavus deformity of his feet. At aged 23 he noted postural and writing tremor in both hands and lateral oscillation of his head, which improved with alcohol. At aged 43, he had rest tremor in both hands, left more than right. This tremor markedly improved with levodopa. On examination he had moderate atrophy of the anterior compartment of both legs. Pes cavus and hammertoe deformities were present in both feet. There was a coarse 8- to 9-Hz flexion–extension tremor in both hands when arms were held in an outstretched position and when writing (Fig. 3). During posture holding of both legs, there was a noticeable tremor in the trunk. He also had a 4- to 5-Hz supinating–pronating rest tremor in both hands, jaw, and tongue. When

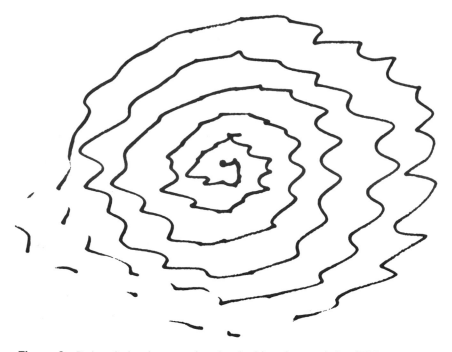

Figure 3 Patient 3 showing tremulous handwriting characteristic of ET.

the effects of levodopa wore off, he had marked hypomimia and bilateral blepharo-spasm. He also had moderate cogwheel rigidity, bradykinesia, and postural instability. Tendon reflexes were absent, and plantar response was flexor. All sensory modalities were diminished in a glove–stocking distribution. Laboratory studies were normal, except for slow NCVs in arms and legs (see Table 4). Sural nerve biopsy showed marked demyelination and "onion bulb" hypertrophy.

The patient's mother, who died at aged 72, had a lifelong history of pes cavus deformity of her feet, gait difficulty, and a postural tremor in both hands. The patient's 55-year-old brother had a pes cavus deformity and slow NCVs in his legs. Also, an 18-year-old son has pes cavus deformity and peripheral neuropathy. Two other children and two sisters are apparently well.

Patient 4.   This was a 79-year-old man, with a history of action tremor since his 20s. He frequently spilled liquids and had very tremulous handwriting. The tremor improved markedly with alcohol, but not with levodopa or amantadine. At aged 69 he noted the gradual onset of a festinating gait and retropulsion. These symptoms improved moderately with levodopa. He also complained of frequent blinking and involuntary eye closure. Examination of his feet showed high arches, hammer toes, atrophy, mild sensory loss, and absent ankle jerks. There was a moderate 4- to 5-Hz rest tremor in his hands and jaw, and an approximately 6- to 7-Hz postural tremor was present when his arms were outstretched or in a wing-beating position. Muscle tone was increased because of cogwheel rigidity. His gait was slow and shuffling, and he needed assistance with ambulation because of severe retropulsion. The essential tremor improved markedly with primidone, and the gait improved with levodopa and amantadine. All blood laboratory studies were normal, and CT and MRI scans showed only mild cerebral atrophy. Electrophysiological studies showed slowing of NCVs, consistent with a de-myelinating peripheral neuropathy. The patient's father has had a long history of bilateral hand tremor.

Charcot and Marie (36) suggested myelopathy, whereas Tooth (37) proposed peripheral neuropathy as pathogenesis for the peroneal muscular atrophy they described simultaneously in 1886. Besides the typical distribution of weakness and atrophy in the legs, the original descriptions also emphasized the presence of pes cavus deformity, and the hereditary nature of the disorder. In 1968, Dyck and Lambert (43,44) correlated nerve conduction changes with nerve biopsy findings and proposed the first useful classification of HMSN. The HMSN type I was characterized by very slow nerve conduction velocities and segmental demyelina-tion, sometimes accompanied by hypertrophic changes. The second type (HMSN II) comprised primarily axonal degeneration, with little or no segmental de-myelination.

Tremor, clinically similar to ET, sometimes accompanies the type I HMSN and less often the type II HMSN. In one series, 67 of 173 (39%) patients with type I HMSN had tremor, ataxia, or both, in upper limbs, and 40 (23%) in the lower limbs (45). In contrast, only 9 of 55 (16%) patients with type II HMSN had tremor or ataxia in upper limbs and 10 (18%) in lower limbs. A reexamination of three patients originally described by Roussy and Levy (38) showed that they had no evidence of cerebellar ataxia and that their tremor was clinically indistinguishable from typical ET (46). In a recent survey of 201 patients with clinically diagnosed HMSN or Charcot–Marie–Tooth disease (CMT), tremor was reported by 43%, involving primarily the hands (100%), arms (29%), legs (28%), and head (17%) (47). Twenty-three percent of all patients reported that at least one of their first-degree relatives demonstrated tremor. Although different genetic abnormalities have been found in families with HMSN, the most common mutation in patients with type I HMSN (or CMTIA) appears to be a large duplication on chromosome 17p11.2 (48–50).

Postural tremor may be seen in a variety of neuropathies (51), particularly the chronic, relapsing inflammatory and the dysgammaglobulinemic polyneuropa-thies (52) and peripheral nerve injuries (53). In contrast with these neuropathic tremors, the tremor encountered in patients with HMSN may be genetically, rather than physiologically, linked to the neuropathy. This notion is supported by the observation that the occurrence of tremor does not seem to correlate with severity of the neuropathy and that postural tremor may be seen in family members of patients with HMSN, who have no clinical nor electrophysiological evidence of neuropathy. Therefore, it is now generally accepted that Roussy–Levy syndrome is not a distinct genetic entity, but rather, a variant of type I HMSN, usually inherited in an autosomal dominant pattern. The families described here are interesting, because the probands, besides having the clinical features of Roussy–Levy syndrome, also have parkinsonian findings and blepharospasm. Although the associations between ET, P, or both, with HMSN have been recognized (36–42,48–50,54,55), the combination of HMSN, ET, P, and blepharospasm present in the four patients described here is unique.

V. ESSENTIAL TREMOR AND OTHER DISORDERS

In addition to the disorders already discussed, ET-like tremor has been reported to occur in patients with essential myoclonus (56). Among 55 living relatives, Korten et al. found myoclonus in 12 and ET in 7; 4 of these subjects had both, myoclonus and tremor (56). In another family with essential myoclonus, some members manifested features consistent with ET (57). Because myoclonus may be rhythmic, it may be difficult to differentiate from ET, thus accounting for the seemingly frequent association between the two disorders. In support of some pathophysiological association is the overlap in clinical features between the two disorders; both share an autosomal dominant pattern of inheritance, are frequently associated with dystonia, and both improve with alcohol. Gait disorders (58,59) and ataxia also have been reported in association with ET. We have also encountered several patients with the restless legs syndrome and ET-like tremor. The ET-like tremor has also been reported in association with hereditary nystagmus, retinitis pigmentosa, familial benign chorea, familial seizure disorder, narcolepsy, migraine, and Klinefelter's syndrome (1–3). However, until definitive diagnostic criteria for ET can be established, these associations must be interpreted cautiously. Finally, it should be emphasized that postural tremors other than ET may be associated with the various neurological disorders.

ACKNOWLEDGMENTS

I would like to express my thanks to Drs. C. Van der Linden, J.-S. Lou, and F. Cardoso for their assistance.

REFERENCES

1. Larsen TA, Calne DB. Essential tremor. Clin Neuropharmacol 1983; 6:185–206.
2. Hubble JP, Busenbark KL, Koller WC. Essential tremor. Clin Neuropharmacol 1989; 12:453–482.
3. Lou JS, Jankovic J. Tremors. Curr Neurol 1991; 11:199–232.

4. Parkinson J. An Essay on the Shaking Palsy. London: Whittingham & Rowland, 1817.
5. Geraghty JJ, Jankovic J, Zetusky WJ. Association between essential tremor and Parkinson's disease. Ann Neurol 1985; 17:329–333.
6. Lou JS, Jankovic J. Essential tremor: clinical correlates in 350 patients. Neurology 1991; 41:234–238.
7. Barbeau A, Pourcher E. New data on the genetics of Parkinson's disease. Can J Neurol Sci 1982; 9:53–60.
8. Roy M, Boyer L, Barbeau A. A prospective study of 50 cases of familial Parkinson's disease. Can J Neurol Sci 1983; 10:34–42.
9. Critchley M. Observations on essential (heredofamilial) tremor. Brain 1949; 72: 113–139.
10. Hornabrook RW, Nagurney JT. Essential tremor in Papua, New Guinea. Brain 1976; 99:654–672.
11. Lang AE, Kierans C, Blair RDG. Family history of tremor in Parkinson's disease compared with those of controls and patients with idiopathic dystonia. Adv Neurol 1986; 45:313–316.
12. Cleeves L, Findley LJ, Koller W. Lack of association between essential tremor and Parkinson's disease. Ann Neurol 1988; 24:23–26.
13. Marttila RJ, Rinne UK. Parkinson's disease and essential tremor in families of patients with early-onset Parkinson's disease. J Neurol Neurosurg Psychiatry 1988; 51:429–431.
14. Schoenberg BS, Anderson DW, Haerer AF. Prevalence of Parkinson's disease in the biracial population of Copiah County, Mississippi. Neurology 1985; 35:841–845.
14a. Jankovic J, Beach J, Schwartz K. Familial tremor in Parkinson's disease. Neurology 1994 (in press).
15. Brooks D, Playford ED, Ibanez V, et al. The association between isolated tremor and disruption of the nigro-striatal dopaminergic system studied with ^{18}F-Dopa and PET. Neurology 1991; 41(suppl 1):360.
15a. Jankovic J, Contant C, Perlmutter J. Essential tremor and PD. Neurology 1993; 43: 1447–1448.
16. Rajput AH, Rozdilsky B, Ang L, Rajput A. Clinicopathologic observations on essential tremor: Report of six cases. Neurology 1991; 41:1422–1444.
17. Gimenez-Roldan S, Mateo D. Cinnarizine-induced parkinsonism. Susceptibility related to aging and essential tremor. Clin Neuropharmacol 1991; 14:156–164.
18. Miller LG, Jankovic J. Metoclopramide-induced movement disorders. Arch Intern Med 1989; 149:2386–2392.
19. Jankovic J, McDermott M, Carter J, et al. Variable expression of Parkinson's disease: a base-line analysis of the DATATOP cohort. Neurology 1990; 40:1529–1534.
20. Simonetta M, Roscol O, Montastruc JL. Orthostatic tremor and Parkinson's disease [abstr]. Mov Disord 1990; 5(suppl 1):14.
21. Couch JR. Dystonia and tremor in spasmodic torticollis. Adv Neurol 1976; 14: 245–258.
22. Baxter DW, Lal S. Essential tremor and dystonia syndromes. Adv Neurol 1979; 24: 373–377.
23. Poewe WH, Lees AJ, Stern GM. Dystonia in Parkinson's disease: clinical and pharmacological features. Ann Neurol 1988; 23:73–78.

24. Katchen M, Duvoisin RC. Parkinsonism following dystonia in three patients. Mov Disord 1986; 1:151–157.
25. LeWitt PA, Burns RS, Newman RP. Dystonia in untreated parkinsonism. Clin Neuropharmacol 1986; 3:293–297.
26. Cohen LG, Hallett M, Sudarsky L. A single family with writer's cramp, essential tremor, and primary writing tremor. Mov Disord 1987; 2:109–116.
27. Rosenbaum F, Jankovic J. Focal task-specific tremor and dystonia: Categorization of occupational movement disorders. Neurology 1988; 38:522–527.
28. Ravits J, Hallett M, Baker M, Wilkins D. Primary writing tremor and myoclonic writer's cramp. Neurology 1985; 35:1387–1391.
29. Klawans HL, Glantz R, Tanner CM, Goetz CG. Primary writing tremor: selective action tremor. Neurology 1982; 32:203–206.
30. Marsden CD, Sheehy MP. Writer's cramp. TINS 1990; 13:148–153.
31. Jankovic J, Ford J. Blepharospasm and orofacial-cervical dystonia: clinical and pharmacologic findings. Ann Neurol 1983; 13:402–411.
32. Jankovic J, Leder S, Warner D, Schwartz PA. Cervical dystonia: clinical findings and associated movement disorders. Neurology 1991; 41:1088–1091.
32a. Chan J, Brin MF, Fahn S. Idiopathic cervical dystonia: Clinical characteristics. Mov Disord 1991; 6:119–126.
32b. Rondot P, Marchand MP, Dellatolas G. Spasmodic torticollis—a review of 220 patients. Can J Neurol Sci 1991; 18:143–151.
32c. Dubinsky RM, Gray CS, Koller WC. Essential tremor and dystonia. Neurology 1993; 43:2382–2384.
33. Jedynak CP, Bonnet AM, Agid Y. Tremor and idiopathic dystonia. Mov Disord 1991; 6:230–236.
34. Rivest J, Marsden CD. Trunk and head tremor as isolated manifestations of dystonia. Mov Disord 1990; 5:60–65.
35. Yanagisawa N, Goto A, Narabayashi H. Familial dystonia musculorum deformans and tremor. J Neurol Sci 1971; 16:125–136.
35a. Conway D, Bain PG, Warner TT, et al. Linkage analysis with chromosome 9 marker in hereditary essential tremor. Mov Disord 1993; 8:374–376.
35b. Dürr A, Stevanin G, Jedynak CP, et al. Familial essential tremor and idiopathic torsion dystonia are different genetic entities. Neurology 1993; 43:2212–2214.
36. Charcot JM, Marie P. Sur une forme particuliere d'atrophie musculaire progressive, souvent familiale, debutant par les pieds et les jambes, et atteignant plus tard les mains. Rev Med (Paris) 1886; 6:97–138.
37. Tooth HH. The peroneal type of progressive muscular atrophy. Thesis, London: HK Lewis, 1886.
38. Roussy G, Levy G. Sept cas d'une maladie familiale particuliere. Troubles de la marche, pieds bots et areflexie tendineuse generalisee avec acessoirement legere maladresse des mains. Rev Neurol 1926; 2:427–450.
39. Lapresle J. Contribution a l'etude de la dystasie areflexique hereditaire. Etat actuel de quatre de sept cas princeps de Roussy et Mlle Levy, treinte ans apres la premiare publication de ces auteurs. Sem Hop Paris 1956; 32:2473–2482.
40. Yudell A, Dyck PJ, Lambert EH. A kinship with Roussy–Levy syndrome: a clinical and electrophysiologic study. Arch Neurol 1965; 13:432–440.

41. Salisachs P, Codina A, Gimenez-Roldan S, Zarranz JJ. Charcot–Marie–Tooth disease associated with "essential tremor" and normal and/or slightly diminished motor conduction velocity. Report of 7 cases. Eur Neurol 1979; 18:49–58.

42. Barbieri F, Filla A, Ragno M, et al. Evidence that Charcot–Marie–Tooth disease with tremor coincides with Roussy–Levy syndrome. Can J Neurol 1984; 11:534–540.

43. Dyck PJ, Lambert EH. Lower motor and primary sensory neuron diseases with peroneal muscular atrophy. I. Neurologic, genetic and electrophysiologic findings in hereditary polyneuropathy. Arch Neurol 1968; 18:603–618.

44. Dyck PJ, Lambert EH. Lower motor and primary sensory neuron diseases with peroneal muscular atrophy. II. Neurologic, genetic and electrophysiologic findings in various neuronal degenerations. Arch Neurol 1968; 18:619–625.

45. Harding AE, Thomas PK. The clinical features of hereditary motor and sensory neuropathy types I and II. Brain 1980; 103:259–280.

46. Salisachs P. Ataxia and other data reviewed in Charcot–Marie–Tooth and Refsum's disease. J Neurol Neurosurg Psychiatry 1982; 45:1085–1091.

47. Cardoso F, Jankovic J. Hereditary motor–sensory neuropathy and movement disorders. Muscle and Nerve 1993; 16:904–910.

48. Bergoffen J, Scherer SS, Wang S, et al. Connexin mutations in X-linked Charcot–Marie–Tooth disease. Science 1993; 262:2039–2042.

49. Hoogendijk JE, Janssen EAM, Gabreëls-Festen AAWM, et al. Allelic heterogeneity in hereditary motor and sensory neuropathy type Ia (Charcot–Marie–Tooth disease type 1a). Neurology 1993; 43:1010–1015.

50. Lupski JR, Chnace PF, Garcia CA. Inherited primary peripheral neuropathies. Molecular genetics and clinical implications of CMT1A and HNPP. JAMA 1993; 270: 2326–2330.

51. Said G, Bathien N, Cesaro P. Peripheral neuropathies and tremor. Neurology 1982; 32:480–485.

52. Dalakas MC, Teravainen H, Engel WK. Tremor as a feature of chronic relapsing and dysgammaglobulinemic polyneuropathies. Incidence and management. Arch Neurol 1984; 41:711–714.

53. Jankovic J, Van der Linden C. Dystonia and tremor induced by peripheral trauma: predisposing factors. J Neurol Neurosurg Psychiatry 1988; 51:1512–1519.

54. Byrne E, Thomas PK, Zilkha. Familial extrapyramidal disease with peripheral neuropathy. J Neurol Neurosurg Psychiatry 1982; 45:372–374.

55. Tandan R, Taylor R, Adesina A, et al. Benign autosomal dominant syndrome of neuronal Charcot–Marie–Tooth disease, ptosis, parkinsonism, and dementia. Neurology 1990; 40:773–779.

56. Korten JJ, Notermand SLH, Frenken CWGM, et al. Familial essential myoclonus. Brain 1974; 97:131–138.

57. Fahn S, Sjaastad O. Hereditary essential myoclonus in a large Norwegian family. Mov Disord 1991; 6:237–247.

58. Larsson T, Sjögren T. Essential tremor. A clinical and genetic population study. Acta Psychiatr Neurol Scand [suppl] 1960; 144:1–176.

59. Singer C, Sanchez-Ramos J, Weiner WJ. Gait abnormality in essential tremor. Mov Disord 1994; 9:193–196.

18

The Pharmacological Management of Essential Tremor

Stefano Calzetti
Institute of Neurology
University of Parma
Parma, Italy

Emilio Perucca
University of Pavia
Pavia, Italy

I. INTRODUCTION

Essential tremor (ET) may be considered a natural model of monosymptomatic chronic motor dysfunction in humans, affecting the upper extremities or other body parts. The pharmacological approach to this disorder provides an unique opportunity to evaluate the antitremor effect of drugs that preferentially act at different sites in both the periphery and in the central nervous system (CNS). This opportunity was first offered in the early 1970s, when it was reported by two different groups that patients with ET had their tremor relieved by the β-adrenoceptor antagonist propranolol (1,2). This discovery initiated a new era in the pharmacological management of this disorder, which up to then was rather unsuccessful and was empirically based on the use of drugs devoid of specific antitremor properties, such as sedatives and tranquilizers. In the following decades, these early reports promoted several clinical studies aimed at understanding not only the mode of action of β-adrenergic blocking drugs in ET, but also the basic pathophysiological mechanism of the disorder.

Interest in this topic was rekindled in 1981, following the reports that primidone, a well-established anticonvulsant, is capable of ameliorating ET and,

263

sometimes, to suppress it completely (3,4). Although other drugs have been subsequently reported to possess tremorolytic properties, their clinical efficacy has been shown only in a limited number of patients or under uncontrolled conditions, so that their role in the management of ET remains to be established.

To date, the therapeutic efficacy of only the β-adrenergic blocking drugs and of primidone has been demonstrated and characterized clearly. In addition, a more widespread application of clinical pharmacological methods in the assessment of drug efficacy and the use of quantitative techniques of tremor recording and measurement, such as surface electromyography (EMG) and accelerometry, coupled with computed analysis of the derived bioelectrical signals, has provided the basis for a more rational approach to the treatment of ET.

Indeed, in spite of the fact that only a limited number of options for the pharmacological control of ET are currently available, there is an increasing demand for medical intervention in this benign, but often disabling, disorder, which in the past had been regarded and accepted as an untreatable condition. In the following paragraphs, the state of the art in pharmacological therapy will be reviewed and the role of β-adrenergic blockers, primidone, and barbiturates in the treatment of ET will be discussed in detail. Finally, guidelines for an integrated approach to the pharmacological treatment of ET will be provided.

II. β-ADRENERGIC BLOCKING DRUGS

The tremorolytic properties and the therapeutic efficacy of β-adrenergic blockers in ET have been documented in a large number of controlled clinical studies (5), and currently these agents represent the first line of pharmacological treatment of this disorder. Propranolol is the compound most extensively investigated, especially for tremor involving the upper extremities, and it represents the reference drug against which the effect of other β-adrenergic blockers can be compared. However, only a limited number of patients (i.e., about 50–70%) show a satisfactory response to the β-adrenergic blockers. The degree of improvement (in terms of percentage reduction in postural hand tremor amplitude, assessed quantitatively by accelerometric testing) varies markedly between patients (on average 40–50% of pretreatment values, with a range between minimal or absent effect, up to a decrease by 60–70%). Unfortunately, this objective reduction in tremor amplitude only rarely corresponds to an equivalent degree of subjective functional benefit in daily-living and occupational activities, especially in the more severe forms. The dominant peak frequency of tremor usually remains unchanged (5).

The reason for the interindividual variability in response to β-adrenergic blockade is unclear, but pharmacokinetic factors (6) and other variables, such as dominant peak frequency and amplitude of tremor, duration of the disorder, pattern of activation of agonist and antagonist muscles (7–11), have been advocated. That ET may not be a single homogeneous entity is also relevant (12). In responders, hand tremor relief becomes apparent within 2 h after a single oral dose of 120 mg propranolol (13,14), on average the reduction in tremor amplitude being similar to that observed for long-term medication at adequate daily drug dosages (5). However, the predictive value of the response to a single dose in individual patients has not yet been adequately assessed. The degree of therapeutic response to propranolol seems to be dose-dependent, at least within the range between 80 and 320 mg/day, optimal efficacy during prolonged treatment being usually achieved at a daily dose of 160–320 mg (15). A lack of correlation between the serum concentration of the drug or its active metabolite 4-hydroxypropranolol and the clinical response is commonly reported, at least in the short-term (10,15).

In spite of the general consensus about the overall tremorolytic action of β-adrenergic blockers, their efficacy in tremor, other than postural, such as the kinetic component involving the upper extremities and in the so-called ET variants, such as primary writing tremor, orthostatic tremor, and kinetic predominant tremor, are controversial. The clinical response in patients with tremors affecting body parts other than the arms (i.e., head, voice, and so on) remains also undefined. Although current opinion favors the view that the tremorolytic effect of β-adrenergic blockers is mainly exerted through blockade of peripheral β_2-adrenoceptors in the striatal muscle (16), the contributions of β_1-mediated mechanisms both in the central nervous system and in the periphery, and of ancillary pharmacodynamic properties, such as membrane-stabilizing action, are unclear.

Since the antitremor effect of the β-adrenergic blockers is solely symptomatic, the crucial question remains of whether or not the initial therapeutic benefit is maintained during long-term treatment. Surprisingly, few studies have assessed the long-term response of ET to the β-adrenergic blockers. Although early reports have shown sustained benefit during maintenance treatment with propranolol (2,8), in a recent prospective study, about 40% of ET patients, over 12 months of continuous medication, required an increase in their daily dose of propranolol to maintain an adequate therapeutic response (17). This was interpreted as indirect evidence of a gradual decline in the tremorolytic effect of the drug, suggesting that tolerance develops during extended treatment. If this is confirmed, a therapeutic approach that is based on intermittent use of these drugs in the long-term management of ET patients would be valuable (see later discussion). Different findings, however, have been reported in another study, which showed that only a small proportion (14%) of patients lost their initial response to propranolol over a 1-year period (18). Differences in the population of patients and study protocol may have accounted for this discrepancy. Further studies are needed to investigate this issue more extensively.

The β-adrenergic blockers should not be administered to patients with certain defined conditions including asthma and other obstructive lung diseases, atrioventricular (AV) heart block, congestive heart failure, and peripheral arterial diseases. In the remaining patients, these drugs are usually relatively well tolerated at the dosages commonly recommended in clinical practice. However, the pulse rate in supine and standing position should be regularly monitored, and an electrocardiogram (ECG) should be performed periodically during extended treatment, especially in the elderly patients.

III. PRIMIDONE AND BARBITURATES

The tremorolytic properties of barbiturates have been reevaluated following the discovery that primidone may prove of remarkable therapeutic benefit in patients with ET (3). Indeed, the symptomatic efficacy of primidone has been substantiated in several studies that have shown a mean degree of clinical response and a proportion of responders comparable with those observed with propranolol, at least in the short-term (19–22). More often than with β-adrenergic blockers, however, complete suppression of postural hand tremor may occasionally be achieved. As with the β-adrenergic blockers, there currently is no reliable way of predicting the degree of individual response to primidone.

The question has been raised about whether the parent drug or its metabolites are responsible for the tremorolytic effect of primidone. Although an effect of the metabolite phenylethylmalonamide (PEMA) has been excluded in a double-blind, placebo-controlled investigation (23), a partial contribution of metabolically derived phenobarbital (PB) to the antitremor efficacy of primidone is generally recognized, based on the results of two separate studies in which the effect of PB has been demonstrated under controlled clinical conditions (24,25). On the other hand, an independent antitremor effect of unchanged primidone is indicated by at least two lines of evidence: (1) there is definite tremor relief following a single oral dose of primidone at a time when serum PB levels are still undetectable (21), and (2) primidone, but not PB, was superior to placebo in a double-blind, crossover study comparing the two drugs, by both clinical and quantitative methods of tremor assessment, in the same group of patients (26,27). Therefore, it is conceivable that the overall tremorolytic effect of primidone results from a combined action of the parent drug itself and of metabolically derived PB.

The tremorolytic effect of primidone, which is unrelated to the serum concentration of either parent compound or derived phenobarbital, seems to be rather specific and not secondary to the sedative action of the drug. The mode of action of primidone and barbiturates in ET is believed to be mediated by an effect on the central nervous system, but the precise site and mechanism is unknown. A mode of action exerted through a change in ionic fluxes across neuronal membranes in the CNS has been postulated (16). As reported in a study of the dose–response relation (21), an optimal therapeutic effect may be achieved with a daily dose of primidone as low as 250 mg, larger doses do not necessarily provide additional benefit.

As with β-adrenergic blockers, there are several unresolved questions concerning the spectrum of the clinical efficacy of primidone. Only a few studies have examined the efficacy of the drug in tremors affecting body parts other than the upper limbs, and the response of ET variants also remains undefined. Also the long-term efficacy of primidone has not been conclusively established. One prospective study has shown that the drug retains its initial tremorolytic effect over 1 year of continuous treatment in about half the patients (18), but these findings have not been replicated by Sasso et al. (28), who found some loss of overall efficacy during long-term administration, as assessed by tests of manual dexterity, clinical evaluation, and patients' self-rating, in the population of patients as a whole. However, the results of these studies are poorly comparable owing to difference in experimental design and statistical analysis. Development of acute and short-term tolerance to the antitremor effect of primidone has been recently reported (22,29) and could account for the lack of response to the drug in some patients. Further studies are required to evaluate the relative frequency of this phenomenon in a population of appropriate size.

Adverse effects represent a major problem with primidone and other barbiturates. Symptoms of acute transient neurotoxicity occur in an high proportion of ET patients at the onset of treatment with primidone, even following a single initial dose as low as 62.5 mg (19). This adverse reaction may account for most of the initial noncompliance. Since early intolerance reactions are less common in patients with epilepsy, it has been suggested that previous exposure to other anticonvulsants may exert a "protecting" effect (30). Dose-related untoward effects, mainly sedation and drowsiness, are commonly observed during maintenance treatment with primidone and other barbiturates. Their occurrence usually requires a dosage adjustment, but only rarely does the drug need to be discontinued. On the other hand, functional tolerance to the sedative effect of these drugs tends to develop during prolonged treatment, leading to improvement in long-term tolerability in most of the patients.

IV. OTHER DRUGS

Although clinical experience has been most extensive with β-adrenergic blockers and primidone, several other drugs have been shown to possess some tremorolytic effects. However, because their efficacy has been documented only by conflicting and isolated reports or by uncontrolled clinical observations, the role of these drugs in the treatment of ET has not yet been established.

A separate comment is required for alcohol. It is well-known that even a small amount of an alcoholic beverage may induce a prompt and marked reduction of hand tremor, an effect that may lead to copious self-prescription in some subjects. The antitremor properties of alcohol have been confirmed in experimental clinical studies and shown to be mediated by an action on the central nervous system (31). The tremorolytic effect is specific for ET, but the precise mechanism has not been clarified (16). The transient nature of the effect, which is followed by a rebound exacerbation of tremor, the toxic potential of the compound, the development of tolerance, and the risk of addiction make a widespread use of alcohol impractical. Occasional situations in which small doses of alcohol may be recommended will be discussed later. Recent studies with mepartynol (methylpentynol), an alcohol derivative, have shown it to be ineffective at subhypnotic doses (200 mg/day) in patients with ET, most of whom were reportedly alcohol-responsive (32).

A. Benzodiazepines

It is generally accepted that benzodiazepines are devoid of specific tremorolytic properties and, therefore, the rationale for their clinical use rests on their ability to prevent or relieve anxiety-induced enhancement of tremor. However, it has been reported recently that clonazepam (1–3 mg/day) may be effective in two ET variants (kinetic-predominant tremor and orthostatic tremor; 5), whereas alprazolam (0.75–2.75 mg/day) was of benefit in patients with ET of the hand and the head in a double-blind, controlled study (33). To what extent sedation could have accounted for the antitremor efficacy of these drugs remains to be clarified.

B. Drugs Acting on α-Adrenoceptors

The α-adrenergic antagonist moxisylyte (thymoxamine; 0.1 mg/kg iv) has been effective in reducing ET in experimental clinical studies (34,35). Its tremorolytic properties are believed to be mediated by inhibition of noradrenergic facilitation of the stretch reflex in the spinal cord (35). However, the clinical use of moxisylyte is limited by its low oral efficacy and poor tolerability. Negative results have been reported for the postsynaptic α-adrenergic blockers phenoxybenzamine (36) and urapidil (37), whereas the efficacy of clonidine, an α_2-adrenoceptor agonist, is controversial (37,38).

C. Serotoninergic Drugs

Whereas the serotonin precursors l-tryptophan and 5-hydroxytryptophan have been ineffective in ET (5), conflicting results have been reported for trazodone, a drug possibly acting by potentiating serotoninergic transmission (39–42).

Other drugs reported to be of benefit in some patients include amantadine, mephenesin, clozapine, glutethimine (5), and linoleic acid (43). Negative results have been reported with the calcium channel blockers verapamil and nifedipine (44) and with progabide, a drug potentiating γ-aminobutyric acid (GABA)ergic transmission (45,46).

V. PRACTICAL GUIDELINES FOR A RATIONAL APPROACH TO THE TREATMENT OF ESSENTIAL TREMOR

The therapeutic strategy in patients with ET depends on a number of factors, such as the severity of the symptom, the age of the patient, the effect of tremor on psychological status, and the possible presence of associated disease(s). The sensitivity of tremor to endogenous and environmental factors, such as emotional stress, and the voluntary habits of the patient may also be important, especially in mild tremors. These factors may contribute to the day-to-day and hour-to-hour intraindividual variability in tremor severity that is commonly observed in untreated subjects. Some patients with mild tremor of the hands, in whom the symptoms cause little or no functional disability except for occasional social embarrassment, often require only reassurance about the "benign" nature of the disorder. In some of these patients, it may be advisable to prescribe the intermittent use of a β-adrenergic blocker (i.e., single or repeated oral doses of 20–40 mg propranolol) alone or associated with an anxiolytic (i.e., a benzodiazepine), to prevent or to treat the possible exacerbation of tremor following exposure to stressful events. The intake of a small amount of alcohol may produce transient relief of tremor and may be useful in special situations of social life. However, because of the potential risk of abuse and decreased efficacy on prolonged use, this practice should not be encouraged. In these patients, the removal of concurrent facilitating factors, such as voluntary habits (caffeine) and drugs known to produce enhancement of tremor, may be necessary.

Whenever tremor interferes significantly with social or occupational activity or causes marked psychological discomfort, institution of maintenance pharmacological treatment is indicated. Under these circumstances, the drug of choice is a nonselective β-adrenergic blocker devoid of intrinsic sympathomimetic activity (ISA). Propranolol may be a suitable choice at an initial dosage of 20–40 mg/day built up gradually, if necessary, to 120–320 mg/day in two to three divided doses. A long-acting formulation of propranolol (up to 320 mg/day once daily in the morning) may provide practical advantages in improving patients' compliance and possibly in minimizing diurnal variability in tremor severity (5). Other nonselective β-adrenergic blockers, such as timolol (10–20 mg/day) and nadolol (120–240 mg/day), are as effective as propranolol (5) and may offer some advantages in terms of better tolerability or more convenient frequency of administration, owing to longer duration of action. β_1-Selective (cardioselective) adrenergic blockers, such as metoprolol (150 mg/day) and atenolol (100 mg/day), are generally less effective than nonselective agents (30) and should be reserved as a second-choice treatment in patients with concurrent bronchospastic disorders or peripheral arterial diseases, who failed to respond to alternative drugs (i.e., primidone and phenobarbital). However, the use of β_1-selective adrenergic agents in these patients must be very cautious because their selectivity is only relative and is partially lost a higher doses with the attendant risk of precipitation of respiratory distress or peripheral ischemia. Theoretically, β_2-selective adrenergic blockers could prove useful in patients with cardiac contraindications, but none of these agents is commercially available and, at least one of those being developed (ICI-118,551) has been withdrawn from clinical investigation. It is extremely improbable that patients failing to respond to propranolol could achieve adequate tremor relief with another β-adrenergic blocker and, under these circumstances, the drug should be discontinued gradually (over not less than 1–2 weeks) to avoid rebound exacerbation of tremor and, possibly, cardiac symptoms.

In patients unresponsive to the β-adrenergic blockers and in patients in whom these drugs are contraindicated, a reasonable alternative is provided by primidone. To minimize initial intolerance reactions, treatment should be started with a very low dose (62.5 mg at bedtime) and increased gradually up to a range of 250–750 mg/day in two to three divided doses, according to clinical response and individual tolerability. Since previous exposure to barbiturates appears to reduce the frequency of early intolerance to primidone, a course of phenobarbital (50 mg/day) might be useful before restarting primidone therapy in patients who have developed these reactions. Phenobarbital itself may be a valuable alternative to primidone in patients unable to tolerate the latter drug. Patients who show little or no response to primidone are not expected to respond to phenobarbital, and prescription of the latter in these patients is not a logical choice.

Only few patients are refractory to either β-adrenergic or primidone and phenobarbital.

When tremor causes marked disability and interferes severely with daily-living activities (eating, drinking, shaving, and so on) and the degree of symptomatic control achieved with a single drug is inadequate, it may be reasonable to try a β-adrenergic blocker and primidone in combination, at dosages adjusted according to clinical efficacy and individual tolerance. However, since it has not yet been established whether the tremorolytic effect of these drugs is additive, the actual advantages of this strategy needs to be investigated. In patients showing a decline in therapeutic efficacy during long-term treatment with β-blockers or primidone, it may be advisable to withdraw the drug temporarily and to reintroduce it after a drug-free period of at least a few weeks in an attempt to restore an adequate clinical responsiveness. Such patients may also be shifted temporarily to an alternative agent (e.g., from a β-blocker to primidone or vice versa). On the other hand, since variability has been reported in the clinical course of the untreated disorder, with occasional long-lasting spontaneous improvement (5), in clinical practice, it may be worthwhile to consider a periodic reduction in dosage and possibly drug withdrawal, even when adequate symptomatic control has been achieved and maintained over time.

REFERENCES

1. Sevitt I. The effect of adrenergic beta-receptor blocking drugs on tremor. Practitioner 1971; 207:677–678.
2. Winkler GF, Young RR. The control of essential tremor by propranolol. Trans Am Neurol Assoc 1971; 96:66–68.

3.   O'Brien MD, Upton AR, Toseland TA. Benign familial tremor treated with primidone. Br Med J 1981; 282:178–280.

4.   Chakrabarti A, Pearce JMS. Essential tremor: response to primidone. J Neurol Neurosurg Psychiatry 1981; 44:650.

5.   Hubble JP, Busenbark KL, Koller WC. Essential tremor. Clin Neuropharmacol 1989; 12:453–482.

6.   Mc Allister RG Jr, Markesbery WR, Ware RW, Howell SM. Suppression of essential tremor by propranolol: correlation of effect with drug plasma levels and intensity of beta-adrenergic blockade. Ann Neurol 1977; 1:160–166.

7.   Dupont E, Hansen HJ, Dalby MA. Treatment of benign essential tremor with propranolol: a controlled clinical trial. Acta Neurol Scand 1973; 69:75–84.

8.   Murray TJ. Long-term therapy of essential tremor with propranolol. Can Med Assoc J 1976; 115:892–894.

9.   Teravainen H, Fogelholm R, Larsen A. Effect of propranolol on essential tremor. Neurology 1976; 26:27–30.

10.   Calzetti S, Findley LJ, Perucca E, Richens A. The response of essential tremor to propranolol: evaluation of clinical variables governing its efficacy on prolonged administration. J Neurol Neurosurg Psychiatry 1983; 46:393–398.

11.   Sabra AF, Hallett M. Action tremor with alternating activity in antagonist muscles. Neurology 1984; 34:151–156.

12.   Marsden CD, Obeso J, Rothwell JC. Benign essential tremor is not a single entity. In: Yahr MD, ed. Current Concepts in Parkinson's Disease. Amsterdam: Excerpta Medica, 1983:31–46.

13.   Calzetti S, Findley LF, Gresty MA, Perucca E, Richens A. Effect of a single oral dose of propranolol in essential tremor: a double-blind controlled study. Ann Neurol 1983; 13:165–171.

14.   Koller WC, Royse V. Time course of a single oral dose of propranolol in essential tremor. Neurology 1985; 35:1494–1499.

15.   Koller WC. Dose–response relationship of propranolol in the treatment of essential tremor. Arch Neurol 1986; 43:42–43.

16.   Guan X-M, Peroutka SJ. Basic mechanisms of action of drugs used in the treatment of essential tremor. Clin Neuropharmacol 1990; 13:210–223.

17.   Calzetti S, Sasso E, Baratti M, Fava R. Clinical and computer-based assessment of long-term therapeutic efficacy of propranolol in essential tremor. Acta Neurol Scand 1990; 81:392–396.

18.   Koller WC, Vetere-Overfield B. Acute and chronic effects of propranolol and primidone in essential tremor. Neurology 1989; 39:1587–1588.

19.   Findley LJ, Calzetti S, Cleeves L. Primidone in essential tremor of the hands and head: a double-blind controlled clinical study. J Neurol Neurosurg Psychiatry 1985; 48:911–915.

20.   Gorman WP, Cooper R, Pocock P, Campbell MJ. A comparison of primidone, propranolol, and placebo in essential tremor, using quantitative analysis. J Neurol Neurosurg Psychiatry 1986; 49:64–68.

21.   Koller WC, Royse VL. Efficacy of primidone in essential tremor. Neurology 1986; 36:121–124.

22. Dietrichson P, Espen E. Primidone and propranolol in essential tremor: a study based on quantitative tremor recording and plasma anticonvulsant levels. Acta Neurol Scand 1987; 75:332–340.

23. Calzetti S, Findley LJ, Pisani F, Richens A. Phenylethylmalonamide in essential tremor. A double-blind controlled study. J Neurol Neurosurg Psychiatry 1981; 44: 932–934.

24. Baruzzi A, Procaccianti G, Martinelli P, et al. Phenobarbital and propranolol in essential tremor: a double-blind controlled clinical trial. Neurology 1983; 33: 296–300.

25. Findley LJ, Cleeves L. Phenobarbitone in essential tremor. Neurology 1985; 35:1784–1787.

26. Sasso E, Perucca E, Calzetti S. Double-blind comparison of primidone and phenobarbital in essential tremor. Neurology 1988; 38:808–810.

27. Sasso E, Perucca E, Fava R, Calzetti S. Quantitative comparison of barbiturates in essential hand and head tremor. Mov Disord 1991; 6:65–68.

28. Sasso E, Perucca E, Fava R, Calzetti S. Primidone in the long-term treatment of essential tremor: a prospective study with computerized quantitative analysis. Clin Neuropharmacol 1990; 13:67–76.

29. Sasso E, Perucca E, Negrotti A, Calzetti S. Acute tolerance to the tremorolytic effect of primidone. Neurology; 1991; 41:602–603.

30. Findley LJ. The pharmacological management of essential tremor. Clin Neuropharmacol 1986; 9(suppl 2):S61–S75.

31. Growdon JH, Shahani BT, Young RR. The effect of alcohol on essential tremor. Neurology 1975; 28:259–262.

32. Teravainen H, Huttunen J, Lewitt P. Ineffective treatment of essential tremor with an alcohol, methylpentynol. J Neurol Neurosurg Psychiatry 1986; 49:198–199.

33. Huber SJ, Paulson GW. Efficacy of alprazolam for essential tremor. Neurology 1988; 38:241–243.

34. Mai J, Olsen RB. Depression of essential tremor by alpha-adrenergic blockade. J Neurol Neurosurg Psychiatry 1981; 44:1171.

35. Abila B, Wilson JF, Marshall RW, Richens A. Differential effects of alpha-adrenoceptor blockade on essential, physiological and isoprenaline-induced tremor: evidence for a central origin of essential tremor. J Neurol Neurosurg Psychiatry 1985; 48:1031–1036.

36. Koller WC. Ineffectiveness of phenoxybenzamine in essential tremor. J Neurol Neurosurg Psychiatry 1986; 49:222.

37. Caccia MR, Osio M, Galimberti V, Cataldi G, Mangoni A. Propranolol, clonidine, urapidil and trazodone infusion in essential tremor: a double-blind crossover trial. Acta Neurol Scand 1989; 79:379–383.

38. Koller WC, Herbster G, Cone S. Clonidine in the treatment of essential tremor. Mov Disord 1986; 1:235–237.

39. McLeod NA, White LE Jr. Trazodone in essential tremor. JAMA 1986; 256:2675–2676.

40. Sanson F, Schergna E, Semenzato D, et al. Therapeutic effect of trazodone in the treatment of tremor. Multicentric double-blind study. Riv Neurol 1986; 56:358–364.

41. Koller WC. Trazodone in essential tremor. Probe of serotoninergic mechanisms. Clin Neuropharmacol 1989; 12:134–137.
42. Cleeves L, Findley LJ. Trazodone is ineffective in essential tremor. J Neurol Neurosurg Psychiatry 1990; 53:268–269.
43. Lieb J. Linoleic acid in the treatment of lithium toxicity and familial tremor. Prostaglandins Med 1980; 4:275–279.
44. Topaktas S, Onur R, Dalkara T. Calcium channel blockers and essential tremor. Eur Neurol 1987; 27:114–119.
45. Mondrup K, Dupont E, Pedersen E. The effect of the GABA-agonist, progabide, on benign essential tremor. A controlled clinical trial. Acta Neurol Scand 1983; 68: 248–252.
46. Koller WC, Rubino F, Gupta S. Pharmacologic probe with progabide of GABA mechanism in essential tremor. Arch Neurol 1987; 44:905–906.

19

Clinical Features of Tremor in Extrapyramidal Syndromes

Ali H. Rajput
University of Saskatchewan
Saskatoon, Saskatchewan, Canada

I. EXTRAPYRAMIDAL SYSTEM

The terms basal ganglia and extrapyramidal system are frequently used interchangeably. Anatomically, the *basal ganglia* are defined as the group of nuclei situated in the diencephalon and mesencephalon—the striatum, pallidum, and substantia nigra being the major structures (1).

Tremor is an involuntary, rhythmic oscillation of a body part and is clinically distinguishable from other involuntary movements (2,3). Physiological tremor is present in everyone, but is not identifiable clinically. When tremor becomes evident or disturbing to the patient, it is considered as pathological tremor (4).

The most important consideration in the clinical assessment of tremor in the extrapyramidal syndromes is the behavioral context during which the tremor manifests itself (2). For the purpose of this chapter, the tremors appearing under different circumstances are briefly outlined.

Resting tremor (RT) is present when the affected part of the body is in repose and is fully supported against gravity—requiring no active muscle contraction (5). Tremor appearing in a body part that is being used for certain physical action (i.e., requiring muscle contraction) is called *action tremor* (AT). The AT is divisible into two subgroups: (1) the AT appearing on positioning against gravity (e.g., holding arms in front perpendicular to the body) is known as *postural tremor* (PT); and (2) the AT evident in a part of body that is involved in active movement (e.g., an attempt to carry a cup from the table to mouth) is called the *kinetic tremor* (KT). A kinetic tremor that appears near the termination of movement is known as the *terminal tremor*. Kinetic tremor present only during specific action, but not with other activities involving the same limb, is called the *task-specific tremor* (6). The most notable example of task-specific tremor is the writing tremor.

In most extrapyramidal syndromes, the tremor is usually intermittent, although, in rare cases, it may be persistent. Any part of the body—head, lips, jaw, tongue, chin, upper limbs, trunk, or lower limbs can be affected by tremor. Tremor frequency, although useful for understanding the pathophysiology, is difficult to measure accurately in the clinical setting. If we consider that the rate of typical RT in Parkinson's disease is 4–5 Hz, the tremor frequency in a patient may be identified as being faster or lower than that. That would provide the approximate frequency of the tremor, which may be useful for clinical purposes.

The final major clinical consideration is the tremor amplitude. The amplitude in the same patient may vary significantly from one to the next assessment, depending on several factors. The tremor amplitude increases if the patient is upset, tired, hungry, or sick owing to a concomitant illness. The amplitude most closely reflects the functional handicap related to tremor (7). Because of the variation in amplitude from one occasion to the next, the description is valid for that given evaluation only. In the event that repeated assessments have been performed, the tremor amplitude noted on the majority of those occasions is considered as the representative one. The amplitude may be clinically divisible into small, medium, or large. The tremor that is barely visible is called fine- or small-amplitude tremor. When the tremor fluctuations are more than 1 cm in a given direction, it is considered a large-amplitude or coarse tremor. The tremor amplitude that falls between the two foregoing extremes is known as medium amplitude. The change in amplitude is also critical for measuring the efficacy of treatment (8).

Considering the characteristics just described, the typical parkinsonian tremor in a patient could be described as an intermittent, flexion–extension, 4- to 5-Hz, medium-amplitude resting tremor at the right wrist.

Since this chapter deals only with clinical aspects of tremor in humans, the naturally occurring or experimentally induced tremor in animals will not be considered. A summary of different forms of tremor in some extrapyramidal disorders is outlined in Table 1.

II. IDIOPATHIC PARKINSON'S DISEASE

The most common extrapyramidal disorder seen in clinical practice is the parkinsonian syndrome (PS). Every large pathological study of parkinsonian syndrome indicates that substantia nigra (SN) neuronal loss and Lewy body (LB) cytoplasmic inclusions constitute the most common pathological findings in these cases. The disorder in this subgroup of patients is usually known as idiopathic Parkinson's disease (IPD) (9). Typical parkinsonian tremor is present at 4–5 Hz during rest (10,11).

Tremor is frequently reported as the initial symptom in IPD (12). It is an easily recognizable symptom, but by contrast, akinesia and rigidity, in our experience, may go unnoticed for a long time in the akinetic–rigid PS patients, thereby considerably delaying the diagnosis. Jankovic contends that only half of the PS patients manifest as tremor (13). When considered retrospectively, in some cases, intermittent tremor may by the only parkinsonian feature for 20–30 years before emergence of other manifestations (2). We have noted that an intermittent stress-related resting tremor may occasionally precede the other IPD manifestations by more than 30 years.

During the early stage, the tremor is intermittent in IPD. With the progression of the disease, the tremor usually becomes more persistent. In some patients, after reaching the peak, the tremor may decline (14), as noted in several of our patients who were followed for a long period.

The absence of tremor during the entire course of IPD is a subject of controversy. Jankovic noted that 15% of patients never manifested tremor (13), and Jenner and Marsden concluded that between 20 and 30% of IPD cases have little or no tremor (15). In the 34 IPD patients whom we followed for several years (median 3.7 years) and confirmed the diagnosis with autopsy studies, every patient manifested RT at some time during the course of illness (16). The reported absence of tremor in IPD by other workers could be explained by the intermittent nature of tremor, the limited number of clinical assessments, the improvement of tremor with treatment, or an inaccurate clinical diagnosis of the PS variant (17).

James Parkinson (18) was so obviously impressed with tremor in the disorder, subsequently named after him, that he called it "the shaking palsy." In our experience, tremor remains an important manifestation in IPD, although the severity varies in different patients.

The most common anatomical site of tremor in IPD patients is the distal parts of the upper limbs. The characteristic upper limb RT includes pronation–supination of the forearm, flexion–extension at the wrist, or pill-rolling thumb movement (2). The pill-rolling tremor is characterized by the thumb producing gliding movements across the first two or three fingers. Tremor may also involve lips, jaw, tongue, or lower limbs. Unlike in essential tremor patients, head tremor is very rare in IPD.

Although in virtually all fully developed, untreated IPD patients, the severity of the tremor is comparable with the severity of bradykinesia and rigidity in some cases, the tremor is more or less pronounced compared with the other two major PS manifestations.

Even though the RT is considered to be the characteristic tremor in IPD, all behavioral types of tremor described in the foregoing—postural and kinetic— may be seen in these patients (11). The postural tremor in IPD is usually of smaller amplitude than the RT, but occurs at a faster rate (approximately 6 Hz) (10,11). Kinetic tremor, although present in some IPD patients, is less common than RT, has a smaller amplitude, and usually produces no significant functional disability.

Table 1 Clinical Aspects of Tremor in Extrapyramidal Diseases

Disorder/disease	The commonness of tremor	Site of tremor in order of frequency	Usual behavioral context, and less frequent tremor type	Some other clinical features	Response to drug therapy
Idiopathic (Lewy body) Parkinson's disease	All cases at some point during the illness; frequently reported as first symptom	UL (distal), LL, jaw, lip, tongue	Rest (4–5 Hz); hand pill-rolling; postural, and kinetic ≥ 6 Hz	Bradykinesia, and rigidity; tremor severity vs akinesia and rigidity, severity varies in different cases	Improves with levodopa and other anti-parkinsonian drugs; when tremor disproportionately more pronounced than bradykinesia and rigidity, the response to drugs is less favorable; β-adrenergic blockers improve tremor
Neurofibrillary tangle parkinsonism	Same as IPD	As above	As above	As above	As above
Parkinsonism due to SN and LC destruction, but no Lewy body	Same as IPD	As above	As above	As above	As above
MPTP-induced parkinsonism	Present in approximately ⅔ cases	Same as IPD	As above	Acute or subacute onset of PS	As above

Postencephalitic parkinsonism	Frequent but not an invariable feature	Upper limbs, LL, jaw, lips, tongue	Rest, action; usually small-amplitude	History of encephalitis; often evidence of other nervous system dysfunction; slow progression; oculogyric crisis	Moderate response to antiparkinsonian drugs
Striatonigral degeneration (only extrapyramidal dysfunction)	None	NA	NA	Akinetic–rigid; rapid progression compared with IPD	Usually no improvement
Multiple system atrophy with dysautonomia (Shy–Drager syndrome)	In approximately ½ cases	UL, lips, tongue, lower limbs	Rest, action (mixed tremor)	Akinesia, rigidity, and clinical evidence of widespread pathology; early bladder dysfunction and sexual potency loss, postural hypotension, rapid progression	With antiparkinsonian drugs; improvement in some patients during early stage
Olivopontocerebellar atrophy	Common	UL, LL	Rest, action (mixed) tremor	Evidence of cerebellar dysfunction frequent	Usually no improvement
Progressive supranuclear palsy	Extremely rare	Upper limb	Action (small-amplitude)	Akinesia, rigidity, and ophthalmoplegia	No improvement
IPD + Alzheimer's disease	Present in most cases with sequential onset of IPD + AD	UL, LL	Rest, action	Dementia	Improvement at early stage only in some patients

Table 1 Continued

Disorder/disease	The commonness of tremor	Site of tremor in order of frequency	Usual behavioral context, and less frequent tremor type	Some other clinical features	Response to drug therapy
Jakob–Creutzfeldt disease	Present in nearly 50% cases	Upper limb	Postural–kinetic; rarely, resting tremor	Dementia, myoclonus, rapid progression	No improvement
Parkinsonism dementia complex of Guam	Only in rare cases	Upper limb	Fine postural and kinetic; rarely resting tremor	Seen only in residents of the endemic region; frequent evidence of motor neuron disease	Poor response
Neuroleptic-induced parkinsonism	Approximately ½ cases	UL, perioral	Resting tremor, postural, kinetic	History of neuroleptic intake	Improves after withdrawing the offending drug and with anticholinergics
Parkinsonism secondary to CO poisoning	Very rare	Upper limb	Small-amplitude resting tremor	History of CO poisoning; akinetic–rigid PS	Usually no improvement
Cyanide-induced PS	Uncommon	UL, tongue, lips	Fine kinetic tremor; rarely, resting tremor	History of cyanide poisoning	Usually no improvement with drugs
PS due to manganese poisoning	Approximately ½ cases	Upper limb	Usually small amplitude; resting; may be kinetic tremor	Mainly akinetic–rigid and behavioral changes	Modest response
PS secondary to ischemia	Rare	Upper limb	Resting	Evidence of arteriosclerosis; mostly akinetic–rigid PS	Usually no improvement with antiparkinsonian drugs

PS secondary to repeated head trauma; "punch drunk syndrome"	Frequent	UL, lips, chin	Small-amplitude; resting, and less often, postural kinetic	Evidence of pyramidal tract and intellectual impairment common	Moderate response to drugs
Wilson's disease	Nearly all cases	UL, LL, jaw, trunk	Kinetic; postural; wing-beating flapping; resting tremor	Behavioral disorder; Kayser Fleischer corneal ring	Penicillamine, zinc sulfate, and, rarely, levodopa may relieve tremor
Dystonic tremor	Common	At the site of dystonia	When dystonic posture is corrected	Dystonia evident	Improves when dystonia improves with levodopa, anticholinergics, or botulinum toxin injection
Dystonia and tremor at different sites	10–85% of dystonia patients have tremor elsewhere	UL, head	Postural and kinetic-like essential tremor	May have family history of essential tremor or dystonia	Improves with β-adrenergic blockers
Dopa-responsive dystonia	Rare 15–30%	Upper limb	Postural tremor (8–10 Hz); resting tremor in some during late stage	Dystonia diurnal fluctuation in 75% of patients	Improves dramatically with small doses of levodopa
Rubral area lesion (rubral tremor)	Always	Upper limb	Kinetic, postural, resting	Cerebellar and midbrain dysfunction	Resting tremor may improve with levodopa

UL, upper limb; LL, lower limb; PS, parkinsonian syndrome; IPD, idiopathic Parkinson's disease; AD, Alzheimer's disease; NA, not applicable.

In some IPD patients, RT is more prominent in the lower than in the upper limbs. Similar to arm tremor, the leg tremor does not interfere with functioning—standing or walking. An independent lower limb RT is helpful in distinguishing IPD from essential tremor (19). Tremor in IPD may change during the course of illness—presumably owing to the evolution of the pathological process.

A.   Neurofibrillary Tangle Type of Parkinsonism

The neurofibrillary tangle type is a rare variant of parkinsonian syndrome (20). The anatomical site of lesions is the same as in IPD, but histologically there are neurofibrillary tangle inclusions and an absence of LB (20). The tremor in these patients is indistinguishable from that in IPD.

We have identified patients who have profound substantia nigra and locus coeruleus cell loss, but no inclusions (21). The tremor in these patients is identical with that in the IPD cases.

B.   Methyl-phenyl-tetrahydropyridine-Induced Parkinsonism

The major clinical features in these patients are the same as in IPD. Although RT is the characteristic tremor, it has been reported absent in three of seven patients (22). The entire course of illness in these cases has not yet been documented.

C.   Postencephalitic Parkinsonism

Tremor is a less prominent manifestation in post-encephalitic parkinsonism (PEP) than is rigidity. Both RT and AT may be seen in these patients, although neither is prominent.

D.   Striatonigral Degeneration

As contrasted with IPD, tremor is an infrequent manifestation of striatonigral degeneration (SND) (23). Since SND is a variant of multiple system atrophy (MSA), the site of pathology is not similar in all patients. Adams and Adams reported tremor in approximately one-half of the SND cases, although they did not clarify the site of lesions in each subgroup. In our SND patients (16,24) for whom the pathology was limited to the SN and the striatum, no RT was noted, but in those with more widespread disfunction, RT was noted in the majority, and in most of these kinetic tremor was also evident.

E.   Multiple System Atrophy with Dysautonomia (Shy–Drager Syndrome)

In approximately one-half of these patients, RT and AT are seen. With evolution of the illness, the tremor characteristic may change in some cases.

F. Olivopontocerebellar Atrophy

Olivopontocerebellar atrophy bears considerable similarity to MSA. Some patients may have resting tremor, as in IPD, but more often there is kinetic and terminal tremor (16,25).

G. Progressive Supranuclear Palsy

Lees (26) concludes that RT is extremely rare in progressive supranuclear palsy (PSP). Tremor in general is extremely rare in PSP (16,27).

H. Idiopathic Parkinson's Disease and Alzheimer's Disease Association

The overlap between IPD and Alzheimer's disease (AD) is extensive (28,29). Most studies have concentrated on the dementia in IPD patients (30–32), on the extrapyramidal signs in AD (33), or on pathological coexistence of IPD and AD (34). However, the information on tremor in patients suffering from both these disorders is limited. Ditter and Mirra reported no tremor in 11 pathologically verified cases of IPD plus AD (28). In the six patients whom we personally followed for a long period and pathologically confirmed the diagnosis of IPD and AD, all manifested RT, which during the early stage was indistinguishable from IPD tremor. With progress of the diseases, RT became less pronounced, and KT became more obvious in these patients (16).

I. Jakob–Creutzfeldt Disease

Tremor is reported in approximately half of these patients. It is usually action tremor—postural and kinetic—although rare cases may have resting tremor.

J. Parkinsonism–Dementia Complex of Guam

Tremor is seldom a prominent feature of the parkinsonian–dementia complex (PDC; 25,27,35,36). When present, it is usually a fine rapid postural and kinetic tremor, although in rare cases, resting tremor has been reported.

K. Neuroleptic-Induced Parkinsonism

In most neuroleptic-induced parkinsonism (NIP) cases, bradykinesia and rigidity are early and dominant manifestations. These patients, in general, are indistinguishable from IPD (37). In rare NIP cases, we have observed RT as the overwhelming clinical manifestation. In some NIP cases, rhythmic tremulousness of the facial muscles and jaw are a prominent feature. This clinical picture has been described as rabbit syndrome. The rationale for this separate label, as distinct from RT has been questioned by some authorities (38).

Lithium may produce action tremor and accentuates essential tremor, although in rare cases, resting tremor has been reported (39).

Neuroleptic malignant syndrome (NMS) is characterized by marked rigidity and akinesia, but small-amplitude resting and action tremor is seen in approximately half the patients (40).

In the parkinsonian syndrome consequent to carbon monoxide, cyanide, manganese, or methyl alcohol poisoning, and in that due to basal ganglia ischemic lesions, tremor is an uncommon manifestation (41–47) (see Table 1).

L. Carbon Monoxide Poisoning

In the PS consequent to carbon monoxide poisoning, akinesia and rigidity are the dominant features although, rarely, small-amplitude RT may be seen (48).

In the cyanide-induced parkinsonism, resting tremor is not a prominent feature (43).

M. Manganese Poisoning

In the PS caused by manganese poisoning, tremor is seen in about half the patients. All varieties—resting, postural, and kinetic—have been reported. In a series of four patients, Wolters et al. noted small-amplitude resting tremor in two cases (42). Huang et al. studied six patients (41). They primarily manifested as akinesia and rigidity, although in three patients (50%) low-amplitude tremor was noted (41).

N. Basal Ganglia Lacunar State

Basal ganglia lacunar state resulting in parkinsonism usually manifests as akinesia and rigidity, but in rare cases, resting tremor may be seen (44).

O. Punch Drunk Syndrome

In traumatic encephalopathy in the professional boxers, 15–20% of them have parkinsonism and widespread central nervous system dysfunction (27). Tremor is frequently seen in these cases. Small-amplitude RT is the most common tremor, but less-pronounced action tremor is also seen.

P. Wilson's Disease

In nearly half of the Wilson's disease patients, the first manifestation is a neurological dysfunction (49). The most common initial symptom (50) and the "most constant feature" of Wilson's disease is tremor (51). The tremor involves upper limbs, lower limbs, head, and trunk (50). During the early stage, there is fine upper limb action tremor that may interfere with writing or feeding. Intermittently, the tremor may become dramatically worse for several minutes. Tremor at the shoulders when the arms are abducted at 90° and flexed at the elbows—known as "wing beating"—is the most characteristic tremor. Some patients may have a flapping tremor at the wrists in the outstretched hands. Although the wing-beating tremor is the most dramatic and is frequently considered to be characteristic of Wilson's disease, resting tremor is probably more common than the other tremor variants in this disease (49). The RT amplitude is usually small, but those postural and kinetic tremors are larger.

III. DYSTONIA AND TREMOR

Association between dystonia and tremor is seen in several clinical situations. These include dystonic tremor, dystonia associated with essential tremor, and dystonia that may evolve into parkinsonism.

A. Dystonic Tremor

Dystonic tremor is triggered when an effort is made to overcome the abnormal posture caused by dystonic muscle contractions. For example, a patient has dystonia that results in pronation of the forearm, if an attempt is made to supinate that arm, it may result in a pronation–supination tremor. Yet if that arm were fully pronated, there would be no tremor. Usually, it is a nonrhythmic jerking movement, although at times, it may acquire the rhythmic character of a tremor (6).

In spasmodic torticollis (ST) patients, in addition to the myoclonic jerks or slow, rhythmic movements that result in deviation of the head, there may also be a rapid, horizontal or vertical head tremor (52). In some patients, the head tremor may precede the spasmodic torticollis by several years.

B. Dystonia Associated with Tremor at Distant Sites

Baxter and Lal noted postural and kinetic tremor in 10% of their dystonia cases (53). Bruyn and Roos reported that 14% of generalized idiopathic dystonia patients have tremor resembling essential tremor (54). Couch noted that 86% of their 30 ST patients had upper limb tremor similar to essential tremor (55).

In levodopa-responsive dystonia, tremor may be seen in 15–30% of cases. The tremor usually emerges after the age of 10 years and responds well to levodopa (56,57). Nygaard et al. reviewed 86 levodopa-responsive dystonic cases and noted that 14% had resting tremor, whereas 22% had postural tremor at the full expression of the disease (59). Some of the levodopa-responsive dystonia patients have additional features of parkinsonism (59). Segawa et al. (56) claim that these DRD patients are different from the early-onset parkinsonism patients, who may have dystonia as the initial manifestation. The juvenile-onset parkinsonian patients, according to these authors (56), have resting tremor, whereas in levodopa-responsive dystonia, the tremor is more postural. In one series of X-linked dystonias, 15% had parkinsonianlike resting tremor (52).

C. Rubral Tremor

Rubral tremor is also known as cerebellar outflow tremor or midbrain tremor. The tremor is present at rest, but becomes more pronounced on maintaining posture and is even more severe during movement (10,60,61). Because of the associated cerebellar and other midbrain neurological signs, this tremor can be distinguished from other forms of kinetic tremor (62). The resting tremor in these patients may improve with levodopa (61).

D. Juvenile Parkinsonism

The first manifestation in about 70% of these patients is gait difficulty. When the onset is younger than age 30, tremor is rare; however, in those with onset after aged 30, tremor is more frequently seen. In only one-third of the patients, the initial symptom is tremor that is present at rest, has faster frequency than the IPD tremor, and accentuates during voluntary activity (63).

E. Akinetic–Rigid Form of Huntington's Disease

The juvenile form of Huntington's disease may be associated with fine action tremor during early stage (64,65).

In benign, hereditary chorea of early onset (also known as chronic juvenile hereditary chorea), less than half the families have upper limb kinetic tremor and, later in the course of illness, they may develop head nodding, and rare cases may develop RT. The picture, on the whole, resembles essential tremor (66).

F. Joseph's Disease

Type II is characterized by slow progression of cerebellar and extrapyramidal dysfunction, and type IV is a form of dominantly inherited parkinsonism, with distal atrophy (27). These patients may manifest resting or mixed tremor.

G. Corticobasal Ganglionic Degeneration

It is also known as corticonigral degeneration or corticodentatonigral degeneration. Tremor is not a dominant feature of this disorder and, when present, is primarily an action tremor.

H. Hallvorden–Spatz Disease

In Hallvorden–Spatz disease, tremor is uncommon (67). When present, it is mainly an action tremor—postural and kinetic—and, less frequently, resting tremor (27).

I. Normopressure Hydrocephalus

In one normopressure hydrocephalus series, 40% of the patients had parkinsonian features (68).

J. Basal Ganglia Calcification

Basal ganglia calcification may be asymptomatic, but some patients will have PS, including resting tremor (27,69). In hyperparathyroidism, the most common extrapyramidal syndrome is parkinsonism (70).

IV. CONCLUSIONS

Tremor is a frequent manifestation in extrapyramidal disorders. The most common is the resting tremor that is characteristic of idiopathic Parkinson's disease. The anatomical and biochemical substrate of the tremor is not fully established. In those disorders in which the pathological process affects the substantia nigra and locus coeruleus, a resting tremor is seen. On the other hand, when the lesions involve the putamen or the globus pallidus, with or without substantia nigra pathology, tremor is not a prominent feature. In the disorders characterized by widespread involvement of the brainstem as well as the substantia nigra (e.g., progressive supranuclear palsy and parkinsonian dementia complex of Guam) tremor is not a prominent feature. In those extrapyramidal disorders, in which cerebellofugal pathways are involved, often there is mixed—resting, postural, and kinetic—tremor. The reasons for the wide variation in the severity of tremor in patients suffering from Lewy body Parkinson's disease remain to be determined.

REFERENCES

1. Weiner WJ, Lang AE. An introduction to movement disorders. In: Weiner WJ, Lang AE, eds. Movement Disorders: A Comprehensive Survey. Mount Kisco, NY: Futura Publishing, 1989:1–22.
2. Hallett M. Differential diagnosis of tremor. In: Vinken PJ, Bruyn GW, Klawans HL, eds. Handbook of Clinical Neurology; Extrapyramidal Disorders. New York: Elsevier Science Publishing, 1986:583–595.
3. Capildeo R, Findley LJ. Classification of tremor. In: Findley LJ, Capildeo R, eds. Movement Disorders: Tremor. London: Macmillan Press, 1984:3–13.
4. Freund HJ, Hefter H, Homberg V, Reiners K. Differential diagnosis of motor disorders by tremor analysis. In: Findley LJ, Capildeo R, eds. Movement Disorders: Tremor. London: Macmillan Press, 1984:27–35.
5. Fahn S. Cerebellar tremor: clinical aspects. In: Findley LJ, Capildeo R, eds. Movement Disorders: Tremor. London: Macmillan Press, 1984:355–363.
6. Fahn S. Atypical tremors, rare tremors and unclassified tremors. In: Findley LJ, Capildeo R, eds. Movement disorders: tremor. London: Macmillan Press, 1984:431–443.

7. Gresty MA, Findley LJ. Definition, analysis and genesis of tremor. In: Findley LJ, Capildeo R, eds. Movement Disorders: Tremor. London: Macmillan Press, 1984:15–26.

8. Gresty MA, McCarthy R, Findley LJ. Assessment of resting tremor in Parkinson's disease. In: Findley LJ, Capildeo R, eds. Movement Disorders: Tremor. London: Macmillan Press, 1984:321–329.

9. Duvoisin R, Golbe LI. Toward a definition of Parkinson's disease. Neurology 1989; 39:746.

10. Marsden CD. Origins of normal and pathological tremor. In: Findley LJ, Capildeo R, eds. Movement Disorders: Tremor. London: Macmillan Press, 1984:37–84.

11. Findley LJ, Gresty MA. Tremor and rhythmical involuntary movements in Parkinson's disease. In: Findley LJ, Capildeo R, eds. Movement Disorders: Tremor. London: Macmillan Press, 1984:295–304.

12. Hoehn MM, Yahr MD. Parkinsonism: onset, progression, and mortality. Neurology 1967; 17:427–442.

13. Jankovic J. Pathophysiology and clinical assessment of motor symptoms in Parkinson's disease. In: Koller WC, ed. Handbook of Parkinson's Disease. New York: Marcel Dekker, 1987:99–126.

14. Stern G. Prognosis in Parkinson's disease. In: Marsden CD, Fahn S, eds. Movement Disorders 2. London: Butterworth & Co. 1987:91–98.

15. Jenner P, Marsden CD. Neurochemical basis of parkinsonian tremor. In: Findley LT, Capildeo R, eds. Movement Disorders: Tremor. London: Macmillan Press, 1984: 305–320.

16. Rajput AH, Rozdilsky B, Ang L. Occurrence of resting tremor in Parkinson's disease. Neurology 1991; 41:1298–1299.

17. Rajput AH, Rozdilsky B, Rajput AH. Accuracy of clinical diagnosis in parkinsonism—a prospective study. Can J Neurol Sci 1991; 18:275–278.

18. Parkinson J. An Essay on the Shaking Palsy. London: Sherwood Neely & Jones, 1817.

19. Rajput AH, Rozdilsky B, Rajput AH. Essential leg tremor. Neurology 1990; 40:1909.

20. Rajput AH, Uitti RJ, Sudhakar S, Rozdilsky B. Parkinsonism and neurofibrillary tangle pathology in pigmented nuclei. Ann Neurol 1989; 25:602–606.

21. Rajput AH, Rozdilsky B, Rajput A, Ang L. Levodopa efficacy and pathological basis of Parkinson syndrome. Clin Neuropharmacol 1990; 13:553–558.

22. Ballard P, Tetrud JW, Langston JW. Permanent human parkinsonism due to 1-methyl-4-phenyl-1,2,3,6-tetrahydropyridine (MPTP): seven cases. Neurology 1985; 35:949–956.

23. Adams RD, Salam-Adams M. Striatonigral degeneration. In: Vinken PJ, Bruyn GW, Klawans HL, eds. Handbook of Clinical Neurology; Extrapyramidal Disorders. New York: Elsevier Science Publishing, 1986:205–212.

24. Rajput AH, Kazi KH, Rozdilsky B. Striatonigral degeneration response to levodopa therapy. J Neurol Sci 1972; 16:331–341.

25. Marshall A. Pathology of tremor. In: Findley LJ, Capildeo R, eds. Movement Disorders: Tremor. London: Macmillan Press, 1984:95–123.

26. Lees AJ. The Steele–Richardson–Olszewski syndrome (progressive supranuclear palsy). In: Marsden CD, Fahn S, eds. Movement Disorders 2. London: Butterworth & Co, 1987:272–287.

27. Weiner WJ, Lang AE. Other akinetic–rigid and related syndromes. In: Weiner WJ, Lang AE, eds. Movement Disorders: A Comprehensive Survey. Mount Kisco, NY: Futura Publishing, 1989:188–189.

28. Ditter SM, Mirra SS. Neuropathologic and clinical features of Parkinson's disease in Alzheimer's disease patients. Neurology 1987; 37:754–760.

29. Gibb WRG. Dementia and Parkinson's disease. Br J Psychiatry 1989; 154:596–614.

30. Rajput AH, Offord KP, Beard CM, Kurland LT. A case control study of smoking habits, dementia and other illnesses in idiopathic Parkinson's disease. Neurology 1987; 37:226–232.

31. Mayeux R, Stern Y, Rosenstein R, et al. An estimate of the prevalence of dementia in idiopathic Parkinson's disease. Arch Neurol 1988; 45:260–262.

32. Brown RG, Marsden CD. How common is dementia in Parkinson's disease? Lancet 1984; 2:1262–1265.

33. Galasko D, Kwo-on-Yuen PF, Klauber MR, Thal LJ. Neurological findings in Alzheimer's disease and normal aging. Arch Neurol 1990; 47:625–627.

34. Jellinger LK. Pathological Correlates of dementia in Parkinson's disease. Arch Neurol 1987; 44:690–691.

35. Chen KM, Chase TN. Parkinsonism–dementia. In: Vinken PJ, Bruyn GW, Klawans HL, eds. Handbook of Clinical Neurology; Extrapyramidal Disorders. New York: Elsevier Science Publishing, 1986:167–183.

36. Hirano A, Malamud N, Kurland LT. Parkinsonism–dementia complex, an endemic disease on the island of Guam. Brain 1961; 84:662–679.

37. Hardie RJ, Lees AJ. Neuroleptic-induced Parkinson's syndrome: clinical features and results of treatment with levodopa. J Neurol Neurosurg Psychiatry 1988; 51:850–854.

38. Tanner CM. Drug-induced movement disorders (tardive dyskinesia and dopa-induced dyskinesia). In: Vinken PJ, Bruyn GW, Klawans HL, eds. Handbook of Clinical Neurology; Extrapyramidal Disorders. New York: Elsevier Science Publishing, 1986: 185–204.

39. Lang AE. Lithium and parkinsonism. Ann Neurol 1984; 15:214.

40. Srinivasan AV, Murugappan M, Krishnamurthy SG, Sayeed ZA. Neuroleptic malignant syndrome. J Neurol Neurosurg Psychiatry 1990; 53:514–516.

41. Huang CC, Chu NS, Lu CS, et al. Chronic manganese intoxication. Arch Neurol 1989; 46:1104–1106.

42. Wolters EC, Huang CC, Clark C, et al. Positron emission tomography in manganese intoxication. Ann Neurol 1989; 26:647–651.

43. Uitti RJ, Rajput AH, Ashenhurst EM, Rozdilsky B. Cyanide-induced parkinsonism: a clinicopathologic report. Neurology 1985; 35:921–925.

44. Murrow RW, Schweiger GD, Kepes JJ, Koller WC. Parkinsonism due to a basal ganglia lacunar state: clinicopathologic correlation. Neurology 1990; 40:897–900.

45. Jellinger K. Degenerations and exogenous lesions of the pallidum and striatum. Handbook of Clinical Neurology, 1968:632–693.

46. Jellinger K. Pallidal, pallidonigral and pallidoluysionigral degenerations including association with thalamic and dentate degenerations. In: Vinken PJ, Bruyn GW, Klawans HL, eds. Handbook of Clinical Neurology; Extrapyramidal Disorders. New York: Elsevier Science Publishing, 1986:445–463.

47. Klawans HL, Stein RW, Tanner CM, Goetz CG. A pure parkinsonian syndrome following acute carbon monoxide intoxication. Arch Neurol 1982; 39:302–304.
48. Jellinger K. Exogenous lesions of the pallidum. In: Vinken PJ, Bruyn GW, Klawans HL, eds. Handbook of Clinical Neurology; Extrapyramidal Disorders. Amsterdam: Elsevier Science Publishers, 1986:465–491.
49. Walshe JM. Wilson's disease. In: Vinken PJ, Bruyn GW, Klawans HL, eds. Handbook of Clinical Neurology; Extrapyramidal Disorders. New York: Elsevier Science Publishing, 1986:223–238.
50. Weiner WJ, Lang AE. Wilson's disease. In: Weiner WJ, Lang AE, eds. Movement Disorders: A Comprehensive Survey. Mount Kisco, NY: Futura Publishing, 1989:257–291.
51. Martin JP. Wilson's disease. In: Vinken PJ, Bruyn GW, eds. Handbook of Clinical Neurology: Diseases of the Basal Ganglia. New York: John Wiley & Sons, 1968: 267–278.
52. Weiner WJ, Lang AE. Movement Disorders: A Comprehensive Survey. Mount Kisco, NY: Futura Publishing, 1989:347–418.
53. Baxter DW, Lal S. Essential tremor and dystonic syndromes. In: Poirier LJ, Sourkes TL, Bedard PJ, eds. Advances in Neurology. New York: Raven Press, 1979:373–377.
54. Bruyn GW, Roos RAC. Dystonia musculorum deformans. In: Vinken PJ, Bruyn GW, Klawans HL, eds. Handbook of Clinical Neurology; Extrapyramidal Disorders. New York: Elsevier Science Publishing, 1986:519–528.
55. Couch JR. Dystonia and tremor in spasmodic torticollis. In: Eldridge R, Fahn S, eds. Advances in Neurology. New York; Raven Press, 1976:245–258.
56. Segawa M, Nomura Y, Kase M. Diurnally fluctuating hereditary progressive dystonia. In: Vinken PJ, Bruyn GW, Klawans HL, eds. Handbook of Clinical Neurology; Extrapyramidal Disorders. New York: Elsevier Science Publishing, 1986:529–539.
57. Nygaard TG, Marsden CD, Fahn S. Dopa-responsive dystonia: long-term treatment response and prognosis. Neurology 1991; 41:174–181.
58. Nygaard TG, Marsden CD, Duvoisin RC. Dopa-responsive dystonia. In: Fahn S, et al. eds. Dystonia 2. Adv Neurol 1988; 50:377–384.
59. Nygaard TG, Duvoisin RC. Hereditary dystonia–parkinsonism syndrome of juvenile onset. Neurology 1986; 36:1424–1428.
60. Koppel BS, Daras M. "Rubral" tremor due to midbrain toxoplasma abscess. Mov Disord 1990; 5:254–256.
61. Findley LJ, Gresty MA. Suppression of "rubral tremor" with levodopa. Br Med J 1980; 281:1043.
62. Weiner WJ, Lang AE. Tremor. In: Weiner WJ, Lang AE, eds. Movement Disorders: A Comprehensive Survey. Mount Kisco, NY: Futura Publishing, 1989:221–256.
63. Narabayashi H, Yokochi M, Iizuka R, Nagatsu T. Juvenile parkinsonism. In: Vinken PJ, Bruyn GW, Klawans HL, eds. Handbook of Clinical Neurology; Extrapyramidal Disorders. New York: Elsevier Science Publishing, 1986:153–165.
64. Bruyn GW. Huntington's chorea; historical, clinical and laboratory synopsis. In: Vinken PJ, Bruyn GW, eds. Handbook of Clinical Neurology; Diseases of the Basal Ganglia. New York: John Wiley & Sons, 1968:298–378.
65. Bruyn GW, Went LN. Huntington's chorea. In: Vinken PJ, Bruyn GW, Klawans HL,

eds. Handbook of Clinical Neurology; Extrapyramidal Disorders. New York: Elsevier Science Publishing, 1986:267–313.

66. Bruyn GW, Myrianthopoulos NC. Chronic juvenile hereditary chorea (benign hereditary chorea of early onset). In: Vinken PJ, Bruyn GW, Klawans HL, eds. Handbook of Clinical Neurology; Extrapyramidal Disorders. New York: Elsevier Science Publishing, 1986:335–348.

67. Seitelberger F. Neuroaxonal dystrophy: its relation to aging and neurologic diseases. In: Vinken PJ, Bruyn GW, Klawans HL, eds. Handbook of Clinical Neurology; Extrapyramidal Disorders. New York: Elsevier Science Publishing, 1986:391–415.

68. Jacobs L, Conti D, Kinkel WR, Manning EJ. "Normal pressure" hydrocephalus. Relationship of clinical and radiographic findings to improvement following shunt surgery. JAMA 1976; 235:510–512.

69. Lowenthal A, Bruyn GW. Calcification of the striopallidodentate system. In: Vinken PJ, Bruyn GW, eds. Handbook of Clinical Neurology; Diseases of the Basal Ganglia. New York: John Wiley & Sons, 1968:703–725.

70. Boller F, Boller M, Gilbert J. Familial idiopathic cerebral calcifications. J Neurol Neurosurg Psychiatry 1977; 40:280–285.

20

Problems in Measurement of Parkinsonian Tremor

Erich Scholz and Michael Bacher
University of Tübingen
Tübingen, Germany

I. INTRODUCTION

Most of the problems encountered in tremor evaluation in Parkinson's disease and other tremor disorders stem from the great variability of this symptom. "Tremor is subject to sudden fluctuations, which seem to be apparently spontaneous and can occur within a short space of time in patients seemingly relaxed and unstimulated" (1). Mental activation (arithmetic, "Stroop test") has been used for clinical differential diagnosis and for tremor activation to establish a standardized reproducible situation and a reliable baseline for the evaluation of treatment effects (1,2). Patient reports, however, indicate that these methods induce an even greater tremor amplitude than that observed in daily life. Attempts to minimize external influences on tremor recording have included requesting the patients to abstain from coffee, tea, and cigarettes; tremor recording at fixed times of the day or in quiet surroundings; and familiarization of patients with the laboratory recording environment. Despite all these efforts, however, no way has yet been found of reliably controlling all the factors influencing tremor. All these factors play a role, not only in all types of short-term tremor evaluation, but in clinical ratings and objective measurement of brief tremor phases as well.

The variability of tremor intensity has been thought to reflect a stochastic process in earlier years; however, it may also reflect changes in a chaotic system. The difference between both models is of importance for tremor evaluation. The assumption of a stochastic process underlying tremor modulation implies that—

provided all factors involved are under control—tremor an be predicted with a certain degree of statistical reliability on the basis of previously measured tremor periods. In a chaotic process, however, the future development of the process is unforeseeable. As a result, future tremor development cannot be predicted from the tremor data at a given time point. One step toward minimizing error in the evaluation of a stochastic as well as a chaotic system is to observe and measure over a long period.

Throughout the years, various efforts have been undertaken to develop methods of objective tremor measurement and were even thought, by some investigators, to make commonly used clinical tremor ratings obsolete. The main criticism concerning these commonly used methods of objective measurement for the evaluation of treatment effects is that short-term recordings usually cover only a few minutes. Because of fluctuations in tremor intensity, such single and short-term tremor measurements may not be representative of the patients' actual disturbances.

Several investigators have explored the usefulness of long-term tremor recording (3–5). Their assumption was that the whole tremor spectrum of a given patient is recorded representatively and unrestrictedly during a longer recording period. Patients are not confined to the laboratory and may even leave the clinic. For unknown reasons, none of these methods has, to our knowledge, yet been used in clinical practice.

We ourselves have developed a method of ambulatory, 24-h electromyographic (EMG) tremor recording that, in our view, is practicable, quick, and easy to use in clinical practice (6,7). This chapter describes results achieved with this method during investigations of the reliability and reproducibility of long-term measurement in de novo patients as well as after treatment. In addition, we compared the results of long-term measurement with those of conventional clinical ratings and patients' self-monitoring of treatment effects.

II. TECHNICAL CONSIDERATIONS

A. Technical Details of 24-Hour Tremor Recording

The tremor EMG signal is recorded by a four-channel Medilog recorder. Two silver–silver chloride pregelled surface electrodes, 1 cm in diameter [commercially available as 24-h electrocardiogram (ECG) electrodes], are placed 10-cm apart over the extensor carpi radialis and flexor carpi ulnaris muscles of each forearm. The electrodes, cables, and recorder do not hinder normal movements. Patients can move freely about on the ward, or even go home, after attachment of the apparatus. The 24-h EMG recordings are stored on tape. This standard equipment amplifies and filters EMG signals with a bandwidth of 0.5–100 Hz.

The recorded tape is replayed on an Oxford PMD12 system (standard EEG recording equipment) at 20 times real-time speed. The EMG signals are A/D-converted and stored on the hard disk of an 80386 PC. The sampling rate is 4000 Hz, corresponding to 200 Hz under real-time conditions. Real-time periods of 5.12 s are sequentially analyzed. Signal quality is monitored automatically against a fixed amplitude range. Segments in which more than 10% of amplitudes exceed the fixed range are withdrawn from further analysis. The final printout gives the percentage of periods containing artifacts, so that the overall quality of the recording can be checked. Low-frequency artifacts are eliminated by means of a digital FIR high-pass filter, with a cutoff frequency of 10 Hz, a length of 75, and a Hamming characteristic. In a second step, the signal is squared and smoothed. The cutoff frequency of the low-pass FIR filter is 20 hz, the length is 51, and a Blackman window is used to calculate the filter coefficients. After filtering, the signal's square root is taken to linearize the data. Power spectra are calculated on the basis of 5.12-s periods, with an FFT-algorithm; hence, the spectrum resolution is 0.1953 Hz. The spectra of three consecutive periods are averaged.

Tremor intensity is estimated by means of the signal/noise ratio (SNR) of the dominant peak of the power spectrum. The peak must be located between 3 and 15 Hz. Three values at the peak (the maximal plus the two neighboring values) are summed. After subtracting the noise level, the sum is divided by the noise level, which is the mean of all spectrum values between 3 and 15 Hz, excluding the three values representing the tremor peak. With this as a relative value for tremor intensity, it is possible to separate tremor from voluntary nonrhythmic activity, independent of the total amount of EMG activity. The frequency of the highest peak value defines the tremor frequency (for further details see Ref. 7).

B. Advantages and Drawbacks of Different Tremor Recording Methods

Methods of objective tremor recording are based either on surface EMG or on movement recordings made with potentiometers, accelerometers, and movement analysis systems (e.g., ELITE). None of these methods has proved superior to the others. Rather, each has its advantages and shortcomings.

1. Accelerometers

Accelerometers are used in most cases (5,8–10). They are much more sensitive to high-frequency vibrations than displacement devices. The acceleration of a limb most directly reflects the underlying muscular contraction. Linear accelerometers on a piezoresistive basis weighing only a few grams are small enough to be fixed to almost any part of the body. Accelerometers seem to be the best choice if the movements of the limb under observation are restricted to those caused by tremor. An accelerometer fixed to the hand, however, will measure all movements of the hand, including those caused by movements of the arm or the whole body. In addition, the influence of gravity will change according to the orientation of the hand. All these factors lead to artifactual low-frequency components that must then be eliminated by a suitable filter. This can affect the tremor signal itself, since the frequency range of the artifacts is close to that of tremor. Therefore, it is customary to restrict the movements of the recorded limb. Another solution may be to use two accelerometers, mounted, for example, on hand and wrist, so that the difference signal is less influenced by other parts of the body. A drawback of accelerometers is that they must be handled with great care. Taken together, these factors may explain why long-term accelerometer recordings under normal daily conditions have not become standard practice.

2. Movement Analysis Systems

The separation of tremor from other signal components is even more complex when movement analysis systems are used. Only restricted movements can be recorded easily, and the recordings are restricted to a laboratory environment. Nevertheless, the effort can be worthwhile if the influence of a special task or limb orientation is to be investigated.

3. Potentiometers

The use of a potentiometer to measure angular displacement (4) offers some advantages over a movement analysis system. In particular, the potentiometer signal is not altered by movements that do not affect the joint angle under observation. Shortcomings of the method are the difficulty in affixing the device and the restriction of the movement under investigation. Although long-term measurements with an average of 2 h are reported, they too are restricted to a laboratory environment.

4. Surface Electromyography

Another approach is to record surface EMG, thus quantifying the muscular activity causing the tremor (11,12). Surface EMG is not affected by passive movements of the limb. Since EMG and limb acceleration are closely related to the muscular force generating the movement, basically the same effects can be studied in EMG and accelerometer recordings (10). Low-frequency artifacts caused by changes of skin resistance or pressure on the electrodes are easily separated from the high-frequency EMG signal itself. Before beginning a spectral analysis, the EMG signal must be rectified or squared. After low-pass filtering, the signal resembles an accelerometer signal. However, problems may arise because tremor is usually not caused by one muscle alone, and it may be difficult to choose the appropriate muscle and recording location. Because of the nature of the signal, the sampling rate for recording must be much higher than for mechanical devices, such as accelerometers. Since it is almost impossible to deduce actual force or acceleration values from EMG signals, absolute EMG values of different patients cannot be compared directly.

C. Spectral Analysis

Fourier analysis is the mathematical method most commonly applied for tremor analysis. A correct understanding of this method requires some consideration of its practical aspects (for details see, e.g., Ref. 13).

Fourier analysis transforms the signal into a sum of sinusoids. A spectrum shows the power that each frequency contributes to the signal. If the signal from a mechanical device consists of only one sinusoid, the spectrum will have one peak at the frequency of that sinusoid, the rest of the spectrum being zero. If the signal is totally random, the power is distributed over the whole frequency range, and no prominent peak appears. Every spectrum calculated represents an estimation of the true spectrum under the distorting effect of different factors. One of these factors is spectral leakage, caused by the sampling period usually not being a multiple of the signal's natural duration. Artificial side lobes in the spectrum owing to spectral leakage can be reduced if drift is eliminated and if the data are smoothly brought to zero at the boundaries. This is achieved by weighting functions, called windows. Classic examples are the Hamming and Blackman windows (see Ref. 14 for a detailed description of windows).

Another distorting factor is the variability of the signal. Changes in frequency and amplitude of the periodic signal typically result in a broader main peak, with additional smaller peaks at multiples of the signal's fundamental frequency (harmonics). The quality of spectrum estimation can be improved by averaging consecutive spectra. However, this basically assumes that tremor is present for the entire duration used for calculation of one spectrum. If, in fact, the tremor episode is shorter, tremor amplitude will be underestimated. Improvement of spectrum estimation, therefore, conflicts with detection of short tremor episodes. Finally, the shape of the periodic signal also influences the spectrum. Deviations from a sinusoidal shape lead to additional peaks at multiples of the signal's fundamental frequency. This is typical for EMG signals, for which pulselike modulations of activity are quite common.

D. Calculation of Tremor Intensity

Most tremor intensity results are derived from spectral values. Every value in a spectrum represents the power that a special frequency contributes to the signal. Intensity may be measured absolutely or relatively. The amplitude of the dominant peak is an example of absolute measurement. The quotient of absolute measurement and a normative value (e.g., the sum of all spectral values) is a relative measurement result. Absolute measurement is suitable for quantifying the amplitude of an otherwise unchanged tremor signal. This approach is very similar to calculation of the mean peak-to-peak amplitude of the signal in the time period.

If the variability, shape or existence of tremor must be quantified, relative measurement should be used. It is not advisable to take only one value of the peak into account. The tremor peak is at least three values wide owing to spectral leakage and may be even wider because of variability caused in the signal by changes in frequency or amplitude of the tremor signal.

Unless the signal amplitude itself is zero, absolute intensity values will decrease, but not approach zero, if the signal changes from periodic to random. Although this is not usually a problem for signals from mechanical devices, the situation is different with EMG signals, which are not smooth and resemble amplitude-modulated noise in appearance. As a consequence, they contain a broadband component in every spectrum of nonzero activity (after rectification) that decreases only slightly in the range between 3 and 15 Hz. If the EMG is modulated periodically, the prominent peak is more variable and less pronounced, and additional peaks are more likely to occur. Therefore, it is more likely that a random signal will be interpreted as tremor. In addition, values for absolute intensity can be compared only for the same person and for a fixed electrode placement. Relative measurement must be used to quantify the variability of tremor. For movement signals, the power concentrated in the peak relative to the total power can be used to quantify the deviations from a sinusoid (10). For EMG signals, however, the broadband component, already mentioned, is always present. Therefore, it is better to use a signal/noise ratio as a relative measure of tremor intensity (11,12). A *signal/noise ratio* can be defined as the power concentrated in the peak area above the mean noise level relative to this noise level (for more details see Ref. 7). The advantage of this approach is that the absence of tremor in the EMG leads to an intensity value of zero, even if other (nonrhythmic) EMG activity is present, so that tremor, and especially the absence of tremor, are quantifiable. Voluntary activity does not affect the calculation of this relative measurement of intensity.

The EMG signals permit a signal/noise ratio to be used as a measure of tremor intensity if rising tremor amplitude leads to an increase in synchronized active motor units. In this situation, decreasing variability can be interpreted as an increase in tremor strength and, as such, can be quantified by a signal/noise ratio. If all active units are synchronized, however, this relative measure will not change, although tremor strength may vary along with the EMG amplitude. As a consequence, a signal/noise ratio is likely to be useful only in the lower range of tremor intensities.

E. Comparison of Intensity Evaluation by Means of Electromyography, Accelerometer, and Angular Displacement (ELITE)

We compared different methods of measuring tremor intensity as follows: angular displacement and acceleration of the hand were measured simultaneously with surface EMG at the extensor carpi radialis muscle in parkinsonian patients. At the same time, angular displacement was measured by an ELITE movement analysis system using markers fixed at the wrist and the proximal joint of the index finger. Finally, a small, lightweight accelerometer was fixed to the back of the hand 5-cm distal to the wrist. We measured tremors of different amplitudes, ranging from mild to coarse, both for rest and postural tremor (Fig. 1). Rest tremor was recorded with the forearm resting on a chair arm. Action or postural tremor was recorded with the arms held horizontally in front of the body. As controls we measured simulated tremor in normal subjects. Spectra were calculated for all signals. Three values of the prominent peak were summed to give an absolute measure of tremor intensity. In addition, the signal/noise ratio of the prominent peak was calculated for EMG. The correlation between intensity values derived from different signals was calculated individually for each subject.

There was a high correlation in normal subjects between the intensities derived from acceleration and from angular movement in both rest tremor and rhythmic movements (in fact, the results were basically equivalent).

Correlation was also high in normal subjects between the intensities derived from movement data (acceleration, angular displacement) and absolute intensities derived from EMG. In parkinsonian patients, however, the correlation was not always significant. The lack of correlation in some patients may have been because we did not record the muscle that was the primary source of the tremor. The slopes of the regression lines differed for each subject owing to the variability of EMG amplitudes.

Although proximal tremor components contribute to both movement signals in action tremor, this contribution is much greater for the acceleration signal than for the angular signal. Some of the correlations found were not significant owing to differences in the influence of proximal tremor components.

There was no correlation between the intensities derived from movement signals (acceleration, angular displacement) and the signal/noise ratio derived from EMG in normal subjects. A few parkinsonian patients, on the other hand, showed a significant correlation. This negative result is not surprising: as mentioned earlier, the signal/noise ratio is useful only if tremor is mild or moderate. The range of intensity values must include small values to produce a significant correlation. Tremor intensities were in the upper range in normal subjects and in most patients. This is shown in Figure 2. A significant correlation was observed in subject D with a wide distribution of tremor intensity values starting nearly at zero.

We can conclude by saying that different signals lead to similar results under restricted and well-controlled conditions when an absolute measure of tremor intensity is used. The EMG is the most reliable signal if movements are unrestricted. Unfortunately, absolute EMG intensities cannot be compared from patient to patient. Relative measurement of tremor intensity is useful for quantifying mild and moderate tremor and demonstrating the existence of tremor in the presence of voluntary activity.

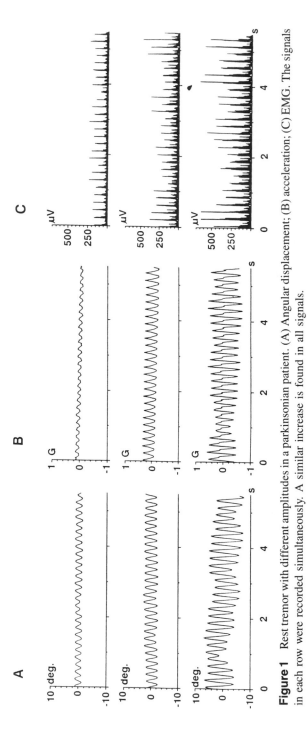

Figure 1 Rest tremor with different amplitudes in a parkinsonian patient. (A) Angular displacement; (B) acceleration; (C) EMG. The signals in each row were recorded simultaneously. A similar increase is found in all signals.

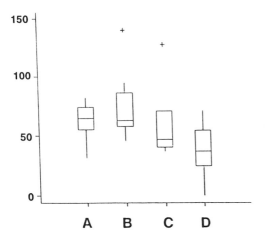

Figure 2 Box and whisker plots for signal/noise ratios derived from EMG spectra in four patients. The horizontal bar gives the median value, the box represents the upper and lower quartile, and the whiskers extend to the whole range. Pluses indicate the outliers. A significant correlation was observed in subject D, with a wide distribution of values starting from almost zero. This relative measure of tremor intensity, therefore, is useful only if tremor is mild or moderate.

III. CLINICAL CONSIDERATIONS

The following data are based on 10 h/day of tremor evaluation, starting at 9 or 10 o'clock AM and thus ranging over the major part of the waking hours. On recording days, each patient was asked to note major daytime events in a diary, as a means of monitoring unusual daytime activities (e.g., longer periods of daytime sleep). Clinical tremor rating was carried out separately for each limb and the head by an experienced neurologist before each tremor recording, using a scale ranging from 0 to 5 for both rest and postural tremor.

A. Variation in Tremor Intensity

In uncomplicated Parkinson's disease (and in essential tremor), tremor intensity changes over time, with no discernible daytime pattern. There is no increase in intensity in the evening, as might be expected from fatigue (Fig. 3A). This random pattern of intensity contains longer time periods with no tremor. Only few parkinsonian patients (i.e., those with wearing-off symptoms) had systematic variations in tremor intensity, with a nearly bell-shaped increase and decrease in intensity during "off." In these patients with a previously "drug-resistant" tremor-dominant Parkinson's disease, tremor vanished for hours during "on." When treatment was kept unchanged, tremor intensity histograms during three consecutive days consistently showed constant distributions.

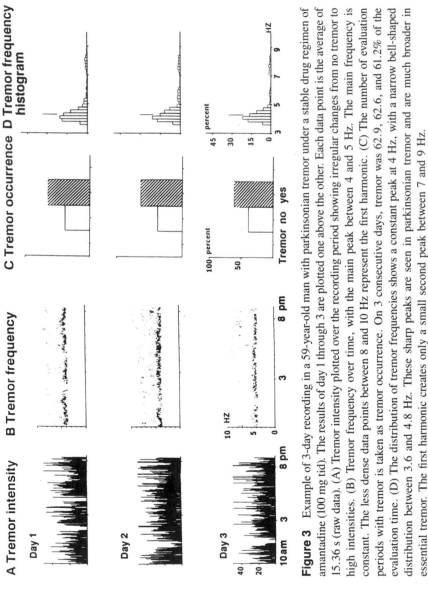

Figure 3 Example of 3-day recording in a 59-year-old man with parkinsonian tremor under a stable drug regimen of amantadine (100 mg tid). The results of day 1 through 3 are plotted one above the other. Each data point is the average of 15.36 s (raw data). (A) Tremor intensity plotted over the recording period showing irregular changes from no tremor to high intensities. (B) Tremor frequency over time, with the main peak between 4 and 5 Hz. The main frequency is constant. The less dense data points between 8 and 10 Hz represent the first harmonic. (C) The number of evaluation periods with tremor is taken as tremor occurrence. On 3 consecutive days, tremor was 62.9, 62.6, and 61.2% of the evaluation time. (D) The distribution of tremor frequencies shows a constant peak at 4 Hz, with a narrow bell-shaped distribution between 3.6 and 4.8 Hz. These sharp peaks are seen in parkinsonian tremor and are much broader in essential tremor. The first harmonic creates only a small second peak between 7 and 9 Hz.

B. Variation in Tremor Frequency

Long-term recording comes up with a normal distribution of frequencies around a constant peak (see Fig. 3D), rather than a single tremor frequency. Frequency varies over a time period, again with no systematic diurnal change (see Fig. 3B). The first harmonic should not be considered as an individual frequency, but as an artifact owing to Fourier analysis of the tremor signal (see foregoing). On 3 consecutive days, the frequency peak, as well as distribution, were for the most part stable (see Fig. 3D). Treatment has no effect on either frequency distribution or the peak frequency. The peak frequency is different in parkinsonian and essential tremor. In most patients, parkinsonian tremor has its peak frequency between 4 and 5 Hz, in essential tremor between 6 and 7 Hz. However, this peak frequency cannot be used for differential diagnosis. In several patients with early-onset parkinsonian tremor (younger than 40 years of age), we observed frequency peaks at about 7 Hz (e.g., the last line on the left in Fig. 4). Conversely, several essential tremor patients have frequency peaks at about 5 Hz. Up to this point, we did not systematically correlate age and tremor frequency.

The broadness of the frequency distribution, however, shows clear-cut differences between parkinsonian and essential tremor (see Fig. 4). We evaluated the broadness of distribution of the dominant peak in 25 histograms in both patient groups. In parkinsonian tremor, the average frequency range (between lowest and highest frequency observed in the main peak of the histogram) was 2.2 Hz, ranging from 1.4 to 2.8 Hz. Essential tremor has a wider range of frequencies, with a mean of 3.4 Hz (range 2.6–4 Hz). The difference was statistically significant ($p < 0.001$; nonparametric two-sample analysis). There was nearly no overlap between both groups. Variability of frequency, therefore, may be an indicator in differential diagnosis.

Several authors have claimed that individual patients can exhibit both tremor forms. In terms of tremor frequency, this should result in two distinct peaks (excluding the first harmonic) in the frequency distribution. We searched through our clinical tremor records and selected parkinsonian patients with clinically observed postural tremor and essential tremor patients with a rest tremor component. In all six parkinsonian patients there was only a single narrow tremor peak. Two of five essential tremor patients showed a bimodal frequency distribution, with one peak about 5 and another about 7 Hz, indicating two distinct tremors.

C. Variability of Tremor Occurrence From Day to Day

Tremor occurrence is the percentage of tremor during the whole evaluation period (see Fig. 3C). It enables us to give a simple value for day-to-day changes in tremor that are either spontaneous, or result from treatment. Since tremor occurrence may change not only from minute to minute, but also from day to day, as shown in the foregoing, we took recordings from 19 tremor patients on three consecutive days:

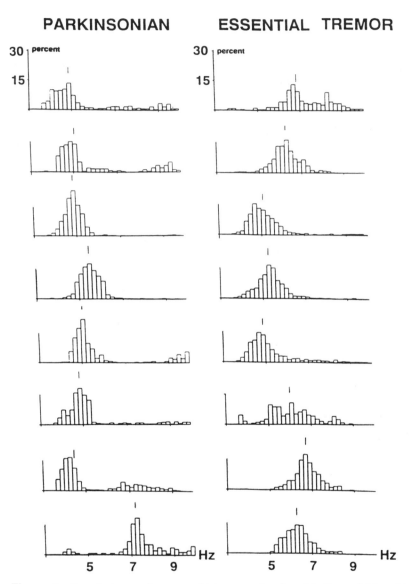

Figure 4 Sample tremor frequency histograms showing data from eight parkinsonian (left row) and eight essential tremor patients (right row). The range of frequencies in the main peak is smaller in parkinsonian than in essential tremor. The left side of each spectrum is about 5 Hz, excluding the lower peak at about 9 Hz, which represents the first harmonic. Frequency variability is significantly greater in essential tremor (see text). Note high-frequency parkinsonian tremor of about 7 Hz in an early-onset patient aged 38 years (lowest line on the left).

16 had parkinsonian tremor and 3 essential tremor. Eleven parkinsonian patients and 2 essential tremor patients were unmedicated, the medication of the remaining patient was kept unchanged during the recording period.

Differences in tremor occurrence of up to ±10% of the 3-day mean were found in individual patients from day to day. For the 19 patients, as a whole, however, the mean values of tremor occurrence remained largely stable (Fig. 5). The test–retest reliability of long-term recording, therefore, must be considered good when treatment remains unchanged, so that group mean values provide a reliable means of measuring treatment effects. In individual patients, however, treatment effects may be enhanced or diminished by this spontaneous variability of ±10%.

D. Influence of Epoch Length on Variability of Tremor Parameters

To estimate tremor variability, we divided the recording time of 10 h into increasingly smaller subsegments. An example was calculated with the raw data presented in Figure 3. All values calculated for these subsegments are plotted in Figure 6. Shortening the evaluation period leads to an increasing range of tremor occurrence values (see Fig. 6A). The same was true of tremor intensity (see Fig. 6B): when evaluation time was shorter, the range of measured values widened and the reliability of quantitative tremor assessment decreased in comparison with long-term measurement.

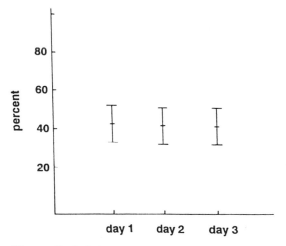

Figure 5 Relatively stable mean values of tremor occurrence in 19 patients over 3 consecutive days (42.4, 41.4, 41.4%; SD 21.2, 21.7, 18.6%). The large standard deviation is due to the large differences in tremor occurrence between patients.

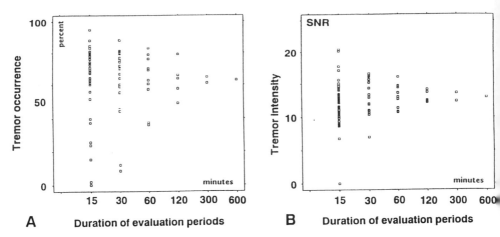

Figure 6 Data from the same patient as in Figure 3, day 1, used here for further calculation of variability in tremor data. Evaluation times were subdivided step by step into shorter segments of 6 h to 15 min. (A) Tremor occurrence values of each segment; (B) mean tremor intensity. The shorter the evaluation time, the more variable were the results obtained in the different subsegments. Evaluation segments of 15 min give the full range of possible values from 0 to 100% of tremor during the evaluation period.

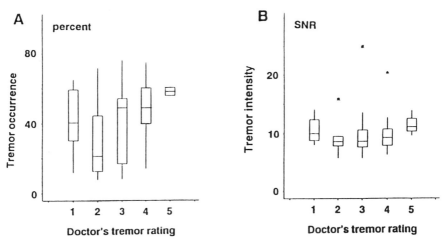

Figure 7 Effects of clinical tremor rating compared with tremor measurement in 19 patients ($n = 57$ records). Tremor was rated before the start of the recording on a clinical scale ranging from 0 to 5. The graphs show box and whisker plots. The horizontal bar gives the median value, the box represents the upper and lower quartile, and the whiskers extend to the whole range. Starts indicate the outliers. Neither tremor occurrence (A, $r = 0.25$; $r^2 = 6.19\%; p = 0.0669$) nor tremor intensity (B, $r = 0.042; r^2 = 0.18\%; p = 0.7586$) show a significant correlation with clinical rating scores in the regression analysis.

E. Comparison Between Clinical Rating and Measurement

Because we did a clinical rating at the start of each recording, we could directly compare clinical rates with recorded data. Clinical rating is still the far most commonly used method of tremor evaluation. It is easily applied, but has two major drawbacks: it is subjective, and it gives only short-term information.

Neither tremor occurrence (Fig. 7A) nor tremor intensity (see Fig. 7B) showed a correlation with clinical rating scores. This may be because clinical rating does not estimate the time during which tremor is present or the intensity is estimated at a time of considerable patient activation (i.e., after the recording device has been attached. Furthermore, clinical intensity evaluation focuses more on the maximum than on the mean tremor intensity.

F. Patients' Self-Monitoring, Physicians' Ratings, and Tremor Measurement in Treatment Evaluation

We compared physician's ratings, patients' self-monitoring, and tremor measurement in evaluating treatment effects in a prospective study including 15 patients. Our hypothesis was that the results of patient self-monitoring would be closer to measurement results than physicians' ratings. Only nondemented patients were included. Patients were asked in a simple, standardized manner for treatment effects. Possible answers were slight or considerable improvement, slight or considerable worsening, or no change in tremor. Treatment effects in the physicians' ratings were calculated as the difference of the rating values before and after treatment. Improvement in tremor measurement was calculated as the difference between tremor occurrence during baseline and treatment divided by the baseline tremor occurrence value (percentage improvement).

Patients' self-monitoring correlated well with measurement values, whereas changes in physician's ratings showed no correlation (Figs. 8 and 9).

IV. CONCLUSIONS

The high variability of tremor makes its evaluation difficult. Since the reasons for this variability are unknown and tremor resists reliable supervision, the best solution at present is long-term measurement (1).

The use of a conventional EEG tape recorder (Oxford Medilog) enables the patient to move around the ward without restraints and even leave the hospital. With this standard equipment, logistics were no problem. Tremor raw data are preserved for visual control and reevaluation in case of conflicting results. Human help is needed only for attachment and removal of the apparatus and amounts to half an hour at most, so that there are no difficulties in practical application. Evaluation of the large amount of data is automatic.

Artifacts of movements other than tremor may technically complicate the use of long-term accelerometer recordings (5), but are easily managed in EMG record-

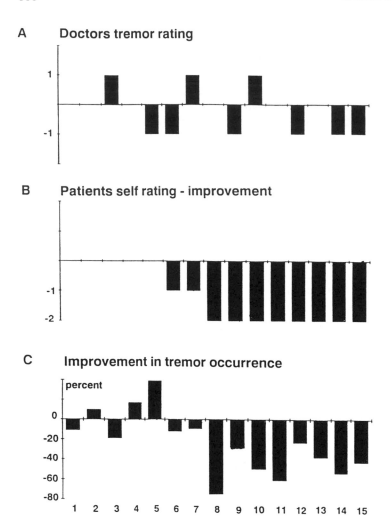

Figure 8 Patient reports on treatment effects compared with clinical ratings and 24-h tremor recording in 15 patients with parkinsonian tremor. The corresponding results of patients 1 through 15 are overlaid. (A) Tremor ratings for each limb on a scale ranging from 0 to 5. The difference in tremor rating is plotted before and during treatment. The differences indicate an improvement of 1 point on the scale (-1) in six, an increase in tremor amplitude of 1 point (± 1) in three, and no change in the remaining six patients. (B) Patients were asked whether their tremor was unchanged (0), better (slightly $= -1$, considerably $= -2$), or worse (slightly $= 1$, considerably $= 2$). (C) Improvement is given as percentage change of the initial premedication tremor occurrence value.

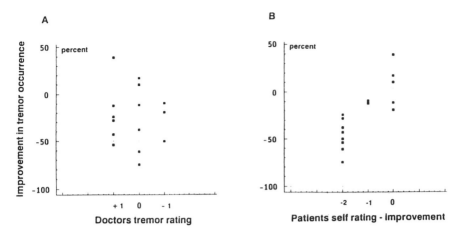

Figure 9 To quantify the relation between the different evaluation procedures, we used Kruskal–Wallis one-way analysis by ranks on the improvement data (see Fig. 8C), using either physicians' rating (see Fig. 8A) or patients' rating (see Fig. 8B) as a classification factor. The calculation revealed no effects for the physicians' rating (significance level $p = 0.9975$), but a significant effect for the patients' rating (significance level $p = 0.0049$). The same significant results were obtained with linear regression analysis.

ing. Within the range of clinically observable tremor amplitudes, tremor intensity values obtained with EMG, accelerometer, and angle displacement recording are correlated in such a way that they yield data of comparable intensity.

Minor problems may arise with both EMG and the accelerometer in that only selected tremulous limbs or muscles can be recorded at a time. This is adequately dealt with by selecting the limb(s) with the clinically most prominent tremor.

Theoretically, tremor variability is a phenomenon that is measurable in terms of minutes, hours, or even days. In practice, however, the tremor occurrence measured in a group of patients on 3 consecutive days remained largely stable. The test–retest reliability of tremor occurrence for group mean values was good. Group effects of treatment, therefore, can also be considered reliable. In individual patients, tremor occurrence varied by ±10%/day from the mean for 3 consecutive days.

Clinical tremor ratings possess two major drawbacks: they are subjective, since intensity estimates of different investigators or centers cannot be compared; and they are based on only short-term information. Compared with long-term tremor measurement, they seem to offer the least reliable results.

Self-monitoring of clinical symptoms by parkinsonian patients is of interest because of its simplicity and the information that thereby becomes available concerning daily activities and environmental factors. However, the data on tremor self-assessment up to now are sparse and conflicting (15–17). In light of our data, the relatively poor agreement between clinical evaluation and patients' physical self-assessment of tremor, especially in the report of Golbe and Pae (15), argue against clinical evaluation. Patients are able to provide an accurate self-report of their global level of disability (16). Ratings of tremor severity have shown test–retest stability over 1 month (17).

The better correlation between measurement and patients' self-monitoring in our treatment evaluation, on the other hand, argues in favor of self-assessment. Contrary to the "one-point tremor assessment" of doctors' ratings, patients can report on long-term changes in tremor, with an integrative overview over a longer period exceeding days or even weeks.

Therefore, we recommend a revision of the priorities presently assigned to certain methods of tremor evaluation in treatment studies. Apart from long-term measurement of parkinsonian tremor, which we consider to be the most reliable, self-monitoring observation methods should be considered as essential and superior to physicians' clinical ratings.

ACKNOWLEDGMENT

The work was in part supported by the Deutsche Forschungsgemeinschaft (SFB 307). We wish to thank Prof. Dr. J. Dichgans for his continuous support and Mrs. B. Guschlbauer for her reliable and sophisticated technical assistance.

REFERENCES

1. Cleeves L, Findley LJ, Gresty M. Assessment of rest tremor in Parkinson's disease. Adv Neurol 1986; 45:349–352.
2. Gresty MA, McCarthy R, Findley LJ. Assessment of resting tremor in Parkinson's disease. In: Findley LJ, Capildeo R, eds. Movement Disorders: Tremor. London: Macmillan Press, 1984:321–329.
3. Cowell TK, Marsden CD, Owen DAL. Objective measurement of parkinsonian tremor. Lancet 1965; 2:1278–1279.
4. Ackmann JJ, Sances A, Larson SJ, Baker JB. Quantitative evaluation of long-term parkinson tremor. IEEE Trans Biomed Eng 1977; 24:49–56.
5. Pimlott RM, Gibson JM, Brown IT, Kennard CA. New ambulatory monitoring system for tremor. Electromyogr Clin Neurophysiol 1983; 56:694–695.
6. Scholz E, Bacher M, Diener HC, Dichgans J. Twenty-four-hour tremor recordings in the evaluation of the treatment of Parkinson's disease. J Neurol 1988; 235:475–484.
7. Bacher M, Scholz E, Diener HC. 24 hour continuous tremor quantification based on EMG recording. Electroencephalogr Clin Neurophysiol 1989; 72:176–183.
8. Dietrichson P, Engebretsen O, Fonstelien E, Hovland J. Quantitation of tremor in man. In: Desmedt JE, ed. Physiological Tremor, Pathological Tremors and Clonus. Basel: S Karger, 1978:90–94.

9. Gresty MA, Findley LJ, Definition, analysis and genesis of tremor. In: Findley LJ, Capildeo R, eds. Movement Disorders: Tremor. London: Macmillan Press, 1984: 15–26.
10. Hömberg V, Hefter H, Reiners K, Freund H-J. Differential effects of changes in mechanical limb properties on physiological and pathological tremor. J Neurol Neurosurg Psychiatry 1987; 50:568–579.
11. Journeé HL. Demodulation of amplitude modulated noise: a mathematical evaluation of a demodulator for pathological tremor EMG's. IEEE Trans Biomed Eng 1983; 30:304–308.
12. Andreeva YA, Ivanova-Smolenskaya IA, Kandel EI, Khutorskaya OY. Envelope EMG spectral analysis in the studies of physiological and pathological tremor. Electromyogr Clin Neurophysiol 1985; 25:273–293.
13. Oppenheim AV, Schafer RW. Digital signal processing. Engelwood Cliffs, NJ: Prentice-Hall, 1975.
14. Harris FJ. On the use of windows for harmonic analysis with the discrete Fourier transform. Proc IEEE 1978; 66:51–84.
15. Golbe LI, Pae J. Validity of a mailed epidemiological questionnaire and physical self-assessment in Parkinson's disease. Mov Disord 1988; 3:245–254.
16. Brown RG, MacCarthy B, Jahanshahi M, Marsden CD. Accuracy of self-reported disability in patients with parkinsonism. Arch Neurol 1989; 46:955–959.
17. Montgomery GK, Reynolds NN. Compliance, reliability, and validity of self-monitoring for physical disturbances of Parkinson's disease. J Nerv Ment Dis 1990; 178:636–641.

21

Some Physiological Aspects of Parkinsonian Tremor

Richard M. Dubinsky
University of Kansas Medical Center
Kansas City, Kansas

I. INTRODUCTION

Tremor is one of the cardinal manifestations of Parkinson's disease. Approximately 75% of patients with Parkinson's disease will have tremor during the course of their illness (1). Despite the widespread prevalence and easy recognition of parkinsonian tremor, there is not yet a universal consensus about its etiology.

The tremor of Parkinson's disease is a resting tremor that begins unilaterally, without a proclivity for the dominant hand. It can present rarely in the cranial musculature. As disease progresses, tremor may be seen in almost any combination of the cranial musculature and the upper and lower extremities. The typical frequency is 3–5 Hz, regardless of location (1–3).

Electromyographic (EMG) recording of parkinsonian rest tremor reveals either alternating or synchronous contraction of antagonist muscles (4; Fig. 1A).

Postural tremor occurs and is symptomatic in 60% of patients with Parkinson's disease (1). The frequency is usually greater than the frequency of the resting tremor (5–12 Hz) and can be indistinguishable from essential tremor. In some patients, the tremor can be at the same frequency as the resting tremor. The postural tremor of Parkinson's disease has many neurophysiological and clinical similarities to essential tremor, and they can be quite difficult to differentiate (see Fig. 1B).

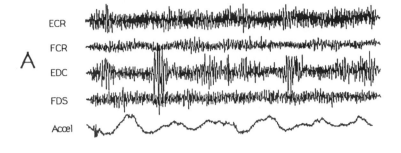

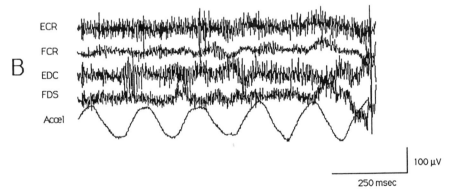

Figure 1   The EMG and accelerometer recording in a 70-year-old woman with Parkinson's disease, Hoehn and Yahr stage II, recorded with surface electrodes and a Grass model SPA-1 accelerometer. Bandpass for EMG was 100–10,000 Hz, bandpass for accelerometer was 1–30 Hz. (A) Resting with the hands on her lap; (B) hands held horizontally at shoulder height. ECR, extensor carpi radialis; FCR, flexor carpi radialis; EDC, extensor digitorum communis; FDS, flexor digitorum sublimis; accel, accelerometer.

II.   POSTULATED MECHANISMS

There are two main mechanisms proposed for the etiology of parkinsonian tremor: *central oscillator* and *stretch reflex mechanisms*. There have been many studies to determine which hypothesis is correct, and the debate is ongoing. The central oscillator hypothesis could be easily integrated into the current theories of motor control and the dysfunction of the basal ganglia that occurs in Parkinson's disease.

On the other hand, it has been well established that basal ganglia dysfunction can lead to disinhibition of spinal reflex mechanisms (5). Disinhibition of spinal reflexes can lead to clinical manifestations of increased tone, but there is no evidence yet that spinal disinhibition can cause the expression of tremor.

A. Stretch Reflex Mechanisms

Oscillations or alterations of the stretch reflexes have long been postulated as an explanation for the resting tremor of Parkinson's disease. Calne and Lader found that prolonged limb ischemia could abolish the resting tremor of Parkinson's disease and that the frequency of tremor in the contralateral limb increased during the period of ischemia (6). Hufschmidt was able to reset the phase of parkinsonian tremor through electrical stimulation (7). However, Lee and Stein (8) and Höberg et al. (9) were unable to reset the phase of parkinsonian rest tremor through the use of limb weighing or mechanical perturbation through a torque motor. There are two other criticisms of the stretch reflex hypothesis: delays have not been found in the latencies of long-loop reflexes to mechanical stretch (5), and there is no correlation between tremor amplitude and the long- or short-latency reflex responses to sudden stretch (10).

Parkinsonian tremor occurs at a uniform frequency in different body parts of the same patient. Hunker and Abbs recorded parkinsonian resting tremor in the lips, jaw, tongue, and digit 2 of three male subjects with Parkinson's disease and compared them with three age- and gender-matched controls (2). Tremor was recorded through EMG and displacement transducers. Long-term spectral averaging was used to determine tremor frequency and magnitude. They found that the tremor was at the same frequency for all four areas in all three parkinsonian subjects, whereas tremor was not recorded in the controls. They concluded that stretch reflex mechanism could not account for parkinsonian rest tremor, since the orofacial muscles have very different innervation than the appendicular muscles. Specifically, muscle spindles have not been found in the lip muscles (11), and the tongue muscle spindles do not appear to project to the hypoglossal motor neurons in the lower brainstem (12). If spindle afferents were involved in the genesis of parkinsonian resting tremor, then the tremor should have different frequencies for the orofacial muscles and the limb muscles (2).

B. Central Oscillator

The central oscillator theory is the stronger of the two theories, yet it remains a theory. It has been known for some time that lesioning of the motor cortex, pyramidal tracts, or thalamus can abolish resting tremor (13–15). These observations do not prove the presence of a central oscillator. Instead they show the involvement of the corticospinal tract and thalamus in the expression of tremor. The pyramidal tract may be acting as the final common pathway of the proposed central oscillator, or it could function as one part of an aberrant transcortical stretch reflex loop.

Stimulation of the cerebral cortex can produce a typical resting tremor in the contralateral limb in both parkinsonian and nonparkinsonian subjects (16). This could be evidence of the activation of a stored motor program for rest tremor. However, the possibility of stimulation of subcortical structures must be taken into account.

Ablation of the thalamus, specifically the nucleus ventral intermedius (Vim) is very effective in the ablation of parkinsonian rest tremor, as well as parkinsonian postural tremor, primary writing tremor, cerebellar outflow tract tremor (rubral tremor), and essential tremor (15,17,18).

Further evidence for a thalamic generator of parkinsonian tremor comes from experimental recordings of the thalamus. Thalamic rhythmicity can be seen in parkinsonian subjects without tremor (19). This inherent rhythmicity may become enhanced in Parkinson's disease, with the result being clinical expression of tremor. Lenz et al. found entrainment of contralateral limb muscles by rhythmically firing thalamic cells (20). They found a high concentration of thalamic cells firing at the same frequency as the tremor recorded from the opposite limb, leading to the conclusion that these groups of cells may be the generator of parkinsonian tremor.

III. EXPERIMENTAL

To further investigate the contributions of abnormalities of segmental reflexes versus a central oscillator, we investigated the integrity of the a transcortical loop by comparing cutaneous long-loop reflexes from subjects with early PD with normal age- and gender-matched controls. The cutaneous long-loop reflex is thought to be transcortical (21). A delay in the early component of the cutaneous long-loop reflex would indicate abnormalities of the afferent portions of the loop or an abnormal delay at the spinal cord level. Delay of the late component of the cutaneous long loop would indicate a delay at a level higher than the spinal cord. The latency of the efferent portion of the loop has proved to be normal by transcranial cortical stimulation (22).

A. Methods

Eight parkinsonian subjects and eight controls (mean age 67.5 ± 3.9 years) were studied. Stimuli were applied to digit 2 of the right hand for 0.2 ms, at a rate of 3 Hz, and an intensity of four times the sensory threshold or at the threshold of pain, whichever was less. The subjects abducted digit 2 at 20% of maximal force. Visual feedback was used to control the force of abduction. The EMG activity was recorded from the first dorsal interosseous muscle, using 10-mm disk electrodes. Bandpass was 10–10,000 Hz. The waveform was sampled for 10 ms before the

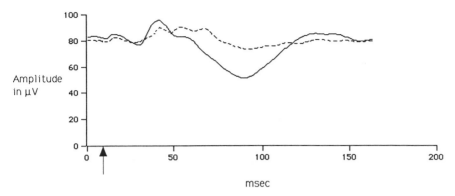

Figure 2 Long-latency reflex responses to cutaneous stimulation. The stimulus (arrow) was applied at 10 ms.

stimulation and 154 ms after the stimulation. Each sweep was rectified and 256 trials were averaged on-line. In addition, each of the parkinsonian subjects had their tremor recorded with a Grass SPA-1 accelerometer for 10-s epochs while at rest and with their arms held outstretched at shoulder height. Tremor frequency and magnitude were determined by fast-Fourier transform (Fig. 2).

The latencies of the first and second excitatory peaks and the first inhibitory peak were the same for both groups. The only difference was in the amplitude of the inhibitory peak (mean latency 51 ms) when compared with the baseline EMG activity. There was a $17.8 \pm 11.2\%$ inhibition for the parkinsonian subjects, whereas the inhibition for the control was $41.6 \pm 15.3\%$ ($p < 0.05$, Student's t test). A correlation was not found between the amount of inhibition and either the tremor frequency or magnitude. The decreased inhibition indicates a loss of a spinal inhibitory mechanism and can be used as a partial explanation of the increased tone in Parkinson's disease (23). As a negative study, this experiment failed to demonstrate an abnormality in one specific type of reflex loop, involving both spinal and presumably cortical segments, that could explain the origin of tremor in Parkinson's disease.

To determine the etiology of parkinsonian tremor further research will be needed, combining peripheral and central neurophysiological recordings perhaps using MPTP animal model of Parkinson's disease.

REFERENCES

1. Lance JW, Scheab RS, Peterson EA. Action tremor and the cogwheel phenomenon in Parkinson's disease. Brain 1963; 86:95–110.
2. Hunker CJ, Abbs JH. Uniform frequency of parkinsonian resting tremor in the lips, jaw, tongue, and index finger. Mov Dis 1990; 5:71–77.

3. Findley LJ, Gresty MA. Tremor. Br J Hosp Med 1981; 26:13–32.
4. Shahani BT, Young RR. Physiological and pharmacological aids in the differential diagnosis of tremor. J Neurol Neurosurg Psychiatry 1976; 39:772–783.
5. Lee RG, Tatton WG. Motor responses to sudden limb displacements in primates with specific CNS lesions and in humans with motor system disorders. Can J Neurol Sci 1975; 2:285–293.
6. Calne DB, Lader MH. Electromyographic studies of tremor using an averaging computer. Electroencephalogr Clin Neurophysiol 1969; 26:86–92.
7. Hufschmidt H-J. Proprioceptive origin or parkinsonian tremor. Nature 1963; 200: 367–368.
8. Lee RG, Stein RB. Resetting of tremor by mechanical perturbations: a comparison of essential tremor and parkinsonian tremor. Ann Neurol 1981; 10:523–531.
9. Hömberg V, Hefter H, Freund H-J. Differential effects of changes in mechanical limb properties on physiological and pathological tremor. J Neurol Neurosurg Psychiatry 1987; 50:568–579.
10. Mortimer JA, Webster DD. Evidence for a quantitative association between EMG stretch responses and parkinsonian rigidity. Brain Res 1979; 162:169–173.
11. Bratzlavsky M, Vander Ecken H. Afferent influences on human genioglossus muscle. J Neurol 1974; 207:19–25.
12. Allum JHJ. Segmental reflex, muscle mechanical and central mechanisms underlying human physiological tremor. In: Findley LJ, Capiledo R, eds. Movement Disorders: Tremor. London: Macmillan Press, 1984; 135–156.
13. Bucy PC. Cortical extirpation in the treatment of involuntary movements. Assoc Res Nerv Ment Dis 1940; 21:551–595.
14. Putnam TJ. The operative treatment of diseases characterized by involuntary movements (tremor, athetosis). Assoc Res Nerv Ment Dis 1940; 21:666–696.
15. Narabayashi H, Ohye C. Importance of microstereoencephalotomy for tremor alleviation. Appl Neurophysiol 1980; 43:222–227.
16. Alberts WW. A simple view of parkinsonian tremor. Electrical stimulation of cortex adjacent to the rolandic fissure in awake man. Brain Res 1972; 44:357–369.
17. Speelman JD, Van Manen J. Stereotactic thalamotomy for the relief of intention tremor of multiple sclerosis. J Neurol Neurosurg Psychiatry 1984; 47:596–599.
18. Narabayashi H. Stereotactic Vim thalamotomy for treatment of tremor. Eur Neurol 1989; 29(suppl 1):29–32.
19. Ohye C, Saito U, Fukamachi A, Narabayashi H. An analysis of the spontaneous rhythmic and non-rhythmic burst discharges in the human thalamus. J Neurol Sci 1974; 22:245–259.
20. Lenz FA, Tasker RR, Kwan HC, et al. Single unit analysis of the human ventral thalamic nuclear group: correlation of thalamic "tremor" cells with the 3–6 Hz component of parkinsonian tremor. J Neurosci 1988; 8:754–764.
21. Tarkka IM. Short and long latency reflexes in human muscles following electrical and mechanical stimulation. Acta Physiol Scand [Suppl] 1986; 557:1–32.
22. Dick JPR, Cowan JMA, Day BL, et al. The corticomotoneurone connection is normal in Parkinson's disease. Nature 310; 1984:407–409.
23. Fuhr P, Hallett M. Cutaneous reflexes in hand muscles in Parkinson's disease. Muscle Nerve 1990; 18:978.

22

MPTP-Induced Parkinsonism and Tremor

James W. Tetrud and J. William Langston
The Parkinson's Institute
Sunnyvale, California

I. INTRODUCTION

In writing his original paper in 1817, James Parkinson chose to refer to the disease that now bears his name as the "shaking palsy" (1), thereby establishing tremor as a veritable signature of Parkinson's disease. As the title implies, tremor was a salient clinical feature of the condition he described. Even at this early date, Parkinson recognized the distinctive character of tremor exhibited by his patients: "In the real Shaking Palsy . . . the agitation continues in full force whilst the limb is at rest and unemployed; and is even diminished by calling the muscles into employment" (1). However, despite major advances in our understanding of the disease over the past 175 years, the underlying pathophysiology of parkinsonian tremor remains poorly understood. Recently, the discovery of a parkinsonian syndrome produced by the neurotoxin 1-methyl-4-phenyl-1,2,3,6-tetrahydropyridine (MPTP; 2) has provided valuable insights into the pathophysiology of Parkinson's disease (3). Because patients with this disorder have exhibited a parkinsonlike tremor, it is reasonable to hope that the MPTP animal model will help unravel some of the mysteries underlying the genesis of parkinsonian rest tremor, a symptom that is often challenging to treat and a source of disability in many patients.

In this chapter, we review studies of tremor in earlier primate models of Parkinson's disease; these models have greatly influenced current concepts about the pathological substrate of parkinsonian tremor. Next, we focus on various studies in primates with MPTP-induced parkinsonism relative to tremor characteristics and associated pathological findings. We then review studies that compare tremor in humans with MPTP-induced parkinsonism and the rest tremor of Parkinson's disease, concluding with a discussion of the possible pathological substrate of parkinsonian tremor.

II. AN EARLY MONKEY MODEL

The earliest animal model of Parkinson's disease actually predated the discovery of dopamine deficiency in the disease. Beginning in the 1940s, several investigators found that lesions placed in the ventral tegmentum of monkeys produce hypokinesia and tremor.

In 1948, Ward and colleagues reported the appearance of hypokinesia and a "rest" tremor in two rhesus monkeys with electrolytic lesions placed in the mesencephalic and pontine tegmentum (4). The following year, Peterson and colleagues, experimenting with the same monkey species, placed electrolytic lesions at eight separate anatomical locations in different monkey groups (5). They found that all of five monkeys with lesions in the ventral tegmentum exhibited hypokinesia and a postural tremor of 6–8 Hz; the tremor had alternating agonist and antagonist contractions, was exacerbated by excitement, and was dampened by movement. In the mid-1950s, Carrea and Mettler published a detailed report (6) of motor manifestations produced by electrolytic lesions in various brainstem sites of rhesus monkeys. Rest tremor was not reported, but in a group of animals that exhibited a postural tremor, lesions were found in the brachium conjunctivum. In 1960, Poirier reported (7) that a "postural tremor or tremor at rest" was associated with combined lesions of the nigral efferent fibers as well as the rubrospinal system and the ventral component of the brachium conjunctivum in eight rhesus monkeys. From these observations, he concluded that tremor in these animals was the result of "concomitant involvement of the nigral outflow and of the corresponding rubrospinal system" (7).

In 1966, Poirier and colleagues reported that rhesus monkeys with lesions confined to the substantia nigra exhibited hypokinesia, but not tremor (8). Although striatal dopamine levels in these animals were significantly depressed, striatal serotonin (5-hydroxytryptamine; 5-HT) levels were normal. In contrast, concentrations of both dopamine and serotonin were significantly depressed in the striatum of three monkeys exhibiting hypokinesia and a 6-Hz postural tremor in which lesions interrupted ascending nigral fibers and the rubrotegmentospinal tract. Given these observations, the authors hypothesized that lesions of "the tegmental part of the rubrotegmentospinal tract" in combination with disruption of nigrostriatal fibers were required to produce a parkinsonian tremor; they also implicated loss of serotonin input to the striatum in the genesis of tremor.

In 1969, Goldstein and colleagues reported on behavioral and pathological findings in African green monkeys with radiofrequency lesions placed in the ventromedial tegmental region of the rostral pons (9). This lesioning approach produced damage in the medial substantia nigra, the dorsomedial region of the cerebral peduncle, and the ventromedial aspect of the red nucleus, with extensive ipsilateral cell loss in the pars compacta and reticularis of the substantia nigra, the third nerve nucleus, and degeneration of neurons in the magnocellular portion of the ipsilateral red nucleus. The behavioral effects noted by these investigators 5–10 days following the radiofrequency lesions included "contralateral hypokinesia" and a *"postural tremor* of the contralateral extremities at a rate of 4–6 cycles/sec." In these monkeys, striatal dopamine was "distinctly lower" on the lesioned side [even in the presence of the monoamine oxidase inhibitor pheniprazine]. In addition, they noted that, although concentrations of serotonin were also lower on the lesioned side, compared with the nonlesioned side, monoamine oxidase inhibition with pheniprazine normalized serotonin levels on the lesioned side. These results suggested that the storage capacity of dopamine, but not serotonin, was affected by these lesions.

In 1976, Goldstein and colleagues reported that a *"resting tremor"* of 4–6 Hz could be produced in some, but not all, African green monkeys, 5–7 days after radiofrequency lesions were placed in the ventromedial tegmentum (10). Clinicopathological comparison revealed that in the monkeys exhibiting tremor, lesions were "larger, involved more medial structures, and extended to a greater extent into the medial substantia nigra and the dorsomedial peduncle areas" than lesions in the monkeys without tremor. They also found that the tremor in these animals was abolished by administering either levodopa or the serotonin precursor L-5-hydroxytryptophan (5-HTP), further suggesting that a combination of dopamine and serotonin deficiency might play a role in the generation of this tremor. Interestingly, other than the mention of rest tremor in rhesus monkeys by Ward and colleagues (4), this is the first reference to explicitly state that a true rest tremor had been produced in nonhuman primates.

The same year, Pechadre and colleagues, using a surgical approach similar to that of Poirier, Goldstein, and others, reported a 7-Hz "postural" tremor in two monkeys (species not specified) in which lesions were found in the red nucleus, cerebellofugal and nigrostriatal tracts (11). In three monkeys with lesions confined to the nigrostriatal tract, no tremor was observed. They concluded that these findings further supported the hypothesis that lesions of the nigrostriatal tract alone were insufficient to generate a parkinsonian tremor, even though the tremor in these animals was described as postural.

Although these early primate models of Parkinson's disease have provided the basis for current concepts concerning the pathophysiology of parkinsonian tremor (12), it is difficult to draw clear-cut conclusions from these studies for a variety of reasons. First, although several of these studies used a similar surgical technique, the results are conflicting in the correlation of behavioral effects caused by these lesions and the underlying histopathological appearance. Second, although at least two reports suggest that a rest tremor can be produced in monkeys by this technique (4,10), objective documentation is lacking; furthermore, in most animals, a postural, rather than rest, tremor has been observed. Third, as pointed out by Rondot and Bathien (13), these primate models exhibit pathological features that differ from those of Parkinson's disease. For example, most of these studies suggest that interruption of the rubro–olivo–dento–rubral loop and nigrostiatal tract are required to generate a tremor in the monkey; however, it is not clear that this loop is affected in Parkinson's disease. Also, the lesions produced by this technique lie close to, and may actually involve, the corticospinal tract as it passes through the midbrain. Interruption of these fibers could mask or alter tremor characteristics in the contralateral upper limb. Thus, as important as they are, these surgically lesioned monkey models do not appear to have provided sufficient information to draw firm conclusions about the pathophysiological substrate of parkinsonian rest tremor.

III. THE MPTP MONKEY MODEL

A. Behavioral Features

The neurotoxin MPTP produces a syndrome in experimental monkeys closely resembling Parkinson's disease. In fact, this syndrome is currently considered to be the best animal model of the disease (14–19). MPTP-induced parkinsonism has been studied in a variety of monkey species, including squirrel (*Saimiri sciureus*; 20), rhesus (*Macaca mulatta*; 16,21–23), macaque (*Macaca fascicularis*, cynomolgus, long-tailed macaque; 19,24–30), common marmoset (*Callithrix jacchus*; 31), and African green (*Cercopithecus aethiops sabaeus*; 3,32). These studies indicate that MPTP consistently produces akinesia, rigidity, and a disturbance of balance (three of the four major cardinal features of Parkinson's disease). However, tremor, if present at all, varies from species to species. For example, in the squirrel monkey, a kinetic or postural tremor has been reported (14) and in the common marmoset, an unusual hind limb postural type tremor has been described (17). The rhesus and long-tailed macaque exhibit a tremor having a regular frequency of 4–6 Hz, although it differs from the typical tremor of Parkinson's disease in being postural, more prominent in the proximal muscles and, in some cases, involving the head and jaw (16,25). On the other hand, in the African green monkey, a tremor more reminiscent of parkinsonian tremor has been reported (32,33). In this species, MPTP induces a regular 4- to 5-Hz tremor in which the amplitude is dampened by movement.

Why rest tremor is the least reproducible feature of MPTP-induced parkinsonism in the nonhuman primate is puzzling, although several possible explanations are worth discussing. First, these animals are probably rarely at rest; usually, the limbs are held in some form of posture when they are being assessed and, quite possibly, this could obscure a true rest tremor if it actually existed. Second, the physical characteristics of monkeys that differ from humans (i.e., relative arm length, body posture, hand and finger position) could influence the character of the tremor. In addition, since monkeys lack the ability to oppose the thumb, they may be incapable of expressing a typical pill-rolling tremor, as seen in humans with Parkinson's disease. Finally, the expression of tremor might depend on the species being studied, as exemplified by the relative absence of tremor in the squirrel monkey and common marmoset, compared with the rhythmic 5- to 6-Hz "postural" tremor observed in the rhesus and African green species. Goldstein and colleagues, who reported a rest tremor in monkeys using the brainstem lesioning technique (10), performed their experiments in the African green monkey, whereas most investigators who observed a postural tremor were using other monkey species. We will return to this issue again when we discuss the effects of MPTP in another species of primate, humans.

B. Pathological Features

The neuropathological changes produced by MPTP appear to vary somewhat among the different monkey species (Table 1). In the squirrel monkey, this toxin produces severe loss of pigmented neurons within the substantia nigra (SN) and, in nearly 50%, lesions in the locus coeruleus (LC); whereas, the ventral tegmental

Table 1 Tremor and Pathological Findings in Various Monkey Species with MPTP-Induced Parkinsonism

Monkey species	Location of lesions[a,b]				Type of tremor	Authors (Ref.)
	A8	A9	A10	LC		
Squirrel	1+	3+	0	2+	Kinetic	Forno et al. (15)
African green	0	3+	2+	0	Postural	Bergman et al. (3)
Cynomolgus	2+	3+	2+	2+	Postural	German et al. (19), Mitchell et al. (24), Schneider et al. (26), Degryse and Colpaert (25)
Rhesus	0	3+	0	0	Postural	Burns et al. (16)
Marmoset	2+	3+	1+	0	Postural	Jenner et al. (17), Gibb et al. (31)
Japanese	0	3+	0	2+	Postural	Miyoshi et al. (27), Tanaka et al. (28)

[a]A8, neurons within the ventral reticular formation located caudal and dorsal to the SNc; A9, neurons within the SNc; A10, neurons medial to the SNc within the VTA; LC, locus coeruleus.
[b]Extent of neuronal damage; 0, none or not reported; 1+, slight to mild; 2+, mild to moderate; 3+, moderate to severe.

area (VTA; A10) is relatively spared in this species (15). In older squirrel monkeys, intracellular eosinophilic inclusion bodies have been observed within the SN, LC, dorsal motor nucleus, basal nucleus of Meynert, dorsal raphe nucleus, and peri-amygdaloid area (15,20). In the rhesus monkey, MPTP causes severe damage to the SN; however, the VTA and LC are both spared, and no inclusion bodies have yet been reported (16,22,23). In the cynomolgus monkey, lesions have been reported in the SN, VTA, LC, and A8 region (neurons within the ventral reticular formation located caudal and dorsal to the SN) (19,24,27,28,30). In the common marmoset, neuronal loss has been observed in the A8 and A9 regions, whereas only a slight loss of neurons was evident in A10 (31). In the African green monkey, MPTP causes extensive damage to the SN and VTA regions (3).

Since the abnormality produced by MPTP in monkeys appears to be limited to a few neuroanatomical areas, the MPTP animal model should be of substantial value in understanding the pathophysiology of tremor in monkeys and, quite possibly, humans with Parkinson's disease. However, it is as yet difficult to draw definitive conclusions from studies because of the variable features of tremor induced by MPTP. Furthermore, the methods of assessing tremor in the various species have not been standardized, nor has there yet been a study specifically designed to investigate tremor and its pathological correlates using the MPTP model.

Nonetheless, it seems quite clear that the dysfunction induced by MPTP in monkeys is selective, with the substantia nigra bearing the brunt of damage. Whether or not the postural tremor observed in several of these monkey species is the behavioral equivalent of parkinsonian rest tremor awaits a well-designed study of tremor in these animals. One hopes that such studies will provide a clearer insight into the pathophysiology of tremor in Parkinson's disease. However, until a more consistent and convincing rest tremor can be demonstrated, concerns must be expressed about the ultimate usefulness of this model.

The African green monkey may be the best candidate for such studies, since the tremor produced by MPTP in this species is quite reminiscent of rest tremor (32,33), and it is also the species reported by Goldstein and colleagues (10) to exhibit rest tremor when surgical lesions were placed in the ventral tegmentum. Perhaps careful neurophysiological measurements of tremor, combined with complete histopathological analysis in the African green monkey, will resolve the issue of whether MPTP produces a true rest tremor in this monkey species and, if so, help establish its neuroanatomical substrate. For the moment, however, we must turn to another species of primate, the human, to address these issues.

IV. MPTP-INDUCED PARKINSONISM IN HUMANS

A. Clinical Features

The clinical features exhibited by humans exposed to MPTP include bradykinesia, rigidity, postural instability, and a tremor resembling parkinsonian rest tremor

(2,34,35). Except for their relative youth and the acute onset of parkinsonism, the clinical features in these individuals are identical with Parkinson's disease. However, since the majority of monkeys administered MPTP exhibited a tremor different from that usually seen in Parkinson's disease (see preceding discussion), there has been some doubt whether MPTP could produce a typical parkinsonian rest tremor (36).

Consequently, we recently undertook a clinical and electrophysiological assessment of tremor in individuals with moderate to severe MPTP-induced parkinsonism (37,38). Of our original seven patients with moderate to severe MPTP-induced parkinsonism (34), four exhibited a parkinsonlike tremor on clinical examination. The demographic profile and clinical features of these patients are shown in Table 2, and tremor characteristics in Table 3. Clinically, tremor in these individuals (1) was most prominent with the limb at rest, (2) dampened with voluntary movement, (3) was higher in amplitude distally, (4) was present in either the upper or lower extremities either unilaterally or asymmetrically, (5) had a frequency of approximately 4–6 Hz, and (6) always improved dramatically with levodopa therapy. In two of these patients, simultaneous EMG activity recorded from the extensor carpi radialis and flexor carpi radialis demonstrated alternating agonist–antagonist discharges of 4.5–5.5 Hz (Fig. 1). Also, a strain-gauge recording of right thumb tremor was carried out in one patient and demonstrated a regular sinusoidal 5.5-Hz rhythm (Fig. 2) (37,38). Thus, out of seven patients with moderate to severe MPTP-induced parkinsonism (34), four exhibited a characteristic parkinsonian rest tremor that dramatically improved with levodopa therapy, and two showed electrophysiological characteristics identical with parkinsonian rest tremor (38). These findings clearly demonstrate that, at least in humans, MPTP can induce a tremor that meets all the clinical and electrophysiological criteria of parkinsonian rest tremor (39).

Table 2 Clinical Features of Patients with Moderate to Severe MPTP-Induced Parkinsonism and Tremor

	Patient number			
Clinical feature	2	5	6	7
Age	30	29	26	31
Sex	F	F	M	F
Rigidity	++	+++	+	++
Bradykinesia	++	+++	++	+++
Resting tremor	++	++	+++	++
Hoehn and Yahr stage	5	5	4	4

+, mild; ++, moderate; +++, severe.

Table 3 Comparison of Tremor in Patients with MPTP-
Induced Parkinsonism and Patients with Parkinson's Disease

Characteristic	PD	Patient number			
		2	5	6	7
Prominent at rest	*	*	*	*	*
Movement suppressed	*	*	*	*	*
Asymmetric	*	*	*	*	*
Greater distally	*	*	*	*	*
Location					
Hand	*	+ +	+ +	+ + +	0
Arm	*	+	+	+ +	0
Foot	*	+	+	+	+ +
Tongue	*	0	+	+ +	0
Lips	*	0	+	+ +	0
Frequency (Hz)	4–5	5–6	5.5	4.5	4–6
Response to L-dopa	*	*	*	*	*

*, present; +, mild; + +, moderate; + + +, severe.

V. DOES REST TREMOR RESULT FROM NIGRAL LESIONS ALONE?

We now turn to the issue of the neuroanatomical substrate of parkinsonian tremor seen in these patients. There are several reasons to suspect that they may have lesions confined to the substantia nigra. First, pathological evidence is available in one patient, a 23-year old man who synthesized and injected a compound that, in retrospect, almost certainly contained MPTP (2,35). He was reported to exhibit bradykinesia, rigidity, and a mild tremor (although whether this was a rest tremor is unclear from the report; 35). He responded to levodopa, but died 18 months later from an apparent drug overdose. At autopsy, the microscopic findings were highly selective and *confined* to the substantia nigra zona compacta (SNc), where extensive neuronal damage, extracellular neuromelanin, and an "intracytoplasmic inclusion body," resembling a Lewy body, were noted. No damage was found in the locus coeruleus or other areas of brain (35). Thus, in this one case of human MPTP-induced parkinsonism, damage to the substantia nigra alone apparently resulted in the four cardinal features characteristic of Parkinson's disease, including tremor. Second, in two patients with moderate to severe MPTP-induced parkinsonism, cerebrospinal fluid (CSF) concentrations of homovanillic acid (HVA) were profoundly depressed, whereas levels of MHPG and hydroxyindole-acetic acid (5-HIAA) were normal (40), suggesting that only dopaminergic neurons had sustained irreversible damage. Finally, levodopa therapy not only

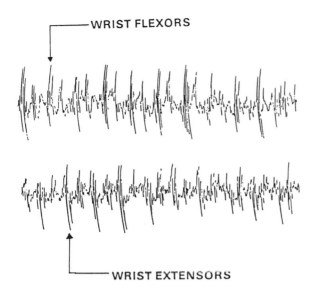

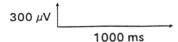

Figure 1 Electromyograms of flexor carpi radialis (top) and extensor carpi radialis (bottom) in patient 6 (34) demonstrating alternating agonist discharge bursts at approximately 5.5 Hz.

reversed bradykinesia, rigidity, and postural instability, but also dramatically suppressed tremor in all of the four individuals with moderate to severe MPTP-induced parkinsonism.

Thus, histological findings in one patient and CSF findings in two others suggest that the SN is selectively damaged in these patients. From these findings, it can be argued that the pathological substrate of rest tremor in humans with MPTP-induced parkinsonism may result from damage to the SN alone.

If one assumes the foregoing is correct, an equally interesting question is why tremor was not present in all of our patients with moderate to severe MPTP-induced parkinsonism (34), since, in all likelihood, they all had extensive damage to dopaminergic SN neurons? There are several possible explanations for this interesting phenomenon. First, since MPTP exposure in our patients was acute (developing over a period of days to weeks), compensatory mechanisms, such as

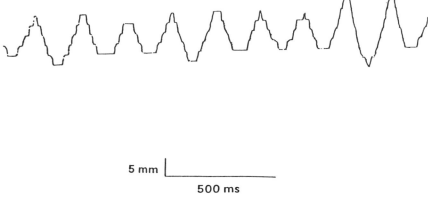

5 mm

500 ms

Figure 2 Strain-gauge recording of the thumb of patient 5, using a Grass force-displacement transducer, demonstrating a rhythmic tremor at approximately 5 Hz.

up-regulation of surviving neurons, axonal sprouting, or dopamine receptor alterations, may have influenced the development of tremor; this process might have easily varied from patient to patient. Second, tremor might depend on the somatotopic distribution of nigral cell damage produced by MPTP. This concept is supported by the findings of Fearnley and Lees (41), who performed age-adjusted regional SN cell counts in ten patients with autopsy-proved striatonigral degeneration (SND) and found that in those patients who developed rest tremor initially (one of ten), or later in the disease course (four of ten), cell loss was more extensive in the ventrolateral regions of the SN, compared with those without tremor. These results suggest that lesions in the ventral regions of the SN might play a role in the development of rest tremor, although this study was not designed to examine the pathological substrate of tremor. Thus, it is possible that variability in the distribution of intranigral MPTP-induced cell loss might explain the variability of tremor expression in our patients.

Chronicity of the MPTP-induced lesion represents another variable that might influence the expression of tremor. One patient who initially presented with tremor in the right hand, now, 8 years later, exhibits a typical rest tremor in all four limbs. In another patient with moderate to severe MPTP-induced parkinsonism, who initially did not exhibit tremor, an intermittent rest tremor has emerged (unpublished observations). Furthermore, one patient who initially presented with mild MPTP-induced parkinsonism has developed a typical unilateral rest tremor, 8 years after exposure to MPTP (unpublished observations).

Although the notion that tremor is a function of nigral cell loss alone is clearly controversial, a recent report by Rajput and colleagues (42) supports this concept. These investigators carried out clinicopathological correlations in a series of patients with parkinsonism over a period of two decades. They found that in 26 patients with autopsy-proved Parkinson's disease, all either presented with a rest tremor or developed rest tremor at some point during the course of their disease. On the other hand, three patients with striatonigral degeneration, two with Shy–Drager syndromes, and three with progressive supranuclear palsy never exhibited tremor during their illness (42). These results suggest that tremor might be present in most, if not all, patients with Parkinson's disease at some point during their illness. Interestingly, in two cases, in which the patients had exhibited a typical rest tremor in life, no Lewy bodies were found at autopsy, and the only cell loss noted was in the SN (42). The authors concluded that "SN pathology alone was sufficient pathology for rest tremor in Parkinson's disease" (43). The strength of this Rajput study derives from its being a thorough clinicopathological correlation performed by the same investigators with expertise in the clinical and pathological features of Parkinson's disease and related syndromes. Similar studies in MPTP-induced parkinsonism and further studies in patients with Parkinson's disease will likely shed more light on this issue in the future.

VI. CONCLUSIONS

There is little doubt that, in humans, MPTP can produce a typical parkinsonian rest tremor. In nonhuman primates, the evidence is less definitive, although at least one species, the African green monkey, exhibits a tremor that is somewhat similar to that seen in Parkinson's disease. The neuropathology in this monkey species appears to be more extensive than in the single human case (35); however, the lesions are less extensive than in Parkinson's disease. Pathological studies in monkeys and the one human case indicate that dopaminergic neurons within the A8, A9, A10 regions, as well as pigmented neurons in the locus coeruleus can be affected by MPTP to a varying degree; yet, the SN is by far the most severely affected region. Clearly, studies specifically designed to investigate the pathological correlates of tremor in the MPTP model are required before drawing conclusions concerning the pathological origin of tremor in Parkinson's disease based on this animal model. However, studies to date, especially in the human cases, at least raise the possibility that the generation of rest tremor in MPTP-induced parkinsonism, and possibly Parkinson's disease, can result from damage to the SN alone. Clarification of this issue is important, since a better understanding of rest tremor pathophysiology should help provide more efficacious pharmacological therapies for this often difficult-to-treat symptom of Parkinson's disease.

ACKNOWLEDGMENTS

The authors wish to thank David Rosner for his assistance in the preparation of this manuscript. This work was supported by the California Parkinson's Foundation, and NIEHS grant 1 RO1 ESO3697-03.

REFERENCES

1. Parkinson J. An Essay on the Shaking Palsy. London: Sherwood, Neeley, & Jones, 1817.
2. Langston JW, Ballard PA, Tetrud JW, Irwin I. Chronic parkinsonism in humans due to a product of meperidine analog synthesis. Science 1983; 219:979–980.
3. Bergman H, Wichmann T, DeLong MR. Reversal of experimental parkinsonism by lesions of the subthalamic nucleus. Science 1990; 249:1436–1438.
4. Ward AA Jr, McCullough WS, Magoun HW. Production of an alternating tremor at rest in monkeys. J Neurophysiol 1948; 11:317–330.
5. Peterson EW, Magoun HW, McCullough WS, Lindsley DB. Production of postural tremor. J Neurophysiol 1949; 12:371–384.
6. Carrea RME, Mettler FA. Function of the primate brachium conjunctivum and related structures. J Comp Neurol 1955; 102:151–322.
7. Poirier LJ. Experimental and histological study of midbrain dyskinesias. J Neurophysiol 1960; 23:534–551.
8. Poirier LJ, Sourkes TL, Bouvier G, Boucher R, Carabin S. Striatal amines, experimental tremor and the effect of harmaline in the monkey. Brain 1966; 89:37–52.
9. Goldstein M, Battista AF, Anagnoste B, Nakatani S. Tremor production and striatal amines in monkeys. In: Gillingham FJ, Donaldson IM, eds. Third Symposium on Parkinson's Disease. Edinburgh: E&S Livingstone, 1969:37–40.
10. Goldstein M, Caesar P. Anagnoste B. Lesions of the nigro-striatal dopamine pathway: effects on the storage and metabolism of striatal dopamine. Pharmacol Ther 1976; 2: 89–95.
11. Pechadre JC, Larochelle L, Poirier LJ. Parkinsonian akinesia, rigidity and tremor in the monkey: histological and neuropharmacological study. J Neurol Sci 1976; 28: 147–157.
12. Jenner P, Marsden CD. Neurochemical basis of parkinsonian tremor. In: Findley LJ, Capildeo R, eds. Movement Disorders: Tremor. New York: Oxford University Press, 1984:305–319.
13. Rondot P, Bathien N. Pathophysiology of parkinsonian tremor. Neurology 1978; 5: 138–149.
14. Langston JW, Forno LS, Rebert CS, Irwin I. Selective nigral toxicity after systemic administration of 1-methyl-4-phenyl-1,2,3,6-tetrahydropyridine (MPTP) in the squirrel monkey. Brain Res 1984; 292:390–394.
15. Forno LS, Irwin I, DeLanney LE, Langston JW. Neuropathology in MPTP-induced parkinsonism in animals. Neuropathology 1991; Suppl 4:67–76.
16. Burns RS, Chiueh CC, Markey SP, Ebert MH, Jacobowitz DM, Kopin IJ. A primate model of parkinsonism: selective destruction of dopaminergic neurons in the pars compacts of the substantia nigra by N-methyl-4-phenyl-1,2,3,6-tetrahydropyridine. Proc Natl Acad Sci USA 1983; 80:4546–4550.
17. Jenner P, Rupniak NMJ, Rose SP, et al. 1-Methyl-4-phenyl-1,2,3,6-tetrahydropyridine-induced parkinsonism in the common marmoset. Neurosci Lett 1984; 50: 85–90.
18. Schwartzman RJ, Alexander GM. Changes in the local cerebral metabolic rate for

glucose in the 1-methyl-4-phenyl-1,2,3,6-tetrahydropyridine (MPTP) primate model of Parkinson's disease. Brain Res 1985; 358:137–143.

19. German DC, Durach A, Askari S, Speciale SG, Bowden DM. 1-Methyl-4-phenyl-1,2,3,6-tetrahydropyridine-induced parkinsonian syndrome in *Macaca fascicularis*; which midbrain dopaminergic neurons are lost? Neuroscience 1988; 24: 161–174.

20. Forno LS, Langston JW, DeLanney LE, Irwin I, Ricaurte GA. Locus ceruleus lesions and eosinophilic inclusions in MPTP-treated monkeys. Ann Neurol 1986; 20: 449–455.

21. Barsoum NJ, Gough AW, Sturgess JM, De La Iglesia FA. Parkinson-like syndrome in nonhuman primates receiving a tetrahydropyridine derivative. Neurotoxicology 1986; 7:119–126.

22. Chiueh CC. Dopamine in the extrapyramidal motor function: a study based upon the MPTP-induced primate model of parkinsonism. Ann NY Acad Sci 1988; 515:226–238.

23. Leenders KL, Aquilonius SM, Bergstrom K, et al. Unilateral MPTP lesion in a rhesus monkey: effects on the striatal dopaminergic system measured in vivo with PET using various novel tracers. Brain Res 1988; 445:61 67.

24. Mitchell IJ, Cross AJ, Sambrook MA, Crossman AR. Sites of the neurotoxic action of 1 methyl-4-phenyl-1,2,3,6-tetrahydropyridine in the macaque monkey include the ventral tegmental area and the locus coeruleus. Neurosci Lett 1985; 61:195–200.

25. Degryse AD, Colpaert FC. Symptoms and behavioral features induced by 1-methyl-4-phenyl-1,2,3,6-tetrahydropyridine (MPTP) in an old Java monkey [*Macaca cynomolgus fascicularis* (Raffles)]. Brain Res Bull 1986; 16:561–571.

26. Schneider JS, Yuwiler A, Markham CH. Selective loss of subpopulations of ventral mesencephalic dopaminergic neurons in the monkey following exposure to MPTP. Brain Res 1987; 411:144–150.

27. Miyoshi R, Kito S, Ishida H, Katayama S. Alterations in the central noradrenergic system in MPTP-induced monkey parkinsonism. Res Commun Chem Pathol Pharmacol 1988; 62:93–102.

28. Tanaka J, Nakamura H, Honda S, Takada K, Kato S. Neuropathological study on 1-methyl-4-phenyl-1,2,3,6-tetrahydropyridine of the crab-eating monkey. Acta Neuropathol 1988; 75:370–376.

29. Unguez GA, Schneider JS. Dopaminergic dorsal raphe neurons in cats and monkeys are sensitive to the toxic effects of MPTP. Neurosci Lett 1988; 94:218–223.

30. Crossman AR, Clarke CE, Boyce S, Robertson RG, Sambrook MA. MPTP-induced parkinsonism in the monkey: neurochemical pathology, complications of treatment and pathophysiological mechanisms. Can J Neurol Sci 1987; 14:428–435.

31. Gibb WRG, Terruli M, Lees AJ, Jenner P, Marsden CD. The evolution and distribution of morphological changes in the nervous system of the common marmoset following the acute administration of 1-methyl-4-phenyl-1,2,3,6-tetrahydropyridine. Mov Disord 1989; 4:53–74.

32. Redmond DE Jr, Roth RH, Sladek JR Jr. MPTP produces classic parkinsonian syndrome in African green monkeys. Soc Neurosci Abstr 1985; 11:166.

33. Tetrud JW, Langston JW, Redmond DE Jr, et al. MPTP-induced tremor in human and non-human primates [Abstr]. Neurology 1986; 36(suppl 1):308.

34. Ballard PA, Tetrud JW, Langston JW. Permanent human parkinsonism due to 1-methyl-4-phenyl-1,2,3,6-tetrahydropyridine (MPTP): seven cases. Neurology 1985; 35:949–956.

35. Davis GC, Williams AC, Markey SP, et al. Chronic parkinsonism secondary to intravenous injection of meperidine analogues. Psychiatr Res 1979; 1:249–254.

36. Jenner P, Marsden CD. MPTP-induced parkinsonism as an experimental model of Parkinson's disease. In: Jankovic J, Tolosa E, eds. Parkinson's Disease and Movement Disorders. Baltimore: Urban & Schwarzenberg, 1988:37–48.

37. Tetrud JW, Langston JW. Early parkinsonism in humans due to MPTP exposure [abstr]. Neurology 1986; 36(suppl 1):308.

38. Tetrud JW, Langston JW. Tremor in MPTP-induced parkinsonism. Neurology 1992; 42:407–410.

39. Findley LJ, Gresty MA. Tremor and rhythmical involuntary movements in Parkinson's disease. In: Findley LJ, Capildeo R, eds. Movement Disorders: Tremor. New York: Oxford University Press, 1984:295–304.

40. Burns RS, LeWitt PA, Ebert MH, Pakkenberg H, Kopin IJ. The clinical syndrome of striatal dopamine deficiency: parkinsonism induced by 1-methyl-4-phenyl-1,2,3,6-tetrahydropyridine (MPTP). N Engl J Med 1985; 312:1418–1421.

41. Fearnley JM, Lees AJ. Striatonigral degeneration. A clinicopathological study. Brain 1990; 113:1823–1842.

42. Rajput AH, Rozdilsky B, Ang L. Occurrence of resting tremor in Parkinson's disease. Neurology 1991; 41:1298–1299.

43. Rajput AH, Rozdilsky B, Ang L. Site(s) of lesion and resting tremor. Neurology 1990; 28:296.

23

Medical Management of Parkinsonian Tremor

Eduardo S. Tolosa and Concepció Marin
Hospital Clínic I Provincial Barcelona
University of Barcelona
Barcelona, Spain

I. INTRODUCTION

Resting tremor, with rigidity and bradykinesia, constitutes one of the cardinal manifestations of Parkinson's disease (PD) and, actually, the most characteristic one. Although both akinesia and rigidity are encountered in practically all forms of secondary parkinsonism, such as progressive supranuclear palsy or multisystem atrophy, a typical tremor occurring only at rest is almost unique to idiopathic PD. Other types of tremor also occur in PD, although most descriptions of the symptomatology of the disorder often do not discuss them. The postural–action tremor of PD is clinically similar to the postural tremor of essential tremor, but it has a different pharmacological profile. Tremor in PD is frequently disabling, interfering with activities of daily living and is typically aggravated by stress and fatigue, constituting a major source of social embarrassment.

Is the medical treatment of tremor in PD that different from the treatment of the other symptoms, particularly of bradykinesia, generally the most disabling symptom, that it justifies a separate chapter in a book? Are some drugs (e.g., the anticholinergics) more effective, and others, such as levodopa, less effective for tremor than for other PD symptoms, as is frequently stated? If this were true, this chapter would indeed be justified and more so if the book is devoted to "tremors."

Several experimental and clinical observations indicate that tremor in PD has some characteristics that separate it from bradykinesia and suggest a different pathophysiology and, possibly, a different treatment. For example, typical resting tremor is a sign difficult to reproduce and, therefore, to study in animal models of PD, including some models in primates. Also, clinically, tremor is a variable symptom easily aggravated by stress and fatigue unlike the bradykinesia of PD. In general, patients with tremor as the predominant feature have a better prognosis than those patients in whom bradykinesia and gait disturbance predominate, and a subset of those tremoric patients are said to be related genetically to essential tremor. In addition, peripheral reflexes might be important in the genesis of the parkinsonian tremor, but not of bradykinesia and, finally, tremor responds far better than bradykinesia to stereotactic thalamotomy.

These differences mentioned here, among others, between tremor and other motor signs of PD make it reasonable to expect that the pharmacology of tremor and, therefore, its medical treatment, might differ from the treatment of the other motor symptoms. After preparing this review we came to the conclusion that the antiparkinsonian drugs in use today, the anticholinergics and the dopaminergic agents, probably are as effective in alleviating resting tremor as in improving other motor symptoms of PD and that no specific tremorolytic drugs exist in the management of PD. However, some drugs (β-adrenergic blockers, benzodiazepines) can improve tremor in PD without modifying other symptoms of the disorder through their peripheral β-adrenergic blocking properties or through an anxiolytic effect.

A brief review on the medical treatment of the tremor of PD is presented in the text that follows. The information available on this topic in the literature is somewhat limited and, at times, contradictory. Tremor, however, is a variable sign with time—a patient may state that he or she has hardly any tremor and, on going to the doctor, may shake like a leaf. It is, therefore, difficult to study, and most drug trials do not specify the effect of the various drugs being evaluated on the different signs and symptoms of the disease. Only rarely, do these studies evaluate the postural–action tremor of the disease.

II. MAJOR ANTIPARKINSONIAN DRUGS IN CURRENT USE

A. Anticholinergics

Ordenstein first described the beneficial effect of the belladonna alkaloids on tremor and other PD symptoms (1), and subsequent investigators (2), at the end of last century and early 20th century, agreed that scopolamine (hyoscine) and hyoscyamine (duboisine) were effective in mitigating tremor and muscular rigidity. For over half a century the belladonna alkaloids formed the mainstay of the medical management of the PD syndrome. These natural products were substituted in the 1960s by a series of synthetic anticholinergics and antihistaminics, several of which are still in use. Anticholinergics exert a modest improvement (3)

(20–30% improvement in functional capacity) in PD, but the percentage of patients reported to improve with these drugs has varied greatly, from 43 to 77% in open trials (2,4) and from 20 to 40% in double-blind studies (5).

It is frequently stated that anticholinergics are more effective in alleviating resting tremor and rigidity than akinesia and that the major benefit derived from their use is precisely from their tremorolytic effects (6,7). Reports to the contrary, however, abound in the literature. Thus, Marshal was of the opinion that anticholinergics "had little or no effect upon the tremor" of PD (8), and Yahr and Duvoisin, in a review on the subject, conclude that the modest improvement achieved in PD with anticholinergics is "derived from a greater effect in relieving muscular rigidity and akinesia rather than tremor" (9).

Although a specific tremolytic effect of the anticholinergics in PD has not been well documented, most investigators report improvement in tremor with anticholinergics monotherapy. A recent double-blind study, using objective evaluation of tremor with accelerometry (10), has clearly shown a reduction in tremor amplitude of about 60% from baseline in a group of ten de novo patients with early parkinsonism, after treatment with trihexyphenidyl.

The differences described in the effect of anticholinergics on tremor and other symptoms of the PD syndrome have been attributed to differences in patient selection, drug dosages, specific drugs studied, and on methods of assessment. Whether patients with early mild disease respond better or worse than those with more advanced parkinsonism, has not been clarified, and it appears that the use of higher doses of anticholinergics does not yield better results than lower doses. Marsden, in a placebo-controlled study, compared different doses of two anticholinergics and found no evidence of increased benefit from higher doses with either of the two (11), a failure that did not seem to be related to the appearance of side effects. Burns et al. also found no evidence of increasing benefit with increasing dosage of trihexyphenidyl in a carefully controlled clinical trial (12). Therapeutic differences among the various synthetic anticholinergics are probably minor, but some patients may tolerate one better than the other. The anticholinergics currently in use are described in Table 1. Development of tolerance to the beneficial effects of anticholinergics is said to occur frequently. Such lack of benefit is indeed a common clinical observation after months of treatment, but should be attributed, at least in part, to progression of the degenerative process. Withdrawal of anticholinergics, even in patients in whom the beneficial effects might have been considered mild or in those in whom it is thought that the drugs are no longer effective, invariably results in worsening of all the parkinsonian symptoms, at times to a level worse than the patients baseline state.

Anticholinergics appear to improve PD tremor through a central anticholinergic effect exerted in the striatum. Duvoisin has shown that anticholinesterase, which can penetrate the brain, increase the severity of PD syndrome (13), an effect that can be reversed by anticholinergics, such as benztropine. This observation

Table 1   Anticholinergic Drugs
Commonly Used to Treat Tremor in
PD

Generic name	Daily dose (mg)
Trihexyphenidyl	1–20
Benztropine	0.5–8
Ethopropazine	100–800
Procyclidine	7.5–20
Diphenhydramine	25–200

provides a rationale for the use of anticholinergics in PD and has led to the suggestion that a state of striatal cholinergic preponderance exists in PD that is secondary to the striatal dopamine (DA) deficiency (14). It is currently believed that antimuscarinic properties of these drugs mediate its tremorolytic properties. Atropine has an antiparkinsonian action, whereas nicotine administered intravenously appears to improve, rather than worsen tremor (15,16). The effectiveness of central anticholinergics might also have been explained through an enhancement of DA activity, by inhibiting its reuptake in the striatum (17).

Peripheral adverse effects of these agents include tachycardia, constipation, urinary retention, blurred vision, and dry mouth (6,18). These effects are all reversible with a decrease or discontinuation of the drug. The usefulness of anticholinergics is also limited by central side effects. These include sedation, confusion, and psychiatric disturbances, such as memory loss and hallucinations (19,20).

Anticholinergics are currently used in the early stages of PD when tremor predominates, in an attempt to delay the introduction of levodopa and to keep the daily dose of dopaminergic drugs to a minimum. In patients receiving long-term levodopa therapy and in more advanced disease, the beneficial effect from adding anticholinergics has been questioned (21), but some authors believe that there is no question that such patients are better when anticholinergics are combined with levodopa (5,10,22).

B.   Amantadine

Amantadine hydrochloride was originally used as an antiviral agent (23) and, only later, used to treat PD (24). Its effects are thought to be mediated by enhancing striatal DA release (25). Other mechanisms of action proposed for amantadine include inhibition of DA reuptake and an anticholinergic effect (26). About 75% of patients treated with amantadine have a 15% overall improvement (27,28). The effect of amantadine on the different elements of the parkinsonian syndrome is still controversial. Schwab et al. (24) and Parkes et al. (29) described a moderate effect on akinesia and a lesser effect on tremor. However, Gilligan et al. (30) and others (5,31) reported greater effects on tremor than on akinesia. Recently, Koller studied the effect of amantadine on resting tremor in nine patients with previously untreated Parkinson's disease (10). Amantadine decreased the amplitude of parkinsonian tremor to about 24% of baseline. A comparison with other drugs was made in this study, showing a greater effect on tremor for anticholinergic drugs or levodopa. The author concludes that amantadine should not be the initial treatment for tremor in PD.

C. Levodopa

Levodopa is the most effective antiparkinsonian agent currently available, more potent, when given at the usual therapeutic doses, than the anticholinergics, amantadine, or the direct DA agonists in its effects on the individual symptoms of PD and in reducing overall disability (32,33). For reasons that are not well understood, the degree of overall response to levodopa is quite variable. Some patients improve dramatically soon after initiation of treatment, whereas, in others, the response is modest, despite progressively higher doses of the drug. The degree of responsiveness of the patients different symptoms also varies. Most studies do not specify the effect of the drug on the different symptoms and, particularly, on tremor, probably because this symptom is difficult to evaluate objectively and because of its variability in time and sensitivity to emotional factors.

1. The First Months of Treatment

The effect of levodopa on tremor and other PD signs and symptoms, at onset and during the first months of treatment, has been detailed in several studies done mostly in the 1970s. Some of these reports contend that bradykinesia and rigidity are more responsive than tremor (34–36), others that each one of the cardinal symptoms of PD responds equally well to levodopa (37,38). In their pioneer studies with dopa in 1967, Cotzias et al. reported a sustained improvement of parkinsonian features in patients treated with 3–16 g/day of D,L-dopa, for a maximum observation period of 1 year (34). As the dose of D,L-dopa was gradually increased, improvement was first noted in rigidity, and only at higher levels was there a decrease or disappearance of tremor. Cotzias et al. later evaluated the therapeutic effects of the L-isomer of dopa (39). Twenty-eight patients were treated with an optimum dose of levodopa (range 4.2–7.5 g/day). Every symptom responded, but not to the same degree in each patient. The time sequence in which the signs of parkinsonism responded was the following: first akinesia, then rigidity, and finally tremor. Tremor reemerged occasionally after rigidity had improved, responding later when the drug was increased further. This last point has been repeatedly observed in several studies (37,38,40), Yahr et al. studied 60 patients for a period between 4 and 13 months (41). They noted that tremor increased in the initial periods of levodopa treatment, but that it improved later and was eventually markedly reduced or completely suppressed. The average reduction of tremor was 66% in comparison with rigidity (72%) and akinesia (56%).

Although the studies just mentioned report that tremor improves later than the other cardinal parkinsonian symptoms, a detailed prospective study (42) on the treatment of 100 patients with levodopa as monotherapy for up to 24 months showed a rapid improvement of tremor after drug initiation. This improvement continued, but at slower rate, until the end of the study period. The maximum effect of levodopa on tremor was less when compared with its maximum effect on rigidity. This study also showed that levodopa was a better antitremor agent than were the anticholinergic drugs.

McDowell et al. described an improvement in tremor (55%) equally to that of akinesia (56%) and, curiously, a less marked improvement of rigidity (39%) in 100 patients receiving levodopa (3–8 g daily) for at least 6 months and some for longer than 1 year (43). Duvoisin et al. also studied in detail the effect of levodopa on the clinical features of PD in 30 patients treated for up to 5 months (44). They noticed that all major clinical features of PD showed improvement and that tremor was suppressed as well as rigidity and akinesia. The average overall improvement was 53%. Tremor was reduced to an average of 53%, rigidity 64%, and akinesia 50%. In this study levodopa also proved to be superior to anticholinergic treatment for all features of parkinsonism, including tremor. The studies just reviewed indicate that levodopa administered at high doses, without a dopa-decarboxylase inhibitor, is already a potent antitremor drug in the early phases of treatment, but indicate that maximal improvement in tremor tends to occur later than in bradykinesia or rigidity. Transient worsening of tremor in the initial weeks of treatment may also occur and might be partly related to the activation of peripheral adrenergic receptors by catecholamines produced during levodopa systemic metabolism. Such a finding has rarely been observed or reported in patients treated with levodopa in combination with a peripheral dopa-decarboxylase inhibitor. In one such study, specifically designed to study drug effects on tremor, Koller evaluated the effect of 300 mg of levodopa combined with carbidopa, administered three times a day, on PD tremor in patients with early parkinsonism (10). Tremor was assessed subjectively by patients self-evaluation and objectively by recording resting tremor with an accelerometer. A 55% reduction in tremor amplitude was observed, slightly less than the one induced by anticholinergics, and tremor aggravation was not detected. The study evaluated drug efficacy during only a 2-week period.

2. Levodopa-Related Motor Fluctuations and Tremor

With the passage of time, the effectiveness of levodopa treatment declines. Levodopa-related motor fluctuations develop in most patients (35) and result in the intermittent reemergence of tremor or other PD signs during the day. The most common types of motor fluctuations are the wearing-off effect and random oscillations (on–off effect). Tremor patients with such fluctuations exhibit recurrent off-period tremor, which can be disabling, but disappears during the period of good control of parkinsonism (on period). In these circumstances, tremor might be the only off-period symptom and the only source of disability, but more commonly, it reemerges in association with akinesia, rigidity, speech or ambulatory disturbances, depending on the clinical picture of the individual patient. The treatment of tremor in these patients is similar to the treatment of other symptoms recurring during the off phases, and consists in administering smaller, but more frequent, doses of levodopa, switching from standard to slow-release levodopa preparations, or adding adjuvant drugs such as amantadine, anticholinergics, deprenyl or DA agonists.

In some patients, resting tremor initially responds well to levodopa and, surprisingly, it does not reappear months or years later. In these patients, other disabling symptoms reemerge, rather than tremor, during off periods, despite the presence of prominent tremor at the beginning of treatment. This "disappearance" of tremor probably occurs independently of treatment.

Although typically recurrent tremor in patients on long-term therapy with levodopa occurs during off periods, it can also reemerge intermittently independent of motor fluctuations (Table 2). In these patients, bursts of tremor occur that appear to be stress- or fatigue-related in most instances, but that sometimes seems to have no obvious explanation. These recurrent tremor bursts can make it difficult to judge whether or not the patient is actually levodopa-underdosed, since the patient may otherwise have an acceptable control of his or her parkinsonism through the day.

Other tremors encountered in patients on long-term levodopa therapy are clearly drug-related. In patients with tremor and diphasic dyskinesias, it is not uncommon that, at the beginning of the effect of a dose of levodopa, tremor appears (at times severe) and later coexists for a time with dyskinesias. These patients find it particularly difficult to describe if the involuntary movements they are having at onset of drug effect represent tremor or dyskinesias from levodopa.

Table 2 Rest Tremor in Patients on Long-Term Levodopa Treatment

1. Intermittent stress or fatigue-related tremor
2. Off-period tremor
3. Levodopa-related tremor–dyskinesia syndrome
4. Levodopa aggravated off-period tremor (rebound effect)
5. Severe nocturnal tremor spells

If, in these patients, an on period eventually does not occur, the patients may experience only a burst of intense tremor followed by dyskinesias and off-period symptoms again. Even intelligent patients find it particularly difficult to describe to their physicians if what they are experiencing is because of an excess, or a defect, in the dosage of levodopa.

Worsening of tremor by levodopa can occasionally be encountered in other circumstances. We have previously mentioned that, in the early phases of treatment, some patients experience a mild worsening of tremor. This aggravation eventually subsides when the dosage of levodopa is further increased. Tremor in patients taking levodopa also can be prominently accentuated in those patients who, on entering the off phase, reach a much worse parkinsonian state (rebound effect) than the one they had at baseline, before taking a levodopa dose. Such levodopa-induced worsening of parkinsonism has been well documented by Nutt et al. (45). Martin et al. also described attacks of generalized tremor in patients on long-term levodopa therapy (42). Such tremor spells have not been described by others as a complication of levodopa treatment, although we have seen occasional patients who experience bursts of tremor, particularly after going to bed or in the early morning, hours after having entered the off phase. They last a variable period (minutes to hours) and are the source of major nocturnal disability.

3. Loss of Benefit of Levodopa and Tremor

After years of chronic levodopa treatment, functional disability tends to worsen in most patients. This progression in disability in levodopa-treated patients has been studied by a number of investigators, who have noticed that it results from worsening of certain, but not all, pretreatment symptoms. Tremor, specifically, is a symptom of PD that generally remains sensitive to levodopa in patients under long-term treatment. In the study of Klawans in 25 patients, tremor remained improved in 53% of patients and unchanged in 47% after 10 years or longer of levodopa treatment (46). Over the same period, improvement in micrographia and rigidity also persisted for most patients, whereas speech, postural stability, and gait disturbances, secondary to akinesia, worsened. Bonnet et al. retrospectively evaluated 193 patients and also showed that the effect of levodopa on tremor remained quite stable during long-term treatment (47). In this study, the main percentage of improvement in tremor after 2 years (29 patients) and 21 years (7 patients) of levodopa treatment was 73 and 85%, respectively. In contrast, symptoms such as speech, gait, and postural stability, progressively worsened, becoming less responsive to levodopa.

4. Levodopa and Postural–Action Tremor

Patients with PD frequently have in addition to the resting tremor an action–postural tremor that can also cause disability. This tremor has been placed in the category of essential tremor or has alternatively been interpreted as an enhanced physiological tremor (48). Action tremor in PD does respond to β-adrenergic blockers (see Sect. III.A) and also lessens with alcohol (49), but can be worsened by levodopa (50,51).

In a recent study, Koller et al. have examined the effect of levodopa therapy on the different types of tremor present in PD (52). In their study, postural tremor was present in 92% and a resting tremor in 76% of patients. Levodopa in association with carbidopa reduced postural tremor in 46% and resting tremor in 58% of patients. This study suggested that postural tremor observed in parkinsonian patients may be equally as responsive to dopaminergic drugs as resting tremor.

D. Direct Dopamine Agonists

Because of the limitations of long-term levodopa therapy, attempts have been made to develop novel and more efficacious antiparkinsonian drugs. Dopamine receptor agonists possess several theoretical advantages over levodopa. By directly stimulating postsynaptic striatal dopamine receptors, they would not be dependent on the metabolic integrity of degenerating presynaptic dopaminergic neurons. In addition, they have the potential to exert more potent and long-lasting effects than levodopa, and specific agonists to dopamine receptor subtypes may produce more specific therapeutic effects and avoid side effects related to generalized dopaminergic activation. Direct dopamine agonists have been used as monotherapy and in association with levodopa.

1. Apomorphine

Apomorphine (APOM) is a direct-acting DA agonist, with affinity for both D_1 and D_2 DA receptors. Sporadic reports on the effect of APOM on PD signs and symptoms have appeared in the literature since 1951, when Schwab (53) drew attention to its effectiveness in PD. In 1970 Cotzias et al. (54) attributed its effects on PD to its dopaminergic properties and drew attention to the similarities between the molecules of APOM and DA. Strian et al. in 1972, also found that APOM, given intravenously or orally, had a marked inhibitory effect on tremor when compared with placebo, in a group of ten patients receiving levodopa (55). The drug inhibited resting tremor, but was felt to worsen action tremor and to be much less effective on rigidity and bradykinesia. More recently, the use of subcutaneous (sc) APOM has been reevaluated for the treatment of off-period disability. Huges et al. have reported an improvement in resting tremor after acute challenges with APOM in 19 of 20 parkinsonian patients taking oral levodopa (56). In 10 of these patients, rest tremor was completely abolished, with mean doses of 2.4 mg (range 1.5–4.5 mg). Some of the patients with fluctuating symptoms and severe off-period tremor were selected for a long-term, intermittent, subcutaneous apo morphine regimen, reaching a reduction in about 50% of tremor-filled hour per day.

The APOM antiparkinsonian effects are strikingly similar to those of levodopa and, from the available data in the literature, one cannot conclude that it is more effective on tremor than on other manifestations of PD. Because of its potent antitremor properties, however, it can be an effective treatment for fluctuating patients with severe breakthrough off-period tremor.

2. Ergot Alkaloids

Bromocriptine (BCT), lisuride (LSD), and pergolide (PGL) are three ergot derivatives with direct DA receptor-activating properties currently in use in the treatment of PD. All three are useful in the treatment of the novo patients and in the treatment of motor fluctuations related to long-term levodopa therapy.

In the novo patients, BCT (57), LSD (58), and PGL (59) have reduced tremor, although extensive studies with PGL monotherapy have not been performed. In these early stages of the illness, however, they are generally not as effective as levodopa, and their beneficial effects appear to have a finite period of 1–3 years. As early therapy, therefore, the ergot agonists are generally preferably combined with levodopa, administered at small doses. The early combination of levodopa and an agonist has also been effective in delaying the appearance of levodopa-related motor fluctuations and dyskinesias (60–62). As adjuvants to levodopa in patients with fluctuations, all three agonists administered orally have also improved tremor as well as other relevant features of the illness (61,63–66).

Lisuride is water-soluble and has been administered intravenously and subcutaneously, and boluses of LSD have been effective in reversing PD tremor (58,67,68). Improvement, objectively measured by an accelerometer, increased to 80% compared with baseline (70% vs placebo) and lasted 2 h (58). Continuous infusions of LSD (12–24 h/day) up to several months has also been highly effective in reducing tremor and other PD manifestations (69).

Although some authors have found a greater effect of BCT (70) and LSD (58) on tremor than on rigidity and hypokinesia, both in the novo patients and in studies in which these drugs were added to levodopa, other studies have not found such a predominant effect on tremor (62), and still others have reported no effect on tremor (71–73).

Few studies have compared the clinical profiles of the different ergot agonists in the same patient. Those available indicate that LSD is equally as effective in controlling tremor as BCT (74). In a study comparing PGL and BCT therapy, in a group of 24 patients, LeWitt et al. (75) found that the clinical usefulness of both drugs in controlling tremor was similar. Despite their different neurochemical profiles, the tremorolytic effect of the various ergot derivates appears to be qualitatively the same.

III. OTHER TREATMENTS

A. β-Adrenergic Blockers

β-Adrenergic blocking drugs may be an effective adjuvant to currently available dopaminergic and anticholinergic therapies for tremor in patients with Parkinson's disease (76,77). It had long been known that anxiety can worsen rest tremor, probably related to β-adrenergic receptor stimulation. Drugs such as isoproterenol and epinephrine may increase rest tremor (78). This increase of parkinsonian tremor can be abolished by adrenergic antagonists (77). The effect of nadolol, a peripherally acting β-adrenergic blocker on resting, postural, and intention tremor was studied by Foster et al. (79). Maximum benefit was achieved with a dose of 240 mg, for which accelerometer readings showed a 54% reduction in resting tremor, 32% in postural tremor, and 54% in intention tremor. Although in some studies, intravenous infusion of propanolol did not alter tremor in parkinsonian patients (80), recently, a beneficial effect of long-acting propanolol (160 mg/day) has been observed with reduction of amplitude of resting tremor by 70% and of postural tremor by 50% (81). No side effects were observed with this drug formulation.

Both central and peripheral mechanisms for the antitremor effect of β-adrenergic blockers have been proposed (77,79). Propanolol penetrates the blood–brain barrier, and central or peripheral actions could account for its effect. However, nadolol does not enter to the central nervous system, and its actions are peripherally mediated.

B. Benzodiazepines

Benzodiazepines are sometimes prescribed for patients with tremor, and they may relieve a sensation of "inner tremor" that some patients have. They have been described as drugs capable of improve PD action tremor. Clonazepam has been effective in diminishing tremors of different causes including PD tremor (82,83). Loeb and Priano (84) reported that clonazepam showed a satisfactory effect in decreasing tremor in 50% of the PD patients when administered either alone or in association with standard antiparkinsonian drugs. Fatigue and drowsiness were the most common side effects found in about half the patients (84). Koller and Herbster, however, did not find a significant effect on tremor (81), suggesting that clonazepam seems to have limited value in the treatment of parkinsonian tremor.

C. Primidone

Primidone is effective in benign essential tremor (85), an effect exerted through an unknown mechanism. It was suggested that primidone's antitremor action was mediated by its metabolite phenylethylmalonamide, but administration of this compound by itself had no effect on essential tremor (86). The lack of effect of primidone in reducing parkinsonian tremor has been recently reported (81).

D. Clozapine

Clozapine is an atypical neuroleptic that does not induce parkinsonian side effects (87), and it has been reported to ameliorate the tremor of PD (88). Friedman and Lannon in an open trial, observed a moderate to marked improvement in tremor with 12.5–25 mg of clozapine in four of five PD patients who had failed to respond to various adjustments of PD medications before starting clozapine (89). The results of this study suggest that clozapine, in small doses, should be considered for the control of disabling parkinsonian rest tremors that do not respond to standard antiparkinsonian medications.

Adverse effects have limited the use of clozapine. The most serious problem is its potential for causing agranulocytosis (90). In PD the doses used are low, and the only major problem has been sedation (91). The mechanism by which clozapine exerts an antitremor effect is unknown.

IV. TREATMENT OF TREMOR IN RECENT-ONSET AND ADVANCED PARKINSON'S DISEASE

The initiation of tremor therapy in recent-onset PD depends on several factors and must be individualized. Mild tremor may require no symptomatic treatment at all. When some symptomatic treatment is needed, anticholinergic drugs might be used. Amantadine, another first-line drug is generally less effective than anticholinergics in the control of tremor in this early stage, but is a reasonable alternative if the anticholinergics fail or bradykinesia is also present (Table 3).

Direct dopaminergic agonists can also be administered for the treatment of parkinsonian tremor of recent onset. Best results, however, have been obtained when the agonists are used in combination with levodopa.

To avoid side effects, anticholinergic agents should not be used in elderly patients. In these patients, treatment with levodopa may be recommended, keeping the dose as low as possible. Elderly PD patients are likely to take longer than young-onset ones to develop fluctuations and dyskinesia after starting levodopa therapy and, when these side effects appear, they are likely to be less functionally disabling.

Tremor is frequent in advanced PD, but is generally less disabling than bradykinesia or other accompanying symptoms (except in severe tremoric cases). Its response to medication is usually no different from the response of other cardinal symptoms of the illness and, therefore, from a therapeutical viewpoint, it is not useful to consider it as a separate or special symptom. Almost all patients at this stage are receiving levodopa, and adjustment of the dosage and schedule of

Table 3 Drug Effects on Parkinsonian Tremor

Drug	Type of tremor[a]	
	Rest tremor	Action tremor
Anticholinergics	+ +	0
Amantadine	+	0
Levodopa	+ + +	0
Dopamine agonists	+ +	0
β-Adrenergic blockers	+	+ +
Benzodiazepines	+	+
Primidone	0	0
Clozapine	+	0

[a]0, no improvement; 1+, mild improvement; 2+, moderate improvement; 3+, marked improvement.

administration of this drug or switching to a slow-release preparation can improve off-period tremor or levodopa-induced tremor worsening (e.g., associated with diphasic dyskinesias). Addition of selegiline or orally administered DA agonists can also attenuated tremor in those patients who are not already receiving these drugs, and intermittent subcutaneous apomorphine administered by Penjet is of help for severe off-period tremor. Clonazepan or clozapine can also be considered for the control of disabling rest tremors that do not respond to standard antiparkinsonian medication. Ansiolitics are also, occasionally, of help in patients in whom stress-aggravated tremor is prominent. If postural tremor is present, propranolol or other β-adrenergic blockers can be tried, but are rarely useful.

REFERENCES

1. Ordenstein L. Sur la Paralysie et al Sclerose en Plaque Generalise. Paris: Martinet, 1867.
2. Strang RR. Orphenadine ("Disipal") in the treatment of parkinsonism: a two year study of 150 patients. Med J Aust 1965; 448–450.
3. Ivanainen M. KR 339 in the treatment of parkinsonian tremor. Acta Neurol Scand 1974; 50:469–477.
4. Corbin KB. Trihexyphenidyl: evaluation of a new agent in treatment of parkinsonism. JAMA 1949; 141:377–382.
5. Parkes JD, Baxter RC, Marsden CD, Rees JE. Comparative trial of benzhexol, amantadine and levodopa in the treatment of Parkinson disease. J Neurol Neurosurg Psychiatry 1974; 37:422–426.
6. Ebling P. The medical management of Parkinson's disease before the introduction of L-dopa. Aust NZ J Med 1971; 1(suppl 1):35–38.

7. Obeso JA, Martinez-Lage M. Anticholinergics and amantadine. In: Koller W, ed. Handbook of Parkinson's Disease. New York: Marcel Dekker, 1987:309–316.
8. Marshall J. Tremor. In: Vinken PJ, Bruyn GW eds. Handbook of Clinical Neurology: Diseases of Basal Ganglia. Amsterdam: Elsevier North-Holland, 1968:809–825.
9. Yahr M, Duvoisin RC. Medical therapy of parkinsonism. In: Vinken PJ, Bruyn GW, eds. Handbook of Clinical Neurology: Diseases of the Basal Ganglia. Amsterdam: Elsevier North Holland, 1968:283–300.
10. Koller WC. Pharmacologic treatment of parkinsonian tremor. Arch Neurol 1986; 43: 126–127.
11. Marsden CD. Extending the use of anticholinergic drugs in Parkinson's disease. In: Gillingham FJ, Donaldson IM, eds. Third Symposium on Parkinson's Disease. Edinburgh, 1969:185–192.
12. Burns D, De Jong D, Solis-Quiroga OH. Effects of trihexyphenidyl hydrochloride (Artane) on Parkinson's disease. Neurology 1964; 14:13–23.
13. Duvoisin RC. Cholinergic-anticholinergic antagonism in parkinsonism. Arch Neurol 1967; 17;124–136.
14. Barbeau A. The pathogenesis of Parkinson's disease: a new hypothesis. Can Med Assoc J 1962; 87:802–807.
15. Velasco F, Velasco M, Romo R. Effect of carbachol and atropine perfusions in the mesencephalic tegmentum and caudate nucleus of experimental tremor in monkeys. Exp Neurol 1982; 78:450–460.
16. Nashold BS. Cholinergic stimulation of globus pallidus in man. Proc Soc Exp Biol Med 1959; 101:68–69.
17. Coyle JT, Snyder SH. Antiparkinsonian drugs: inhibition of dopamine uptake in the corpus striatum as a possible mechanism of action. Science 1969; 166:899–901.
18. Duvoisin RC. A review of drug therapy in parkinsonism. Bull NY Acad Med 1965; 41:898–910.
19. Porteous HB, Ross DDN. Mental symptoms in parkinsonism following benzhexol hydrochloride therapy. Br Med J 1956; 2:138–140.
20. Koller WC. Disturbance of recent memory functions in parkinsonian patients on anticholinergic therapy. Cortex 1984; 20:307–311.
21. Martin WE, Lowenson RB, Resch JA, Baker AB. A controlled study comparing trihexyphenidyl hydrochloride plus levodopa with placebo plus levodopa in patients with Parkinson's disease. Neurology 1974; 24:912–919.
22. Tourtellotte WW, Potvin AR, Syndulko K, et al. Parkinson's disease: Congentin with Sinemet, a better response. Prog Neuropsychopharmacol Biol Psychiatry 1982; 6: 51–55.
23. Davies WL, Grunert RR, Haff RF, et al. Antiviral activity of 1-adamantamine (amantadine). Science 1964; 144:862–863.
24. Schwab RS, England AC, Poskanzer DC, Young RR. Amantadine in the treatment of Parkinson's disease. JAMA 1969; 208:168–1170.
25. Scatton B, Cheramy A, Besson MJ, et al. Increased synthesis and release of dopamine in the striatum of the rat after amantadine treatment. Eur J Pharmacol 1970; 13:131–133.
26. Gerlak RP, Clark R, Stump JM, et al. Amantadine–dopamine interaction. Science 1970; 169:203–204.

27. Blutzer JF, Silver DE, Sahs AL. Amantadine in Parkinson's disease: a double-blind placebo-controlled crossover study with long-term follow-up. Neurology 1975; 25: 603–606.

28. Timberlake WH, Vance MA. Four-year treatment of patients with parkinsonism using amantadine alone or with levodopa. Ann Neurol 1978; 3:119–128.

29. Parkes JD, Baxter RCH, Curzon G, et al. Treatment of Parkinson's disease with amantadine and levodopa. Lancet 1970; 1:1083–1087.

30. Guilligan BS, Veale J, Wodak J. Amantadine hydrochloride in the treatment of Parkinson's disease. Med J Aust 1970; 2:634–637.

31. Bauer RB, Mc Henry JT. Comparison of amantadine, placebo and levodopa in Parkinson's disease. Neurology 1974; 24:715–720.

32. Fahn S, Calne DB. Considerations in the management of parkinsonism. Neurology 1978; 28:5–7.

33. Boshes B. Sinemet and the treatment of parkinsonism. Ann Intern Med 1981; 94: 364–370.

34. Cotzias GC, Van Woert MH, Schiffer LM. Aromatic amino acids and modification of parkinsonism. N Engl J Med 1967; 276:374–379.

35. Jankovic J, Fahn S. Physiologic and pathologic tremors. Diagnosis, mechanism and management. Ann Intern Med 1980; 93:460–465.

36. Koller WC, Hubble JP. Levodopa therapy in Parkinson's disease. Neurology 90; 40(suppl 3):40–47.

37. Yahr MD. Results of long-term administration of L-dopa. In: Monoamines, Noyaux Gris Centraux et Syndrome de Parkinson (Symposium Bel Air IV, Geneve). Paris: Masson & Cia, 1970:403–410.

38. Boudin G, Castaigne P, Lhermitte F, et al. Traitement des syndromes parkinsoniens par la L-dopa. In: Monoamines, Noyaux Gris Centraux et Syndrome de Parkinson (Symposium Bel Air IV, Geneve). Paris: Masson & Cia, 1970:411–418.

39. Cotzias GC, Papavasiliou PS, Gellene R. Modification of parkinsonism—chronic treatment with L-dopa. N Engl J Med 1969; 28:337–345.

40. Barbeau A. L-Dopa therapy in Parkinson's disease. A critical review of nine years experience. Can Med Assoc J 1969; 101:59–68.

41. Yahr MD, Duvoisin RC, Schear MY, Barret RE, Hoehn MM. Treatment of parkinsonism with levodopa. Arch Neurol 1969; 21:343–354.

42. Martin WE, Lowenson RB, Bilek MK, Resch JA, Baker AB. Long-term treatment of Parkinson's disease with levodopa. J Chronic Dis 1974; 2:77–93.

43. Mc Dowell F, Lee JE, Swift T, Sweet RD, Ogsbury SS, Kessler JT. Treatment of Parkinson's syndrome with L-dihydroxyphenylalanine (levodopa). Ann Intern Med 1970; 72:29–35.

44. Duvoisin RC, Barret R, Schear M, Hoehn MM, Yahr MD. The use of L-dopa in parkinsonism. In: Gillingham FJ, Donaldson IM, eds. Third Symposium in Parkinson's Disease. Edinburgh, 1969:185–192.

45. Nutt JG, Gaucher ST, Woodward WR. Does an inhibitory action of levodopa contribute to motor fluctuations? Neurology 1988; 38:1553–1557.

46. Klawans HL. Individual manifestations of Parkinson's disease after ten or more years of levodopa. Mov Dis 1986; 1:187–192.

47. Bonnet AM, Loria Y, Saint-Hilaire MH, Lhermitte F, Agid Y. Does long-term aggravation of Parkinson's disease result from nondopaminergic lesions? Neurology 1987; 37:1539–1542.
48. Fahn S. Pharmacological differentiation of tremor. In: Findley LJ, Capildeo R, eds. Movement Disorders: Tremor. London: Macmillan Press, 1984:85–93.
49. Rajput AH, Jamieson H, Hirsh S, Quraishi A. Relative efficacy of alcohol and propanolol in action tremor. Can J Neurol Sci 1971; 2:31–35.
50. Shahani BT, Young RR. Physiological and pharmacological aids in the differential diagnosis of tremor. J Neurol Neurosurg Psychiatry 1976; 39:772–778.
51. Young RR, Shahani BT. Pharmacology of tremor. Clin Neuropharmacol 1979; 4: 139–156.
52. Koller WC, Veter-Overfield B, Baxter R. Tremors in early Parkinson's disease. Clin Neuropharmacol 1989; 12:293–297.
53. Schwab RS, Amador LV, Levine JY. Apomorphine in Parkinson's disease. Trans Am Neurol Assoc 1951; 76:251–253.
54. Cotzias GC, Papavasiliou PS, Fehling C, Kaufman B, Mena I. Similarities between neurological effects of L-dopa and apomorphine. N Engl J Med 1970; 282:31–33.
55. Strian F, Micheler E, Benkert O. Tremor inhibition in Parkinson syndrome after apomorphine administration under L-dopa and decarboxylase-inhibitor basic therapy. Pharmakopsychiatr Neuro-Psychopharmakol 1972; 5:198–205.
56. Hughes AJ, Lees AJ, Stern GM. Apomorphine in the diagnosis and treatment of parkinsonian tremor. Clin Neuropharmacol 1990; 13:312–317.
57. Riopelle RJ. Bromocriptine and the clinical spectrum of Parkinson's disease. Can J Neurol Sci 1987; 14:455–459.
58. Agnoli A, Ruggieri S. Baldassarrw M, Stochi F, Denaro A, Falaschi P. Dopaminergic ergots in parkinsonism. In: Calne DB, Horowski R, McDonald RS, Wuttke W, eds. Lisuride and Other Dopamine Agonists. New York: Raven Press, 1983:407–417.
59. Rinne UK. New ergot derivates in the treatment of Parkinson's disease. In: Calne DB, Horowski R, McDonald RJ, Wuttke W, eds. Lisuride and Other Dopamine Agonists. New York: Raven Press, 1983:431–432.
60. Lees AJ, Stern GM. Sustained bromocriptine therapy in previously untreated patients with Parkinson's disease. J Neurol Neurosurg Psychiatry 1981; 44:1020–1023.
61. Calne DB, Rinne UK. Controversies in the management of Parkinson's disease. Mov Disord 1986; 1:159–162.
62. Tolosa E, Blesa R, Bayés A, Forcadell F. Low-dose bromocriptine in the early phases of Parkinson's disease. Clin Neuropharmacol 1987; 10:169–174.
63. Rinne UK. Combined bromocriptine–levodopa therapy in Parkinson's disease. Neurology 1985; 35:1196–1198.
64. Caraceni T, Giovannini P, Parati E, Scigliano G, Grassi MP, Carella F. Bromocriptine and lisuride in Parkinson's disease. Adv Neurol 1984; 40:531–535.
65. Jankovic J. Controlled trial of pergolide mesylate in Parkinson's disease and progressive supranuclear palsy. Neurology 1983; 33:505–507.
66. Jankovic J. Long-term study of pergolide in Parkinson's disease. Neurology 1985; 35: 296–299.

67. Quinn N, Marsden CD, Schachter M, Thompson C, Lang AE, Parkes JD. Intravenous lisuride in extrapyramidal disorders. In: Calne DB, Horowski R, McDonald RJ, Wuttke WS, eds. Lisuride and Other Dopamine Agonists. New York: Raven Press, 1983:383–393.

68. Parkes JD, Schachter M, Marsden CD, Smith B, Wilson A. Lisuride in parkinsonism. Ann Neurol 1981; 9:48–52.

69. Obeso JA, Luquin MR, Martinez-Lage JM. Intravenous lisuride corrects oscillations of motor performance in Parkinson's disease. Ann Neurol 1986; 19:31–35.

70. Rinne UK, Marttila R. Brain dopamine receptor stimulation and the relief of parkinsonism: relationship between bromocriptine and levodopa. Ann Neurol 1978; 4:263–267.

71. Lieberman A, Zolfaghari M, Boal D, et al. The antiparkinsonian efficacy of bromocriptine. Neurology 1976; 26:405–409.

72. Parkes JD, Marsden CD, Donaldson I, et al. Bromocriptine treatment in Parkinson's disease. J Neurol Neurosurg Psychiatry 1976; 39:184–193.

73. Sage IJ, Duvoisin RC. Pergolide therapy in Parkinson's disease: a double-blind, placebo-controlled study. Clin Neuropharmacol 1985; 8:260–265.

74. LeWitt PA, Gopinathan G, Ward CD, et al. Lisuride versus bromocriptine treatment in Parkinson's disease: a double blind study. Neurology 1982; 32:69–72.

75. LeWitt PA, Ward CD, Larsen TA, et al. Comparison of pergolide and bromocriptine therapy in parkinsonism. Neurology 1983; 33:1009–1014.

76. Herring AB. Action of pronethalol on parkinsonian tremor. Lancet 1964; 2:892.

77. Owen DAL, Marsden CD. Effect of adrenergic beta-blockade on parkinsonian tremor. Lancet 1965; 2:1259–1262.

78. Barcroft H, Peterson E, Schwab RS. Action of adrenaline and noradrenaline on the tremor in Parkinson's disease. Neurology 1952; 2:154–160.

79. Foster NL, Newman RP, Le Witt PA, Gillespie MM, Larsen TA, Chase TN. Peripheral beta-adrenergic blockade treatment of parkinsonian tremor. Ann Neurol 1984; 16:505–508.

80. Vas CJ. Propanolol in parkinsonian tremor. Lancet 1966; 1:182–183.

81. Koller WC, Herbster G. Adjuvant therapy of parkinsonian tremor. Arch Neurol 1987; 44:921–923.

82. Biary N, Koller WC. Kinetic predominant tremor: effect of clonazepam. Neurology 1987; 37:471–474.

83. Heilman KM. Orthostatic trunkal tremor. Arch Neurol 1984; 41:880–881.

84. Loeb C, Priano A. Preliminary evaluation of the effects of clonazepam on parkinsonian tremor. Eur Neurol 1977; 15:143–145.

85. O'Brien MD, Upton AR, Toseland PA. Benign familiar tremor treated with primidone. Br Med J 1981; 282:178–180.

86. Calzetti S, Findley LJ, Pisani F, Richens A. Phenylethylmalonamide in essential tremor. A double-blind controlled study. J Neurol Neurosurg Psychiatry 1981; 44:932–934.

87. Gerlach J, Kappelhus P, Helweg E, et al. Clozapine and haloperidol in a single crossover trial. Acta Psychiatr Scand 1974; 50:410–424.

88. Pakkenberg H, Pakkenberg B. Clozapine in the treatment of tremor. Acta Neurol Scand 1986; 73:295–297.
89. Friedman JH, Lannon MC. Clozapine-responsive tremor in Parkinson's disease. Mov Disord 1990; 225–229.
90. Idanpaan-Heikkila S, Alhara E, Olkinuora M, Palva I. Clozapine and agranulocytosis. Lancet 1975; 2:611.
91. Wolters EC, Hurutz TA, Peppard RF, Calne DB. Clozapine: an antipsychotic agent in Parkinson's disease. Clin Neuropharmacol 1989; 12:83–90.

24

Normal and Abnormal Tremor in the Elderly

James Kelly
Frne Hospital
Enniskillen, Northern Ireland

Hugh McA. Taggart and Paul McCullagh
Queen's University of Belfast
Belfast, Northern Ireland

I. INTRODUCTION

A. Historical Aspects of Tremor in the Elderly

Tremor is the most common movement disorder seen in clinical practice. Most members of the public are familiar with the terms "shaking with fright" or "trembling with fear" as a manifestation of tremor. Unfortunately, many people, even within medical circles, associate the presence of tremor with either a serious nervous disorder or advanced senility. Terms such as senile tremor have added to the myth that tremor is a normal accompaniment of old age. It is not known who first described the association of tremor with age, but there are biblical references such as that in Ecclesiastes (XII. 3.) "the keepers of the house shall tremble," a remark interpreted as referring to tremor of the hands of an elderly gentleman. Charcot (1), as long ago as 1876, pointed out that tremor was not necessarily an unavoidable feature of old age, as was generally believed at the time. In a review of 2000 elderly patients he identified only "about 30" with tremor. Tremor is more common in the elderly, but this is due to the increased incidence of Parkinson's disease and essential tremor in this aged group.

The association between the tremor of Parkinson's disease and age has been well recognized for many years. Uncertainty exists about whether Parkinson's disease, as described by James Parkinson in 1817 (2), existed before the 19th century, but it has been suggested that the innkeeper in Rembrandt's 1630 sketch *The Good Samaritan* was a Parkinson's disease sufferer. Guiseppe Longhi (3), the late 18th and early 19th century engraver, wrote that the innkeeper in the picture is in "an attitude which can only be found in one who has constant tremor so that . . . , he really seems to shake." Whether or not this is a true example of Parkinson's disease, it is clear in the picture that the man is stooped and very elderly.

Charcot, in 1888 (4), identified Parkinson's disease as the fifth most common disease treated at the Salpêtrière, and confirmed the age of onset to be older than 40 or 50 years of age. Gower, in his 1893 book *Diseases of the Nervous System* reviewed his experience of over 80 patients with paralysis agitans (5). He emphasized the age distribution of the condition and commented that it was "essentially a disease of the degenerative period of life, not of extreme senility."

Essential tremor, the most common movement disorder, has long been closely associated with age and has even gained the term "senile tremor" when it appears in older-aged groups. Trousseau, in 1885, mentioned that "senile tremor" was not necessarily confined to old people and could appear in middle life or even in adolescence (6). However, the first detailed description of this "hereditary tremor" is from Dana in 1887 (7). It was known as Minor's disease, at the turn of the century, named after the Russian neurologist, L. Minor, who published five papers on the condition (8). The tremor was later defined by age groups so that such terms as "infantile tremor," "juvenile tremor," "presenile tremor," and "senile tremor" became commonplace. Unfortunately, such artificial separation tends to imply tremors of different origins and with different treatment options, which is not so.

Part of the reason that these misconceptions continue is the lack of detailed study of tremor in the elderly, both in terms of neurophysiological mechanisms and in the effects and efficacy of antitremor agents.

The first significant attempt to treat tremor comes from Charcot (1879) when, using belladonna alkaloids in the form of hyoscine (scopolamine), he successfully ameliorated tremor (9). This was almost certainly the first documented use of an antitremor pharmacological agent. Duvoisin (10) has identified Ordenstein, a student of Charcot, as the person who suggested this therapeutic approach. This group of drugs and the newer synthetic anticholinergic drugs have been the mainstay of treatment of parkinsonian tremor ever since.

The treatment of tremor is often thought of with a nihilistic attitude, and this is especially so for elderly patients in whom the therapeutic approach is greatly limited by the increased incidence of side effects of drugs, such as the β-adrenergic blockers and anticholinergics. Tremor gives rise to more problems in elderly patients; when present in young patients, it rarely causes more than social embarrassment, but in older patients, it often results in considerable disability, with functional impairment. Despite this, there has been little study of antitremor agents, new or old, in this aged group.

This chapter aims to review current knowledge of physiological tremor and the common abnormal or pathological tremors in the elderly. Some relevant aspects of therapeutic approaches to tremor in the elderly will also be discussed.

II. PHYSIOLOGICAL TREMOR IN THE ELDERLY

Physiological tremor is the normal, generally invisible, small-amplitude, whole-body vibration that can be readily recorded with sophisticated transducing devices. Although there has been much research into physiological tremor, there have been relatively few studies of this tremor in older-aged groups. This is despite the fact that many researchers have suggested that there are important changes in physiological tremor with increasing age (11,12).

A. Studies in Variation With Age

After Schäfer (13) first identified a 10-cycle/s vibration in the normal human myogram, many researchers have since shown this to be the 10-Hz physiological tremor found in adults. Marshall, using a 65-g double-diode accelerometer, recorded physiological tremor in 600 subjects aged between 2 and 96 years (14, 15). With use of visual analysis of the output, he discovered that the dominant frequency increased from 5–6 Hz in children to 8–12 Hz in adults, with a gradual decrease to 6–7 Hz in patients between 40 and 70 years of age.

The development of computed spectral analysis of tremor signals enabled more objective studies of physiological tremor to be carried out. Marsden and co-workers (11) were the first to study variation with age using this technique. They analyzed finger tremor recorded with an accelerometer strapped to the terminal interphalangeal joint of the index finger. Eighty-eight subjects, aged 3–85 years, were studied with the limb supported to the wrist. Children and adults had similar dominant frequency of 8–9 Hz, but in patients older than 60 years, this frequency appeared to decrease to a mean of 7.7 Hz.

Both these studies assessed tremor in what was termed a postural position. A further analysis of physiological tremor in the postural position was carried out by Wade et al. (16). They performed a normative study of amplitude, frequency, and variability of postural tremor in 97 subjects between 15 and 80 years. With a 6-g piezoresistive accelerometer, mounted on the dorsum of the hand, they recorded and analyzed 60 s of tremor signal. They found that the peak frequency was stable at 7.0 Hz in patients up to aged 70 years. Older than this age the tremor frequency decreased to a mean of 6 Hz.

Birmingham and colleagues (12), recognizing that previous studies of tremor variation with age used different recording techniques and differing recording positions, carried out a detailed analysis of finger tremor in various aged groups. They recorded finger tremor, in three different positions, using a 15-g accelerometer.

Analysis of 190 subjects between 7 and 77 years of age revealed a shift in the dominant frequency with increasing age. For rest and postural tremor, frequency rose throughout childhood to reach its highest levels in adult life, with a tendency to fall again in later life.

Differences between these four studies almost certainly relate to problems with methodology, in particular, the different recording methods, positions, and modes of analysis used.

Unfortunately, the equipment used to record tremor can introduce perturbations into the system. The use of large bulky accelerometers must introduce some mechanical effects on the tremor-oscillating system; therefore, the tremor signal may well represent a form of activated tremor, rather than pure physiological tremor (12). Marshall's results may well suffer from this problem, as the accelerometer used weighed about 65 g. Birmingham and co-workers (12) were aware of this problem, and even with a lighter accelerometer (15 g), commented on how this could represent a mass effect for children. A similar argument can be made for frail, elderly persons.

Nevertheless, one pattern that emerged in all these studies, was the decrease in physiological tremor frequency in the older-aged groups. Marsden made the point that the decrease appeared to continue with advancing years and that, although various mechanical and neuronal factors have been identified, the exact pathogenesis of this tremor remains unknown (17). The significance of possible changes in physiological tremor with age is also uncertain.

In an attempt to address these difficulties, we carried out a detailed investigation of physiological tremor in an elderly population, looking at both the changes in dominant frequency and in amplitude that occur in the elderly (18).

The physiological tremor was recorded in three positions using an ultralight accelerometer (0.45 g) attached to the middle finger. The recordings were analyzed using computed spectral analysis, and the results compared with anthropometric data to elucidate some of the important factors in the genesis of physiological tremor in the elderly.

B. Methods

The subjects were a random sample of 94 well elderly patients with an age range of 65–98 years (mean age 79.5 years): 26 subjects were men and 68 women. All subjects were right-handed.

1. Tremor Recording

All measurements were taken with the subject seated in a quiet room, free from extraneous vibrations or electrical interference. Finger tremor was recorded from both right and left hands, using a lightweight (0.45 g) piezoelectric accelerometer attached to the terminal phalanx of the middle finger. Recordings were taken in three positions: (1) with the forearm supported to the wrist and the hand relaxed in a flexed posture over the edge of a tremor platform (rest position), (2) with the limb supported to the wrist and the hand extended horizontally beyond the tremor platform (modified postural position), (3) with the arm and hand fully outstretched horizontally at shoulder level (postural position). All recordings were performed under standardized conditions (19). Tremor was recorded for 64 s in each of the three positions. The tremor signal was amplified and stored on an on-line microcomputer for subsequent spectral analysis, as described in detail elsewhere (20).

2. Anthropometric Measurements

The height and weight and midarm circumference (cm) of each subject were measured. Triceps skinfold thickness (mm) was measured in the standardized fashion using Harpenden calipers. Grip strength (mmHg) was measured using a "Boots gripmeter." From this anthropometric data, the arm muscle area and total body muscle mass were mathematically derived by using the modified equations of Heymsfield and co-workers (21).

3. Statistical Analysis

The dominant frequency and root mean squared (RMS) amplitude were compared for selected aged groups by analysis of variance. Right and left hands were compared with paired t-tests, and men were compared with women by unpaired t-tests. Multiple linear regression analysis was used to assess the relative effects of age, height, weight, body mass index, and grip strength on tremor frequency and amplitude.

C. Results

Patients were divided into four aged groups: 65–69 years, 70–79 years, 80–89 years, and 90+ years. Mean dominant tremor frequency for each aged group in the different tremor recording positions for both left and right hands are shown in Table 1. There was a significant ($p < 0.01$ for right hand, $p < 0.001$ for left hand) decrease in postural frequency with increasing age (Fig. 1). Resting frequency and modified postural frequency, however, were unrelated to age.

For the three positions, the mean RMS amplitude in each of the aged groups showed no significant age-related changes. Amplitude values were very much higher for both the modified postural and the postural recordings than in resting position. There was no correlation between tremor amplitude and the dominant frequency.

The anthropometric data is displayed in Table 2. Midarm circumference and triceps skinfold thickness did not change significantly with age. Grip strength ($p < 0.001$; see Fig. 1), height ($p < 0.005$), and weight ($p < 0.001$), all decreased significantly with increasing age.

By multiple linear regression analysis, arm muscle area and total body mass

Table 1 Dominant Frequency for Selected Aged Groups

	Population (N = 94)	65–69 (n = 15)	70–79 (n = 35)	80–89 (n = 30)	90+ (n = 14)
Right hand					
Rest frequency (Hz)	8.37	7.90	8.35	8.34	9.00
	(8.12–8.62)	(7.41–8.39)	(7.96–8.74)	(7.80–8.88)	(8.46–9.46)
Modified postural frequency (Hz)	8.17	8.02	8.16	8.40	7.89
	(7.86–8.48)	(7.62–8.42)	(7.68–8.64)	(7.77–9.03)	(6.85–8.93)
Postural frequency (Hz)	6.81	7.60	6.89	6.62	6.16[a]
	(6.51–7.11)	(7.05–8.15)	(6.39–7.39)	(6.06–7.18)	(5.46–6.86)
Left hand					
Rest frequency (Hz)	8.46	8.33	8.56	8.38	8.52
	(8.16–8.76)	(7.68–8.98)	(8.01–9.11)	(7.82–8.94)	(7.95–9.09)
Modified postural frequency (Hz)	8.15	8.66	8.10	8.22	7.57
	(7.83–8.47)	(7.78–9.54)	(7.56–8.64)	(7.73–8.71)	(6.72–8.42)
Postural frequency (Hz)	6.69	7.78	6.75	6.44	5.89[b]
	(6.38–7.00)	(7.25–8.31)	(6.29–7.21)	(5.85–7.03)	(5.16–6.62)

Figures in parentheses represent the mean ± 95% confidence intervals.

[a] $p < 0.01$.

[b] $p < 0.001$ using analysis of variance to compare across the aged groups.

Source: Ref. 18.

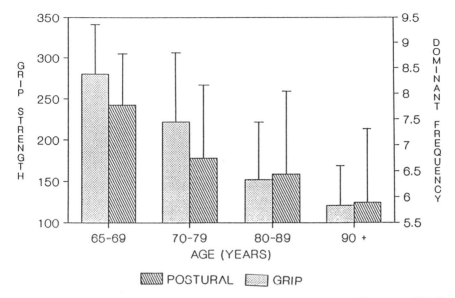

Figure 1 Left hand mean grip strength (mmHg) and mean postural frequency (Hz) for selected age groups. Grip strength and postural frequency decreased significantly with age ($p < 0.005$, $p < 0.001$, respectively).

were found to contribute significantly to the decrease in dominant frequency with increasing age ($p < 0.05$). Grip strength, however, proved to be the most significant variable ($p < 0.005$).

There was no difference between left and right hands for dominant frequency, amplitude, or anthropometric data, whether comparisons were made for the whole population, or for the individual aged groups.

There was no significant difference in tremor amplitudes between the men and women, but postural frequencies were significantly lower in the women ($p < 0.01$).

D. Discussion

These results not only confirm the decrease in frequency of physiological tremor in the postural position with increasing age, but also demonstrate, for the first time, that this decrease continues into advanced old age.

Measuring physiological tremor in the three positions has helped clarify some of the conflicting results of earlier studies. Marshall (14,15) measured tremor in the postural position, finding a change in tremor frequency with age. Marsden and co-workers (11) recorded tremor in a position akin to the modified postural position and did not find a direct change with increasing age, although they did identify a

Table 2 Anthropometric Data Measured in Both Right and Left Arms for Selected Aged Groups

	Population (N = 94)	65–69 (N = 15)	70–79 (N = 35)	80–89 (N = 30)	90+ (N = 14)
Right hand					
Grip strength (mmHg)	195.8	262.0	227.3	163.9	114.6
(mean ± SD)	(108.0–273.6)	(197.3–346.7)	(149.5–294.9)	(90.7–237.1)	(64.3–164.7)
Mean arm circumference (cm)	26.8	30.0	27.7	24.0	27.3
(mean ± SD)	(21.1–32.5)	(26.5–33.5)	(23.3–32.1)	(20.1–27.9)	(17.4–37.2)
Triceps skinfold thickness (mm)	15.0	19.5	17.8	10.3	13.1
(mean ± SD)	(7.5–22.5)	(10.2–28.8)	(10.9–27.7)	(5.4–15.2)	(7.6–18.6)
Left hand					
Grip strength (mmHg)	193.8	280.1	222.0	151.7	121.1
(mean ± SD)	(105.5–282.1)	(217.4–340.8)	(138.9–305.1)	(81.8–221.6)	(72.9–169.3)
Mean arm circumference (cm)	26.1	29.5	27.5	23.8	24.4
(mean ± SD)	(21.8–30.4)	(25.6–33.4)	(23.6–31.4)	(20.0–27.6)	(21.2–27.6)
Triceps skinfold thickness (mm)	14.8	19.4	17.9	10.2	11.3
(mean ± SD)	(7.4–22.2)	(9.8–29.0)	(11.1–24.7)	(5.8–14.6)	(7.6–15.0)

Source: Ref. 18.

difference in tremor frequency between young and old patients. Birmingham and associates (12) used recording positions similar to those in the present study, along with a recording while the finger performed a simple work task. Only in the postural position was a decrease in tremor frequency with age identified.

The amplitude of physiological tremor did not change significantly with age, and no direct relation with frequency was identified. Stiles, however, found a negative correlation between tremor frequency and amplitude (22). This is most likely explained by the fact that the experiments of Stiles involved fatiguing the patients. This is now a recognized cause of enhanced physiological tremor. We avoided this problem by using a short recording time and an ultralightweight accelerometer.

That physiological tremor frequency decreases only in the postural position suggests that mechanical factors are of importance. This is supported by the finding of a highly significant effect of grip strength on the changes in tremor frequency with age. Viitasalo et al. compared various anthropometric data in different-aged groups and found that grip strength was the variable most strongly correlated with age (23). They found that the grip strength was one of the few anthropometric measurements not influenced by the different amounts of exercise and training subjects undertake. Grip strength relates mostly to the muscle mechanics of the limb, suggesting that changes in muscle components with aging may be important in tremor frequency changes. The finding that body muscle mass and arm muscle area both contributed significantly to the change in frequency with age supports this suggestion. Other workers (24,25) have shown that human skeletal muscle undergoes a striking reduction in muscle volume and muscle strength with increasing age. Lexell and colleagues reported that this decline starts at about the age of 25 years (26), so that by the age of 50 years, 10% of muscle area is lost. The process accelerates in the elderly so that by 80 years of age, 50% of muscle is lost. Aniansson and co-workers (27) showed that myopathic changes in aging muscle were rare, suggesting that neuropathic factors, as identified by Tomonaga (28), are important in the muscle decline in elderly subjects. Changes in tetanic fusion frequency described by Newton and Yemm (29) in elderly subjects, although relevant, do not entirely explain the changes in tremor frequency, as a decrease in contraction time would also influence amplitude.

Further research to elucidate these mechanisms is required and might include electromyographic (EMG) spectral analysis and long-latency reflex studies.

III. PARKINSONIAN TREMOR

Tremor is one of the most frequent presenting features of Parkinson's disease (30). Some patients even report a sense of inner tremulousness before the appearance of their tremor (31). Lakie and Mutch have confirmed this in 20 elderly patients (mean age 75.3 years) with idiopathic Parkinson's disease and have suggested that the measurement of this invisible, early parkinsonian tremor may have diagnostic significance in some patients (32). The clinical and spectral analysis characteristics of the resting parkinsonian tremor in the elderly are similar to those found in younger patients. The presence of additional postural, clonuslike, and action tremors is also recognized in older parkinsonian patients (33). There is no evidence to suggest any differences due to age in parkinsonian tremor genesis.

The major area in which parkinsonian tremor differs between younger and older patients is in the therapeutic options available for tremor management. Many antitremor or antiparkinsonian agents used routinely in younger patients have an unacceptably high side effect profile in the elderly.

Anticholinergic agents, such as trihexyphenidyl (benzhexol), orphenadrine, and benztropine, all reduce parkinsonian resting tremor (34). It has been suggested that when tremor is the predominant symptom the use of an anticholinergic drug is preferable (35). Unfortunately, enthusiasm for these drugs must be tempered with caution, as they are associated with side effects, such as dry mouth, constipation, blurred vision, confusion, and memory impairment (36,37). In elderly patients these side effects are particularly common and troublesome and almost prohibit the use of such drugs in this aged group (38,39).

The use of β-adrenergic blocking drugs, such as propranolol, shown to be effective in some patients with parkinsonian tremor (40), also has an unacceptably high side effect profile in the elderly.

Dopamine agonists, such as bromocriptine, pergolide, and lisuride, although reducing tremor by about 35% (41), frequently cause hypotension and nausea. There is a high frequency of these side effects in the elderly, again making these drugs unsuitable for elderly patients (42). Apomorphine, the first dopamine agonist to be used in Parkinson's disease (43), has been rediscovered for use in subcutaneous infusions and for "Penject" injections (44). The use of domperidone, a peripheral dopamine antagonist, to counteract the side effects of apomorphine has permitted more widespread use of this agent. Stibe and co-workers, suggested that apomorphine particularly reduced tremor (45). There have been no studies as yet of its use in elderly patients, but there seems no reason to deny them this new therapeutic development.

The monoamine oxidase inhibitors (MAOIs), especially the selective type B agent selegiline, have become very important in the management of Parkinson's disease. Birkmayer, first reported the benefits of adding this agent to levodopa therapy and then suggested, on a 9-year follow-up study, that the agent improved survival (46,47). The role of selegiline in blocking the oxidative stages of the toxin 1-methyl-4-phenyl-1,2,3,6-tetrahydropyridine (MPTP) emphasized the importance of this drug in future management of Parkinson's disease (48). Evidence now exists that selegiline can slow progression of Parkinson's disease, and it is now administered at time of diagnosis, rather than late in the disease process (49,50).

The MAOIs have a good side effect profile and can be safely given to elderly patients. There have been no trials, as yet, looking specifically at how this group of drugs affects tremor or at their use in the elderly. From our own pilot study, a double-blind, placebo-controlled assessment of levodopa with selegiline versus levodopa with matched placebo in six elderly patients (mean age 80.0 years) with Parkinson's disease, we identified a significant mean percentage reduction in resting tremor over baseline recordings of 60.2% ($p < 0.05$) (51). The drug was also well tolerated in this group of elderly patients. It is possible that the observed benefits were due to the potentiation of the levodopa; hence, further study of selegiline in de novo tremor-dominated Parkinson's disease patients is required to ascertain its true effectiveness.

Despite their widespread use, the effect of levodopa preparations on tremor has not been studied using objective-recording techniques. Estimates of the tremor-reducing properties of levodopa range from 43 to 79% (52,53) with subjective scoring methods. These rating scales have been shown to be unreliable in such assessments (54).

We have studied the effect of levodopa combined with benserazide (Madopa) on parkinsonian tremor in a double-blind, placebo-controlled fashion. The efficacy of this drug was measured for both the resting and postural tremor found in Parkinson's disease. The technique of computed spectral analysis was used to quantify this effect. Subjective means of assessing tremor were compared with this objective recording techniques.

A. Methods

1. Calculations

Mean values of amplitude and frequency for active and placebo treatments were compared using Student's t test for paired data. Changes in the North Western University Disability (NWUD) and Webster rating scales, tremor scoring, and performance test scores were analyzed using a nonparametric coefficient test (Wilcoxon matched pairs signed-rank test). The relation between the response to placebo or to active drug and the various rating scales, tremor scoring, and performance tests was calculated by Spearman's rank correlation coefficient.

2. Subjects

Twelve patients, 6 men and 6 women, with tremor-dominated, idiopathic Parkinson's disease and an average age of 78.3 years (range 69–85) were included. The mean duration of their symptoms was 5.2 years (range 1.25–12).

All patients had stable, nonfluctuating, moderate or severe parkinsonian rest tremor. Patients had their tremor assessed, both objectively, with full-tremor recording, and subjectively, on six occasions in each wing of the study.

B. Results

Figure 2 shows the percentage improvement for each of the 12 patients. A considerable placebo effect was observed in 5 of the patients (range 33.1–76.6,

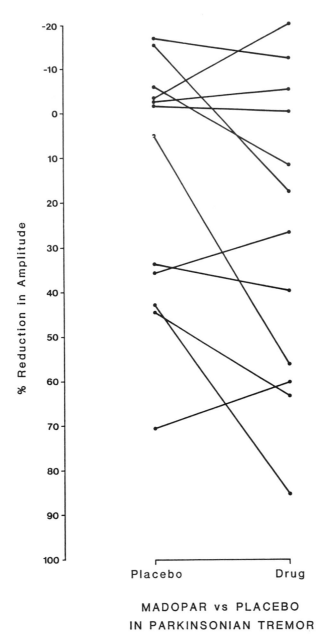

Figure 2   Percentage reduction in resting tremor amplitude for active and placebo agents. There is a significant mean reduction of 25.5% in tremor amplitude ($p < 0.006$).

mean 51.6). Four patients showed a clear improvement on active drug when compared with placebo (mean difference = 25.5%). Seven patients showed no marked difference between placebo and drug, whereas one patient's tremor worsened. Statistical comparison of all the amplitude values for each wing of the study revealed a significant ($p = 0.006$) reduction in tremor amplitude with the active drug.

The results for postural tremor in the 12 patients studied were that 4 showed improvement, 4 had larger tremor amplitudes, and 4 remained unchanged on active drug therapy. There was no statistically significant difference between the two treatment groups for postural tremor amplitude.

There were no obvious differences in the Webster and NWUD scores between the placebo and drug regimens. Statistical analysis using Wilcoxon-signed rank test failed to demonstrate any significant difference between the two groups.

Patient self-rating when compared for the treatment groups as a whole did reveal a significant ($p < 0.01$) difference. Assessing separately individual visit scores for all 12 patients also revealed a significant correlation between patients self-assessment and reduction in tremor ($p < 0.05$).

C. Discussion

The results of this study, the first double-blind, placebo-controlled study using objective recording methods to assess the effect of Madopa on tremor in Parkinson's disease, show that the drug exerts a variable effect. For rest tremor, there was a significant improvement for the active treatment group as a whole, although only four patients showed a beneficial response to the drug, representing a response rate of 33.3%. This response rate and the mean percentage improvement of 53.9, for the four patients, is slightly less than earlier studies (55). This may reflect the lower doses used in this study or, more likely, that the tremor was objectively quantified and not open to errors caused by subjective rating. Although the results show a significant effect of levodopa and benserazide on parkinsonian rest tremor, there appears to be no method of identifying the 33.3% of patients likely to produce a large enough response to gain functional benefit.

There was no useful response of tremor to active therapy when measured in the postural positions. The four patients in whom resting tremor improved showed no reduction in the postural and modified postural tremor. This difference in response could be considered as indirect evidence for postural tremor having a different pathophysiology from resting tremor, as proposed by Findley and co-workers (33).

The possibility still exists that the low response to active therapy, albeit still significant, could be due to the active drug being administered in too small a dose. The maximum dosage of 300 mg levodopa may appear small in comparison with the early studies using levodopa in Parkinson's disease. However, given the elderly population studied and the long-term problems associated with levodopa therapy, high-dose treatment for tremor-dominated Parkinson's disease could not be recommended.

The lack of change in the Webster and NWUD scales with tremor response may be explained by the overall low level of disability in the selected patients, most patients being Hoehn and Yahr grade II. Alternatively, it may reflect the inadequacy of using these types of scales to detect a monosymptomatic response.

The failure of a range of subjective tremor assessments by the physician to identify changes quantified by the tremor-recording system confirms the rather unreliable nature of this type of assessment. Interestingly, the patients' self-assessment, based on a simpler scoring system, did reflect the tremor response.

This study represents the first placebo-controlled, double-blind crossover design study to specifically assess the effect of levodopa therapy on parkinsonian tremor. Furthermore, the tremor-recording system accurately allowed the magnitude of response to therapy to be analyzed objectively and was easily applicable to elderly patients.

IV. BENIGN ESSENTIAL TREMOR

Essential, or senile, tremor is common in the elderly, with a mean age of onset between 40 and 50 years. Prevalence studies in the older than 40-year aged group give values between 0.4 and 5.6% (56,57). Rautakorpi and co-workers estimated the prevalence may be as high as 12.9% in those aged 75–79 years. The clinical features of this condition are well reviewed by Critchley (58) and do not require expansion in this chapter.

Many agents have been used in the treatment of essential tremor, and what has now emerged is that there is still no entirely satisfactory pharmacological treatment, particularly when the elderly are concerned.

Alcohol, in small quantities, provides temporary relief for many patients, but the possibility of a rebound effect and the dangers of predisposing the patient to alcoholism make it an unsuitable therapeutic agent in any aged group (59).

The mainstay of treatment for this condition remains β-adrenergic blockers, with oral propranolol, 120–240 mg, the most widely used therapeutic regimen (60). Although suitable for younger patients, unfortunately, these drugs are frequently unacceptable to older patients.

Reports of beneficial response to an anticonvulsant agent, primidone, have opened a new therapeutic opportunity (61). Findley and co-workers studied 22 patients with moderately severe essential tremor and found that all but 1 of the 16 patients completing the study had a beneficial response (62). The response was said to be equivalent to that achieved by 240 mg of propranolol.

Unfortunately, primidone often causes significant side effects, such as dizziness, nausea, vomiting, and postural hypotension. Of the patients studied, 25–35% show this acute toxic reaction. It has been proposed that inducing liver enzymes by pretreatment with phenobarbitone for 1–2 weeks may alleviate this toxicity (62). Alternatively, the administration of low-dose primidone, such as 62.5 mg, has been almost as effective, while minimizing the toxic reactions (63).

We have investigated the efficacy and side effect profile of ultra–low-dose primidone in the treatment of elderly patients with severe essential tremor (64). Preliminary results of this study are presented in the following.

A. Method

Ten patients (mean age 78.4 years) with moderate to severe essential tremor were studied in a randomized, double-blind, placebo-controlled fashion. The mean duration of tremor was 12.8 years. Primidone or matched placebo was administered in incremental stages, from 50 mg to 250 mg. Two baseline recordings and five further tremor recordings were taking for each patient during each phase of the study. Computed spectral analysis and statistical analysis of results were performed in a fashion similar to that already outlined for the parkinsonian tremor study.

B. Results

One patient out of the ten suffered early toxicity and could not complete the study. Five patients showed improvement when taking active drug, but in only two cases was this statistically significant. The improvement in tremor amplitude was apparent both for postural and resting tremor recordings. Tremor frequencies did not alter with treatment. No direct correlation between blood primidone levels and tremor reduction could be identified.

The primary finding of this study is that low-dose primidone can be safely administered, with a low frequency of toxic reactions, as a treatment for essential tremor in elderly patients. The study also showed that those patients responsive to primidone tend to show an immediate first-dose effect (63). The low incidence of toxic reactions has led us to use low-dose primidone as first-line therapy for elderly patients with essential tremor.

A striking feature of both the Parkinson's disease tremor study and the low-dose primidone in essential tremor study is the large placebo effect observed (mean = 28%). The placebo effect was observed at the beginning of each treatment period and lasted for the duration of the study. This shows the importance of using placebo controls in all therapeutic trials of drugs for tremor.

V. CEREBELLAR TREMOR

The early recognition of action tremor by Galen probably represents an early description of cerebellar tremor. Holmes (65), studied cases of intention tremor, particularly in World War I victims with cerebellar gunshot injuries. In his

Croonian lectures he delineated the clinical signs of cerebellar disease, noting hypotonia, coexisting postural tremors, and titubation. Over subsequent years, he added others to the list, such as pendular reflexes and rebound phenomena. This tremor is not infrequently seen in elderly patients and, when present, it causes severe functional difficulties. The characteristics of the tremor are similar to those found in younger patients.

Despite advances in the understanding of cerebellar tremors, very little knowledge has been gained about treatment, although Holmes recognized that weighting the limb dampened the tremor oscillations (66). Various therapeutic agents including, alcohol, propranolol, and isoniazid have as yet proved of minimal benefit and are not suitable for elderly patients (67).

VI. DRUG-INDUCED TREMORS

The drug-induced tremors are common in elderly patients, but only in exceptional circumstances do they become troublesome. In many patients they are a transient phenomenon. Pinder gives a detailed review of the major drug groupings producing tremor (68).

Drug-induced parkinsonian tremor does occur and presents as the typical rest tremor (69). Findley and Gresty pointed out that most drugs acting on the central nervous system were capable of inducing tremor (70). This is a particularly common cause of tremor in the elderly, with neuroleptics being the main offender (71).

Further study of this group of tremors is important, as it will almost certainly shed light on some neurophysiological mechanisms of tremor.

VII. CONCLUSIONS

Tremor in the elderly remains a challenge to all physicians. Accurate diagnosis, with or without computer-assisted spectral analysis, remains paramount. We must abandon the nihilistic approach to therapy and actively seek out new treatment regimens. All such treatment regimens must be subjected to placebo-controlled, objective analysis of the tremor response.

Improving our knowledge of the neurophysiological changes in physiological tremor that occur through aging, will almost certainly assist in future understanding of the mechanisms involved in the genesis of pathological tremors.

ACKNOWLEDGMENT

The authors wish to thank Research into Ageing for financial support with studies outlined in this chapter. A special thanks to Miss Vivienne Crawford for her assistance with statistical analysis of data.

REFERENCES

1. Charcot JM. Du tremblement senile. Prog Med 1876; 1:815.
2. Parkinson J. An essay on the shaking palsy. Reprinted in: Critchley M, ed. James Parkinson (1755–1824). London: Macmillan Press, 1955:145–218.
3. Longhi G. La Calcographia Propriamante Detta Ossia l'Arte d'Incidere in Rame Co'aqua-forte. Milano: Stamperia Reale, 1980:135–140.
4. Charcot JM. Policilinique du Mardi. Paris: Lecons de Mardi. 1888:563–566.
5. Gower WR. A Manual of Diseases of the Nervous System. Vol. 2. 2nd ed. Philadelphia: Blakiston, 1893.
6. Trousseau A. Tremblement senile et paralysis agitans. Clin Med Hotel Dieu Paris 1885; 47:280–292.
7. Dana CL. Hereditary tremor, a hitherto undescribed form of motor neurosis. Am J Med Sci 1887; 94:386–393.
8. Minor L. Uber hereditaren tremor. Zentralbl Gesampta Neurol Psychiat 1922; 28: 514–516.
9. Charcot JM. Clinical Lectures on the Diseases of the Nervous System. 2nd ed. Vol. 1. [transl Sigerson G]. Philadelphia: Henry C Lea, 1879.
10. Duvoisin RC. Cholinergic–anticholinergic antagonism in parkinsonism. 1967; 17: 124–136.
11. Marsden CD, Meadows JC, Lange GW, Watson RS. Variations in human physiological finger tremor with particular reference to changes with age. Electroencephalogr Clin Neurophysiol 1969; 27:169–178.
12. Birmingham AT, Wharrad HJ, Williams EJ. The variation of finger tremor with age in man. J Neurol Neurosurg Psychiatry 1985; 48:788–798.
13. Schäfer EA, Canney HE, Tynstall JO. On the rhythm of muscular response to volitional impulses in man. J Physiol 1886; 7:111–117.
14. Marshall J. Physiological tremor in children. J Neurol Neurosurg Psychiatry 1959; 22:33 35.
15. Marshall J. The effect of ageing upon physiological tremor. J Neurol Neurosurg Psychiatry 1961; 24:14–17.
16. Wade P, Gresty MA, Findley LJ. A normative study of postural tremor of the hand. Arch Neurol 1982; 39:358–362.
17. Marsden CD. Origins of normal and pathological tremor. In: Findley LJ, Capildeo R, eds. Movement Disorders: Tremor. London: Macmillan Press, 1984:37–84.
18. Kelly JF, Taggart HMcA, McCullagh PJ. Physiological tremor in an elderly population. In: Bartko D, Gerstenbrand F, Turcani P, eds. Neurology in Europe 1. London: John Libbey & Co, 1990:541–545.
19. Taggart HMcA, Kelly JF. Objective assessment of tremor and antitremor drug efficacy. Geriatr Med 1989; 19:17–18.
20. McAllister HG, McCullagh PJ, Kelly JF. Automated classification of peripheral movement disorder. J Micro Appl 1990; 13:281–290.
21. Heymsfield SB, McManus C, Smith J, Stevens V, Nixon DW. Anthropometric measurement of muscle mass: revised equations for calculating bone-free arm muscle area. Am J Clin Nutr 1982; 36:680–690.

22. Stiles RN. Frequency and displacement amplitude relations for normal hand tremor. J Appl Physiol 1976; 40;44–54.

23. Viitasalo JT, Era P, Leskinen AL, Heikkinen E. Muscular strength profiles and anthropometry in random samples of men aged 31–35, 51–55 and 71–75 years. Ergonomics 1985; 28:1563–1574.

24. Grimby G, Saltin B. The ageing muscle. Clin Physiol 1983; 3:209–218.

25. Vandervoort AA, Hayes KC, Belanger AY. Strength and endurance of skeletal muscle in the elderly. Physiother Can 1986; 38:167–173.

26. Lexell J, Taylor CC, Sjöström M. What is the cause of the ageing atrophy? Total number, size and proportion of different fiber types studied in whole vastus lateralis muscle from 15–83 year old men. J Neurol Sci 1988; 84:275–294.

27. Aniansson A, Grimby G, Hedberg G, Krotkiewski M. Muscle morphology, enzyme activity and muscle strength in elderly men and women. Clin Physiol 1981; 1:73–86.

28. Tomonaga M. Histochemical and ultrastructural changes in senile human skeletal muscle. J Am Geriatr Soc 1977; 25:125–131.

29. Newton JP, Yemm R. Changes in the contractile properties of the human first dorsal interosseous muscle with age. Gerontology 1986; 32:98–104.

30. Mutch WJ, Strudwick A, Roy SK, Downie AW. Parkinson's disease: disability, review and management. Br Med J 1986; 293:675–677.

31. Martilla RJ. Diagnosis and epidemiology of Parkinson's disease. Acta Neurol Scand [Suppl] 1983; 95:9–17.

32. Lakie M, Mutch WJ. Finger tremor in Parkinson's disease. J Neurol Neurosurg Psychiatry 1989; 52:392–394.

33. Findley LJ, Gresty MA, Halmagyi GM. Tremor, the cogwheel phenomena and clonus in Parkinson's disease. J Neurol Neurosurg Psychiatry 1981; 44:534–546.

34. Onuaguluchi G. Clinical and pharmacological studies in post-encephalitic parkinsonism. PhD dissertation, Glasgow University, Glasgow, Scotland, 1961.

35. Calne DB. The role of various forms of treatment in the management of Parkinson's disease. Clin Neuropharmacol 1982; 5(suppl 1):38–43.

36. Newman RP, Calne DB. Diagnosis and management of Parkinson's disease. Geriatrics 1984; 39:87–96.

37. Koller WC. Disturbance of recent memory functions in parkinsonian patients on anticholinergic therapy. Cortex 1984; 20:307–311.

38. DeSmet Y, Ruberg M, Serdaru M, Dubois B, Lhermitte F, Agid Y. Confusion, dementia, and anticholinergics on Parkinson's disease. J Neurol Neurosurg Psychiatry 1982; 45:1161–1164.

39. Miller E, Berrios GE, Politynska B. The adverse effect of benzhexol on memory in Parkinson's disease. Acta Neurol Scand 1987; 76:278–282.

40. Koller WC, Herbster G. Adjuvent therapy of parkinsonian tremor. Arch Neurol 1987; 44:921–923.

41. Tolosa E, Blesa R, Bayes A, Forcadell F. Low-dose bromocriptine in the early phases of Parkinson's disease. Clin Neuropharmacol 1987; 10:169–174.

42. Hardie RJ, Lees AJ, Stern GM. The controversial role of bromocriptine in Parkinson's disease. Clin Neuropharmacol 1985; 8:150–155.

43. Schwab R, Amador LV, Lettvin JY. Apomorphine in Parkinson's disease. Trans Am Neurol Assoc 1951; 76:251–253.

44. Frankel JP, Lees AJ, Kempster PA, Stern GM. Subcutaneous apomorphine in the treatment of Parkinson's disease. J Neurol Neurosurg Psychiatry 1990; 53:96–101.

45. Stibe CMH, Lees AJ, Kempster PA, Stern GM. Subcutaneous apomorphine and lisuride in the treatment of parkinsonian on–off fluctuations. Lancet 1988; 1: 403–406.

46. Birkmayer W, Riederer P, Youdim MBH, Linauer W. The potentiation of the anti-kinetic effect after L-dopa treatment of MAO-B deprenyl. J Neural Transm 1975; 36:303–326.

47. Birkmayer W, Knoll J, Riederer P, Youdim MBH, Hars V, Marton J. Increased life expectancy resulting from the addition of L-deprenyl to Madopar treatment in Parkinson's disease: a long term study. J Neural Transm 1985; 64:113–127.

48. Tetrud JW, Langston JW. R-(−)-Deprenyl as a possible protective agent in Parkinson's disease. J Neural Transm 1987; 25(suppl):69–79.

49. Parkinson Study Group. Effect of deprenyl on the progression of disability in early Parkinson's disease. N Engl J Med 1989; 321:1364–1371.

50. Tetrud JW, Langston JW. The effect of deprenyl (selegiline) on the natural history of Parkinson's disease. Science 1989; 245:519–522.

51. Kelly JF. A clinical study of physiological and pathological tremor in the elderly. M.D. dissertation, Queen's University, Belfast, Ireland, 1988.

52. Rinne UK, Sonninen V, Siirtola T. Treatment of Parkinson's disease with L-dopa and decarboxylase inhibitor. Neurology 1972; 202:1–20.

53. Agnoli A, Cassachia M, Fazio C, et al. Comparison between the therapeutic effects of L-dopa and L-dopa plus decarboxylase inhibitors in Parkinson's disease. In Yahr MD, ed. Current Concepts in the Treatment of Parkinsonism. New York: Raven Press, 1974:87–94.

54. Ginanneshi A, Degl'Innocenti F, Magnolfi S, et al. Evaluation of Parkinson's disease: reliability of the three rating scales. Neuroepidemiology 1988; 7:38–41.

55. Martinez-Lage JM, Marti Masso JF, Carrera N, et al. A single blind comparative study with the combination of carbidopa and L-dopa in Parkinson's disease treatment. In Yahr MD, ed. Current Concepts in the Treatment of Parkinsonism. New York: Raven Press, 1974:3–11.

56. Haerer AF, Anderson DW, Schoenberg BS. Prevalence of essential tremor in the biracial adult population of Copiah County, Mississippi. Ann Neurol 1981; 10:93–94.

57. Rautakorpi I, Takala J, Martilla RJ, Sievers K, Rinne UK. Essential tremor in a Finnish population. Acta Neurol Scand 1982; 66:58–67.

58. Critchley E. Clinical manifestations of essential tremor. J Neurol Neurosurg Psychiatry 1972; 35:365–372.

59. Growdon JH, Shahani BT, Young RR. The effect of alcohol on essential tremor. Neurology 1975; 25:259–262.

60. Wilson JF, Marshall RW, Richens A. Essential tremor; treatment with beta-adrenoceptor blocking drugs. In: Findley LJ, Capildeo R, eds. Movement Disorders: Tremor. London: Macmillan Press, 1984:245–260.

61. O'Brien MD, Upton AR, Toseland PA. Benign essential tremor treated with primidone. Br Med J 1981; 282:178–180.

62. Findley LJ, Cleeves L, Calzetti S. Primidone in essential tremor of the hands and head: a double blind controlled clinical study. J Neurol Neurosurg Psychiatry 1985; 48:911–915.

63. Koller WC, Royse VL. Efficacy of primidone in essential tremor. Neurology 1986; 36:121–124.

64. Kelly JF, Taggart HMcA, McCullagh P. Low dose primidone in the treatment of essential tremor [abstr]. Age Ageing 1990; 19(suppl 2):P8.

65. Holmes G. Clinical symptoms of cerebellar diseases. [The Croonian Lectures]. Lancet 1922; 1:1177–1182, 1231–1237; and 2:59–65, 111–115.

66. Holmes G. The cerebellum of man. Brain 1939; 62:1–30.

67. Koller WC. Pharmacologic trials in the treatment of cerebellar tremor. Arch Neurol 1984; 2:499–514.

68. Pinder RM. Drug induced tremor. In: Findley LJ, Capildeo R, eds. Movement Disorders: Tremor. London: Macmillan, 1984:445–461.

69. Stephen PJ, Williamson J. Drug induced parkinsonism in the elderly. Lancet 1984; 2:1082–1083.

70. Findley LJ, Gresty MA. Tremor. Br J Hosp Med 1981; 26:16–32.

71. Simpson GM, Pi EH, Sramek JJ. Adverse effects of antipsychotic drugs. Drugs 1981; 21:139–151.

25

Cerebellar Tremors: Physiological Basis and Treatment

P. Rondot and N. Bathien
Centre R. Garcin—CHSA
Paris, France

I. INTRODUCTION

The main anomaly of cerebellar movement is its discontinuity (1). "Instead of being continuous, tonic as in normal states," wrote Thomas and Durupt (2), "it is discontinuous, clonic, epileptoid." From Holmes (1), "delay in starting movement and slowness and irregularity in its acceleration are probably fundamental disturbances." When this discontinuity in movement becomes rhythmic we are in the presence of cerebellar tremor (CT). Two types of tremor have been observed in cases of cerebellar lesions: Kinetic tremor, appearing either from the beginning or exclusively at the end of movement; and postural tremor, appearing when a position is being held, or during isometric contractions, as, for example, when constant pressure is maintained (3,4).

Other than these two types of tremor there are rhythmic activities provoked by lesions of the dentate nucleus. These rhythmic activities, most often called *myoclonus*, appear at rest and are usually localized at the pharyngeal muscles; but they also may involve muscles of the limbs, most often the proximal muscles (5). Recordings indicate rhythmic activity isolated in a muscular group or synchronization of activity in agonist–antagonist muscles. Alternation of activity in these muscles, as in a tremor, may also appear. This is why they are classified alongside the tremors.

II. SYMPTOMATOLOGY

The clinical and electromyographic characteristics of each of these tremors (CT) are reviewed:

A.   Cerebellar Kinetic Tremor

Kinetic tremor of cerebellar origin is the most frequent. It occurs during voluntary movement and is characterized by jerky movements as the limb approaches its target. These movements are accompanied by oscillations of variable amplitude that are perpendicular to the direction of the movement. They cause the hand or the foot to deviate from the axis of the movement, as if the direction of the movement has not been preserved, although it has been, in spite of the jerkiness (6).

This tremor sometimes sets in at the beginning of the movement. When it appears only at the approach to the target it is designated *intention tremor* so characteristic of cerebellar lesions.

The amplitude and frequency of this tremor are quite variable. Usually the frequency is low (3–5 Hz). Its amplitude is at times quite intense, making each jerk of the limb resemble a myoclonus; this is the hyperkinetic tremor (7) that is frequently seen in cases of multiple sclerosis and as a sequela to cranial trauma. The specific amplitude of this tremor is due to the rhythmic contraction of the shoulder muscles—the abductors–adductors and the internal–external rotators—that provokes large oscillations of the limb and increases the amplitude and the complexity of the tremor. *Oppositional* tremors have also been observed, when the movement is carried out in the direction opposed to that of the command. This anomaly is relatively rare (7). Electromyographic (EMG) traces indicate that the first burst of activity is in the agonists.

This tremor is easily revealed by the classic tests: finger-to-nose and heel-to-knee. It can be facilitated if the movement necessitates the contraction of other muscular groups; thus, when the finger-to-nose test is applied in sitting position there is sometimes no tremor, since only the forearm flexors are activated from the beginning to the end of the movement. On the other hand, the test may be accompanied by tremor when executed by a subject lying on his or her back: the forearm flexors are the active muscles until the forearm reaches a 90° angle; after this angle has been reached, the weight of the forearm enforces the flexors, and the movement must be stalled by the brachial triceps. Delay in command of the triceps often results in tremor in this second part of the movement.

The tremor may also be visible in writing, when the patient tries to join two parallel vertical lines by horizontal lines. The lines drawn are wavy, and either overstep the vertical lines, or do not reach them. Phonation may also be disturbed by the tremor: rhythmic contraction of the laryngeal muscles causes the voice to be choppy, produced in bursts.

Kinetic tremor is predominant either in the upper limbs or in the lower limbs;

it is not yet possible to determine the anatomical correlations accounting for this predominance. It is often more marked in the lower limbs during olivopontocerebellar atrophies, whereas in multiple sclerosis the CT is usually more ample in the upper limbs.

1. Electromyography

Electromyographic examinations allow us to specify the time sequence of activation of the different muscles during the movement, and to quantify the speed of the movement.

The principal characteristics of cerebellar movement are found during the CT. The anomalies in cerebellar movement involve its reaction time, the mode of activation of the first burst of the agonists, and the speed of the movement (Table 1). The reaction time is 60–80 ms longer than that of control subjects. A "triphasic pattern" characterizes normal voluntary contraction: there is an initial burst of muscle activity in the agonist, followed by a burst of the antagonist muscle, then the resumed activity of the agonist. This is disturbed in cerebellar movement (8). The first burst of the agonist muscle occurs after a longer period than normally observed, and is prolonged. The first burst of the antagonist is difficult to systematize in human subjects (8). It either alternates with the two first bursts of the agonist or occurs in synchrony. Hore and Flament (9) observed these same anomalies in monkeys in which the dentate nuclei had been cooled. The antagonist's burst lasts longer in the cerebellar subject than in the normal subject (8); this facilitates dissymmetry in the cerebellar subject. The second burst of activity of the agonist is not any easier to systematize than the first burst of the antagonist. The anomaly in the first burst of activity in the agonist is all the more interesting, given that the triphasic component of the movement is considered to be programmed, unvarying according to peripheral input.

Table 1 Changes in Reaction Times in a Patient With a Unilateral Cerebellar Syndrome[a]

	Reaction time (ms)		
Type of movement	Control side	Affected side	p Value
Extension, $n = 15$	171.89 ± 9.07	253.53 ± 15.18	$p < 0.001$
Flexion	178.16 ± 10.92	238.53 ± 15.55	$0.04 < p < 0.01$

[a]Reaction time was measured from the warning visual signal to the onset of the EMG activity in the agonist muscle. Triceps was recorded during extension and biceps during flexion. Values are mean $\pm$ SEM. The p value are two-tailed significance levels of the comparison of reaction time in affected side against controlled.
Source: Ref. 12.

A change in the pattern of the beginning of the movement affects the kinetics of the movement: instead of being symmetric, the velocity curve of the cerebellar movement is asymmetric (Fig. 1): the magnitudes of acceleration decreased and magnitudes of deceleration increased (10,11). Even if the speed of the cerebellar movement can be modified as a function of its amplitude, as in normal subjects, the asymmetry of the movement's velocity curves is more marked when its amplitude and duration increase, at least when the cerebellar syndrome is of moderate intensity (11).

The tremor does not modify the delay in the first burst of activity of the agonist (12). The tremor itself is recorded in the form of bursts lasting 50–300 ms, succeeding one another at a frequency of 3–7 Hz (Fig. 2). The bursts are recorded earlier in the movement when the cerebellar syndrome is more intense, or when the movement is of greater velocity (Figs. 2 and 3). The number of bursts decreases with decrease in speed, as the movement becomes regular.

If it occurs at the beginning or the end of a kinetic tremor, actualizing an intention tremor (see Figs. 2, 3, and 4), the first burst of the tremor is brief and phasic. The first activity of the antagonist appears at various points: sometimes, as in the triphasic pattern, it follows the first burst of the agonist, followed by other rhythmic bursts that alternate with bursts from the agonists. This is not the most frequent pattern. A synchronous agonist–antagonist activity has also been observed during the movement (see Figs. 2 and 4). There may even be no rhythmic

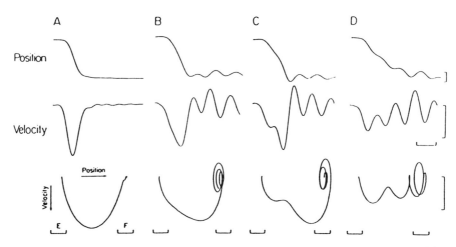

Figure 1 Discontinuous movement and terminal tremor in elbow flexion produced by cerebellar nuclear cooling (monkey DU). Position, velocity, and phase-plane trajectory for four representative single, movements. (A) Control; (B–D) during cerebellar nuclear cooling. Calibrations: position, 11°; velocity, 200°/s; time, 200 ms. (From Ref. 10.)

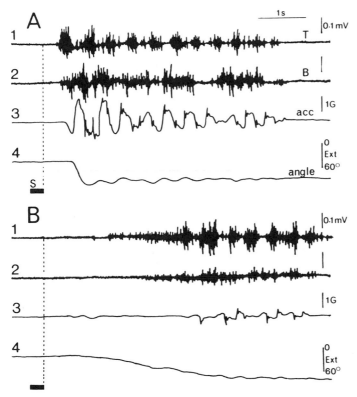

Figure 2 Tremor with severe cerebellar atrophy. Elbow extension. Movement of 60° angle with an initial peak acceleration (A) of 1.0 G; and (B) 0.1 G. Traces are: 1, 2, EMG recordings from triceps (T) and biceps (B) muscles; 3, accelerometric recordings (acc); 4, position of the elbow (angle).

activity of the antagonist, or its activity may take on a rhythmic quality only at the end of a movement, even though the contractions of the agonist are rhythmic from the beginning (see Fig. 2B).

When the movement is spontaneous, the proximal muscles are also frequently the seat of rhythmic activity, in particular, the rotators (infraspinatus and teres major muscles). The tremor becomes more intense when the activity of these muscles becomes rhythmic (Fig. 5). It is possible to compare, in the same patient, slow movement without tremor and rapid movement with tremor (see Fig. 2A,B). The difference between the two appears at the very first burst of the agonist, which is much more developed in tremor, and is followed by a period of silence or weak activity; the second burst of the agonist is delayed (200–250 ms) in comparison

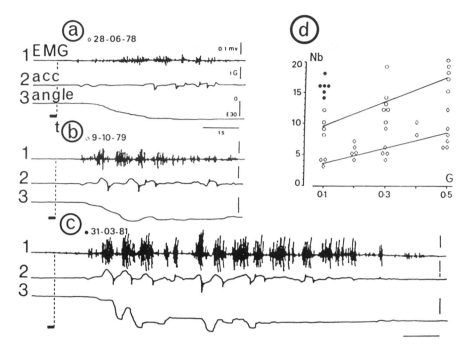

Figure 3 Cerebellar tremor from a patient with a cerebellar atrophy. Tremor activity was recorded three times during 33 months: (a) open squares, data collected on June 28th 1978; (b) open circles, on October 9th, 1979; and (c) filled circles, on March 31th 1981. Traces compare tremor initiated by extension movements of the elbow with a similar peak of initial acceleration. Graphs (d) show the relation between the number of bursts in EMG activity from the triceps muscle to the peak amplitude of initial movement acceleration. Same abbreviations as Fig. 2.

with that observed in the normal subject (50–100 ms). The first burst of the antagonist usually does not alternate with that of the agonist: most often, they are synchronous (see Figs. 4 and 5).

For movements with identical acceleration at the onset, recordings made in a patient at different points during his or her progressive evolution (see Fig. 3) initially reveal a nearly normal recording, 16 months later bursts of abnormal intensity in the agonist produce a tremor that intensifies; 17 months later there is a succession of ample bursts of the agonists at intervals varying from 300 to 500 ms. In both cases, we observed two main anomalies: the increase in time between the first and second burst of activity of the agonist, and the phasic aspect of the bursts.

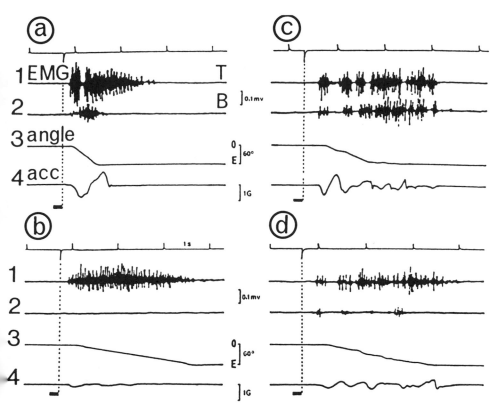

Figure 4 Elbow extension from a patient with unilateral cerebellar deficit. EMG activity from triceps (T) and biceps (B), position (angle) and acceleration (acc) for single movements with an initial peak acceleration of 1.0 G (a,c) and 0.1 G (b,d); control side (a,b); affected side (c,d). (From Ref. 12.)

This is quite different from what is usually noted in cerebellar movements; the fragmentation of the first agonist burst being a common finding (8).

B. Cerebellar Postural Tremor

Holmes (13) mentions the postural tremor during which "the patient attempts to maintain the limb accurately in certain positions as in posture necessary for the performance of some act." Gilman et al. (14), Rondot et al. (3), and Marsden (15) have also stressed this type of tremor that is so often neglected in descriptions of cerebellar syndrome. Nonetheless, one frequently observes that cerebellar patients have trouble keeping their outstretched upper limb in front of a target without

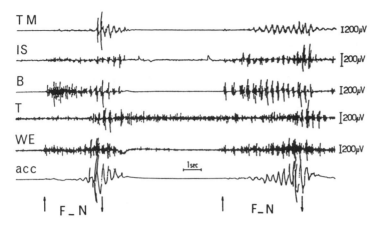

Figure 5   Kinetic tremor: bursting activity recorded during the finger–nose movement (FN). EMG recordings from teres major, infra spinatus, biceps, triceps, and wrist extensor.

touching it. Here, the postural tremor has followed the kinetic tremor. But it may appear independently when, after passively positioning the outstretched upper limb, the patient is requested to maintain this posture without moving. A postural tremor, sometimes a head tremor, may be the first sign of a kinetic cerebellar syndrome that will become apparent only several months after the onset of the postural tremor.

A specific type of postural tremor has been described by Cole et al. (4). They requested the patient to maintain constant pressure on a typewriter key connected to a strain-gauge. Under these conditions, with unilateral cerebellar lesions (in presence or absence of clinical evidence of tremor), there is a significant decrease in stability contralateral to the lesions. One might record a tremor with a frequency of 5–10 Hz, variable according to localization of the lesion in the cerebellum or the brainstem.

On EMG recordings of tremor in the outstretched limb, one frequently observes that rhythmic activity persists after the end of the movement when the finger is kept in position in front of a target (Fig. 6). The frequency of this tremor is 2–4 Hz; it is only inconsistently characterized by alternating agonist–antagonist rhythmic bursts.

C.   Rhythmic Activities Caused by Lesions in the Dentoolivary System

Rhythmic movements caused by lesions of the dentoolivary system are most often localized in the laryngopharyngeal muscles. They appear in the form of muscular

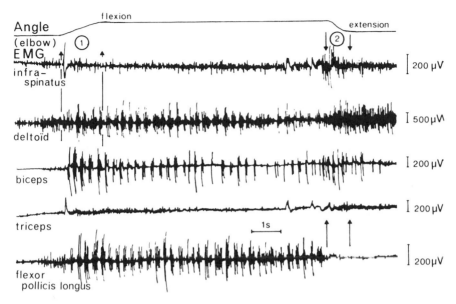

Figure 6 Postural tremor from a patient with cerebellar deficit: bursting activity recorded during the elbow-flexion posture.

jerks of relatively low frequency, 100–160 cycles/min. The diaphragm is also sometimes affected by these movements; they are constant, observed at rest, and during voluntary contraction, which does not cause them to increase. They may even persist during sleep. The muscles of the limbs may also be affected by these movements, which have been called "myoclonies squelettiques" by Guillain and Mollaret (16,17). They appear independently of or simultaneously with the movements of the pharynx and larynx, the rhythms of which are not identical (5). The state of tonic contraction of the muscles where the rhythmic movements are observed modifies their amplitude. Sometimes they appear clinically only when the limb is placed in certain positions. In this sense, they are related to the postural tremors.

The EMG recordings of these rhythmic activities show bursts of activity of short duration, either isolated or accompanied by constant tonic activity. When voluntary contraction is moderate, it is possible to observe the persistence of this rhythmic activity against a background of interferential contraction. Thus, this rhythmic activity behaves differently from the parkinsonian tremor at rest which, at the beginning of the disease, disappears during voluntary movement.

If, in the limbs, the muscle that is the site of the tremor, or the nerve that innervates it, is stimulated, the silent phase that follows the burst of activation is short, 80–100 ms, as in essential tremors. It is followed by an acceleration of the rhythm, which returns to its preceding frequency 2–3 min later.

III. PATHOPHYSIOLOGY OF CEREBELLAR TREMOR

Cerebellar lesions disturb the execution of movement causing dysmetria and tremor. This effect is most likely due to the absence of the modulation that the cerebellum normally exercises over the motor cortex by way of a circuit that runs from the cerebellum to the thalamus and the motor cortex. Discharges of the dentate nucleus during movement precede those of the motor cortex (18). Shibasaki et al. have demonstrated the decrease of premotor potentials in human subjects with nuclear cerebellar lesions (19).

What factors cause cerebellar tremor? The interaction between the dentate nucleus and the precentral neurons has been explored in animals in which a cerebellar syndrome was reproduced by destruction or cooling of the dentate nuclei (20–23). Unfortunately, these studies often did not distinguish the "cerebellar movement" from the "cerebellar tremor": in the few studies that did specify the type of movement caused by the lesion, great differences have been observed (10,21).

One of the major effects of destruction of dentate nuclei is to lengthen the latency of movement-related responses after sensory stimuli (20) and, more specifically, after visual or auditory stimuli, but not after somesthetic stimuli (23). This anomaly is similar to the delay noted in cerebellar movement in human subjects (1). It is clearly revealed in unilateral cerebellar syndrome by the delay for the forefinger on the cerebellar side in the finger-to-nose test; Thomas and Durupt (2) have called this phenomenon *dyschronometry*. This increase in reaction time is not due to an increase in transmission time between the precentral neurons and the muscle, since the time between neuronal activation and the beginning of the movement is not modified after cooling. On the other hand, the period between sensory stimulation and the start of neuronal activity is increased, and this represents the totality of the delay in reaction time. These characteristics are specific for cerebellar movement, with or without tremor (10).

The main cerebellar functions act on the motor system: sensory responses of the precentral neurons remain normal after cerebellar lesions (22).

What differences have been noted between cerebellar movement with and without tremor at the level of neuronal discharge? Spontaneous discharges of motor cortex neurons are not modified by cerebellar lesions (23). Nonetheless, motor cortex discharges preceding the cerebellar movement without tremor are different after cerebellar nuclear cooling: they lose their phasic characteristic and are prolonged (10,20); this explains the decrease in speed and longer duration of the movement. However, it is not due to an overall depression of neuronal activity, since the tonic discharge that precedes the movement is increased (9) and, even if the initial accelerations of the movement are diminished, its peak velocities are not lowered during dentate nucleus cooling (9). The pattern of neuronal discharges changes with the onset of tremor: they become strongly phasic, in close correlation to the tremor. Not all of the neurons manifest this type of activation: some continue to have tonic discharges during the tremor. According to Hore and Flament (9), the neurons that react in relation to the cerebellar tremor also have strong responses to disturbances in the contralateral limb.

Why does the neuronal activity become phasic again, and why does EMG activity in the agonist break up into bursts separated by silent intervals of 200–250 ms? There are questions as yet unresolved for cerebellar tremor.

Is the discontinuous activity of the agonist caused by discharges from a central oscillator? Is it due to inhibition caused by extension of the antagonist? Is it a phasic servoassistance response to the deviation in trajectory, or are there other factors involved?

Is the cerebellar tremor caused by a thalamic or cortical central oscillator? The rhythmic discharges would then be due to either a defect in timing of the efferent command, or to a defect in the error-detecting mechanisms which would no longer allow the cortex to readjust the movement toward the target, thereby facilitating the oscillations. Although the peripheral limb perturbations activate the same neurons that discharge strongly in relation to the tremor (9), sectioning of the posterior roots (14) neither stops nor diminishes the tremor. In humans, lesions of the posterior funiculus appreciably aggravate cerebellar tremor. On the other hand, stimulation of Ia fibers by application of vibrations to the tendon diminishes the tremor (12). It is thus highly unlikely that the hypothetical oscillator is maintained by peripheral feedback.

According to another hypothesis, the cerebellar tremor comes from a series of stretch reflexes that cause alternate inhibition of the agonist or of the antagonist by means of a short loop or a long transcortical loop (9). The first burst of activity of the agonist causes an extension reflex in the antagonist that inhibits the agonist. This causes a slowing in the trajectory, followed by a second burst of the agonist that has the properties of a servolike response and also generates stretch of the antagonist. This presents us with a series of phases that are inhibitory to the agonist, and oscillations that form a tremor, similar to the clonus in spasticity. The cortical neurons would be particularly sensitive to peripheral perturbations, especially those that cause extension.

This hypothesis evokes several objections. In effect, cerebral lesions depress the fusimotor system (24). Cerebellar nuclear cooling causes the disappearance of the discharges observed in the precentral neurons during extension of the forearm, and these neurons are predominantly related to flexion (25). The mechanism just described could only be taken into consideration in instances when the movement starts in a triphasic pattern. However, observation of the beginning of a cerebellar tremor, when the movement is rapid, frequently shows a simultaneous contraction of the agonists and the antagonists (see Figs. 4 and 5) (12,26). Under these conditions, one cannot single out the role of the stretch reflex, since the antagonist is in a state of contraction. Therefore, it appears highly improbable that, in humans, the cerebellar tremor is influenced at the beginning of the movement by a proprioceptive feedback. But it is possible that such a mechanism might be responsible for the tremor that sets in at the end of the movement, since stretching the antagonist facilitates and increases the contraction of this muscle, resulting in deviation instead of adjustment of the trajectory.

What other factors, on the motor cortex level, cause cerebellar tremor at the beginning of the movement in certain severe forms of lesions? One of the anomalies most frequently observed by Hallett et al. (8) is the lengthening of the first burst of the agonist. The triphasic pattern characteristic of the ballistic movement is, on the contrary, rarely present in cerebellar movement, with or without tremor (8,12). In fact, the first burst of the antagonist often coincides with that of the agonist. Meyer-Lohmann et al. have observed in monkeys that biceps–triceps cocontraction was more frequent after cooling of the dentate nucleus (25). However, the two first bursts of the agonist and the antagonist are not involved in any peripheral feedback; they are generated by a central program. Perhaps these anomalies are related to an affection of the Purkinje cells? Smith et al. (27) and Frysinger et al. (28) have shown that they may play a role in the selection or alternation between inhibition or antagonist coactivation.

Another important anomaly has been observed during the kinetic cerebellar tremor: the first burst of the EMG activity of the agonist is too ample and phasic (see Figs. 2 and 3). Miller and Freund (29) have already remarked, in cerebellar dyssynergia in humans, that both peak acceleration and peak velocity were increased with affected limbs; the lack of increase in mean velocity was thought to reflect cessation of movement and not a progressive decrease in velocity. In the monkey, Meyer-Lohmann (25) noted increased peak values of acceleration and discharge intensity during dentate nucleus cooling, the precentral unit activity appearing more as dense bursts. A marked increase in motor cortex neural discharges accompanied cerebellar cooling in movements of monkeys in which tremor occurred (9). On the contrary, the cerebellar movement without tremor is accompanied by a lengthening of the EMG activity of the first burst of the agonist (8), the tonic characteristics of which are related to the usual decrease in phasic activity of the cortical motor neurons (9). A shift was observed in the timing of neuronal discharge from an accelerationlike discharge under control conditions, to a velocitylike discharge during cerebellar cooling. It is important not to be too hasty in assigning the anomalies observed in the cerebellar movement without tremor to the cerebellar tremor, since the activity of the agonists at the beginning of movement are different in the two cases.

In conclusion, cerebellar tremor relates to different mechanisms than does cerebellar movement without tremor. Two mechanisms in particular are at the origin of tremor in the cerebellar subject. The first is a delay in the appearance of contraction of the antagonist which, at the end of the movement, usually allows adjustment of the movement in relation to the target by slowing the limb down during approach. This results in an overstepping of the target, which then is badly corrected by a contraction of the agonist, causing the intention tremor during the last phase of the movement.

The second deficiency at the origin of kinetic tremor when it appears at the beginning of movement is a fault in programming of the movement. This disorder involved the intensity of the movement, frequently causing a contraction that is too ample; it also affects the timing of the movement, resulting in a delay in the first contraction of the agonist and, above all, in badly adapted timing of antagonist contraction. What follows is a bad regulation of the movement, which is made up of a series of jerks during which the agonists and the antagonists often contract simultaneously. Does this disorder come from the cerebellum itself—we now know that the cerebellar nuclear cells discharge in strict relation to the force of the movement (30)—or does it come from a fault in choice of program?

IV. TREATMENT

In the absence of precise data on the origins of cerebellar tremors and possible dysfunctioning of neurotransmitters, treatment of this tremor remains highly undefined.

The importance of the neurotransmitter γ-aminobutyric acid (GABA) at the level of the Purkinje cells has evoked treatment with isoniazid, which raises the GABA level in the cerebrospinal fluid (CSF) (31). Several authors (32–34) reported favorable, although variable, results in the treatment of postural tremor in cases of multiple sclerosis. Isoniazid is administered in doses of 900–1200 mg daily, associated with 100 mg of pyridoxine. It is necessary to supervise transaminase levels, given the hepatotoxicity of this product. 5-Hydroxytryptophan has also been recommended for this type of tremor (35).

Attempts at surgical treatment by coagulation of cerebellar efferent pathways to the thalamic relay centers produced positive results (7,36) in major forms of cerebellar tremor. Such treatment should be applied only in multiple sclerosis if the disease is in a stable phase and when the functional discomfort caused by the tremor is considerable. The amplitude of the kinetic tremor is decreased, reducing it to an intention tremor.

REFERENCES

1. Holmes G. The cerebellum of man. The Hughlings Jackson Memorial Lecture. Brain 1939; 62:1–30.
2. Thomas A, Durupt A. Localisations cérébelleuses. Paris: Vigot 1914:151–155.

3. Rondot P, Bathien N, Toma S. Physiopathology of cerebellar movement. In: Massion J, Sasaki K, eds. Cerebro-cerebellar Interactions. Amsterdam: Elsevier/North-Holland Biomedical Press, 1979:203–230.
4. Cole JD, Philip HI, Sedwick EM. Stability and tremor in the fingers associated with cerebellar hemisphere and cerebellar tract lesions in man. J Neurol Neurosurg Psychiatry 1988; 51:1558–1568.
5. Rondot P, Ben Hamida M. Myoclonies du voile et myoclonies squelettiques. Etude clinique et anatomique. Rev Neurol 1968; 119:59–83.
6. Babinski J. Oeuvre Scientifique. Paris: Masson et Cie, 1934.
7. Rondot P, Said G, Ferrey G. Les hyperkinésies volitionnelles. Etude électrologique. Classification. Rev Neurol 1972; 126:415–426.
8. Hallett M, Berardelli A, Matheson JN, Rothwell J, Marsden CD. Physiological analysis of simple rapid movements in patients with cerebellar deficits. J Neurol Neurosurg Psychiatry 1991; 53:124–133.
9. Hore J, Flament D. Changes in motor cortex neural discharge associated with the development of cerebellar limb ataxia. J Neurophysiol 1988; 60:1285–1302.
10. Hore J, Flament D. Evidence that a disordered servo-like mechanism contributes to tremor in movements during cerebellar dysfunction. J Neurophysiol 1986; 56: 123–136.
11. Brown SH, Hefter H, Mertens M, Freund HJ. Disturbances in human arm movement trajectory due to mild cerebellar dysfunction. J Neurol Neurosurg Psychiatry 1990; 53:306–313.
12. Rondot P, Bathien N. Motor control in cerebellar tremor. In: Findley LJ, Capildeo R, eds. Movement Disorders: Tremor. London: Macmillan Press, 1984:366–376.
13. Holmes G. Clinical symptoms of cerebellar disease and their interpretation. The Croonian lectures II. Lancet 1922; 1:1231–1237.
14. Gilman S, Carr D, Hollenberg J. Kinematic effects of deafferentation and cerebellar ablation. Brain 1976; 99:311–330.
15. Marsden CD. Origins of normal and pathological tremor. In: Findley LJ, Capildeo R, eds. Movement Disorders: Tremor. London: Macmillan Press, 1984.
16. Guillain G, Mollaret P. Deux cas de myoclonies synchrones et rythmées vélo-pharyngo-laryngo-oculo-diaphragmatiques. Le problème anatomique et physiologique. Rev Neurol 1931; 11:545–566.
17. Guillain G, Mollaret P. Le syndrome myoclonique synchrone et rythmé vélo-pharyngo-laryngo-oculo-diaphragmatique. Presse Méd 1935; 43:57–60.
18. Thach WT. Timing of activity in cerebellar dentate nucleus on cerebral motor cortex during prompt volitional movement. Brain Res 1975; 88:233–241.
19. Shibasaki H, Shima F, Kuroiwa Y. Clinical studies of the movement-related cortical potential (MP) and the relationship between the dentato-rubro-thalamic pathway and readiness potential (RP). J Neurol 1978; 219:15–25.
20. Meyer-Lohmann J, Hore J, Brooks VB. Cerebellar participation in generation of prompt arm movements. J Neurophysiol 1977; 40:1038–1050.
21. Vilis T, Hore J. Central neural mechanisms contributing to cerebellar tremor produced by limb perturbation. J Neurophysiol 1980; 43:279–291.
22. Lamarre Y, Busby L, Spidalieri G. Fast ballistic arm movements triggered by visual,

auditory and somesthetic stimuli in the monkey. I. Activity of precentral cortical neurons. J Neurophysiol 1983; 50:1343–1358.

23. Spidalieri G, Busby L, Lamarre Y. Fast ballistic arm movements triggered by visual, auditory and somesthetic stimuli in the monkey. II. Effects of unilateral dentate lesion on discharge of precentral cortical neurons and reaction time. J Neurophysiol 1983; 50:1359–1379.

24. Gilman S. The nature of cerebellar dyssynergia. In: Williams D, ed. Modern Trends in Neurology. London: Butterworths, 1972:60–79.

25. Meyer-Lohmann J, Conrad B, Matsunami K, Brooks VB. Effects of dentate cooling on precentral unit activity following torque pulse injections into elbow movements. Brain Res 1975; 94:237–251.

26. Hallett M, Shahani BL, Young RR. EMG analysis of patients with cerebellar deficits. J Neurol Neurosurg Psychiatry 1975; 38:1163–1169.

27. Smith AM, Frysinger RC, Bourbonnais D. Discharge pattern of cerebellar cortical neurons during the co-activation and reciprocal inhibition of forearm muscles. Exp Brain Res 1983; 7(suppl):298–308.

28. Frysinger RC, Bourbonnais D, Kalaska JF, Smith AM. Cerebellar cortical activity during antagonist cocontraction and reciprocal inhibition of forearm muscles. J Neurophysiol 1984; 51:32–49.

29. Miller RG, Freund HJ. Cerebellar dyssynergia in humans. A quantitative analysis. Ann Neurol 1980; 8:574–579.

30. Wetts R, Kalaska JF, Smith AM. Cerebellar nuclear activity during antagonist cocontraction and reciprocal inhibition of forearm muscles. J Neurophysiol 1985; 54:231–244.

31. Manyam EV, Katz L, Hare TA, et al. Isoniazid-induced elevation of CSF GABA levels and effects on chorea in Huntington's disease. Neurology 1979; 29:370–375.

32. Sabra A, Hallett M, Sudarsky L, Mullally W. Treatment of action tremor in multiple sclerosis with isoniazid. Neurology 1982; 32:912–913.

33. Bozek CB, Kastrukoff LF, Wright J, Perry T, Paty DW. A double-blind crossover trial of isoniazid (INH) in the treatment of action tremor associated with multiple sclerosis. Neurology 1984; 34(suppl):128.

34. Hallett M, Lindsey JW, Adelstein BD, Riley PO. Controlled trial of isoniazid therapy for severe postural cerebellar tremor in multiple sclerosis. Neurology 1985; 35:1374–1377.

35. Rascol A, Clanet M, Montastruc JL, Delage W, Guiraud-Chaumeil B. LSH tryptophan in the cerebellar syndrome treatment. Biomedicine 1981; 35:112–113.

36. Narabayashi H. Surgical approach to tremor. In: Marsden CD, Fahn S, eds. Movement Disorders. Butterworth's International Medical Reviews: Neurology, 2. London: Butterworth Scientific, 1982:292–299.

26

Primary Orthostatic Tremor

P. D. Thompson
Institute of Neurology
National Hospital for Neurology and Neurosurgery
London, England

I. INTRODUCTION

The term *orthostatic tremor* was introduced by Heilman (1) to describe the clinical phenomenon of tremor of the legs and trunk during stable (*static*) standing in an upright posture (*ortho*). In a strict literal sense, this definition encompasses any tremor of the legs or trunk when standing. A differential diagnosis of the variety of conditions that may give rise to involuntary movements of the legs is shown in Table 1 (2). The electromyographic (EMG) characteristics of some of these are illustrated in Figures 1, 2, and 3. Accordingly, the term orthostatic tremor has been used in the literature to describe a variety of different conditions. Conversely, the clinical syndrome of orthostatic tremor also had been described and illustrated previously as a "disorder of standing" (3). We have suggested previously (4,5) that several clinical, electrophysiological, and pharmacological features of the clinical syndrome described by Heilman (1) allow the identification of *primary orthostatic tremor* as a distinct entity (Table 2). These features and the absence of other complaints or physical signs distinguish this syndrome from the other conditions listed in Table 1.

II. PRIMARY ORTHOSTATIC TREMOR

The leg and trunk tremor of primary orthostatic tremor can vary from a "quivering" sensation of the legs, to shaking of the whole body. The original and subsequent case reports emphasized that leg and trunk tremor was accompanied by a sensation of unsteadiness (1,4–16). Indeed, the presenting symptoms of many

387

Table 1 Conditions That May Produce
Involuntary Movements of the Legs or Trunk
When Standing

Orthostatic tremor
Benign essential tremor
Parkinson's disease
Action myoclonus (e.g., postanoxic myoclonus)
Clonus (in spasticity)
Spastic ataxia (e.g., multiple sclerosis)
Cerebellar degeneration

Source: Modified from Ref. 2.

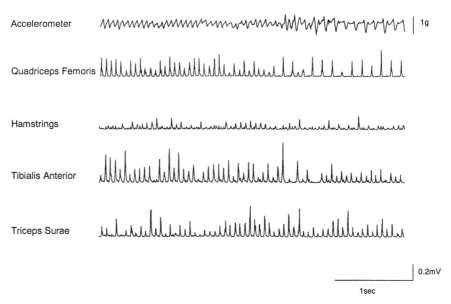

Figure 1 Accelerometer (attached over right quadriceps muscle) and rectified and filtered surface EMG recordings from muscles of the right leg in a patient with primary orthostatic tremor while standing. A tremor of 16 Hz frequency is evident in the muscles shown. Note the change in tremor frequency in the quadriceps from 16 to 8 Hz. Tremor frequency remained constant in other muscles. The muscle bursts responsible for the tremor were alternating in antagonist muscle pairs. (From Ref. 4.)

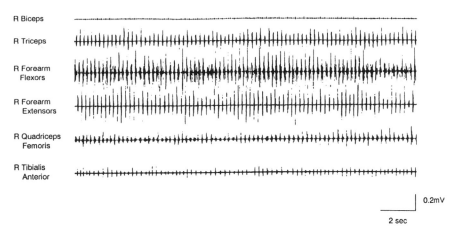

R Biceps

R Triceps

R Forearm Flexors

R Forearm Extensors

R Quadriceps Femoris

R Tibialis Anterior

0.2mV

2 sec

Figure 2 Surface EMG recordings from muscles of the right upper and lower limbs in a patient with Parkinson's disease. A 4- to 5-Hz tremor is evident in the arms and legs.

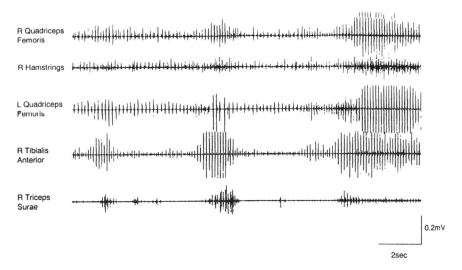

R Quadriceps Femoris

R Hamstrings

L Quadriceps Femoris

R Tibialis Anterior

R Triceps Surae

0.2mV

2sec

Figure 3 Surface EMG recordings from muscles of the right and left lower limbs in a patient with hereditary spastic paraplegia and clonus due to spasticity. The clonus was sufficiently troublesome when standing for the patient to complain of shaking of the legs when he attempted to stand still, although he did not report unsteadiness. Rhythmic, alternating EMG bursts are evident in antagonist muscle pairs at a frequency of 6–8 Hz. Note the fluctuation in the amplitude of the bursts with time, presumably reflecting differences in the amount of stretch applied to the muscles with changes in body position and sway.

Table 2 Summary of Clinical Features, Family History and Response to Therapy in Cases From the Literature With a 16-Hz Orthostatic Tremor of the Legs[a]

Author (Ref.)	Case	Age (yr)	Sex	Duration (yr)	FH tremor	Leg tremor Occurrence	Leg tremor Frequency (Hz)	Leg tremor EMG patterns	Tremor at other sites Location	Tremor at other sites Frequency (Hz)	Drugs
Heilman (1)	1	63	F	20	Yes	Standing	NS	NS	UL[b]	NS	Clonazepam
	2	78	M	10	No	Standing	NS	NS	None		No response
	3	79	M	10	No	Standing	NS	NS	None		Clonazepam
Pazzaglia et al. (3)	1	70	M	NS	No	Standing	14–16	Alternating	UL	16	NS
Wee et al. (6)[c]	2	70	F	15	ET	Standing/Action	15–17	Synchronous	UL	7–8	Clonazepam
Deuschl et al. (7)	1	48	F	6	ET	Standing/Action	16	Synchronous	UL	NS	Primidone
Papa and Gershanik (9)	13	63	F	7	No	Standing/Action	16/6–8	Alternating or Synchronous	UL[b]	6–8/15–16	Clonazepam
	14	68	F	1.5	No	Standing/Action	16/6–8	Synchronous	UL[b]	6–8/15–16	Phenobarbitone
	15	72	F	NS	ET	Standing/Action	16/6–8	Synchronous	UL[b]	6–8/15–16	
Taly et al. (10)	1	66	M	3	No	Standing	14–15	Synchronous	UL[b]	10–11	No response
Uncini et al. (11)	1	64	F	2	NS	Standing/Action	16	Alternating	UL[b]	NS	No response
Gabellini et al. (12)	1	68	F	NS	No	Standing	14–16	Synchronous	UL[b]	NS	NS
	2	56	F	NS	Yes	Standing	14–16	Synchronous	UL[b]	NS	NS
	3	45	F	NS	No	Standing	14–16	Synchronous	Cranial	NS	NS
Vieregge and Kompf (13)	1	70	M	3	No	Standing	16	Synchronous	UL	8	Clonazepam
Brunotte and Porburski (14)	1	66	F	14	No	Standing	16	Synchronous	UL	NS	Clonazepam
Walker et al. (15)[d]	1	79	M	NS	No	Standing/Action	15	Synchronous	UL	15	Clonazepam/primidone

Reference	Case	Age	Sex	Duration (yr)	Family history	Type	Age at onset (yr)	Timing[a]	Upper limb[b]	Frequency (Hz)	Treatment
Fitzgerald and Jankovic (16)	1	60	M	35	Yes	Standing	18–20	NS	UL[b]	8–9	Primidone/clonazepam
	2	46	M	8	Yes	Standing	12–14	Synchronous	UL[be]	8–9	Primidone/clonazepam
	3	70	M	5	Yes	Standing	12	NS	UL[b]	8–9	? Clonazepam
	4	56	F	5	Yes	Standing/Action	14	NS	UL	14	Clonazepam
Thompson et al. (4)	1	55	M	4	No	Standing	16	Alternating	UL[bf]	10/16	No response
Britton et al. (5)	1	63	F	5	No	Standing	16	Synchronous	UL[bf]	8/16	None tried
	2	25	F	4	No	Standing	16	Alternating	None	16	No response
	3	68	M	15	No	Standing/Action	16	Synchronous	UL[b]	16	No response
	4	47	F	4	No	Standing/Postural	16	Alternating	UL[f]	16	No response
	5	57	F	5	No	Standing/Postural	16	Alternating	UL[bf]	8/16	No response
	6	64	M	4	Yes	Standing/Postural	14–16	Alternating	UL[b]	15–16	? Propranolol
Present report	1	44	M	4	No	Standing/Action	16	Synchronous	UL[b]	16	No response
	2	72	M	8	No	Standing/Postural	14	Synchronous	UL[f]	14–15	No response
	3	60	F	4	No	Standing	15	Alternating	UL[f]	15	No response
	4	52	F	6	No	Standing	16–17	Alternating	UL[bf]	16	? Clonazepam

ET, essential tremor; UL, upper limb; NS, not stated.

[a] Postural leg tremor refers to positions of the legs other than standing where the body weight is supported by the legs such as crouching on all four limbs. Action tremor of the legs refers to tremor during any activation of leg muscles by moving the legs when seated. The drugs listed are those that the authors reported to be of benefit.

[b] Tremor of outstretched upper limbs.

[c] The two cases reported by Wee et al. (6) were mother and daughter. Only case 2 is listed in the table, since information about leg tremor was given only for this case.

[d] The case reported by Walker et al. (15) exhibited leg tremor when standing or pressing the legs against a wall when supine, but not during knee extension while seated.

[e] Case 2 of Fitzgerald and Jankovic (16) had tremor of the upper limbs, lip and voice in addition to leg tremor.

[f] Tremor of upper limbs when engaged in postural support such as crouching on all fours or leaning against a wall.

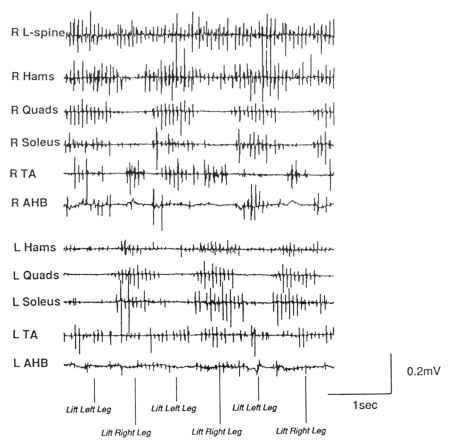

Figure 4 Surface EMG recordings from a patient with primary orthostatic tremor from right lumbar paraspinal muscles (R,L-spine), and various muscles of the right (R) and left (L) legs and feet (hamstrings, Hams; quadriceps femoris, Quads; tibialis anterior, TA; and abductor hallucis brevis, AHB) while "walking on the spot." The tremor is modified by the action of stepping. Immediately upon lifting the left foot to step with the left leg, the tremor is abolished in the left leg but continues in the weight-bearing right leg. On returning the left foot to the floor to commence a step with the right leg, the left leg tremor reappears as the foot is placed back onto the floor and tremor disappears in the stepping right leg. The tremor in paraspinal muscles is relatively unaffected by stepping. (From Ref. 5.)

patients with this condition have been related to unsteadiness when standing and leg stiffness rather than leg tremor. The leg and trunk tremor has a rapid frequency of about 16 Hz (see Fig. 1). It produces a fine-amplitude rippling movement of the quadriceps, which often is better appreciated by palpation than visual inspection. Occasionally the tremor frequency may halve to about 8 Hz (see Fig. 1), resulting in more vigorous contraction of the quadriceps muscles, and visible oscillation of the patella. This often is accompanied by worsening of the sensation of unsteadiness. In spite of this, tremor may still be less conspicuous than the dramatic compensatory maneuvers adopted by the patient in an effort to minimize the symptoms of unsteadiness when standing. Patients may stand in a slightly stooped posture on a widened stance base, with their legs stiffly extended and claw at the floor with their toes or shuffle their feet in an attempt to steady themselves. Finally, they may reach to grasp at nearby secure objects for further support. Both the leg tremor and the sensation of unsteadiness appear a few seconds after standing still, and are relieved by walking, sitting down, or leaning against a support (Fig. 4). One striking finding is that the tremor is abolished by lifting the patient off the floor so that the feet are no longer in contact with the floor. Tremor is most pronounced in leg and trunk (cervical, thoracic, and lumbar paraspinal) muscles, but can also be detected in upper limb muscles during certain postural maneuvers. Arm tremor is rarely accompanied by complaints of shaking and varies in frequency depending on arm posture (Fig. 5). With the arms held outstretched the frequency may be 16 Hz (as in the legs and trunk) or 8 Hz. If the arms are used in a postural mode by supporting body weight when standing on all fours, a 16-Hz arm tremor also may be seen.

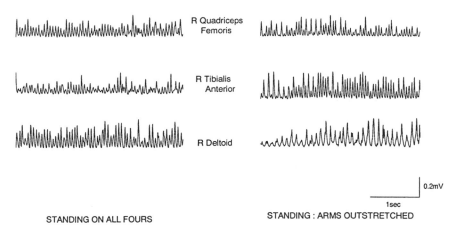

Figure 5 Surface EMG recordings from muscles of the upper and lower limbs when crouching on all fours (left panel) and when standing with the arms outstretched (right panel) in a patient with primary orthostatic tremor. When crouching on all fours (i.e., using both upper and lower limbs for postural support), a 16-Hz tremor is evident in both upper and lower limbs. A rapid tremor with a frequency of 16 Hz also is evident in the lower limbs when standing, but in this position there is an 8-Hz tremor of the upper limbs (deltoid) when the arms are held outstretched. (From Ref. 5.)

Physiological studies have revealed that agonist and antagonist muscle pairs may exhibit an alternating or cocontracting relation during tremor. The tremor is highly regular, and the order of muscle activation, both within and between limbs, tends to be stereotyped (4,5). This stability of the tremor is illustrated by the high degree of synchrony between motor unit discharges in the right and left tibialis anterior muscles (Fig. 6). Furthermore, the timing of motor unit discharge between the upper and lower limb muscles also shows a high degree of synchrony (Fig. 7). The tremor cannot be reset by a peripheral nerve stimulus, unlike some examples of essential tremor (Fig. 8). These features all suggest a central origin for orthostatic tremor. Interestingly, the interval between the timing of discharge of motor units in deltoid and tibialis anterior in the primary orthostatic tremor cycle

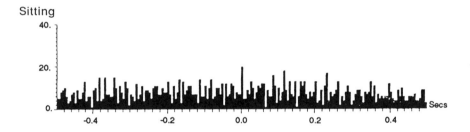

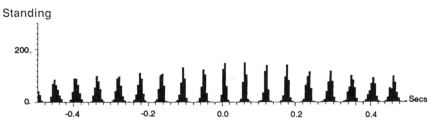

Figure 6 Cross-correlogram (5-ms bin width) of the timing of single motor unit discharges in left and right tibialis anterior during activation of the units by voluntary dorsiflexion of the feet (upper panel) and during quiet standing (lower panel) in a patient with primary orthostatic tremor. The timing of unit discharge in each muscle was recorded by a neuron pulse sorter over a series of 1-s epochs of tremor. For the cross-correlogram, the timing of the left tibialis anterior unit discharge in relation to the unit discharge in the right tibialis anterior (over a 1-s period) was denoted by a count in the histograms. During activation of the muscle by voluntary dorsiflexion of the feet while seated (upper histogram) there was no clear relation between the unit discharges in each leg. During tremor when standing (lower histogram) the relation of the left tibialis anterior unit discharge was closely correlated with that of the right tibialis anterior unit at a number of intervals, corresponding to the tremor cycle. The unit discharges were not absolutely synchronous, since the peak at $t = 0$ ms is shifted slightly by one or two bin widths. (From Ref. 5.)

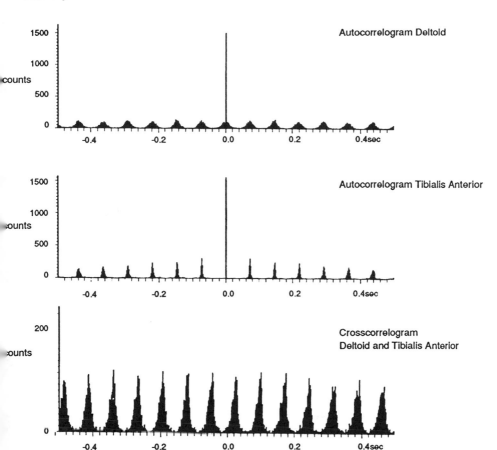

Figure 7 Auto- (upper two panels) and cross-correlograms (lower panel) (2-ms bin width) of the timing of single motor unit discharges in right deltoid and tibialis anterior muscles in a patient with primary orthostatic tremor while standing with the arms outstretched. The correlograms were constructed over a series of 1-s epochs of tremor during which time the discharge of the motor unit was recorded by a neuron pulse sorter. In the autocorrelograms, the timing of motor unit discharge in both the deltoid (upper panel) and tibialis anterior (middle panel) fell into well-defined periods throughout the tremor cycle. In the cross-correlogram, the timing of the deltoid unit discharge is shown in relation to the discharge of the tibialis anterior unit (at $t = 0$ ms). There was a close correlation of the timing of unit discharge in these muscles, since the deltoid unit fired at certain periods in relation to the unit in tibialis anterior. Note that the units in each muscle did not discharge synchronously. The deltoid unit fired some 20 ms before the tibialis anterior unit (at $t = 0$ ms). (From Ref. 5.)

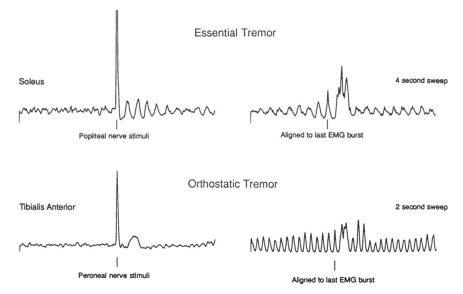

Figure 8 Phase resetting of leg tremor in essential tremor (upper traces) and primary orthostatic tremor (lower traces). Rectified surface EMG records from the soleus (upper traces) in a patient with essential tremor during supramaximal stimulation of the popliteal nerve (in the popliteal fossa) and from tibialis anterior in a patient with primary orthostatic tremor during peroneal nerve stimulation (at the head of the fibula). Note the difference in sweep times. The traces are aligned to the stimulus (left panels) and to the last EMG bust of the ongoing tremor before the stimulus. Stimuli were given at random timings throughout the tremor cycle. The averages of 50 trials are shown. Essential tremor is modulated by the stimulus in contrast with primary orthostatic tremor, which is unaffected by the peripheral stimuli (see text for further details).

is of the order of 20 ms (see Fig. 7). This figure closely approximates the difference in latency between these muscles following magnetic or electrical stimulation of the motor cortex in intact humans. Accordingly, it could be argued that the interval between tremor in the upper and lower limbs is related to time taken for signals descending from higher levels within the nervous system to reach the appropriate spinal levels. The striking postural sensitivity of the tremor is more difficult to explain, although it suggests that the tremor generator is engaged by mechanisms within the central nervous system that are involved in, and activated during, the maintenance of body posture during quiet standing or supporting the trunk with either upper or lower limbs. The nature of the generator and its relation to the structures concerned with postural maintenance is unknown.

A total of 28 cases of primary orthostatic tremor, defined as a 14- to 16-Hz leg tremor when standing, have now been described in the literature (1,3–16), to which we can add a further 4 new cases, bringing the total to 32 (see Table 2). There is no clear sex preponderance, and the age at onset of symptoms ranged from 21 to 67 years, with most patients developing symptoms in the sixth and seventh decades (mean 61 years). These patients present a stereotyped clinical picture of unsteadiness and shaking of the legs and trunk when standing, and relief of symptoms on sitting or movement. In addition to the 14- to 16-Hz leg and trunk tremor when standing, tremor on holding the arms outstretched (frequency 6–11 Hz) was present in 13. Fifteen patients also had a rapid (14- to 16-Hz) tremor of the arms when the upper limbs were engaged in postural support, such as crouching on all fours (some of these patients also had an action tremor of the arms).

III. RELATION BETWEEN ESSENTIAL TREMOR AND ORTHOSTATIC TREMOR

Essential tremor predominantly affects the arms and most commonly presents with symptoms related to hand and arm tremor. Leg tremor has been reported to occur in 15–30% of patients (17–19) with this condition, but it is unusual for patients to describe a profound sensation of unsteadiness when standing. However, patients with essential tremor may complain of leg tremor when standing still, as was the case in the reports of Wee et al. (case 1) (6) and Cleeves et al. (19). Interestingly, the latter patient had a family history of essential tremor, typical 7-Hz upper limb and 6.4-Hz lower limb tremors, and described relief of tremor when walking or leaning against a support. On clinical examination, essential tremor of the legs appears as an action tremor on standing and also is evident during the activation of leg muscles in any posture, irrespective of whether the patient is seated or walking. Essential tremor has a frequency of approximately 6–8 Hz, which occasionally can be reset by a peripheral stimulus, unlike primary orthostatic tremor (see Fig. 8).

The relation of orthostatic tremor to familial benign essential tremor has been discussed by several authors (6,8,9,19–21). In the report by Wee (6) of a family with essential tremor of the arms, two patients were identified who exhibited trunk and leg tremor only when standing, in addition to their arm tremor. In the case illustrated in Figure 2, 15- to 16-Hz EMG activity is evident in tibialis anterior muscle and intermittently in the paraspinal muscles during quiet standing. Activation of the legs when seated was accompanied by a 6- to 7-Hz leg tremor (6). These authors concluded that orthostatic tremor was a "static postural tremor" and a variant of essential tremor. Papa and Gershanik (9) reported three patients with a 6- to 8-Hz postural tremor of all limbs and a 16-Hz tremor of both upper and lower limbs during standing and when the feet were pressed against the floor while seated, or against a hard surface when lying supine with their legs extended. In the same paper these authors described 12 patients with essential tremor of both legs and arms (frequency 5–8 Hz), 7 of whom had complaints of unsteadiness while standing and 5 who did not. These observations lead the authors to conclude that "orthostatic tremor is a variant within the spectrum of essential tremor." In a review of 200 patients with essential tremor, Martinelli et al. (8) included 5 with orthostatic leg tremor as a "peculiar form of essential tremor"; tremor frequency was not mentioned. Gabellini et al. (12) reported eight patients with "essential and symptomatic" orthostatic tremor; three had tremor frequencies of 14–16 Hz, one of whom had a family history of tremor. Overall, a family history of tremor has been reported less frequently in primary orthostatic tremor (approximately 30%) than in essential tremor, for which approximately 50% of affected individuals have a family history of the condition (22). However, four of the 5 patients with difficulty standing and leg tremor reported by Fitzgerald and Jankovic (16) (included in the analysis of primary orthostatic tremor in Table 2) had a family history of tremor.

This analysis suggests there may be some overlap between primary orthostatic tremor and essential tremor, but as emphasized in the foregoing, there also are many clinical and neurophysiological differences between these tremors. From the pharmacological point of view, primary orthostatic tremor and essential tremor appear to respond to different medications. Alcohol or β-adrenergic blocker responsiveness is not a feature of primary orthostatic tremor, yet both these drugs may produce dramatic improvement in essential tremor. Only clonazepam and primidone have been reported to improve primary orthostatic tremor. In our experience, the benefit gained from these and many other drugs has been minimal.

Finally, it is acknowledged that there are several difficulties in using tremor frequency analysis as the sole arbiter in distinguishing between tremulous conditions (23). Resolution of the question on the relation of these two tremors may have to await molecular genetic identification of the gene defect in essential tremor.

REFERENCES

1. Heilman KH. Orthostatic tremor. Arch Neurol 1984; 41:880–881.
2. Thompson PD, Marsden CD. Walking disorders. In Bradley WG, Daroff RB, Fenichel GM, Marsden CD, eds. Neurology in Clinical Practice. Boston: Butterworth, Heinemann, 1991:369–380.
3. Pazzaglia P, Sabattini L, Lugaresi E. Su di un singolare disturbo della stazione eretta (osservazione di tre casi). Riv Freniatria 1970; 96:450–457.
4. Thompson PD, Rothwell JC, Day BL, et al. The physiology of orthostatic tremor. Arch Neurol 1986; 43:584–487.
5. Britton TC, Thompson PD, van der Kamp W, et al. Primary orthostatic tremor: further observations in six cases. J Neurol 1992; 239:209–217.
6. Wee AS, Subramony SH, Currier RD. "Orthostatic tremor" in familial essential tremor. Neurology 1986; 36:1241–1245.
7. Deuschl G, Lucking CH, Quintern J. Orthostatischer tremor: Klin Pathophysiol Ther. EEG-EMG 1987; 18:13–19.

8. Martinelli P, Gabellini AS, Gulli MR. Lugaresi E. Different clinical features of essential tremor: a 200-patient study. Acta Neurol Scand 1987; 75:106–111.
9. Papa SM, Gershanik OS. Orthostatic tremor: an essential tremor variant. Mov Disord 1988; 3:97–108.
10. Taly AB, Nagaraja D, Vasanth A. Trunkal tremor: orthostatic or essential? J Assoc Physicians India 1989; 37:539–541.
11. Uncini A, Onofrj M, Basciani M, Cutarella R, Gambi D. Orthostatic tremor: report of two cases and an electrophysiological study. Acta Neurol Scand 1989; 79:119–122.
12. Gabellini AS, Martinelli P, Gulli MR, Ambrosetto G, Ciucci G, Lugaresi E. Orthostatic tremor: essential and symptomatic cases. Acta Neurol Scand 1990; 81:113–117.
13. Vieregge P, Kompf D. Orthostatischer tremor. Akt Neurol 1990; 17:69–72.
14. Brunotte P, Poburski R. Orthostatischer tremor. Akt Neurol 1991; 17:36.
15. Walker FO, McCormick GM, Hunt VN. Isometric features of orthostatic tremor: an electromyographic analysis. Muscle Nerve 1990; 13:918–922.
16. Fitzgerald PM, Jankovic J. Orthostatic tremor: an association with essential tremor. Mov Disord 1991; 6:60–64.
17. Critchely E. Clinical manifestations of essential tremor. J Neurol Neurosurg Psychiatry 1972; 35:365–372.
18. Gerstenbrand F, Klingler D, Pfeiffer B. Der essentielle tremor, phaenomenologie und epidemiologie. Nervenarzt 1982; 53:46–53.
19. Cleeves L, Cowan J, Findley LJ. Orthostatic tremor: diagnostic entity or variant of essential tremor. J Neurol Neurosurg Psychiatry 1987; 52:130–131.
20. Findley LJ, Koller WC. Essential tremor: a review. Neurology 1987; 37:1194–1197.
21. Koller WC, Glatt S, Biary N, Rubino FA. Essential tremor variants: effects of treatment. Mov Disord 1987; 4:342–350.
22. Larson TA, Calne DB. Essential tremor. Clin Neuropharmacol 1983; 6:185–206.
23. Elble RJ. Physiologic and essential tremor. Neurology 1986; 36:225–231.

27

Primary Writing Tremor

Rajesh Pahwa
University of Kansas Medical Center
Kansas City, Kansas

I. INTRODUCTION

Task-specific tremor may be defined as tremor that is produced mainly by the act of performing certain specific motor tasks. When produced with writing, it is called primary ·writing tremor.

II. CLINICAL FEATURES

In 1979, Rothwell et al. described a patient who, at the age of 12 years, developed shaking and jerking movements of his right hand while using a pen, or of either hand when using a knife or holding a cup (1). After electrophysiological studies it was determined that these movements were tremors and, as the major disability involved writing, they called it "primary writing tremor." Since this initial report, there have been several cases reported of patients whose sole complaint is of tremor while writing or performing a few other skilled manual tasks. The tremor is often not produced by posture or goal-directed movement. In most patients, it is asymmetric and focal (2). It is not associated with other neurological disturbances.

Primary writing tremor has been reported between the ages of 11 and 72 years in both sexes (1,3–5). It is mainly a pronation–supination tremor, with a frequency of 5–6 Hz (4). The cardinal feature is the limited range of action during which the tremor is present (4). Although writing is the motor task that commonly provokes the tremor, other tasks that have been reported include golf club swinging, clenching fist, shaving, combing, using a screwdriver, sewing, cutting with scissors, holding a glass or cup, and protruding the tongue (1,4–6). In some patients the tremor could be provoked either by taps with a tendon hammer to supinate or pronate the forearm (4). Postural tremor is present in approximately 41% of these patients (7). None of the patients have been reported to have a resting tremor. There are usually no other neurological signs or symptoms. Although most of the patients reported having a negative family history for movement disorders, there are a few patients with a family history of essential tremor, primary writing tremor, dystonia, and Parkinson's disease (3,5,8).

III. ETIOLOGY AND PATHOLOGY

The cause of this condition is unknown. There have been reports of hand injuries, meningitis, and perinatal hypoxia in some patients (3,4). No autopsy studies have been performed; hence, the primary abnormality of the condition is unknown.

IV. ELECTROPHYSIOLOGY

In most patients, there is an alternating pattern of electromyographic (EMG) activity in the agonist and antagonist muscles, but a few patients have a synchronous pattern (6,9). Stretch reflex amplitudes, duration, and latencies are normal (4,6).

V. PATHOPHYSIOLOGY

Rothwell et al. proposed that primary writing tremor resulted from an abnormal hyperactive response to muscle spindle input from the pronator teres (1). The tremor was abolished by anesthesia of the motor point of the pronator teres. This blocked the proprioceptive spindle afferent impulses, which was indicated by the abolition of the stretch reflex, but did not affect the motor efferent impulses, as the normal voluntary activity was preserved. However, Ravits et al. had different physiological findings and found no evidence of the abnormal hyperactive response to the muscle spindles (6).

VI. TREATMENT

Various medications, including ethanol, propranolol, primidone, and anticholinergic agents have been tried with variable results. Klawans et al. tried levodopa, propranolol, and neuroleptics with no beneficial effects (3). Four of their patients improved after receiving scopolamine and benztropine. However, other authors have reported improvement in primary writing tremor with ethanol, propranolol, and primidone (4,5,10). Ohye et al. successfully treated three patients with primary writing tremor by stereotactic selective thalamotomy centered mainly on the ventralis intermedius nucleus (11). To date, there have been no reported cases of the use of botulinum toxin in primary writing tremor.

VII. PRIMARY WRITING TREMOR AND WRITER'S CRAMP

There is controversy whether primary writing tremor is a variant of essential tremor, or whether it has some relation with focal dystonia. The clinical and neurophysiological characteristics of primary writing tremor suggest it might be a variant of essential tremor. Kachi et al. raised the possibility that primary writing tremor was a variant of essential tremor because the tremor frequency and the response of the patients to alcohol and propranolol, were similar to essential tremor (4). Similarly, Koller and Martyn reported the efficacy of primidone in primary writing tremor (12), further indicating that this entity could be a sub-type of essential tremor. Rosenbaum and Jankovic studied 28 patients with focal task-specific movement disorders (5). They subgrouped the patients according to the presence of focal tremor alone, dystonia alone, or a combination of tremor–dystonia, suggesting that in a subgroup of patients both conditions may coexist.

There are certain similarities between primary writing tremor and writer's cramp. Both these disorders are task-specific, asymmetric, focal, with no associated neurological abnormalities and responsive to anticholinergics (13). Furthermore, although patients with essential tremor frequently have a family history of tremor, primary writing tremor and writer's cramp are usually sporadic. Cohen et al. reported on a family with essential tremor, primary writing tremor, and writer's cramp (8), further suggesting a possible link.

Elble and co-workers (14) described five patients with primary writing tremor and found EMG and clinical evidence of dystonia in each patient. The dystonic posturing was subtle and was often overshadowed by the tremor; however, EMG showed definite evidence of dystonia. They suggested that patients with primary writing tremor may exhibit varying proportions of tremor and focal dystonia. Similarly, Lang reported a mother and son who had tremor, mainly while writing and who later developed focal dystonia (14).

In conclusion, although patients may have varying degrees of tremor and dystonia, unless we know more about the pathophysiology of these conditions, clinical observations will be only speculative.

REFERENCES

1. Rothwell JC, Traub MM, Marsden CD. Primary writing tremor. J Neurol Neurosurg Psychiatry 1979; 42:1106–1114.
2. Hallet M. Classification and treatment of tremor. JAMA 1991; 266:1115–1117.
3. Klawans HL, Glantz R, Tanner CM, Goetz CG. Primary writing tremor: a selective action tremor. Neurology 1982; 32:203–206.
4. Kachi T, Rothwell JC, Cowan JMA, Marsden CD. Writing tremor: its relationship to benign essential tremor. J Neurol Neurosurg Psychiatry 1985; 48:545–550.
5. Rosenbaum F, Jankovic J. Focal task-specific tremor and dystonia: categorization of occupational movement disorders. Neurology 1988; 38:522–527.

6. Ravits J, Hallet M, Baker M, Wilkins D. Primary writing tremor and myoclonic writer's cramp. Neurology 1985; 35:1387–1391.
7. Weiner WJ, Lang AE. Tremor. In: Movement Disorders, A Comprehensive Survey. New York: Futura Publishing, 1989:221–256.
8. Cohen LG, Hallet M, Sudarsky L. A single family with writer's cramp, essential tremor, and primary writing tremor. Mov Disord 1987; 2:109–116.
9. Elble RJ, Koller WC. Unusual Forms of Tremor. In: Tremor. Baltimore: Johns Hopkins University Press, 1990:143–157.
10. Koller WC, Glatt S, Biary N, Rubino FA. Essential tremor variants: effect of treatment. Clin Neuropharmacol 1987; 10:342–350.
11. Ohye C, Miyazaki M, Hirai T, Shibazaki T, Nakajima H, Nagaseki Y. Primary writing tremor treated by stereotactic selective thalamotomy. J Neurol Neurosurg Psychiatry 1982; 45:988–997.
12. Koller WC, Martyn B. Writing tremor: its relationship to essential tremor. J Neurol Neurosurg Psychiatry 1986; 49:220.
13. Sheehy MP, Marsden CD. Writer's cramp—a focal dystonia. Brain 1982; 105: 461–480.
14. Elble RJ, Moody C, Higgins C. Primary writing tremor. A form of focal dystonia? Mov Disord 1990; 5:118–126.
15. Lang AE. Writing tremor and writing dystonia [letter]. Mov Disord 1990; 5:354.

28

Tremor and Dystonia

Richard M. Dubinsky
University of Kansas Medical Center
Kansas City, Kansas

I. INTRODUCTION

Dystonia is defined as "sustained muscle contraction frequently causing twisting or abnormal posture of the body parts" (1). Dystonia can have many associated movement abnormalities, including myoclonus and tremor. The first description of dystonia, by Oppenheim, mentions tremor associated with the dystonic movements (2). Because of the rhythmic clinical manifestations of dystonia, dystonic tremor is described in many series of patients with dystonia. Marsden and Harrison reported that 14% of 42 patients with generalized dystonia had tremor as a clinical feature (3). Tremor may also be the initial manifestation of focal dystonia. Both Rivest and Marsden (4) and Hughes et al. (5) have described cases of focal tremor preceding focal dystonia by several months to years.

Jedynak et al. (6) studied 45 patients with idiopathic dystonia who had a complaint of tremor. They were able to classify the tremor as a dystonic tremor using the following criteria: postural tremor, frequently associated with myoclonus; localized, irregular in amplitude and frequency; disappears when the involved muscles are relaxed; and the tremor appears with muscle contraction sufficient to maintain a posture or movement, but not while exerting great force. Included in this group of patients were eight subjects, five with primary writing tremor and three with a head-nodding tremor, who were felt to have dystonia based upon the presentation of the tremor under specific tasks. Current thought in the field of movement disorders is that primary writing tremor and task-specific tremors are forms of focal dystonia (7–9).

Jankovic et al. described associated movement disorders in 300 patients with cervical dystonia (10). Besides cervical dystonia, 48% of the group had other dystonias. Of the 271 patients with available clinical information concerning tremor, they found that 71% had tremor, with 60% having associated head and neck tremor. One-third had tremor outside the head and neck region, with 23% having essential tremor or postural hand tremor, 5% having truncal tremor, and 4% having tremor of the voice, lips, or legs. Twelve percent of the patients had a relative with cervical dystonia, 8% reported another type of familial dystonia, and 32% had relatives with essential type tremor. The overlap between the patients with a family history of essential tremor and the group with clinical essential tremor was not specified. Lou and Jankovic reported associated movement disorders in 350 consecutive patients with essential tremor (11). They found that 47.1% had associated dystonia, with cervical dystonia being the most common in 26.8% and dystonic writer's cramp in 13.7%. Seventy-one patients (20.2%) were found to have cardinal manifestations of Parkinson's disease. These last two studies have an obvious bias in that they were performed at a tertiary movement disorder research center; thus, they may overrepresent the true extent of overlap between focal dystonia and tremor.

II. INCIDENCE OF TREMOR IN A DYSTONIA CLINIC

Because some of the prior studies were flawed because of ascertainment bias, among other factors, the database of the Dystonia Clinic at the University of Kansas Medical Center, Kansas City, Kansas, was examined for possible relation between tremor and dystonia. The Dystonia Clinic serves as a regional referral center for dystonia throughout the state of Kansas, western portions of Missouri, northern Oklahoma, and southern Nebraska. All patients with the diagnosis of dystonia who were examined in the clinic from July 1, 1988 through July 31, 1992, were entered sequentially into the database. At the time of entry all patients were examined for coexistent neurological disease, with special emphasis being placed on movement disorders. At subsequent visits the database was updated to reflect new information (e.g., a family history of tremor, spread of dystonia). Dystonia was categorized by the body portion(s) involved (12). *Parkinsonian tremor* was defined as a resting tremor in the presence of bradykinesia or rigidity of the involved limb, a history of progression, and responsiveness of the bradykinesia and rigidity to levodopa. *Tremor* was defined as a rhythmic, kinetic, or postural tremor of one or more limbs, or involving the head and neck or voice. *Essential tremor* was defined as a tremor present with sustained posture or with kinesis, without a marked resting tremor. For the purposes of this study, a family history of a kinetic or postural tremor was not required for the diagnosis of essential tremor. Alcohol responsiveness was not used as a diagnostic criterion because of the low use of alcohol in some segments of our referral population. All patients were questioned concerning their family's medical history, with emphasis being placed on the presence of movement disorders.

A total of 308 patients with dystonia have been followed in the Dystonia Clinic. After excluding those with psychogenic dystonia ($n = 6$), paroxysmal kinesogenic dystonia ($n = 2$), secondary to structural lesions (1 with post hemiplegic dystonia and 1 with a Chiari type I malformation and syringomyelia), tardive dystonia ($n = 1$), possible 1-methyl-4-phenyl-1,2,3,6-tetrahydropyridine (MPTP)-induced parkinsonism and dystonia ($n = 1$), there were 296 patients with idiopathic dystonia. Of these, 24 had generalized dystonia, 26 had blepharospasm, 35 had facial dystonias or Meige's syndrome, 193 had cervical dystonia, 2 had cervical and brachial dystonia, 26 had focal limb dystonia manifested as a writer's or typist's cramp, 4 had crural dystonia, 3 had hemidystonia, and 4 had spasmodic dysphonia. There was overlap between the facial dystonia subgroup and the subgroups with cervical and spasmodic dysphonia.

Thirty-two (10.18%) of the dystonia patients had tremor. Twenty patients with cervical dystonia had an isolated head-nodding tremor in a "no–no" pattern, 2 patients with writer's cramps had isolated ipsilateral hand tremor, and 2 patients with generalized dystonia had arm tremor. These 24 patients had tremor present in a body part affected by the dystonia, thus meeting the diagnostic criteria for dystonic tremor (6). Only eight patients, all with cervical dystonia, had essential tremor. In all eight cases, the tremor preceded the onset of their dystonia by at least 5 years. One patient had coexisting Parkinson's disease.

Thirty-three patients (11.15%) had a family history positive for essential tremor. This group included 30 patients with cervical dystonia, 2 with writer's cramp (including 1 patient with focal tremor of the involved arm), and 1 with blepharospasm. All 8 of the cervical dystonia patients with essential tremor had a positive family history of essential tremor in at least one first-degree relative.

The incidence of essential tremor in the general population of North America is estimated to up to 1.7% in the general population and as high as 5.55% in the population 40 years old or older (13). Applying this to our study population, there should have been five patients with essential tremor in our study group (not significant by χ^2 test).

III. CONCLUSIONS

Essential tremor and dystonia are similar from a physiological standpoint, in both disorders there is excessive cocontraction of antagonist muscles, and both disorders can be only minimally suppressed (6,14,15). In essential tremor, there is rhythmic cocontraction of antigravity agonist and antagonist muscles. Most commonly, this is simultaneous cocontraction. Less common muscle activation patterns include alternating antigravity agonist and antagonist contraction, and antigravity agonist contraction alone. In cervical dystonia there is cocontraction of antagonist muscles, with the results being deviation of the head and neck away from the midline. The muscle activation pattern can be either tonic or spasmodic, resulting in a rhythmic jerking of the head toward one side (16,17). Two percent of patients with essential tremor and 10% of patients with focal dystonias can suppress the movements, but only with significant effort (15).

The precise etiologies of essential tremor and primary, nonheriditary, dystonia are unknown. Peripheral neuropathies, primarily involving large fibers, have been reported to cause intention tremor (18). Peripheral nervous system damage can also induce both dystonia and tremor (19–22). Toxic exposure to 2,3,7,8-tetrachlordibenzo-p-dioxin has been reported to cause both action-induced dystonia (writer's cramp) and intention tremor in 22 railroad workers exposed while cleaning up a railroad car spill (23). The postulated mechanisms include peripheral neuropathy, since 43 of the 45 exposed workers had histories and physical examinations consistent with this disorder. Central nervous system trauma can cause both focal dystonias and tremor (20).

This study has demonstrated that the prevalence of essential tremor is no greater in a large population of dystonic patients, seen at a regional referral center, than in the general population. This result contradicts several prior studies (10,11, 24), yet agrees with the low incidence of tremor in dystonia reported by others (3,25). Martinelli et al. found a 1% incidence of dystonia in their study of 200 consecutive patients with essential tremor seen in a movement disorders clinic (25). The major difference may be found in the study population. Unlike the studies of Jankovic and Lou, the patient population was taken from a regional referral center for movement disorders instead of a quaternary referral center. Tertiary and quaternary referral centers may have a patient population skewed more toward unusual manifestations of movement disorders. The same ascertainment bias may be applied to this study. Yet, as a primary and secondary referral center, our statistics may be closer to the true population. The best way to overcome this problem would be with a true population-based survey for neurological disease. However, with the relatively rare incidence of dystonia, compared with essential tremor and Parkinson's disease, the study population would need to be larger than 1 million, with a mixture of rural and urban origins. Another possible conflict is in the definition of tremor. This study used a rigid, narrow definition for the diagnosis of essential tremor. A more liberal definition would have allowed the inclusion of dystonic tremor patients into the group defined as having essential tremor. The rate of positive family history of essential tremor is twice what would be expected. This may be due to the imprecise nature of diagnosing a relative solely from the patient's description and without any opportunity to examine the relative. Thus, some of these first-degree relatives may have had Parkinson's disease, medication-induced tremor, or other tremor disorders.

REFERENCES

1. Jankovic J, Fahn S. Dystonic syndromes. In: Jankovic J, Tolosa E, eds. Parkinson's Disease and Movement Disorders. Baltimore: Urban & Schwarzenberg, 1988:283–314.

2. Oppenheim H. Uber eine eigenartige Kramfkrankheit des kindlichen und jungendichen Alters (Dysbasia lordotica progressiva, dystonia musculorum deformans). Neurologie Centralblatt 1911; 30:1090–1107.

3. Marsden CD, Harrison MJG. Idiopathic torsion dystonia (dystonia musculorum deformans). A review of forty-two patients. Brain 1974; 97:793–810.

4. Rivest J, Marsden CD. Trunk and head tremor as isolated manifestations of dystonia. Mov Disord 1990; 5:60–65.

5. Hughes AJ, Lees AJ, Marsden CD. Paroxysmal dystonia head tremor. Mov Disord 1991; 6:85–86.

6. Jedynak CP, Bonnet AM, Agid Y. Tremor and idiopathic dystonia. Mov Disord 1991; 6:230–236.

7. Lang AE. Writing tremor and writing dystonia. Mov Disord 1990; 5:354.

8. Elbe RJ, Moody C, Higgins C. Primary writing tremor: a form of focal dystonia? Mov Disord 1990; 5:518–526.

9. Rosenbaum F, Jankovic J. Focal task-specific tremor and dystonia: categorization of occupational movement disorders. Neurology 1988; 38:522–527.

10. Jankovic J, Leder S, Warner D, Schwartz K. Cervical dystonia: clinical findings and associated movement disorders. Neurology 1991; 41:1088–1091.

11. Lou JS, Jankovic J. Essential tremor: clinical correlates in 350 patients. Neurology 1991; 41:234–238.

12. Fahn S. Concept and classification of dystonia. Adv Neurol 1988; 50:1–9.

13. Hubble JP, Busenbark K, Koller WC. Essential tremor. Clin Neuropharmacol 1989; 12:453–482.

14. Sabra AF, Hallet M. Action tremor with alternating activity in antagonist muscles. Neurology 1984; 34:151–156.

15. Koller WC, Biary N. Volitional control of involuntary movements. Mov Disord 1989; 4:153–156.

16. Thompson PD, Stell R, Maccabe JJ, Day BL, Rothwell JC, Marsden D. Electromyography of neck muscles and treatment in spasmodic torticollis. In: Berardelli A, Benecke E, Manfredi M, Marsden CD, eds. Motor Disturbances II. London: Harcourt, Brace, Jovanovich, 1990:289–304.

17. Dubinsky RM, Gray C. Electromyographic patterns in torticollis. Muscle Nerve 1989; 12:770.

18. Said G, Bathien N, Cesaro P. Peripheral neuropathies and tremor. Neurology 1982; 32:480–485.

19. Truong DD, Dubinsky R, Hermanowicz N, Olson WL, et al. Post traumatic torticollis. Arch Neurol 1991; 48:221–223.

20. Koller WC, Wong GF, Lang A. Post traumatic movement disorders: a review. Mov Disord 1989; 4:20–36.

21. Scherokman B, Husain F, Cuetter A, Jabbari B, Maniglia E. Peripheral dystonia. Arch Neurol 1986; 43:830–832.

22. Schott GD. Induction of involuntary movements by peripheral trauma: an analogy with causalgia. Lancet 1986; 2:712–715.

23. Klawans HL. Dystonia and tremor following exposure to 2,3,7,8-tetrachlor-dibenzo-*p*-dioxin. Mov Disord 1987; 2:255–261.

24. Lang AE, Kierans C, Blair RD. Family history of tremor in Parkinson's disease compared to those of controls and patients with idiopathic dystonia. Adv Neurol 1987; 45:313–316.

25. Martinelli P, Gabellini AS, Gulli MR, Lugaresi E. Different clinical features of essential tremor: a 200-patient study. Acta Neurol Scand 1987; 75:106–111.

29

Trauma and Tremor

Terry G. Curran
Vernon Jubilee Hospital
Vernon, British Columbia, Canada

Anthony E. Lang
The Toronto Hospital
University of Toronto
Toronto, Ontario, Canada

I. INTRODUCTION

Interest in trauma and abnormal involuntary movements (AIMs) has had a recent resurgence in the medical literature, especially with respect to peripheral trauma. Trauma causing AIMs has traditionally been divided into central (head), peripheral, (usually an extremity), emotional, and "physiological" (e.g., cold exposure). The role of psychological and medicolegal factors must always be considered in cases for whom trauma is being blamed as the cause of tremor, particularly when the trauma was mild or remote. In our experience, this diagnosis accounts for a large proportion of cases referred with "posttraumatic tremor." "Psychogenic tremor" is discussed in Chapter 36.

Head trauma as a cause of tremor is now relatively well established, with a small number of cases providing good clinicopathological correlation. Other related tremor disorders (e.g., cerebellar tremor, midbrain tremor, hemisphere lesions and tremor) are covered in other chapters and, therefore, will be mentioned only briefly here. Peripheral trauma as a precipitant of AIMs is also becoming increasingly recognized, even for entities that were once thought to be purely centrally generated (e.g., dystonia). Peripheral trauma resulting in tremor, however, has not received as much attention, but this may change as our understanding of other peripherally induced AIMs evolves.

II.   HISTORICAL REPORTS OF TRAUMA AND TREMOR

The earliest reports of trauma and tremor were those associated with parkinsonism (Pm). James Parkinson, in his 1817 *Essay on the Shaking Palsy*, was the first to implicate trauma as a cause of Parkinson's disease (PD), although none of his patients reported trauma (1). The real interest in the role of trauma occurred in Europe in the 1870s with workmen's compensation legislation. During this period, peripheral trauma received more attention than central trauma (2). Charcot believed that a peripheral injury could induce an inflammatory reaction in the peripheral nerve that could then ascend along the nerve to involve the central nervous system ("ascending neuritis hypothesis"; cited in Ref. 2). Teillet, in 1952 (3), summarized the literature dealing with peripheral trauma as a cause of parkinsonism and provided a rather ambivalent conclusion, ruling neither for or against this hypothesis. Physiological trauma (e.g., cold exposure) and emotional trauma were also touted as precipitants of PD in the early 19th century (4,5). However, several subsequent reviews denounced them as precipitants of PD. This was largely supported by the absence of increase in frequency of PD following World War I, when peripheral and emotional traumas were abundant (2,6).

Other than James Parkinson's reference to central trauma causing tremor, this association went relatively unrecognized until 1904. Holmes (7) then described tremor in a patient with brainstem injury and attributed it to damage to the red nucleus or the superior cerebellar peduncle. In 1928, Martland drew attention to the parkinsonian symptoms associated with a chronic encephalopathy seen in boxers and called it the "punch drunk" syndrome (8). Crouzon and Justin-Besancon published the first review of head trauma (single or isolated) and parkinsonism in 1929 and set the following criteria (6); firstly, trauma had to be sufficiently violent to cause a concussion; secondly, the time between trauma and onset of parkinsonism had to be short; and finally, an uninterrupted course of parkinsonism should follow. Grimberg (2) came to similar conclusions in his 1934 review of 86 cases, stating that parkinsonism developed only if significant head and cerebral injury had occurred. In 1947, Kremer et al. (9) reported three adult patients in whom head trauma induced tremor, and the authors emphasized the associated midbrain clinical abnormalities.

Therefore, by the end of the 1950s, it was recognized that severe head trauma could precipitate tremor, with or without associated parkinsonism, and that repeated less severe head trauma could also cause tremor, with associated parkinsonism. The earlier belief that peripheral, emotional, and physiological trauma could cause various forms of tremor had fallen into disrepute.

III.   RECENT REPORTS OF TRAUMA AND TREMOR

A.   Central Trauma

In this chapter we will limit our discussion to *extrinsic* (e.g., head injury) as opposed to *intrinsic* trauma (e.g., cerebrovascular accident, ateriovenous malformation), although the final mechanisms of tremorogenesis may be identical. Rarely, is tremor secondary to head trauma seen in isolation, and more often it occurs within a spectrum of other neurological abnormalities. There are a variety of different types of central trauma reported to precipitate tremor, and likely there is some pathophysiological overlap, but we have chosen to discuss them separately for convenience and simplicity.

1. Severe Head Trauma and Tremor

In this chapter severe head trauma implies significant brain injury, with a variable period of coma. Most cases of tremor resulting from severe head trauma are believed to result from damage to the midbrain; thus, the common term *midbrain tremor*. There are many synonyms for this type of tremor (e.g., rubral tremor, cerebellar outflow tremor, and "red and black" tremor; 10) that are less accurate and thereby create confusion. The term "rubral tremor" should be avoided, as other neighboring structures in the midbrain may be equally, if not more, important in tremorogenesis and, indeed, the red nucleus may not have to be involved at all to produce midbrain tremor (11). The term "cerebellar outflow tremor" places too much emphasis on the cerebellar fibers as being the only source of tremor. However, there is a distinct form of cerebellar tremor that is discussed in Chapter 25 and will not be considered further here. The term "red and black" tremor comes from the suggestion that both the red nucleus and the dopaminergic system originating from the substantia nigra (SN) need to be involved for this tremor to develop.

In its classic form, a preponderantly unilateral rest tremor is present, with a progressive increase in amplitude with the maintenance of a posture, and a further accentuation with any attempted movement (i.e., resting < postural < kinetic tremor) (12). This type of tremor usually causes marked functional disability (13) and most often affects the upper extremity more than the lower. There is frequently a "myoclonic component" believed to be due to exaggerated or large-amplitude tremor bursts (14,15). Less often, the movement is more complex and may even resemble chorea (13), possibly owing to additional injury to the subthalamic nucleus. The frequency of the tremor is usually 1.5–3 Hz (13), and it commonly involves both proximal and distal muscles. In children and young adults, it typically follows a recovering hemiparesis (14,16,17). The insult is usually a closed head injury, with the resulting coma lasting 1 week to 5 months (14), and the tremor beginning 1–19 months later (13,14). Even in the absence of an initial hemiparesis, the tremor onset is often delayed by many weeks after the insult. The tremor usually begins insidiously, but occasionally, quite abruptly and, in some patients, it may be accentuated or even precipitated by dopamine receptor-blocking agents (13). It appears to be reported more often in children than in adults, and this likely reflects the higher morbidity and mortality seen with midbrain injuries in adults (18). Posttraumatic midbrain tremor seems to have a variable outcome, with some cases reported to progressively worsen (13), others remaining static (14,19), and a small proportion improving spontaneously (13).

There are several reported cases describing both palatal myoclonus (or similar orolingual rhythmic movements) and midbrain tremor following severe head trauma. It is now generally believed that the term "palatal myoclonus" is a misnomer and that this movement disorder should be reclassified as a subgroup of tremor. Denny-Brown reported (20) two patients with this combination and another with facial "myoclonus" and ipsilateral limb tremor. Samie et al. (13) reported three cases of severe head trauma and midbrain tremor in which two of the patients later developed palatal myoclonus, with a frequency similar to the limb tremor. One potential source of confusion or overlap, when considering abnormal rhythmic movements of the limb caused by brainstem injury, is a disorder termed *myorthythmia*. This term was first used by Hertz in 1931 (21) to distinguish this slower, irregular tremor from the tremor of Parkinson's disease. Myorhythmia most often occurs in association with intrinsic brainstem disease, such as hemorrhage or ischemic stroke, and is often accompanied by branchial myoclonus. But in the report by Masucci et al. (22) of 24 cases, only one had associated palatal myoclonus. The proper nosological placement of this movement disorder relative to midbrain tremor and palatal myoclonus is uncertain. Most likely it represents the limb version of palatal myoclonus, but there are some clinical differences (e.g., it lacks persistence in sleep, which is common in palatal myoclonus). There are also many similarities between this type of tremor and classic midbrain tremor, including delayed onset from the time of insult and the rest component that increases with posture and action. Also, both have a relatively slow frequency (2–3 Hz), but myorhythmia may be slower and more complex. Further clinical–electrophysiological–pathological correlative studies are needed to help unravel this confusion.

Finally, Keane described two patients with severe head trauma, who later developed isolated paroxysmal tongue movements, which he referred to as "galloping tongue" (23). There was a 3–4 week delay in the onset of rhythmic movements that lasted 10 s and recurred every 20 s. They started in the midline as a full contraction and had a frequency of 3 Hz. Additional clinical findings suggested a pontine origin. Keane distinguished this disorder from that reported by Troupin and Kamm (24), who described a case of posttraumatic rapid tongue movements that they considered a form of branchial myoclonus. How these cases relate to isolated classic palatal myoclonus and palatal myoclonus associated with midbrain tremor or myorhythmia is uncertain. Further reference to these overlapping AIMs will be made in our discussion of pathophysiology (see Sect. IV.A).

The topic of posttraumatic parkinsonism should be mentioned for completeness in discussing severe head injury and tremor. The parkinsonism occasionally seen in this clinical setting is usually associated with other midbrain abnormalities. Lindenberg, in 1964 (25), described three patients with posttraumatic parkinsonism, who also had cranial nerve or pyramidal dysfunction. The pathological assessment revealed hemorrhagic lesions in the midbrain, centered in the SN and tegmentum. In 1985, Nayernouri (26) described a 37-year-old man, who developed parkinsonism after moderate head injury. This patient also had a left third nerve lesion and right hemiparesis. The computed tomography (CT) scan revealed a low-density lesion in the area of the SN bilaterally, with extension into the left cerebral peduncle.

There have also been rare cases with isolated parkinsonism following head trauma. Bruetsch and DeArmond (27) described a 60-year-old man who developed this disorder 8 months after falling and striking the back of his head on a concrete floor. At autopsy a residual fracture was seen in the occipital bone. The SN was depigmented, but Lewy bodies were absent. As well, small petechial hemorrhages were seen in the striatum. In the 1988 review by Factor et al. of trauma and parkinsonism, they concluded that severe head trauma can cause a syndrome in which parkinsonian features are present, but there is no evidence that a condition mimicking idiopathic PD can result from either minor or severe head trauma (28).

2. Recurrent Head Trauma and Tremor

Recurrent head trauma (usually mild to moderate severity), as occurs in boxers, can result in a chronic encephalopathy, with a typical parkinsonian rest tremor. This entity is often referred to as the *punch drunk* syndrome (8) or dementia pugilistica (29). More common features include cerebellar and pyramidal signs, other parkinsonian signs, mental status changes, and dysarthria. Critchley in 1957 (29) and, more recently, Roberts (30), have delineated the different neurological syndromes that can be seen and have reemphasized that the severity of encephalopathy is proportional to the number of fights. Symptoms may not appear until many years after retiring, and the parkinsonian rest tremor is typically a late manifestation.

3. Minor Head Trauma and Tremor

Minor head trauma as a cause or precipitant of tremor is less well established. Minor head trauma refers to injury causing only brief or no loss of consciousness (LOC), with minimal or no neurological sequelae. Biary et al. recently reported four cases of tremor following minor head trauma in which two patients had brief LOC and the others had none (19). The tremor began 1–4 weeks following trauma and clinically resembled essential tremor, with postural and kinetic components. The tremor was present mostly in the upper extremities and was asymmetric. Similarities to tremor following severe head trauma included a "myoclonic-like" component in two of the four patients, and one patient had rhythmic tongue movements on protrusion, which could have been similar to palatal myoclonus, but may simply have represented a postural tongue tremor. Imaging studies were normal, and a psychogenic cause was thought unlikely.

Andrew et al. (31) described a single case of "minor head trauma" in a 33-year-old man, who fell from his motorbike and twisted his neck to avoid hitting his head. Two weeks later he developed a sudden left hemiparesis, and over the following 3 months as the motor symptoms improved, he developed a coarse rest tremor in the left upper extremity. This increased progressively with maintenance of posture and action, as is seen in midbrain tremor. The authors believed that the mechanism of brain injury was an embolic event from a carotid dissection. A CT scan demonstrated a lucency in the contralateral white matter, close to the roof of the body of the lateral ventricle. Although this case could be classified under minor head trauma and tremor, it represents an unusual mechanism and an equally unusual site of brain injury, if indeed this was the source of the tremor. This case might be more appropriately considered an example of intrinsic hemispheric injury causing tremor, which may have a different mechanism than the previously mentioned cases and is discussed further in chapter 30.

4. Perinatal Head Injury and Tremor

In contrast with the occasional occurrence of delayed-onset dystonia (32), there have been no reported cases of isolated tremor (immediately or delayed in onset) following traumatic birth, although a "dystonic tremor" may be present in patients with delayed-onset dystonia. Tremor is a feature of the hemiparkinsonism–hemiatrophy syndrome (HPHA), for which traumatic birth histories are often noted (33). These patients most often present at a relatively young age with unilateral rest tremor, and there is usually also a history of dystonia antedating the use of levodopa therapy. Other features include additional parkinsonian signs, a slow progression, and a relatively good response to levodopa. The severity of hemiatrophy varies considerably and may be quite subtle. Giladi et al. recently presented their experience with 11 patients in whom 5 had tremor as the presenting symptom (rest tremor in 4, action tremor in 1) (34). They noted that some of their cases progressed more rapidly than previously reported, and some did not have body hemiatrophy, but did have brain hemiatrophy on imaging studies. In addition, their cases differed from earlier reports in that none had an abnormal perinatal history, and only 3 of the 11 had any significant history of head trauma. However, they did conclude that this syndrome most likely represents another example of delayed-onset movement disorder, possibly caused by perinatal asphyxia.

B. Spinal Trauma and Tremor

There are no reports of isolated spinal cord injury and tremor. Spinal segmental myoclonus may occur after spinal cord injury (35), and this is often a rhythmic movement that might be confused with tremor.

C. Peripheral Trauma and Tremor

The number of movement disorders reported to be induced or precipitated by peripheral trauma is steadily increasing, with dystonia being the most recent addition to the list (36). However, it is often difficult to prove cause and effect. Unlike the case with central trauma, there is often a less well-defined history of injury. It is also unclear how long the delay can be between trauma and the onset of tremor. Finally, it is not certain whether repeated performance of a task (i.e., "overuse") constitutes peripheral trauma, which may then result in certain task-specific movement disorders (including tremor), or whether these disorders result from a primary disturbance of the nervous system (or a combination of the two).

Isolated tremor induced by peripheral trauma is rarely reported. More often, tremor is associated with other abnormalities, such as dystonia or reflex sympathetic dystrophy (RSD). It might be useful to divide peripheral trauma according to severity, as we have done in central trauma. Theoretically, electrophysiological testing could be used to grade severity (e.g., denervation versus no denervation), but in practice, this may be quite difficult, since such studies often have not been performed in reported cases. However, this separation may be moot, since the underlying pathophysiology of the tremor may, in contrast with CNS trauma, be identical, regardless of the severity of the peripheral trauma. Electrophysiological studies are, however, particularly useful in distinguishing the rare cases in whom other forms of rhythmic abnormal movements (e.g., myokymia, myoclonus) induced by peripheral trauma may mimic isolated focal tremor (37,38).

1. Isolated Tremor and Peripheral Trauma

Jankovic and Van Der Linden described 23 patients with a variety of AIMs following peripheral trauma (39). Five developed tremor in the injured limb with a variable latency of 1 day to 9 months. The tremor was most often present in the upper extremity, but occasionally in the leg, and was clinically similar to essential tremor. The types of trauma included complicated laminectomy, vibration trauma, neck injury, electric shock, and wrist laceration. Electrophysiological testing was carried out in four patients and demonstrated an ulnar neuropathy only in the patient with the wrist laceration. In two patients, symptoms remained static and, in the remainder, other AIMs developed, including parkinsonism, cervical dystonia, and segmental myoclonus. The authors emphasized that a significant proportion (> 65%) of their cases had some potential underlying predisposition (e.g., genetic, birth injury, other) to the development of AIMs. In support of this concept is the report by Cole et al. describing a 62-year-old man, with a past history of a mild postural tremor, who fell and fractured his right wrist and required casting for 6 weeks (40). Immediately after removal of the cast, there was a 7-Hz postural tremor in the right hand, which was quite positional in nature. Over the subsequent 4 years, the tremor remained static and localized to the right hand. Herbaut and Soeur described two cases of peripheral trauma followed by tremor (41). The first patient also had a past history of mild postural tremor in both upper extremities as well as a family history of essential tremor. This patient suffered a fractured fifth metacarpal bone that required splinting for a short period.

Upon removal of the splint a high-amplitude 7-Hz postural tremor was noted in that hand. An EMG revealed evidence of a slight compression of the ulnar nerve at the elbow. The second patient experienced a whiplash injury that was immediately followed by a high-amplitude 6-Hz tremor of the right arm that was very positional. Both patients were followed over a year with no change or spread of the tremor. In our experience with similar cases of sudden-onset tremor immediately following minor injury or whiplash, most if not all patients have demonstrated very strong evidence for a principal diagnosis of psychogenic tremor (42). This may apply even if there is a preceding history of a milder tremor, in which case, a psychogenic tremor may be superimposed on an underlying organic tremor (43).

2. Peripheral Trauma, Dystonia, and Tremor

As was mentioned earlier, there is growing evidence that peripheral trauma can be associated with a variety of AIMs, including focal dystonias. Clinical differences that exist between posttraumatic and idiopathic dystonia support the suggestion that these disorders have differing pathophysiologies (44). It is known that postural tremor can be seen in some 15–20% of patients with idiopathic dystonias (45), and it appears that dystonia following peripheral trauma may also be associated with tremor. For example, Jankovic and Van Der Linden noted that 4 of their 23 patients developed a combination of focal dystonia and tremor (39). Three developed focal dystonia in the area injured and, then later, developed tremor that affected a different site from that initially traumatized. One patient developed a focal foot dystonia and tremor simultaneously. Electrophysiological testing was done in three and was normal. Schott described ten patients with a variety of AIMs occurring after peripheral trauma (46). One of these patients lacerated his right forearm at the age of 47, and 3 years later he developed right hand dystonia. Fifteen years after this, he developed a tremor in the right upper extremity. Schott noted that this prolonged latent interval made a casual relation tenuous.

Occupational dystonia (task-specific dystonia) is one type of idiopathic focal dystonia, with writer's cramp being the most common example. Trauma, as a single isolated event, or more commonly as repeated overuse, is frequently reported in writer's cramp and in other allied conditions, thereby encouraging the term *overuse syndromes* (e.g., as seen in performing musicians) (47). Tremor is reported in 30% of patients with writer's cramp, either only with writing or with postural maintenance (47). The nosology of these disorders becomes even more complicated when primary writing tremor is considered. Some authors have emphasized the relation between this condition and writer's cramp, whereas others classify it as a variant of essential tremor (48).

3. Peripheral Trauma and Parkinsonism

Schott's recent report (46) of AIMs following peripheral trauma has reopened the question of peripheral trauma as a cause of parkinsonism. He described three patients in whom mild peripheral injury was followed 2–28 days later by the development of parkinsonism. The site of onset of symptoms was the same as the location of injury. Two of these began with focal rest tremor, and the other with foot dystonia, followed by resting tremor. Over the ensuing months to years further typical parkinsonian symptoms evolved that responded to levodopa in all three. The initial trauma caused a significant amount of pain in two of these patients, and this may have some pathophysiological importance. Schott emphasized the similarities between his patients and cases of RSD relative to pain, latency, the trivial nature of the injury, and subsequent progression. Jankovic and Van Der Linden (39) described a 38-year-old man with a complicated laminectomy who, 9 months later, developed tremor in both legs and then, subsequently, parkinsonism. This patient was, however, human immunodeficiency virus (HIV)-positive. Despite these and earlier cases mentioned at the beginning of this chapter, reviews concerning trauma and parkinsonism (28,42) provide little or no reliable evidence supporting a role of peripheral trauma as a cause of any type of parkinsonian syndrome, with the possible exception of rare examples of psychogenic parkinsonism (Lang AE, personal observation).

4. Peripheral Trauma, Reflex Sympathetic Dystrophy, and Tremor

An assortment of involuntary movements have been noted to accompany RSD, including tremor, dystonia, "spasms," and other less well-defined abnormal movements (49–51). Reflex sympathetic dystrophy (RSD) may be precipitated by a wide variety of events, with peripheral trauma, usually of a minor nature, being the most common (52). Schwartzman and Kerrigan recently presented 43 cases of RSD complicated by a variety of AIMs (51). In 38 of their patients, a history of peripheral injury was given, and often this was as minor as a simple foot sprain. The most pronounced movement abnormality was that of painful dystonic posturing. In addition, a fine tremor was noted in the affected extremity of all patients who could move the limb. This was usually a 3- to 6-Hz resting flexion–extension tremor of the fingers that increased with postural maintenance. One patient had an unusual 4- to 5-Hz flexion–extension tremor of the ankle that was quite variable in amplitude, depending on the posture. Two other patients had large-amplitude intentionlike tremors of the upper extremity. All tremors were diminished (or abolished) by sympathetic blockade. In Jankovic and Van Der Linden's series of peripheral trauma and AIMs, ten patients had associated RSD (39). One of these patients had isolated tremor, whereas the remainder had dystonia, with or without tremor (39). Yokota et al. recently presented four interesting cases (53) of motor paresis following minimal or no trauma, who later developed pain and a fine postural tremor of the involved limb. The authors referred to this as a "sympathetic motor paresis" and suggested that this was a form of RSD. The importance of the sympathetic nervous system and its influence on the motor system was stressed.

Two additional abnormal movement syndromes that share similarities with RSD should be mentioned here. The first is the painful legs and moving toes syndrome (now more appropriately referred to as the painful limb and moving digits syndrome; PLMD) in which there is often minimal peripheral trauma or some other source of peripheral nerve dysfunction leading to a causalgic-type pain and writhing movements of the digits (54). These movements can occasionally resemble tremor (55). The second related syndrome encompasses the motor sequelae that occasionally occur in the stump after limb amputation ("stump dyskinesias"; SD). Pain is often a significant factor, and a variety of motor phenomena have been described, including repetitive jerking, spasms, chorea, and tremor (56,57).

These three entities (RSD, PLMD, SD) appear to have a common theme of peripheral trauma, which is frequently minimal, a significant component of pain, and often, a delayed onset of AIMs, with tremor occasionally being a prominent feature. The possible link between peripheral injury, the sympathetic nervous system, pain, and AIMs (including tremor) will be discussed under pathophysiology (see Sect. IV.B).

D. Physiological or Emotional Trauma and Tremor

There are few contemporary reports of physiological or emotional trauma precipitating tremor in isolation or in disease-associated states. However, it is common for these types of "trauma" to cause transient exacerbations of preexisting tremor. In addition, the earliest symptoms of occult disease may first appear in these circumstances. For example, patients with PD will occasionally recall that their tremor first appeared in an emotionally stressful situation. Laboratory studies confirm the role of stress in precipitating motor symptomatology in asymptomatic animals with severe degrees of dopamine depletion (58). Apart from these examples it is unlikely that such trauma can *cause* irreversible tremor states (28).

IV. PATHOPHYSIOLOGY

As with most disorders in neurology, the traditional approach is to search for an anatomical basis to help explain the underlying pathophysiology. Clinicopathological correlation is possible in many cases of tremor following head trauma, thanks to postmortem assessments and modern imaging techniques. Unfortunately, this understanding is still lacking in most cases when tremor follows peripheral trauma. We have chosen to discuss central trauma and peripheral trauma separately, although in many instances the distinction is artificial, given the intimate interactions between the central and the peripheral nervous systems.

A. Central Trauma and Tremor

There are several areas within the brain that are capable of generating oscillatory behavior (59). To what extent these play a role in generating and maintaining tremor after head trauma remains uncertain. There is likely considerable overlap between the traumatic and nontraumatic tremor states; however, underlying mechanisms for most of these are far from clear. We will consider the different types of central trauma individually, as we have done in our clinical discussion.

1. Severe Head Trauma and Tremor

The tremor most often associated with severe head injury is believed to occur as a consequence of damage to the rostral midbrain. Experiments in animals have supported this by producing similar tremors with lesions placed in this location (59). The midbrain appears to be highly susceptible to damage from severe head trauma through a variety of mechanisms (18).

However, it is likely that tremor can occur with lesions in areas of the brainstem other than the midbrain. Both branchial myoclonus and myorhythmia are believed to be caused by damage to the dentatorubroolivary pathway (Guillain–Mollaret triangle). This disconnection may occur in the ipsilateral dentate nucleus, superior cerebellar peduncle, or contralateral central tegmental tract (60). Pseudohypertrophy of the inferior olive (a pathological hallmark of palatal myoclonus) occurs only when extremity myorthymia is accompanied by palatal myoclonus (22). The reports mentioned earlier of coexisting midbrain tremor and palatal myoclonus suggest a link between the two. Supporting this theory is the report by Samie et al. (13) of "midbrain tremor," revealing the lesion in one case to be similar in location to that of classic palatal myoclonus. Furthermore, the frequent association of myorhythmia and palatal myoclonus may suggest a common mechanism for midbrain tremor and myorhythmia. Unfortunately, the confusion that exists with proper identification and classification of midbrain tremor and myorthythmia makes any further discussion of pathophysiology difficult. Finally, the report by Maki et al. of posttraumatic hemorrhage in the putamen producing tremor in a child (61) invokes another area with potential tremorogenic importance in cases of tremor following severe head injury.

Posttraumatic parkinsonian tremor likely occurs because of damage to the SN or its efferents as has been demonstrated in a small number of cases at necroscopy (25,26). The possible role of nigral dysfunction in the resting component of midbrain tremor has been mentioned earlier. The CT scan in posttraumatic parkinsonism may show low-density abnormalities in the mesencephalon (26). The use of magnetic resonance imaging (MRI) and positron emission tomography (PET) promises greater insight into the location and mechanisms accounting for these clinical features.

In summary, the location of dysfunction in most cases of tremor following severe head trauma is in the midbrain tegmentum. However, it is likely that other areas within the brainstem and mesencephalon are also capable of generating and maintaining posttraumatic tremor. Our current understanding of the location of the tremor generators and how these oscillatory circuits are maintained or disinhibited after severe head injury remains extremely rudimentary.

2. Recurrent Head Trauma and Tremor

The parkinsonian rest tremor seen in the punch drunk syndrome is identical with the rest tremor of idiopathic PD. Histologically, one sees petechial hemorrhages and focal scarring in the cortex, cerebellum, and brainstem, with degeneration of the SN and extensive neurofibrillary tangles throughout these structures (29,30). These changes are believed to occur as a consequence of linear and rotational acceleration movements from repeated head trauma (62), with shearing forces acting at a variety of levels, including the midbrain (63,64). Therefore, in cases of repeated head trauma (usually mild to moderate severity) causing tremor, the likely site of abnormality is the SN. However, there are other areas of diffuse brain injury, including the cerebellum, which may also play a role.

3. Minor Head Trauma and Tremor

Minor head trauma-induced tremor has only rarely been reported. Therefore, it is difficult to draw definitive conclusions about its very existence, let alone its potential pathophysiology. The tremor reported in the four cases of Biary et al. (19) had some similarities to that seen after severe head trauma (asymmetry and associated myoclonus; 15). One of these patients also had rhythmic tongue movements, suggesting a similarity to branchial myoclonus. These features may suggest some overlap in anatomicopathophysiological mechanisms between tremors induced by minor and severe head injury.

4. Perinatal Birth Trauma and Tremor

It is uncertain whether the hemiparkinsonism–hemiatrophy syndrome is due to extrinsic injury, such as trauma in utero at the time of birth, or to a primary intrinsic brain disorder (e.g., asphyxia, with or without ischemia), or to a combination of both. The actual location of injury remains uncertain, but levodopa responsiveness in most cases supports a possible role of the SN or its efferents. Further clinical and, particularly, pathological correlative studies are needed for a better understanding of this entity.

B. Peripheral Trauma and Tremor

Because of the rarity of reports of peripheral trauma and tremor, the following paragraphs will concentrate on other peripherally induced AIMs, with extrapolation to the question of peripheral trauma and tremor. This is appropriate, since most cases of tremor following peripheral trauma have been associated with other syndromes. However, it is uncertain if isolated tremor, as occurs rarely after peripheral trauma, has the same pathophysiological basis as tremor associated with other syndromes, such as RSD or peripherally induced dystonia.

Hemifacial spasm (HFS) is probably the most common movement disorder believed to be peripherally initiated and maintained. Because of its frequency, most of the proposed pathophysiological explanations for other peripherally induced AIMs are based on this entity. However, there is still much controversy concerning the principal site of neuronal injury and, therefore, the mechanism(s) underlying the abnormal movements (65). Three theories have been proposed: peripheral, central, and combined. The *peripheral hypothesis* attributes the movement disorder to ectopic excitation and ephaptic transmission at the site of the peripheral injury. In HFS, this is most commonly believed to be at the root entry zone of the seventh nerve secondary to compression from a "vascular loop" (66). The concept of peripheral nerve injury giving rise to abnormal motor activity is not new, and there are a variety of other examples, such as fasciculations, myokymia (67), and plexus lesions causing myoclonus (38). The *central hypothesis* suggests that plasticity occurring within the facial nucleus, and possibly even further rostrally, may result in the abnormal movements secondary to hyperexcitability (possibly by disinhibition) or denervation supersensitivity (68). Finally, the *combined hypothesis* proposes a combination of peripheral and central mechanisms. This is likely the most accurate mechanism whereby central changes may develop as a consequence of abnormal afferent input (69).

These same hypotheses can be applied to other syndromes, such as RSD, PLMD, and SD, which are thought to be peripherally initiated in most cases and are associated with variety of AIMs, including tremor. However, they are likely heterogeneous and, therefore, no one single theory will explain all cases. For example, Schoenen et al. (70) recently presented evidence that PLMD could be divided into two general categories, a central oscillatory group and a peripheral oscillatory group. The peripheral trauma (often mild) associated with these three conditions is believed to generate abnormal neuronal activity in the periphery. With time, this appears to be associated with central neuronal changes (i.e., the combined hypothesis), and there is now good evidence that trauma to peripheral nerves can induce central plasticity, both at the segmental and suprasegmental levels (50,71). The resultant central neuronal hyperexcitability may then be reflected in increasing anterior horn cell activity and abnormal movements (72).

Two additional features common to these three entities (but not found in HFS) are prominent pain and alterations in function of the sympathetic nervous system (SNS). The potential interaction and influence of these factors on the motor system are only recently becoming recognized. For example, there are many neurotransmitters common to motor and pain pathways. Spinal dopaminergic neurons may be involved in pain modulation, autonomic nervous system functioning, and motor response, thus allowing a common link between pain and AIMs (73). In addition, substance P has now been shown to have a significant effect on sensory and motor neuronal function (74), and the SNS is also known to have profound effects on primary C fiber afferents, muscle spindles, as well as the muscle itself (75). Supporting these concepts are the observations by Schwartzman and Kerrigan (51) that pain and AIMs, including tremor, in their RSD patients abated with sympathetic blockade. These authors proposed an interaction between substance P and the anterior horn cells (by way of the SNS) to account for the motor abnormalities seen in RSD. Additional support for this hypothesis is the report by Yokota et al. (53) that paresis and tremor increased with sympathetic stimulation and decreased with sympathetic ganglionic blockade in their four cases of "sympathetic motor paresis."

In conclusion, it is hypothesized that peripheral trauma initiates local neuronal activity, with subsequent increase in afferent input to the spinal cord (including substance P-containing neurons). The SNS neurons may subsequently be activated with the potential to excite anterior horn cells. This, rarely, may then result in the development of a variety of abnormal involuntary movements, including tremor. Because substance P and SNS neurons are often involved, pain and symptoms of local dysautonomia are often present. Why this cascade of events occurs in only a few patients is uncertain. The occurrence of a delay between the trauma and the onset of these neurological symptoms suggests a role for plasticity, occurring either peripherally or more likely centrally. This does not explain those AIMs (specifically tremor) that are rarely reported to occur immediately following trauma (41,46). If organic tremor can truly occur immediately following peripheral trauma (especially minor trauma), then mechanisms different from those outlined in the foregoing discussion will have to be invoked.

V. TREATMENT

Midbrain tremor, limb myorhythmia, and branchial myoclonus are notoriously resistant to drug therapy. Numerous medications have been reported, with variable success in lessening tremor resulting from severe head injury. Ellison reported benefit with propranolol in two cases of midbrain tremor (17), whereas Obeso et al. found the combination of propranolol and valproic acid better than either alone (15). Samie et al. obtained a marked response with anticholinergics in two patients, and another had an excellent response with levodopa (13). The same patients were unresponsive to propranolol, primidone, and amantadine. Clonazepam has also been reported rarely effective for midbrain tremor unrelated to traumatic brain injury (19), as has isoniazid (76). Finally, it may also be worth trying 5-hydroxytryptophan in resistant cases, in view of the beneficial response occasionally obtained in patients with palatal myoclonus (77).

Stereotactic thalamotomy (nucleus ventralis intermedius; Vim) has also been used successfully for posttraumatic midbrain tremor. Andrew et al. reported eight cases treated with thalamotomy (14). The rest tremor was completely abolished in all eight, and in seven the postural and kinetic tremors also greatly improved. Seven of the patients required a second thalamotomy, and five required a third, with extension into the nucleus oralis externus or more medially and superiorly in the Vim. The overall functional improvement in these patients was striking. Side effects included transient worsening of dysarthria, ataxia, and hemiparesis. The authors concluded that the presence of these clinical features before surgery should be used as a relative contraindication to thalamotomy. They also recommended waiting for 1 year after the onset of symptoms before undertaking surgery because of the possibility of spontaneous improvement. Others have also reported similar responses too thalamotomy (78), including the case described by Andrew and his colleagues in whom the lesion was in the subcortical white matter (31).

In general, conventional medication used for other types of tremor (e.g., essential tremor) has not been helpful in the various forms of tremors induced by peripheral trauma (19). In patients with RSD, sympathetic blockade has been reported to improve the tremor and other involuntary movements, as well as the causalgic symptoms (51,53); however, this has not been uniformly successful (39).

Botulinum toxin injections may show some promise in the management of these refractory forms of tremor (39). This therapy needs to be more carefully assessed in a variety of tremors before its place in the management of these disorders can be defined. The development of more effective therapy for the various types of posttraumatic tremor may have to await further advances in the understanding of their complex pathophysiologies.

REFERENCES

1. Parkinson J. Essay on the Shaking Palsy. London: Whittingham & Rowland, for Sherwood, Neely & Jones, 1817.
2. Grimberg L. Paralysis agitans and trauma. J Nerv Ment Dis 1934; 79:14–42.
3. Teillet R. Traumatismes des membres et syndromes parkinsoniens. These de Toulouse, Faculte de medecine, Universite de Toulouse, France, 1952.
4. Eulenburg A. Lehrbuch Functionellen Nervenkrankheiten auf Physiolgischer Basis. Berlin: Hirschwald, 1871.
5. Boucher A. De la maladie de Parkinson et en particulier de la forme fruste. These de Paris, Faculte de medecine, Universite de Paris, France, 1877.
6. Crouzon O, Justin-Besancon L. Le parkinsonisme traumatique. Presse Med 1929; 37: 1325–1327.
7. Holmes G. On certain tremors in organic cerebral lesions. Brain 1904; 27:327–375.
8. Martland HS. Punch drunk. JAMA 1928; 91:1103–1107.
9. Kremer M, Ritchie RW, Smyth GE. A midbrain syndrome following head injury. J Neurol Neurosurg Psychiatry 1947; 10:49–60.
10. Fahn S. Differential diagnosis of tremors. Med Clin North Am 1972; 56:1363–1375.
11. Marsden CD. Origins of normal and pathological tremor. In: Findley LJ, Capideo R, eds. Movement Disorders, Tremor. London: Macmillan Press, 1984:37–84.

12. Findley LJ, Gresty MA. Tremor. Br J Hosp Med 1981; 26:16–32.
13. Samie MR, Selhorst JB, Koller WC. Post-traumatic midbrain tremors. Neurology 1990; 40:62–66.
14. Andrew J, Fowler CJ, Harrison MJG. Tremor after head injury and its treatment by stereotaxic surgery. J Neurol Neurosurg Psychiatry 1982; 45:815–819.
15. Obeso JA, Narbona J. Post-traumatic tremor and myoclonic jerking. J Neurol Neurosurg Psychiatry 1983; 46:788.
16. Szelozynska K, Zmamironski R. Extrapyramidal syndrome in post-traumatic hemiparesis in children. Neurol Neurochir Pol 1974; 8:167–170.
17. Ellison PH. Propranolol for severe post-head injury action tremor. Neurology 1978; 28:197–199.
18. Rosenblum WL, Greenberg RP, Seelig JM, Becker DP. Midbrain lesions: Frequent and significant prognostic feature in closed head injury. Neurosurgery 1981; 9: 613–620.
19. Biary N, Cleeves L, Findley L, Koller W. Post-traumatic tremor. Neurology 1989; 39:103–106.
20. Denny-Brown D. The Basal Ganglia and Their Relation to Disorders of Movement. London: Oxford University Press, 1962; 65–67.
21. Hertz E. Die amyostatischen unruheerscheinungen. Klinisch kinematographische analyse ihre kennzeichen und beleiterscheinungen. J Psychol Neurol 1931; 43:146–163.
22. Masucci EF, Kurtzke JF, Saini N. Myorhythmia: a widespread movement disorder. Clinicopathological correlations. Brain 1984; 107:53–79.
23. Keane JR. Galloping tongue: post-traumatic, episodic, rhythmic movements. Neurology 1984; 34:251–252.
24. Troupin AS, Kamm RF. Lingual myoclonus: case report and review. Dis Nerv Syst 1974; 35:378–380.
25. Lindenberg R. Die schadigungsmechanismen der substantia nigra bei hirntraumen und das problem des posttraumatischen parkinsonismus. Dtsch Z Nervenheilkd 1964; 185:637–663.
26. Nayernouri T. Posttraumatic parkinsonism. Surg Neurol 1985; 24:263–264.
27. Bruetsch WL, DeArmond M. The parkinsonian syndrome due to trauma. A clinico-anatomical study of a case. J Nerv Ment Dis 1935; 81:531–543.
28. Factor SA, Sanchez-Ramos J, Weiner JW. Trauma as an etiology of parkinsonism: a historical review of the concept. Mov Disord 1988; 3:30–36.
29. Critchley M. Medical aspects of boxing, particularly from a neurological standpoint. Br Med J 1957; 1:357–362.
30. Roberts AH. Brain Damage in Boxers. London: Pitman Medical Scientific Publishing, 1969.
31. Andrew J, Fowler CJ, Harrison MJG, Kendall BE. Post-traumatic tremor due to vascular injury and its treatment by stereotactic thalamotomy. J Neurol Neurosurg Psychiatry 1982; 45:560–562.
32. Burke RE, Fahn S, Gold AP. Delayed-onset dystonia in patients with "static" encephalopathy. J Neurol Neurosurg Psychiatry 1980; 43:789–797.
33. Klawans HL. Hemiparkinsonism as a late complication of hemiatrophy: a new syndrome. Neurology 1981; 31:625–628.

34. Giladi N, Burke RE, Kostic V, et al. Hemiparkinsonism–hemiatrophy syndrome: clinical and neuroradiological features. Neurology 1990; 40:1731–1734.

35. Jankovic J, Pardo R. Segmental myoclonus. Clinical and pharmacologic study. Arch Neurol 1986; 43:1025–1031.

36. Schott GD. The relationship of peripheral trauma and pain to dystonia. J Neurol Neurosurg Psychiatry 1985; 48:698–701.

37. Streib EW. Distal ulnar neuropathy as a cause of finger tremor: a case report. Neurology 1990; 40:153–154.

38. Banks G, Nielsen VK, Short MP, Kowal CD. Brachial plexus myoclonus. J Neurol Neurosurg Psychiatry 1985; 48:582–584.

39. Jankovic J, Van Der Linden C. Dystonia and tremor induced by peripheral trauma: predisposing factors. J Neurol Neurosurg Psychiatry 1988; 51:1512–1519.

40. Cole JD, Illis LS, Sedgwick EM. Unilateral essential tremor after wrist immobilisation: a case report. J Neurol Neurosurg Psychiatry 1989; 52:286–287.

41. Herbaut AG, Soeur M. Two other cases of unilateral essential tremor, induced by peripheral trauma. J Neurol Neurosurg Psychiatry 1989; 52:1213.

42. Koller WC, Wong GF, Lang A. Posttraumatic movement disorders: a review. Mov Disord 1989; 4:20–36.

43. Ranawaya R, Riley D, Lang A. Psychogenic dyskinesias in patients with organic movement disorders. Mov Disord 1990; 5:127–133.

44. Truong DD, Dubinsky R, Hermanowicz N, et al. Posttraumatic torticollis. Arch Neurol 1991; 48:221–223.

45. Baxter DW, Lal S. Essential tremor and dystonic syndromes. Adv Neurol 1979; 24: 373–379.

46. Schott GD. Induction of involuntary movements by peripheral trauma: an analogy with causalgia. Lancet 1986; 2:712–716.

47. Marsden CD, Sheehy MP. Writer's cramp. TINS 1990; 13:148–153.

48. Rothwell JD, Traub MM, Marsden CD. Primary writing tremor. J Neurol Neurosurg Psychiatry 1979; 42:1106–1114.

49. Marsden CD, Obeso JA, Traub MM, et al. Muscle spasms associated with Sudeck's atrophy after injury. Br Med J 1984; 28:173–176.

50. Robberecht W, Van Hees J, Adriaensen H, Carton H. Painful muscle spasms complicating algodystrophy: central or peripheral disease? J Neurol Neurosurg Psychiatry 1988; 51:563–567.

51. Schwartzman RJ, Kerrigan J. The movement disorder of reflex sympathetic dystrophy. Neurology 1990; 40:57–61.

52. Schwartzman RJ, McLellan TL. Reflex sympathetic dystrophy. Arch Neurol 1987; 44:555–561.

53. Yokota T, Furukawa T, Tsukagoshi H. Motor paresis improved by sympathetic block. A motor form of reflex sympathetic dystrophy? Arch Neurol 1989; 46:683–687.

54. Spillane JD, Nathan PW, Kelly RE, Marsden CD. Painfull legs and moving toes. Brain 1971; 94:541–556.

55. Montagna P, Cirignotta F, Sacquegna T, et al. "Painfull legs and moving toes" associated with polyneuropathy. J Neurol Neurosurg Psychiatry 1983; 46:399–403.

56. Russell WR. Neurological sequelae of amputation. Br J Hosp Med 1970; 6:607–609.

57. Marion MH, Gledhill RF, Thompson PD. Spasms of amputation stumps: a report of 2 cases. Mov Disord 1989; 4:354–358.

58. Zigmond MJ, Acheson AL, Bergmann MJ, Stricker EM. Neurochemical compensation after partial injury of the nigrostriatal bundle in an animal model of preclinical parkinsonism. Arch Neurol 1984; 41:856–861.

59. Lamarre Y. Tremorgenic mechanisms in primates. Adv Neurol. 1975; 10:23–34.

60. Lapresle J. Palatal myoclonus. In: Fahn S, Marsden CD, Van Woert eds. Myoclonus. Adv Neurol 1986; 43:265–273.

61. Maki Y, Akimoto H, Enomoto T. Injuries of basal ganglia following head trauma in children. Child's Brain 1980; 7:113–123.

62. Corsellis JAN, Bruxton CJ, Freeman-Brown D. The aftermath of boxing. Psychol Med 1973; 3:270–303.

63. Holborn AHS. The mechanisms of brain injury. Br Med Bull 1945; 3:147–149.

64. Peerless SJ, Newcastle NR. Shear injuries of the brain. Can Med Assoc J 1967; 96: 577–582.

65. Adams CBT, Chir M. Microvascular compression: an alternative view and hypothesis. J Neurosurg 1989; 57:1–12.

66. Nielsen VK. Electrophysiology of the facial nerve in hemifacial spasm. Ectopic/ephaptic excitation. Muscle Nerve 1985; 8:545.

67. Medina JL, Chokroverty S, Reyes M. Localized myokymia caused by peripheral nerve injury. Arch Neurol 1976; 33:587–588.

68. Bratzlavsky J, Van der Eecken H. Altered synaptic organization in facial nucleus following facial nerve regeneration. A electrophysiological study in man. Ann Neurol 1977; 2:71–73.

69. Esteban A, Molina-Negro P. Primary hemifacial spasm. A neurophysiological study. J Neurol Neurosurg Psychiatry 1986; 49:58.

70. Schoenen J, Gonce M, Delwaide PJ. Painfull legs and moving toes: a syndrome with different physiopathologic mechanisms. Neurology 1984; 34:1108–1112.

71. Kaas JH, Merzenich MM, Killackey HP. The reorganization of somatosensory cortex following peripheral nerve damage in adult and developing animals. Annu Rev Neurosci 1984; 6:325–356.

72. Loeser JD, Ward AA. Some effects of deafferentation on neurons of the cat spinal cord. Arch Neurol 1967; 17:629–636.

73. Lindvall O, Bjorklund A, Skagerberg G. Dopamine-containing neurons in the spinal cord: anatomy and some functional aspects. Ann Neurol 1983; 14:255–260.

74. Henry JL. Effects of substance P on functionally identified units in cat spinal cord. Brain Res 1976; 114:439–451.

75. Grassi C, Possatore M. Action of sympathetic system on skeletal muscle. Ital J Neurol Sci 1988; 9:23–28.

76. Hallett M, Lindsey JW, Adelstein BD, Riley PO. Controlled trial of isoniazid therapy for severe postural tremor in multiple sclerosis. Neurology 1985; 35:1374–1377.

77. Batt M, Snow B, Varelas M, Calne D. Palatal myoclonus: treatment with 5-hydroxytryptophan and carbidopa. Mov Disord 1990; 5:339–340.

78. Scott MR, Brody JA. Benign early onset Parkinson's disease: a syndrome distinct from classic postencephalitic parkinsonism. Neurology 1971; 21:366–368.

30

Hemisphere Lesions and Tremor

J. D. Cole
Southampton General Hospital
Southampton, England

I. INTRODUCTION

Damage at most levels of the neuraxis concerned with movement is known to lead to abnormal tremor. For instance, within the present volume, studies are detailed of tremor following neurological lesions of peripheral nerve, basal ganglia, brainstem, and cerebellum, as well as tremors in which the central areas of involvement are less well defined anatomically. The generation of tremor under such conditions has been ascribed to an unbalancing within control loops and to a disinhibition of central generators.

The cerebral hemispheres are not usually invoked in such a litany, because lesions of this area do not commonly lead to tremor. This may initially surprise, since the movement area of cerebral cortex is so involved with the other areas of the nervous system concerned with movement. For instance, the main output of the basal ganglia is through the cerebral cortex movement area and there are strong connections between that area and the cerebellum.

Not only are there anatomically important connections between the cerebral cortex and subcortical movement areas in which lesions lead to tremor, but there is evidence that the cortex is essential for the clinical expression of some tremors for which the main damage is thought to originate elsewhere. Parkinson noted that after a classic middle cerebral artery stroke, leading to hemiparesis, the tremor of paralysis agitans was relieved (see Ref. 1). There is also some evidence that the reduction in tremor associated with cortical lesions in experimentally induced parkinsonism in primates can be dissociated from the weakness. Thus, Cordeau reported that light mechanical pressure on the motor cortex of monkeys stopped

429

reversibly a parkinsonian type tremor, without necessarily weakening the limb (2). Essential tremor may also disappear after cerebral stroke (3), and after cerebellar stroke (4).

A corollary of such work is that the cerebral cortex is involved in the propagation at least of some of the tremors following lesions elsewhere. Experimental work provides support for such ideas. Hore and Flament found some motor cortex neurons that discharged strongly in relation to the cerebellar tremor produced by cooling of cerebellar nuclei (5). These cells also responded to peripheral inputs. Although there was no implication from this work that the motor cortex was the generator of cerebellar tremor in this situation, these studies have shown an involvement of precentral cells in cerebellar tremor. Such work would not have surprised Hughlings Jackson, for whom the effects of a central lesion were always explained in terms of residual function in other parts of the brain.

Tremor associated with damage to the cerebral hemisphere may be divided into that caused by discharges originating from that area, and that expressed following removal of a cortical influence on other areas. As will be seen, there is some evidence for both of these.

In this chapter, by a physiologist admittedly, there will be little detailed neuroanatomical discussion on the origin of tremor following cortical damage. Lesions may not be so accurately localized that it is possible to say whether the primary motor cortex or premotor areas are involved. Even the recent powerful imaging techniques have tended to reveal lesions far larger and more diffuse than expected from classic clinical neurological deduction.

This also raises the question of whether an anatomical approach is sufficient. What, for instance, of the inputs and outputs of the cortex movement area through the thalamus and internal capsule? Schlitt et al. described a severe tremor as a late complication of an intracerebral hemorrhage of the right thalamus (6). Duncan et al. reported a person with essential tremor in whom the tremor was cured following thalamic infarction (7). In Ohye et al.'s sample of eight cases, in whom thalamotomy relieved their poststroke tremor, two had originally suffered a stroke of the thalamus (8).

Massey et al. have also described asterixis, lapses of posture when the arms were outstretched, after hemiplegic strokes associated with posterior capsule lesions (9). They recorded electromyographic (EMG) activity during these tests and showed that the lapses were associated with cessation of EMG activity for 35–200 ms or so on each occasion. This would suggest that the motor cortex outflow may be involved, not only in movements, but in postural maintenance as well.

Although the involvement of inputs and outputs from the movement cortex in these tremors cannot be assumed, these examples do serve to show that effects immediately down- and upstream from the cortex should also be considered.

The remainder of this short chapter, however, will review evidence for tremor following damage primarily to the cerebral hemispheres.

II. ABNORMAL MOVEMENTS FOUND CONTRALATERAL TO CEREBRAL CORTEX DAMAGE

A cardinal sign of cortical lesions is an abnormality of movement in the contralateral side. These may go from slight clumsiness and lack of fine control, to the complete lack of movement seen in a dense hemiplegia. It is not a common experience that with degrees of hemiparesis there is an associated tremor. However, some such cases have been reported.

Contralateral (and unilateral) involuntary movements and shaking have been described after cerebral ischemia in the carotid territory (10,11). These authors showed small infarcts in the appropriate hemisphere on computed tomography (CT) scanning. Nagaratam et al. described a single case of a 78-year-old man who presented with uncontrollable rapid shaking movements of the hand at 3–5 Hz, associated with weakness of that hand (12). A CT scan showed two small infarcts in the left posterior parietal area and another deep in the left frontal area. The movement disorder was not described as a tremor because it was irregular and coarse. Although electroencephalograms (EEGs) showed an abnormal pattern suggesting a focal lesion, it was not epileptiform (such a record does not exclude epilepsy entirely). The cases of Baquis et al. did not show epileptiform features either (11). Thus, limb shaking can occur contralateral to small hemispheric ischemic events, which are not usually considered to be epileptic.

III. FOCAL EPILEPSY AFTER CORTICAL LESIONS

Focal epilepsy in this context is a comparatively rare condition in which an abnormality of the motor cerebral cortex area leads to repetitive movement of the contralateral limb because of synchronous discharge of cortical cells. For this to occur, the damage presumably has to be large enough to allow such firing and overcome local and distant inhibitory mechanisms, but not large enough to prevent such firing of motor cortex cells at all.

Harrington et al. described three such cases (13). One was a young woman who presented with grand mal fits during pregnancy, followed by major and minor seizures after delivery. The minor episodes consisted of episodes of rhythmic tremor of the right arm, with parasthesia of this area and mutism. An EEG was normal at rest, but showed focal spikes in the left rolandic area during drowsiness. A large frontal astrocytoma was found at surgery. The second subject had developed seizures after a head injury, with both major and minor attacks. Again, an EEG taken at rest was normal, but showed left-sided spikes during drowsiness. During one recording, she had an attack that manifested as tremor of the right arm moving to the jaw and lasting 70 s. The EEG showed a left temporal slow-wave abnormality. Pneumoencephalography showed dilation of the temporal horn of the lateral ventricle, presumed to be due to sclerosis, and matters were taken no further. The third case's history began with a severe headache and 15-min period of lost consciousness some years before. He presented with a more recent onset of partial and generalized seizures. An EEG at rest again was normal. An attack was witnessed with tremor of the right arm at 8–9 Hz and, during these attacks, an EEG showed temporal rhythmic slow waves at 4–5 Hz. A left carotid angiogram showed a left middle cerebral artery aneurysm.

In these three cases, tremor was seen at the onset of the epileptic attack. The authors concluded that the source of the tremor may have been not the motor cortex, but the supplementary motor area, and cited experiments by Penfield and Jasper in which stimulation of this area led to contralateral arm movement.

They also make the point that the cause of the tremor was different in each of the subjects, so that no clue to the type of abnormality can be gained from the seizure.

IV. EPILEPSIA PARTIALIS CONTINUA

Epilepsia partialis continua may be described as a continuous focal epilepsy. I have seen two cases in which continuous tremor of the hand and arm were associated with contralateral cortical lesions. They are shown in Figure 1.

The first subject had presented with partial sensory seizures and had been found to have a right frontoparietal convexity meningioma. After partial removal, she was left with a left hemiparesis, episodic incontinence, and sensory seizures. On examination she had reduced joint position sense, and a mild weakness on the left, but normal tone and reflexes. However, there was a profound inability to use the left arm, so much so that the question of functional loss was raised at one time, by a surgeon. Use of a test of fine motor control of the finger (14), showed a clear left-sided tremor (see Fig. 1), which was not apparent clinically. The EEG showed a right frontoparietal focal discharge, and a diagnosis of epilepsia partialis continua was made. Penfield (15), wrote:

> the effect of the [cortical stimulating] electrode is to interfere with the patient's ability to make voluntary employment of the cortex near the electrode. Sometimes the electrode produces no movement and then this interference is the only effect of the stimulating current.

Presumably sensory epilepsy has a similar effect.

The second case was startlingly similar. She too presented with sensory epilepsy and was found to have a meningioma in the right parietal area. After surgery, she was left with a mild and transient weakness and sensory parasthesia. An EEG showed a right parietal sharp wave discharge, and tests of tremor showed a 6-Hz peak in the contralateral index finger.

In these cases, the EEG showed a sharp wave discharge at a frequency similar to the contralateral tremor. However, the tremor was rhythmic, whereas the cortical

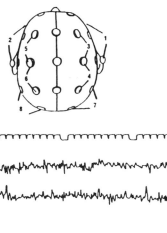

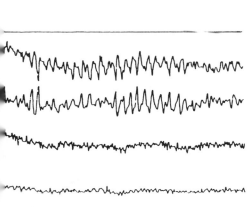

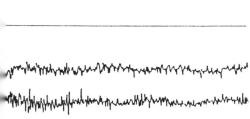

Left index finger 100g/V

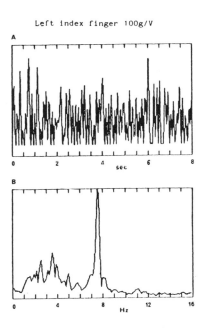

Figure 1 Epilepsia partialis continua in a patient with a right parietal meningioma. On the left of the figure is shown an EEG with a right parietal focal sharp-wave disturbance (electrodes 3 and 4). On the right results from measurement of stability in the left index finger. Above raw data from *XY* plot, below fast Fourier transform (FFT) showing subclinical 7.6-Hz tremor. (Cole, unpublished.)

discharge, viewed from the scalp, at least, was irregular. For this and other reasons (EEG and tremor tests were not synchronized), it is not possible to say that the discharge was time-locked to the tremor. However, it would seem reasonable in these patients to suggest that the tremor arose from the cortex. A voluntarily produced repetitive movement mimicking a tremor in a control subject does not lead to any EEG synchrony.

In the remainder of this chapter examples of tremors associated with cortical damage will be given in which the site of origin of the tremor is much less clear.

V. FRONTAL TUMORS AND TREMOR

There is an extensive literature on the relation between frontal tumors and tremor, of both ipsilateral and contralateral sides. The tumors usually present late and so are quite large. Both Foy (16) and Garfield (17), in their chapters in Northfield describe such cases. Foy describes the asterixis and tremor that may accompany massive frontal tumors. Garfield writes of massive tumors that may be of the frontal lobe or situated more deeply in its posterior part, which can give arise to a parkinsonian-type tremor.

In possibly the largest study of its kind, Biemond (18), described tremor in 22 of 108 frontal tumors. The tremor was found unilaterally in 12 (7 ipsilateral and 5 contralateral), and bilaterally in 10. In some, there was an associated parkinsonianlike syndrome and, in others, autonomic problems. He discussed the etiology of tremor in this situation, mentioned direct compression and compromised blood supply.

However such lesions do not have to be large. Andrew et al., in a short paper on thalamic tremor (19), mentioned three cases of parkinsonian-type tremor with rigidity, associated with small frontal tumors on or near the surface of the brain.

These accounts suffer from two difficulties. The tremors are merely described and not quantified and, second, the lesions causing them have not been located with the newer-imaging techniques, nor related to functional areas. There is clearly a need to investigate this field further so that the mechanism and prevalence of this type of tremor may become better understood.

VI. IPSILATERAL ABNORMALITIES ASSOCIATED WITH CEREBRAL HEMISPHERE DYSFUNCTION

The conventional functional division of the brain's movement area about the midline, with one side controlling the opposite limb only, has been known to be an oversimplification for some time. Small ipsilateral, as well as the more obvious contralateral, deficits have been described following lesions of one cerebral hemisphere if the sensorimotor test requires enough skill. Thus, ipsilateral deficits have been described in pegboard and groove steadiness (20,21). These tests have often been in the psychological domain, but the concept has been part of clinical teaching for some time.

In a general medical textbook, Growden and Young (22) describe how, in hemiplegia, the paretic side may worsen when the contralateral motor system is affected by disease. One of the classic accounts of this phenomenon came from introspective clinical acumen. The Norwegian neuroanatomist, Brodal (23), suffered a pure motor stroke, leading to a left hemiplegia, and wrote of his experience.

He found that, in the acute stages of the illness, although there was no dysgraphia or other parietal symptoms and signs (these terms being synonyms in such a man), his writing with the dominant unaffected hand was affected. He thought that there must be a bilateral representation of movement of the hand within the nervous system and concluded that this might involve the cerebellum. Since the original problem was a stroke, pressure effects within the cranial vault, with effects across the midline, may be excluded. Since then, there have been several accounts in which effects on movement have been found ipsilateral to lesions localized to one cortical hemisphere.

Conventional studies of tremor have been conducted with an accelerometer, or by interruption of a light beam to minimize the inertia that is inevitable if a device is attached to a moving part. Tremor has been measured at rest, during postures, and during movement. For some patients, however, the first difficulties they notice with disabilities of movement are during fine tasks, such as buttoning clothes or holding pens. For these tasks, small accurate movements are made with minimal movement and maximal accuracy.

Cole et al. devised a task that they hoped would be similar to such fine tasks (14). A strain-gauge connected to a typewriter key was set into the top of a flat box. The aim was to keep the strain-gauge still with the index finger, with feedback given from a milliammeter dial. The task was difficult because the movement allowed was 0.1–1.0 mm, and the forces employed were low (10–100 gwt). The task was achieved only with small perturbations or tremor, which were seen on-line with an *XY* plotter (Fig. 2) and stored for subsequent fast Fourier transform (FFT) analysis.

Of relevance to the present review was the study on two groups of patients with frontoparietal lesions. In the first were 16 subjects with minimal signs of such lesions. Five had no signs, having presented with sensory epilepsy, 4 had no motor signs, and the remainder had minimal weakness (down to MRC grade 4).

In this latter group, it was found that stability was greater contralateral to the lesions (see Fig. 2). When compared with control subjects, the most significant factor was that stability was decreased in the side ipsilateral to the lesion, and that contralateral stability was not significantly different from controls.

This unexpected finding was compounded when a second group of patients were assessed, in whom the signs of frontoparietal disturbance were more severe.

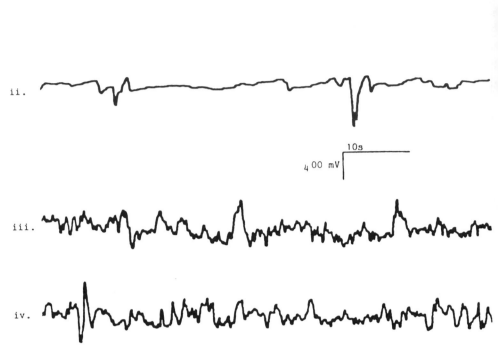

Figure 2 An *XY* plot of index finger stability in a patient with a right middle cerebral artery stroke leading to hemiparesis. (i) left finger, eyes open; (ii) left, eyes shut; (iii) right finger, eyes open; (iv) right, eyes shut. (From Ref. 14.)

In this group of 13, 3 had evidence of moderate midline shift on CT scan, 7 a minimal such shift, and 3 had no such effect. There was still an ipsilateral instability compared with controls. In addition, however, there was a clear peak in tremor frequency at 6–7 Hz ipsilaterally that was not seen in controls (Fig. 3). This was unlikely to be due to a pressure effect, since it was seen in patients with completed hemiplegic strokes, when it occasionally became a sine wave tremor, which was subclinical (Fig. 4). These findings, even in those tremors found with mature strokes, were not reported clinically and were seen in approximately half of those patients so tested.

The mechanism of these effects cannot be deduced by the techniques used in those experiments. However, it would seem most likely that there is a subcortical component in the genesis of the tremor, and instability, as Brodal suggested.

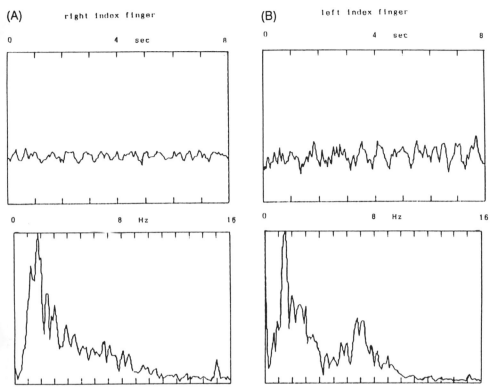

Figure 3 Fast Fourier transform (FFT) and *XY* plots of tremor in a patient with a left middle cerebral artery stroke. (A) *XY* plots, (B) FFT plots. Note the peak in tremor at 6–7 Hz ipsilaterally. (From Ref. 14.)

Although all subjects had CT scans, it was not considered possible to relate the effects to lesions of any particular cortical area.

There is, however, other evidence that the ipsilateral arm is not normal after unilateral stroke. Jones et al. performed a battery of integrated sensorimotor tests on human subjects with unilateral cerebral hemisphere stroke (24). The tests included joint movement sense, object perception, range of movement, grip strength, reaction time, speed, and steadiness. The symptomatic arm was grossly affected. However, they also found that the asymptomatic arm was impaired when compared with controls, even though clinically the asymptomatic arm was normal.

They tested at 11 days and as 12 months after the stroke. Most of the ipsilateral effects, although they remained, did improve with time. However, among the tests that did not improve in the ipsilateral arm over a year was steadiness. This was an

0   4   sec   8

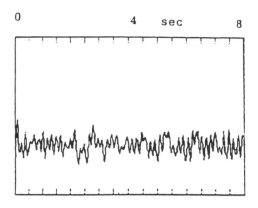

0   8   Hz   16

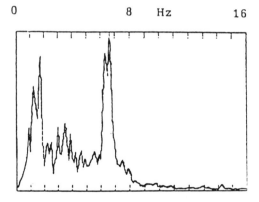

Figure 4   Fast Fourier transform and *XY* plots from the right index finger of a man with a completed stroke affecting the right hemisphere and leading to a dense left hemiplegia. (From Ref. 14.)

apparent anomaly that they questioned. However, this was a not dissimilar paradigm for testing movement to that used by Cole et al. (14). The latter authors found the most impressive ipsilateral sine-wave tremors in completed strokes only, so this phenomenon may develop with time and be resistant to recovery in the arm ipsilateral to unilateral stroke.

These two groups have provided evidence that steadiness may be a function for which localization of central control is rather different from that of other postures or movements. With the aid of physiological tools, they may have found what Stewart (25) reported following clinical observation in 1906, for he wrote in his account of frontal tumors that, when the motor cortex is affected, there is a homolateral tremor that is fine, rapid, and vibratory. With the arms extended horizontally, the hands facing down, and the fingers extended, he described a fine tremor seen only in the homolateral hand, which could be felt if one's palm was placed gently on the back of the subject's hand.

Yet there are other motor functions in which an ipsilateral effect may be shown following cortical lesions. Colebatch and Gandevia, measured the distribution of weakness in 12 muscle groups in the arm of subjects with upper motor lesions that were unilateral, both subjectively and to routine clinical examination (26). Sensory loss in this group was variable, but rarely marked. When strength in paretic muscles was compared with the opposite side, a certain distribution of weakness was then found. However, as they said, this use of the stronger side as a reference assumed that there was no ipsilateral effect. So they compared a group of severely affected hemiplegics with age-matched controls in their strength ipsilateral to the stroke. Most of the muscles on the spared side were weaker than in controls, with a mean reduction of 12%. Both proximal and distal muscles were affected, with shoulder adduction and wrist extension the most severely so.

They discussed the physiological and anatomical evidence for bilateral projections from each cerebral hemisphere, with possible different densities of projections from each hemisphere to each muscle group. Jones et al. (24) also considered, in some detail, the organization of motor control and its dependence on peripheral feedback, which might underlie the effects they had observed. An ipsilateral projection to motoneurons affecting proximal arm muscles was also suggested by physiological experiments (27).

In subhuman primates, there is some evidence that, in the primary motor cortex (M1), there are cells with direct influences on ipsilateral hand muscles. Aizawa et al. recorded from single cells in M1 (28) and related their discharge to pressing of a key by the ipsilateral or contralateral hand in conscious cooperative monkeys. They recorded from an area of M1 medial to the face area and rostrolateral to the digit area. In an sample of 81 cells, they found 15 that responded only if the contralateral hand was used, and 14 responded if the ipsilateral hand was moved. Intracortical microstimulation with recording from intramuscular electrodes also showed ipsilateral movements following stimulation. The premotor areas of the cortex are known to be involved in bilateral movement coordination. Perhaps some of this occurs through M1. Thus, there is evidence of ipsilateral, as well as the larger contralateral, cortical influence on movement of the hand and arm.

The physiological and anatomical origin of this instability and tremor may not be determined by such studies alone. It may, however, be possible to study this further with the use of positron emission tomography techniques. Recently, Colebatch et al. studied several persons with essential tremor (29). They found that, during periods of involuntary tremor, increased blood flow was observed in the contralateral cerebral cortex, both lateral premotor regions, and in both cerebellar hemispheres. In normal controls, who held a posture without movement, and in subjects with essential tremor, who had passive wrist movement imposed on them, only the cerebellum was not activated. Therefore, they concluded that the cerebellum may be involved in tremor generation. This technique obviously has great potential for investigating other problems of localization of tremor generators.

VII. CONCLUSION

The involvement of the cerebral hemispheres in the generation of tremor is rare and, in some cases, can be determined with techniques allowing the measurement of subclinical movement disorders. Apart from the obvious, but infrequent, focal epilepsies, tremor has been described accompanying frontal lesions that are presumed to compromise motor or premotor areas, although some effect on subcortical structures cannot be excluded in some of these cases. There is also a need for more analysis of the phenomenology of these tremors.

Tremor has also been ascribed in some situations, both contra- and ipsilaterally to lesions of the movement cortex, although in the latter, this is a rare, poorly understood, and subclinical event.

Why tremor should be so uncommon after lesions of the cortex compared with other structures concerned with movement remains so unclear that it is possible only to speculate. Possibly, the subcortical structures are concerned with postural and preprogrammed movements that, when unbalanced, lend themselves to tremor, whereas despite the existence of transcortical loops (e.g., see Ref. 30), the cortex is more concerned with superimposition onto such programs of alterations in movement as a result of peripheral feedback and conscious control. That damage to the cerebral cortex does not commonly lead to tremor tells us something about the physiology of this part of the brain's movement area. Our task is to determine what that something is.

REFERENCES

1. DeLong MR, Georgopoulos AP. Motor functions of the basal ganglia. In: Brooks VB, ed. Handbook of Physiology, Bethesda MD: American Physiological Society, 1981: 1017–1061.
2. Cordeau JP. Microelectrode studies in monkeys with a postural tremor. Rev Can Biol 1961; 20:147–157.
3. Mylle G, van Bogaert L. Etudes anatomo-cliniques de syndromes hypercinetiques complexes. 1. Sur le tremblement familial. Monatsschr Psychiatr Neurol 1940; 103: 28–43.
4. Dupuis MJ, Delwaide PJ, Boucquey D, Gonsette RE. Homolateral disappearance of essential tremor after cerebellar stroke. Mov Disord 1989; 4:183–187.

5. Hore J, Flament D. Changes in motor cortex neural discharge associated with the development of cerebellar limb ataxia. J Neurophysiol 1988; 60:1285–1302.

6. Schlitt M, Brown JW, Zeiger HE, Galbraith JG. Appendicular tremor as a late complication of intracerebral hemorrhage. Surg Neurol 1986; 25:181–184.

7. Duncan R, Bone I, Melville ID. Essential tremor caused by infarction adjacent to the thalamus. J Neurol Neurosurg Psychiatry 1988; 51:591–592.

8. Ohye C, Shibasaki T, Hirai T, Kawashima Y, Hirato M, Matsuma M. Plastic change of thalamic organisation in patients with tremor after stroke. Appl Neurophysiol 1985; 48:288–292.

9. Massey EW, Goodman JC, Stewart C, Brannan WL. Unilateral asterixis: motor integrative dysfunction in focal vascular disease. Neurology 1979; 29:1188–1190.

10. Baquis GD, Passin MS, Scott RM. Limb shaking—a carotid TIA. Stroke 1985; 16: 444–448.

11. Yanagihara T, Klass DW. Rhythmic involuntary movement as a manifestation of transient ischemic attacks. Trans Am Neurol Assoc 1981; 106:46–48.

12. Nagaratnam N, Ghougassian DF, Lewis-Jones M. The shaking limb—a lacunar syndrome. Postgrad Med J 1988; 64:311–312.

13. Harrington RB, Karnes WE, Klass DW. Ictal tremor. Arch Neurol 1966; 14:184–189.

14. Cole JD, Philip HI, Sedgwick EM. The effect of frontoparietal lesions on stability and tremor in the finger. J Neurol Neurosurg Psychiatry 1988; 51:1411–1419.

15. Penfield W. The Excitable Cortex in Conscious Man. Liverpool: Liverpool University Press, 1967.

16. Foy PM. The meningiomas: haemangioblastoma. In: Miller JD, ed. Northfield's Surgery of the Central Nervous System. 2nd ed. Oxford: Blackwell, 1987.

17. Garfield JS. Malignant intracranial tumours. In: Miller JD, ed. Northfield's Surgery of the Central Nervous System. 2nd ed. Oxford: Blackwell, 1987.

18. Biemond A. Brain Diseases. Amsterdam: Elsevier, 1970.

19. Andrew J, Fowler CJ, Harrison MJG, Kendall BE. Post-traumatic tremor due to vascular injury and its treatment by stereotactic thalamotomy. J Neurol Neurosurg Psychiatry 1982; 45:560–567.

20. Vaughan HG, Costa LD. Performance of patients with lateralised cerebral lesions. II. Sensory and motor tests. J Nerve Ment Dis 1962; 134:237–243.

21. Haarland KY, Delaney HD. Motor deficits after left or right hemisphere damage due to stroke or tumour. Neuropsychology 1981; 19:17–27.

22. Growden JH, Young RR. Paralysis and other disorders of movement. In: Braunwald E, Isselbacher KJ, Petersdorf RG, Wilson JD, Martin JB, Fauci AS, eds. Harrison's Principles of Internal Medicine. 11th ed. New York: McGraw-Hill, 1987.

23. Brodal A. Self-observations and neuroanatomical considerations after a stroke. Brain 1973; 96:675–694.

24. Jones RD, Donaldson IM, Parkin PJ. Impairment and recovery of ipsilateral sensory–motor function following cerebral infarction. Brain 1989; 112:113–132.

25. Stewart TG. The diagnosis and localisation of tumours of the frontal regions of the brain. Lancet 1906; 2:1209–1211.

26. Colebatch JG, Gandevia SC. The distribution of muscular weakness in upper motor neuron lesions affecting the arm. Brain 1989; 112:749–763.

27. Colebatch JG, Rothwell JC, Day BL, Thompson PD, Marsden CD. Cortical outflow to proximal muscles in man. Brain, 1990; 113:1843–1856.
28. Aizawa H, Mushiake H, Inase M, Tanji J. An output zone of the monkey primary motor cortex specialized for bilateral hand movement. Exp Brain Res 1990; 82: 219–221.
29. Colebatch JG, Findley LJ, Frackowiak RSJ, Marsden CD, Brooks DJ. Preliminary report: activation of the cerebellum in essential tremor. Lancet 1990; 2:1028–1030.
30. Matthews PBC, Farmer SF, Ingram DA. On the localisation of the stretch reflex of intrinsic hand muscles in a patient with mirror movements. J Physiol 1991; 428: 561–578.

31

Tremor in Peripheral Neuropathy

Ian Stewart Smith
Leeds General Infirmary
Leeds, England

I. INTRODUCTION

Tremor associated with certain types of peripheral neuropathy is increasingly recognized as a cause of disability, in addition to that imposed by the neuropathy itself. The association between tremor and hereditary motor and sensory neuropathy (HMSN), chronic inflammatory demyelinating polyneuropathy (CIDP), and immunoglobulin M (IgM) chronic paraproteinemic demyelinating polyneuropathy (IgM CPDP) is now well recognized, and this review is mainly concerned with these three conditions. Tremor can also be seen in the Guillain–Barré syndrome, particularly the recovery stages (1) and has been reported in a few cases of peripheral neuropathy associated with diabetes, uremia, and porphyria (2,3). Amiodarone, a drug used to treat cardiac dysrhythmias, can cause both tremor and peripheral neuropathy (4,5), as can alcohol.

Tremor was defined by Holmes as a "clinical phenomenon consisting in the involuntary oscillation of any part of the body around any plane" (6). Tremor should be distinguished from other types of movement disorder that can be found in patients with peripheral neuropathy, such as sensory ataxia, choreiform movements, or pseudoathetosis.

II. CHRONIC DEMYELINATING POLYNEUROPATHY WITH BENIGN IMMUNOGLOBULIN M PARAPROTEINEMIA

Immunoglobulin M CPDP is a chronic sensorimotor neuropathy, usually starting in the sixth or seventh decades, in which motor nerve conduction velocities are markedly reduced (7–10). The patients all have IgM paraproteinemia, usually without any evidence of malignant immunocytic dyscrasia, such as Waldenström's macroglobulinemia. The pathological changes found in peripheral nerve biopsy specimens are those of a demyelinating neuropathy. This has been generally assumed to be a primary demyelinating neuropathy, but there has been one postmortem study that showed changes in peripheral nerves suggestive of a primary axonal neuropathy, with secondary demyelination (11). Electron microscopy often shows widening of the spaces between the major dense lines of the outer and inner lamellae of the myelin sheaths, owing to splitting at the intraperiod line. The paraproteins in the sera of these patients are made up of monoclonal IgM antibodies that can specifically bind to myelin-associated glycoprotein and other glycoproteins and glycolipids, all of which are present in normal peripheral nerves (12). Monoclonal IgM antibodies are found in the peripheral nerves of these patients. They are localized to the outer and sometimes inner parts of surviving myelin sheaths. Intraneural injection of serum from these patients into a feline peripheral nerve causes extensive demyelination (13,14). The evidence suggests that the neuropathy is caused by the monoclonal IgM antibodies that enter peripheral nerves and bind to myelin-associated glycoprotein and, possibly, other glycoproteins and glycolipids.

Tremor is a common finding in these patients (7). There are at least 26 clinical reports that among them describe a total of 66 cases of IgM CPDP. Tremor in the hands was present in 31 of these 66 cases (7,11,15–24). The proportion of patients reported to have tremor varies considerably. Thus, some have found that most patients in their series have tremor (7,11,22), whereas others have not reported tremor in any of their patients (25,26). This may be partly due to the variation in length of follow-up in these reports, since tremor is almost always one of the later symptoms of this condition. This was the case in 20 of 21 patients for whom data are available, the interval between the onset of neuropathy symptoms and the onset of tremor varying from 1.5 to 12 years (mean 4.7 years). This may explain why Powell et al. (25) did not report tremor in their five cases, as the duration of their symptoms ranged from 1 to 5 years. They would not all be expected to have developed tremor at this stage. Smith et al. (7) detected tremor in 10 of 12 of their cases, and the histories ranged from 3 to 18 years in duration, with a mean of 9.8 years. Another reason for the variation in the reporting of tremor may be that it is often mild and, thus, easily overlooked (7).

The clinical characteristics of the tremor in the 31 cases who have been reported are fairly consistent. No patient had titubation or voice tremor. Only two patients had tremor in the legs (16,24). Six patients had rest tremor in the hands (7,17,19, 24). In three it was of the "pill-rolling" type, which is often seen in Parkinson's disease (7,19,24). Tremor was usually present in the hands on maintaining a posture, such as outstretched arms, and during actions, such as the finger-to-nose test. Tremor was often of greater amplitude during movement than during a postural contraction (7,11,15,16). The amplitude of tremor varied greatly. In some, it was mild [cases 5–7,9,10, and 12 of Smith et al. (7), cases 4 and 5 of Mendell et al. (11), and both cases of Jensen et al. (23)], and in others it was quite marked [cases 1–3, and 8 of Smith et al. (7), cases 2 and 3 of Mendell et al. (11), the case of Spencer and Moench (16), cases 2 and 4, Table 2 of Dalakas et al. (18), and case 6 of Nobile-Orazio et al. (22)]. The patients with marked tremor were significantly disabled, having great difficulty in feeding or dressing themselves or writing legibly because of tremor. Although weakness and sensory loss were sometimes contributing to their disability, it was clear that tremor was greatly increasing this disability. In general, the tremor was similar to that found in patients with benign essential tremor. Theirs is mainly a postural and action tremor, but some patients also have rest tremor. The severity of tremor in different patients varies considerably (27).

No clear relation between amplitude of tremor and weakness or sensory loss has been established (7,18). Power in the muscles responsible for the tremor can be normal [the case of Spencer and Moench (16) and case 2, Table 2 of Dalakas et al. (18)], and sometimes no sensory loss can be demonstrated in the tremulous hand.

Recordings of tremor frequency in the thumb, using a force transducer, have been made in 18 patients with various types of peripheral neuropathy (28). In the 10 patients with IgM CPDP, frequency varied from 3.3 to 8 Hz (mean 5.1 Hz). Their ulnar motor nerve conduction velocities varied from 9 to 48 m/s (mean 19.7 m/s). Both in these 10 patients and in the whole group of 18, there was a direct relation between frequency of tremor and ulnar motor nerve conduction velocity, such that patients with low-conduction velocities had low-frequency tremor and vice versa. There was no clear relation between amplitude and frequency of tremor.

There have been many reports on the results of treatment. The treatments that have been used include corticosteroids, cytotoxic agents (chlorambucil, melphalan, cyclophosphamide, and azathioprine), intravenous immunoglobulin (29), and plasma exchange. Although there have been reports of improvement in the neuropathy following treatment, especially when a combination of corticosteroids, a cytotoxic drug, and plasma exchange has been used (18,21,25,29–35), many other patients have shown no improvement (17,18,26,29,31,32,36,37). Similarly, such treatment has been found to improve tremor (16), or else not to affect it (17,18). Tremor in two patients responded to propranolol (18). Dyck (38) has concluded that the efficacy of any treatment regimen is as yet uncertain.

A. Other Types of Paraproteinemic Neuropathy

Peripheral neuropathy is also associated with benign IgG and IgA paraproteinemia and with benign IgM paraproteins, without antimyelin-associated glycoprotein activity (10). The patients have a chronic progressive neuropathy. The neuropathy in patients with IgG paraproteinemia often responds to treatment with cortico-steroids. Two cases with tremor have been described. Dalakas et al. reported one patient with an IgG paraproteinemia and slow motor conduction velocities, who had postural tremor (18). Both the neuropathy and the tremor responded to treatment with prednisone and azathioprine. Provinciali et al. reported a patient with IgA paraproteinemia and disabling postural and action tremor both in the hands and feet (24). Tremor appeared some years after the neuropathy, over a period when conduction velocities fell from the normal range to 10 m/s. There was no response to prolonged treatment with azathioprine.

III. CHRONIC INFLAMMATORY DEMYELINATING POLYNEUROPATHY

A chronic sensorimotor neuropathy, CIDP, may follow either a relapsing–remitting or a progressive course. Motor nerve conduction velocities are reduced, and peripheral nerves show demyelination, sometimes with focal accumulations of inflammatory cells. It is thought to have an autoimmune pathogenesis (39).

Tremor has often been observed in this condition, and the proportion of patients reported to have tremor varies from 3 (39) to 84% (40), other workers having found intermediate values [Prineas and Mcleod (41) 12%, Dalakas and Engel (42) 24%, Ormerod et al. (43) 30%, Gigli et al. (44) 33%]. The reason for this variation is unclear.

In the relapsing–remitting form of the neuropathy, tremor sometimes appears in the first attack, but more commonly does so in the second or third attacks (18). There is a tendency for the tremor to appear during a relapse and improve when the symptoms remit, either spontaneously or in response to treatment (18,45,46).

One patient has been found to have rest tremor (45). It resembled the pill-rolling tremor of Parkinson's disease. Most patients have a postural and action tremor in the hands (18,40,43,45–47). The presence of tremor was not related to the degree of proprioceptive loss or weakness (18,42). In one series, there was no difference between motor nerve conduction velocities in those patients with or without tremor (42).

The frequency of tremor in the hands varied from 3.3 to 6.4 Hz in one series of seven patients (18). The frequency could vary in some patients, but in those patients with high-amplitude tremor, the frequency was very constant. Other workers have found frequencies of 6–8 Hz in two patients (48) and 6 Hz in one patient (45).

The neuropathy usually responds to corticosteroid therapy, either alone or in conjunction with a cytotoxic drug. Plasma exchange may also improve it. Gener-ally, if the neuropathy responds to treatment, then tremor also improves (18). Propranolol has not been effective in controlling tremor (18,46).

IV. HEREDITARY MOTOR AND SENSORY NEUROPATHY

Hereditary Motor and Sensory Neuropathy, or Charcot–Marie–Tooth disease, is a chronic neuropathy that is genetically determined. There are two main types. Type 1 patients have low motor nerve conduction velocities (less than 38 m/s in the arms), with segmental demyelination present in peripheral nerves. Type 2 patients have normal or slightly reduced velocities, with axonal degeneration, but very little demyelination in peripheral nerves (49).

Tremor has been found in both types of HMSN, but it is more common in type 1 (49). Such cases constitute the Roussy–Lévy syndrome. Yudell et al. described four patients with tremor in the outstretched arms, absent at rest, and accentuated by finger–nose testing (50). One of these patients had voice tremor and another had titubation, facial and voice tremor, and slight action tremor in the legs. All had mild weakness in the intrinsic hand muscles, but no sensory loss was detected in the arms. None of the patients were conspicuously disabled by the disorder. Salisachs described seven patients with HMSN and tremor (51). Four were significantly disabled by tremor. The tremor usually appeared after the neuropathy. It was present at rest in the hands of one patient, and all had tremor in the outstretched arms. In the patient with the most severe tremor, it was much worse on action than during a postural contraction; the frequency was 4 Hz. One patient had voice tremor, and three had tremor in the legs. All had distal weakness in the arms, but most had no loss of sensation. Motor conduction velocities were significantly reduced (13.5–33 m/s) in all except one of the seven patients, but were normal or only slightly reduced in seven similar patients reported by Salisachs et al. (52), all of whom had tremor in the hands. The HMSN tremor often responds to treatment with propranolol (46). Several authors have emphasized the similarity of this type of tremor to benign essential tremor (46,50–52).

V. DISCUSSION

The association between tremor and IgM CPDP is well established. Nearly half the cases reported in the literature have tremor, and this may well be an underestimate of the prevalence of tremor in these patients (7). Some authors have found that a high proportion of CIDP patients have tremor (40–43). The association of HMSN and tremor has long been recognized, and such cases constitute the Roussy–Lévy syndrome (49). The association between tremor and other types of neuropathy is less well established.

The similarity between peripheral neuropathy tremor and benign essential tremor has often been observed (7,46,50,51). Like essential tremor, the tremor in peripheral neuropathy patients is mainly seen in the hands during posture and action and, occasionally, at rest. Sometimes tremor is found in the legs. The range of frequencies found in peripheral neuropathy tremor and essential tremor are very similar (18,27,28). Unlike essential tremor, titubation is very uncommon and has been reported in only two patients (41,50). The possibility has been considered that the association between HMSN and tremor is due to the combination of two separate dominant genes, one for HMSN and the other for essential tremor. The observations of the frequency of HMSN and essential tremor in a single large kinship did not support this conclusion (50).

Other reasons for the association between peripheral neuropathy and tremor that have been considered include the selective loss of proprioceptive fibers from muscles (46), the neuropathy specifically affecting the spinocerebellar pathways (53), and the presence of muscle weakness (2). These suggestions are not supported by the observation that many patients with peripheral neuropathy and tremor in the hands do not have weakness or sensory loss in the hands (7,16,18, 21,50,51). Furthermore, most patients with weakness and sensory loss due to various types of peripheral neuropathy do not have tremor.

Another possibility that has been considered is that an abnormality in the central nervous system, associated with peripheral neuropathy, might cause tremor. Some cases of CIDP have shown pathological changes in the brainstem, cerebellum, and spinal cord (54). Visual-evoked responses are often abnormal in patients with HMSN (55), IgM CPDP (56), and CIDP (44,57). Brainstem auditory-evoked potentials may also be abnormal in patients with CIDP (44,57). Somato-sensory-evoked potentials showing abnormal central conduction have been found in HMSN (58). Patients with CIDP can have increased central motor conduction times (43). Magnetic resonance imaging studies have shown abnormalities suggestive of demyelination in the brains of patients with CIDP (40,43,59,60), IgM CPDP (24,60), and IgG paraproteinemic neuropathy (24,60). Some of these patients have tremor.

There are several observations which suggest that central nervous system damage could occur in patients with IgM CPDP. Myelin-associated glycoprotein is present in normal brain. The monoclonal IgM antibodies from IgM CPDP patients will react with certain neurons in the human brain (61). They will also bind to certain components of the cerebral cortex and cerebellar molecular layer (20). The IgM antibodies can be taken up peripherally by normal nerve fibers and transported centrally to neuronal cell bodies in the brain (62). Cells secreting antimyelin-associated glycoprotein antibodies can be found in the cerebrospinal fluid of patients with IgM CPDP (63). In vivo demyelination of mammalian optic nerve has been produced by intraneural injection of antimyelin-associated glycoprotein antibodies (64). Thus, there is evidence to suggest that the IgM monoclonal antibodies present in the serum of these patients could affect the central nervous system. However, efforts to demonstrate the presence of IgM antibodies in neural tissues of the brains of patients with IgM CPDP have so far been unsuccessful (11,23). Pathological changes in the central nervous system causing the tremor is an attractive hypothesis, as it would explain the presence of tremor in a limb that does not show any sign of weakness or sensory loss.

Most patients with peripheral neuropathy and tremor have demyelinating neuropathies with reduced nerve conduction velocities. This has led to the consideration that tremor may be related to slowing of nerve conduction in the stretch reflex (1,48). Physiological tremor may be partly due to the stretch reflex acting as a negative-feedback servomechanism (65). Delay in such mechanisms can lead to oscillation in the system. The slowing of nerve conduction would increase the delay in the stretch reflex, and it may be that this would lead to enhancement of tremor so that it becomes symptomatic. This theory does not explain why many patients with slowing of nerve conduction do not have tremor and, conversely, why some patients with near normal conduction velocities do have tremor (1,7,42,48,52,66).

Despite the lack of correlation between slowing of nerve conduction and presence of tremor, a correlation between slowing of conduction and frequency of tremor has been found, showing that patients with the lowest velocities have the lowest tremor frequencies and vice versa (28,67). A clear relation between conduction velocity and amplitude of tremor was not established. Tremor was studied in three patients with severe polyneuropathy who recovered (65). Their conduction velocities increased from a mean of 27 to 45 m/s, and their tremor peak frequency increased from 7.0 to 8.7 Hz. These results suggest that the tremor frequency is partially determined by the conduction velocities in peripheral nerves, but they do not necessarily explain why tremor is present. However, the results do have implications for any theory of a central generator of tremor. They imply that a central oscillator is not producing the tremor, as the frequency generated peripherally by a central oscillator would not be affected by slowing of peripheral nerve conduction. The frequency at which nerve impulses arrive at a muscle is not altered by changes in the speed at which they are conducted. The relation between conduction velocity and tremor frequency instead suggests that the stretch reflex may be playing a part in the production of tremor, because an increase in the delay around the stretch reflex loop, caused by slowing of nerve conduction, would be expected to reduce the frequency of tremor, if it were a consequence of oscillation in the stretch reflex.

A unifying hypothesis for the generation of tremor in peripheral neuropathy has been proposed (67). The tremor may be due to an abnormality in the central nervous system, but when it appears, the frequency is influenced by the degree of slowing of conduction in peripheral nerves. This would explain why tremor is not related to weakness or sensory loss and why not all patients with demyelinating neuropathies have tremor. If there is no central abnormality, then there is no tremor. Why certain patients should have a central abnormality is unclear, but the relation between conduction velocity and frequency suggests that oscillation in the stretch reflex may take part in the generation of tremor.

This combined central–peripheral hypothesis on the generation of tremor requires that the stretch reflex is still functioning in these patients. Although tendon reflexes in the arms are usually absent, they can sometimes be normal in patients with peripheral neuropathy and obvious tremor. This does not necessarily mean the stretch reflex is intact, but does suggest that it could be. There have been no published studies on the stretch reflex in peripheral neuropathy, but it may be relevant to consider peripheral neuropathy patients with severe proprioceptive loss, in whom it is likely that the stretch reflex is impaired. In a series of 12 patients with IgM CPDP, the 2 who, on subsequent follow-up, had the most severe deafferentation and the slowest conduction velocities were also the only 2 patients in that series without tremor (7). They were very ataxic. A study on tremor in three patients with neuropathy and severe proprioceptive loss showed that none developed enhanced physiological tremor on fatigue, unlike five normal subjects (68). It may be that impairment of the stretch reflex was responsible for the lack of tremor in these patients. They may be similar to three severely deafferented tabetic patients who did not show a normal peak tremor frequency (69). Five less severely affected tabetic patients all had normal or enhanced tremor peaks.

VI. CONCLUSION

The observations on patients with peripheral neuropathy and tremor suggest that their tremor may be caused by an abnormality in the central nervous system, but that the frequency of this tremor is partly determined by the degree of conduction slowing in peripheral nerves. This hypothesis would be in accord with tremor being a manifestation of oscillation in the stretch reflex, as has been suggested for enhanced physiological tremor (65). The clinical characteristics of the tremor and the range of tremor frequencies encountered in peripheral neuropathy patients are very similar to those of benign essential tremor.

REFERENCES

1. Thomas PK. Clinical features and differential diagnosis. In: Dyck PJ, Thomas PK, Lambert EJ, eds. Peripheral Neuropathy. Philadelphia: WB Saunders, 1975:495–512.
2. Said G, Bathien N, Cesaro P. Peripheral neuropathies and tremor. Neurology 1982; 32:480–485.
3. Ridley A. The neuropathy of acute intermittent porphyria. Q J Med 1969; 38:307–333.
4. Pellissier JF, Pouget J, Cros D, et al. Peripheral neuropathy induced by amiodarone chlorhydrate. A clinicopathological study. J Neurol Sci 1984; 63:251–266.
5. Coulter DM, Edwards IR, Savage RL. Survey of neurological problems with amiodarone in the New Zealand Intensive Medicines Monitoring Programme. NZ Med J 1990; 103:98–100.
6. Holmes G. On certain tremors in organic cerebral lesions. Brain 1904; 27:327–375.

7. Smith IS, Kahn SN, Lacey BW, et al. Chronic demyelinating neuropathy associated with benign IgM paraproteinaemia. Brain 1983; 106:169–195.

8. Kelly JJ. Peripheral neuropathies associated with monoclonal proteins: a clinical review. Muscle Nerve 1985; 8:138–150.

9. Meier C. Polyneuropathy in paraproteinaemia. J Neurol 1985; 232:204–214.

10. McLeod JG, Pollard JD. Peripheral neuropathy associated with paraproteinaemia. In: Matthews WB, ed. Handbook of Clinical Neurology. Vol. 7. Neuropathies. Amsterdam: Elsevier, 1987:429–444.

11. Mendell JR, Sahenk Z, Whitaker JN, et al. Polyneuropathy and IgM monoclonal gammopathy: studies on the pathogenetic role of anti-myelin-associated glycoprotein antibody. Ann Neurol 1985; 17:243–254.

12. McGinnis S, Kohriyama T, Yu RK, Pesce MA, Latov N. Antibodies to sulfated glucuronic acid containing glycosphingolipids in neuropathy associated with anti-MAG antibodies and in normal subjects. J Neuroimmunol 1988; 17:119–126.

13. Hays PA, Latov N, Takatsu M, Sherman WH. Experimental demyelination of nerve induced by serum of patients with neuropathy and an anti-MAG IgM M-protein. Neurology 1987; 37:242–256.

14. Willison HJ, Trapp BD, Bacher JD, Dalakas MC, Griffin JW, Quarles RH. Demyelination induced by intraneural injection of human antimyelin-associated glycoprotein antibodies. Muscle Nerve 1988; 11:1169–1176.

15. Fitting JW, Bischoff A, Regli F, de Crousaz G. Neuropathy, amyloidosis and monoclonal gammopathy. J Neurol Neurosurg Psychiatry 1979; 42:193–202.

16. Spencer SS, Moench JC. Progressive and treatable cerebellar ataxia in macroglobulinemia. Neurology 1980; 30:536–538.

17. Melmed C, Frail D, Duncan I, et al. Peripheral neuropathy with IgM kappa monoclonal immunoglobulin directed against myelin-associated glycoprotein. Neurology 1983; 33:1397–1405.

18. Dalakas MC, Teräväinen H, Engel WK. Tremor as a feature of chronic relapsing and dysgammaglobulinemic polyneuropathies. Arch Neurol 1984; 41:711–714.

19. Julien J, Vital C, Vallat JM, Lagueny A, Ferrer X, Leboutet MJ. Chronic demyelinating neuropathy with IgM-producing lymphocytes in peripheral nerve and delayed appearance of "benign" monoclonal gammopathy. Neurology 1984; 34:1387–1389.

20. Meier C, Vandevelde M, Steck A, Zurbriggen A. Demyelinating polyneuropathy associated with monoclonal IgM-paraproteinaemia. J Neurol Sci 1984; 63:353–367.

21. Pollard JD, McLeod JG, Feeney D. Peripheral neuropathy in IgM kappa paraproteinaemia: clinical and ultrastructural studies in two patients. Clin Exp Neurol 1985; 21:41–54.

22. Nobile-Orazio E, Marmiroli P, Baldini L, et al. Peripheral neuropathy in macroglobulinaemia: incidence and antigen-specificity of M proteins. Neurology 1987; 37:1506–1514.

23. Jensen TS, Schrøder HD, Jønsson V, et al. IgM monoclonal gammopathy and neuropathy in two siblings. J Neurol Neurosurg Psychiatry 1988; 51:1308–1315.

24. Provinciali L, Di Bella P, Logullo F, Vesprini L, Pasquini U, Scarpelli M. Evidence of central nervous system involvement in chronic demyelinating neuropathies with "benign" gammopathies. Riv Neurol 1989; 59:36–44.

25. Powell HC, Rodriguez M, Hughes RAC. Microangiopathy of vasa nervorum in dys-
     globulinemic neuropathy. Ann Neurol 1984; 15:386–394.
26. Hafler DA, Johnson D, Kelly JJ, Panitch H, Kyle R, Weiner HL. Monoclonal
     gammopathy and neuropathy: myelin-associated glycoprotein reactivity and clinical
     characteristics. Neurology 1986; 36:75–78.
27. Marsden CD, Obeso J, Rothwell JC. Benign essential tremor is not a single entity. In:
     Yahr MD, ed. Current Concepts in Parkinson's Disease. Amsterdam: Excerpta Medica,
     1983:31–46.
28. Smith IS. Tremor associated with peripheral neuropathy. Electroencephalogr Clin
     Neurophysiol 1989; 72:41P.
29. Cook D, Dalakas M, Galdi A, Biondi D, Porter H. High-dose intravenous immuno-
     globulin in the treatment of demyelinating neuropathy associated with monoclonal
     gammopathy. Neurology 1990; 40:212–214.
30. Latov N, Sherman WH, Nemni R, et al. Plasma-cell dyscrasia and peripheral neurop-
     athy with a monoclonal antibody to peripheral-nerve myelin. N Engl J Med 1980;
     303:618–621.
31. Dalakas MC, Engel WK. Polyneuropathy with monoclonal gammopathy: studies of
     11 patients. Ann Neurol 1981; 10:45–52.
32. Bosch EP, Ansbacher LE, Goeken JA, Cancilla PA. Peripheral neuropathy associated
     with monoclonal gammopathy. Studies of intraneural injections of monoclonal immu-
     noglobulin sera. J Neuropathol Exp Neurol 1982; 41:446–459.
33. Meier C, Steck RA, Hess C, Miloni E, Tschopp L. Polyneuropathy in Waldenström's
     macroglobulinaemia: reduction of endoneurial IgM-deposits after treatment with
     chlorambucil and plasmapheresis. Acta Neuropathol 1984; 64:297–307.
34. Sherman WH, Olarte MR, McKiernan G, Sweeney K, Latov N, Hays AP. Plasma
     exchange treatment of peripheral neuropathy associated with plasma cell dyscrasia. J
     Neurol Neurosurg Psychiatry 1984; 47:813–819.
35. Ernerudh J, Brodtkorb E, Olsson T, Vedeler CA, Nyland H, Berlin G. Peripheral
     neuropathy and monoclonal IgM with antibody activity against peripheral nerve
     myelin; effect of plasma exchange. J Neuroimmunol 1986; 11:171–178.
36. Stefansson K, Marton L, Antel JP, et al. Neuropathy accompanying IgM lambda
     monoclonal gammopathy. Acta Neuropathol 1983; 59:255–261.
37. Busis NA, Halperin JJ, Stefansson K, et al. Peripheral neuropathy, high serum IgM,
     and paraproteinemia in mother and son. Neurology 1985; 35:679–683.
38. Dyck PJ, Intravenous immunoglobulin in chronic inflammatory demyelinating poly-
     radiculoneuropathy and in neuropathy associated with IgM monoclonal gammopathy
     of unknown significance. Neurology 1990; 40:327–328.
39. McCombe PA, Pollard JD, McLeod JG. Chronic inflammatory demyelinating poly-
     radiculoneuropathy. A clinical and electrophysiological study of 92 cases. Brain
     1987; 110:1617–1630.
40. Feasby TE, Hahn AF, Koopman WJ, Lee DH. Central lesions in chronic inflammatory
     demyelinating polyneuropathy: an MRI study. Neurology 1990; 40:476–478.
41. Prineas JW, McLeod JG. Chronic relapsing polyneuritis. J Neurol Sci 1976; 27:
     427–458.
42. Dalakas MC, Engel WK. Chronic relapsing (dysimmune) polyneuropathy: patho-
     genesis and treatment. Ann Neurol 1981; 9(suppl):134–145.

43. Ormerod IEC, Waddy HM, Kermode AG, Murray NMF, Thomas PK. Involvement of the central nervous system in chronic inflammatory demyelinating polyneuropathy: a clinical, electrophysiological and magnetic resonance imaging study. J Neurol Neurosurg Psychiatry 1990; 53:789–783.

44. Gigli GL, Carlesimo A, Valente M, et al. Evoked potentials suggest cranial nerves and CNS involvement in chronic relapsing polyradiculoneuropathy. Eur Neurol 1989; 29:145–149.

45. Matthews WB, Howell DA, Hughes RC. Relapsing corticosteroid-dependent polyneuritis. J Neurol Neurosurg Psychiatry 1970; 33:330–337.

46. Shahani BT, Young RR. Action tremors: a clinical neurophysiological review. In: Desmedt JE, ed. Physiological Tremor, Pathological Tremors and Clonus. Prog Clin Neurophysiol 1978; 5:129–137.

47. Thomas PK, Lascelles RG, Hallpike JF, Hewer RL. Recurrent and chronic relapsing Guillain-Barrè polyneuritis. Brain 1969; 92:589–606.

48. Adams RD, Shahani BT, Young RR. Tremor in association with polyneuropathy. Trans Am Neurol Assoc 1972; 97:44–48.

49. Harding AE, Thomas PK. Genetically determined neuropathies. In: Asbury AK, Gilliatt RW, eds. Peripheral Nerve Disorders. Boston: Butterworths, 1984:215–242.

50. Yudell A, Dyck PJ, Lambert EH. A kinship with Roussy–Levy syndrome. Arch Neurol 1965; 13:432–440.

51. Salisachs P. Charcot–Marie–Tooth associated with "essential tremor." J Neurol Sci 1976; 28:17–40.

52. Salisachs P, Codina A, Giminez-Roldan S, Zarranz JJ. Charcot–Marie–Tooth disease associated with "essential tremor" and normal and/or slightly diminished motor conduction velocity. Eur Neurol 1979; 18:49–58.

53. Hallett M. Differential diagnosis of tremor. In: Vinken PJ, Bruyn GW, Klawans HL, eds. Handbook of Clinical Neurology. Vol. 5. Extrapyramidal Disorders. Amsterdam: Elsevier, 1986:583–595.

54. Dyck PJ, Lais AC, Ohta M, Bastron JA, Okazaki H, Groover RV. Chronic inflammatory polyradiculoneuropathy. Mayo Clin Proc 1975; 50:621–637.

55. Carroll WM, Jones SJ, Halliday AM. Visual evoked potential abnormalities in Charcot–Marie–Tooth disease and comparison with Friedreich's ataxia. J Neurol Sci 1983; 61:123–133.

56. Barbieri S, Nobile-Orazio E, Baldini L, Fayoumi Z, Manfredini E, Scarlato G. Visual evoked potentials in patients with neuropathy and macroglobulinemia. Ann Neurol 1987; 22:663–666.

57. Pakalnis A, Drake ME, Barohn RJ, Chakeres DW, Mendell JR. Evoked potentials in chronic inflammatory demyelinating polyneuropathy. Arch Neurol 1988; 45:1014–1016.

58. Jones SJ, Carroll WM, Halliday AM. Peripheral and central sensory nerve conduction in Charcot–Marie–Tooth disease and comparison with Friedreich's ataxia. J Neurol Sci 1983; 61:135–148.

59. Mendell JR, Kolkin S, Kissel JT, Weiss KL, Chakeres DW, Rammohan KW. Evidence for central system demyelination in chronic inflammatory demyelinating polyradiculoneuropathy. Neurology 1987; 37:1291–1294.

60. Hawke SHB, Hallinan JM, McLeod JG. Cranial magnetic resonance imaging in

chronic demyelinating polyneuropathy. J Neurol Neurosurg Psychiatry 1990; 53: 794–796.

61. Gregson NA, Leibowitz S. IgM paraproteinaemia, polyneuropathy and myelin-associated glycoprotein. Neuropathol Appl Neurobiol 1985; 11:329–347.

62. Fabian RH. Uptake of antineuronal IgM by CNS neurons: comparison with antineu-ronal IgG. Neurology 1990; 40:419–422.

63. Baig S, Yu-Ping J, Olsson T, Cruz M, Link H. Cells secreting anti-MAG antibody occur in cerebrospinal fluid and bone marrow in patients with polyneuropathy associated with M component. Brain 1991; 114:573–583.

64. Sergott RC, Brown MJ, Lisak RP, Miller SL. Antibody to myelin-associated glyco-protein produces central nervous system demyelination. Neurology 1988; 38:422–426.

65. Marsden CD. The mechanisms of physiological tremor and their significance for pathological tremors. In: Desmedt JE, ed. Physiological Tremor, Pathological Tremors and Clonus. Prog Clin Neurophysiol 1978; 5:1–16.

66. Harding AE, Thomas PK. Autosomal recessive forms of hereditary motor and sen-sory neuropathy. J Neurol Neurosurg Psychiatry 1980; 43:669–678.

67. Smith IS, Furness P, Thomas PK. Tremor in peripheral neuropathy. In: Findley LF, Capildeo R, eds. Movement Disorders: Tremor. London: Macmillan Press, 1984: 399–406.

68. Sanes JN. Absence of enhanced physiological tremor in patients without muscle or cutaneous afferents. J Neurol Neurosurg Psychiatry 1985; 48:645–649.

69. Halliday AM, Redfearn JWT. Finger tremor in tabetic patients and its bearing on the mechanism producing the rhythm of physiological tremor. J Neurol Neurosurg Psychiatry 1958; 21:101–108.

32

Midbrain Tremor

Kurt J. Hopfensperger, Karen Busenbark, and William C. Koller
University of Kansas Medical Center
Kansas City, Kansas

Midbrain, or "rubral," tremor, is a distinct, but uncommon, clinical entity caused by a lesion involving the cerebellar outflow pathways or the area around the red nucleus. Although the red nucleus itself is often involved, destruction of this nucleus is not required for the syndrome to occur (1,2).

Holmes, in 1904, described tremor associated with a midbrain lesion—a fluid tremor—associated with independent tremors of the fingers, rotation at the wrist and elbow, and imposition of intention tremor with voluntary movement. The tremor was described as mainly postural, because movement stopped only when the affected limb was completely at rest (3).

Benedikt described a syndrome consisting of contralateral tremor and an ipsilateral oculomotor nerve palsy, resulting from a lesion in the tegmentum of the midbrain that involved the red nucleus and the third cranial nerve fibers traversing this structure (4). Benedikt did not fully describe the characteristics of the tremor, except that it increased with action. His autopsied case was a 4-year-old boy, with multiple tuberculomas, including one in the right cerebral peduncle, causing destruction of the oculomotor nerve. This patient had a left hemiparesis and a left-sided tremor, plus the right oculomotor palsy.

CLINICAL FEATURES

Midbrain tremor is typically described as a combination of rest, postural, and kinetic tremor (2). The resting tremor worsens on adopting posture and becomes uncontrollable on attempting movement (5); the kinetic tremor is, thus, the most severe of the three positions (1). The tremor at rest can be quite large and irregular and increases markedly during intended movement or with certain sustained postures (6). During active movement, there is typically a dramatic terminal accentuation (2,6).

The frequency of the tremor has been variously reported to be 2–5 or 3–5 Hz and commonly involves both proximal and distal muscles. Proximal muscles may be more affected than distal muscles, and the head and trunk may also be involved (7). The low frequency, coarseness, and presence at rest of the tremor has even led to the misdiagnosis of focal motor epilepsy (2). It is one of the least common types of tremors, and one of the most difficult to treat.

Patients with midbrain tremor usually have other signs of midbrain damage, such as a third cranial nerve palsy and hemiparesis (2).

PHYSIOLOGY OF MIDBRAIN TREMOR

The term *rubral* tremor has been used since Holmes stated that the rubrospinal tract played a role in this tremor, on the basis of one case with tremor in whom the lesion involved the rubrospinal tract in the pons (3). However, there is no direct evidence that lesions of the red nucleus result in a tremor unique from that resulting from lesions of the brachium conjunctivum or other portions of the cerebellar outflow system (6). Marsden states that red nucleus involvement is not necessary for the development of midbrain tremor (8); the red nucleus per se has not been shown to be a source of abnormal oscillation (2). For these reasons, the term *midbrain* tremor is preferable to rubral tremor.

Laboratory studies in rhesus and macaque monkeys demonstrate that midbrain tremor is caused by combined lesions of the red nucleus and its neighboring structures (9,10). There also must be concomitant damage to the cerebellothalamic fibers and nigrostriatal dopaminergic fibers (2); most clinicopathological correlations of midbrain tremor have described lesions in the upper brain stem that involve the dentatothalamic and dentatoolivary systems (6). Since the brachium conjunctivum traverses the red nucleus, midbrain tremor may be due to involvement of this pathway, rather than the red nucleus itself (11). That the tremor can involve limbs either ipsilateral or contralateral to the causative lesion reflects the anatomical relations of cerebellar outflow pathways (6).

The principal role of the red nucleus in the production of tremor is probably by virtue of its participation in the rubroolivocerebellorubral loop (2). Lesions of other fiber pathways that traverse the midbrain tegmentum, such as the ascending serotonergic fibers from the median raphe of the midbrain and pons and the dopaminergic nigrostriatal fibers, may be involved in tremor. These lesions may interrupt the rubroolivocerebellorubral loop and the rubrotegmentospinal fibers (11).

Poirier et al. suggested that slow tremors, such as those seen in midbrain disease, occur from the release of a thalamocortical oscillator owing to alteration of either the pallidal dopaminergic pathway or the cerebellorubral thalamic tract to the ventrolateral thalamus (12).

Midbrain tremor most likely is due to interruptions of a combination of pathways in the midbrain tegmentum; namely, that rubroolivocerebellorubral loop, rubrospinal fibers, dopaminergic nigrostriatal fibers, and the serotoninergic brain stem telencephalic fibers.

ETIOLOGY

Infarction and contusion of the midbrain are probably the most common causes of midbrain tremor, but other focal midbrain lesions, such as tumor, abscess, and demyelination, are occasionally responsible (2).

Vascular

Blood is supplied to the red nucleus and the medial substantia nigra by the paramedian arteries, derived from the posterior communicating artery and the proximal portions of the posterior cerebral arteries. Occlusion of these vessels, or hemorrhage from these arteries, is the most common cause of midbrain lesions resulting in tremor.

Infection

Benedikt's description of a midbrain syndrome with tremor was from a patient with multiple tuberculomas. Koppel et al. described a patient with rubral tremor, caused by a presumed toxoplasmal abscess of the midbrain, that persisted unchanged despite computed tomography (CT) evidence of resolution of the lesion following appropriate therapy (6). It is likely that any localized infection or abscess in the midbrain affecting the appropriate structures can produce tremor.

Demyelination

Midbrain tremor is commonly found in multiple sclerosis with widespread midbrain involvement (9).

Trauma

Brain trauma has long been known as a cause of tremor (13). Critchley, in 1957, reported several cases described variously as "striatal," "cerebellar," and "striatocerebellar" punch-drunkenness in professional and amateur boxers. These cases exhibited postural or intention tremors, with dysdiadochokinesia in two cases (14). Patients with posttraumatic midbrain tremor have had generalized brain stem dysfunction, or few other signs, with normal radiographic studies (5).

PHYSIOLOGICAL STUDIES

Physiological studies in midbrain tremor are few. Andrews and associates (13) studied ten patients with athetosis, one of whom had suffered a midbrain thrombosis, resulting in a right third nerve palsy and a coarse left-sided postural tremor, described as "wing-beating" or "red nucleus" tremor. The tremor was absent when the arm was supported and appeared on abduction of the shoulder or during isometric voluntary contraction. The accelerometer recording at the forearm revealed a tremor that fluctuated in frequency (2.5–3.0 cycles/s) and amplitude. The electromyograms (EMGs) of biceps and triceps were, at times, similar to those seen in patients with athetosis (15). Hallett remarks that EMG studies show bursts of activity lasting 125–150 ms, with alteration of antagonist muscles (7).

TREATMENT

Symptomatic treatment of midbrain tremor is usually unsuccessful (2). Owing to destruction of the nigrostriatal dopaminergic neurons believed to be involved in the production of this tremor, levodopa and dopaminergic agonists may be beneficial. Drugs used in the treatment of essential tremor are worth trying, but usually are not helpful. Gradual spontaneous improvement may occur.

Findley and Gresty reported the case of a 51-year-old man, with a fixed midbrain lesion following a vascular accident. The patient developed a large-amplitude, violent resting tremor of the affected body side. Administration of the dose of levodopa diminished the amplitude of his tremor to 1/80 of its initial value, and the patient was successfully treated with long-term levodopa therapy (16).

Samie et al. reported a dramatic response to levodopa therapy in one of their three patients with posttraumatic midbrain tremor. In the other two patients, tremor was controlled with anticholinergics and apparently worsened with neuroleptics (5). Propranolol has been reported to reduce tremor in several patients with head injury (17). The combination of propranolol and valproate controlled tremor in one patient with a suspected midbrain tremor (5). Clonazepam is reportedly effective in some patients (18).

Patients with long-standing tremor and stable medical illness can be considered for stereotaxic thalamotomy. Andrew et al. performed stereotaxic thalamotomy in eight patients with tremor after severe closed head injury. Five of the eight patients had clinical lesions in the midbrain. The patients had action tremor of the affected side limbs, with a postural component in seven; the tremor was intractable and severe. Ablation of the ventrolateral nucleus and, in some cases, the ventralis anterior nucleus, was performed. The tremor was greatly improved in seven of the eight cases (19).

REFERENCES

1. Koller WC. Evaluation of the tremor disorders. Hosp Prac (Off) 1990; May: 23, 26–7, 30–1.
2. Elble RJ, Koller WC. Tremor. Baltimore: John Hopkins University Press, 1990.
3. Holmes G. On certain tremors in organic cerebral lesions. Brain 1904; 27:327–375.
4. Benedikt M. Translated in Wolf JK: The Classical Brain Stem Syndromes. Springfield, IL: Charles C Thomas, 1991.
5. Samie MR, Selhorst JB, Koller WC. Post-traumatic midbrain tremors. Neurology 1990; 40:62–66.
6. Koppel BS, Daras M. "Rubral" tremor due to midbrain toxoplasma abscess. Mov Disord 1990; 5:254–256.
7. Hallett M. Differential diagnosis of tremor. In: Vinken PJ, Bruyn GW, Klawans HL, eds. Handbook of Clinical Neurology. Vol. 49. New York: Elsevier Science Publishing, 1986:583–595.
8. Marsden CD. Origins of normal and pathological tremor. In: Findley LJ, Capideo R, eds. Movement Disorders, Tremor. London: Macmillian Press, 1984:37–84.
9. Carpenter MB. A study of the red nucleus in the rhesus monkey. J Comp Neurol 1956; 105:195–249.
10. Ohye C, Shibazaki T, Hirai T, et al. Special role of the parvocellular red nucleus in lesion-induced spontaneous tremor in monkeys. Behav Brain Res 1988; 28:241–243.
11. Fahn S. Differential diagnosis of tremor. Med Clin North Am 1972; 56:1363–1375.
12. Poirier LJ. Experimental and histological study of midbrain dyskinesias. J Neurophysiol 1960; 23:534–551.
13. Kremer M, Russel R, Smythe GE. A midbrain syndrome following head injury. J Neurol Neurosurg Psychiatry 1947; 10:49–60.
14. Critchley M. Medical aspects of boxing, particularly from a neurological standpoint. Br Med J 1957; 1:357–362.
15. Andrews CJ, Burke D, Lance JW. The comparison of tremors in normal, parkinsonian and athetotic man. J Neurol Sci 1973; 19:53–61.
16. Findley LF, Gresty MA. Suppression of "rubral" tremor with levodopa. Br Med J 1980; 28:1043.
17. Ellison PA. Propranolol for severe post-head injury action tremor. Neurology 1978; 28:197–199.
18. Biary N, Cleeves L, Findley LJ, Koller WC. Post-traumatic tremor. Neurology 1989; 39:103–106.
19. Andrew J, Fowler CJ, Harrison MJ. Tremor after head injury and its treatment by stereotaxic surgery. J Neurol Neurosurg Psychiatry 1982; 45:815–819.

33

Head Tremor

Stuart Mossman
Wellington Hospital
Wellington South, New Zealand

Leslie J. Findley
Regional Centre for Neurology and Neurosurgery
Oldchurch Hospital and Harold Wood Hospitals
Romford, Essex
and Institute of Neurology
London, England

DEFINITION

Tremor may be defined as a involuntary, rhythmic, oscillating movement of a body part, with the implication of a relatively fixed periodicity and amplitude, and a waveform that, to some extent, is variable over time (1). *Tremor of the head* is usually a postural tremor occurring, in general, in well-defined clinical conditions in which the specific diagnosis is often made from the associated clinical signs. Tremor, thus, may be an expression of a variety of underlying neuropathological processes. Head tremor has been recognized by clinicians who have experience in dealing with patients with tremors that although it may not, of itself, produce functional deficits and disability, it can produce a profound handicap from the social and psychological stress it produces. This is further complicated by the fact that, in general, head tremors are less responsive to drugs than tremors of other body parts, in particular, the hands.

Head tremor may occur with oscillations confined strictly to yaw, which is a "no–no" tremor, or with oscillations confined preponderantly to pitch, which is a "yes–yes" tremor. Alternatively, it may be a combination of both and, in more complex tremors, there may be fluctuations between an obvious no–no and an obvious yes–yes tremor. Indeed, on clinical grounds, it may not be possible to separate tremor of the head from other movement disorders, such as chorea (1).

The overall frequency spectra of head tremor, for example, in essential tremor, may show well-defined peaks, indicating sustained sinusoidal tremor of fairly constant and consistent frequency. However, other patients with a similar amplitude of essential tremor of the head, may have broad peaks, indicating high-frequency deviations, waveform distortion, or intermittency of the tremulous movement (1). Head tremor may occur with or without synchronization of tremor of other body parts.

COMMON CAUSES OF THE HEAD TREMOR

Essential Tremor

The most common cause of tremor of the head, is essential tremor (ET). This disorder can now be clearly divided into the syndrome of inherited essential tremor and that of sporadic essential tremor(s) (2). In a recent study, 7 out of 20 index patients, who had inherited or familial essential tremor, exhibited head tremor. Seventeen percent of the 71 affected relatives of these 20 index patients also had head tremor. All patients with inherited essential tremor had hand tremors (2). Massi and Paulson (3) showed that, in 10% of patients with essential head tremor, the head tremor was the sole manifestation of the disease, although in most, it occurred in association with hand or voice tremor. Essential tremor of the jaw, tongue, and trunk tends to be associated with head tremor (1). Essential head tremor is usually considered to be a postural tremor; however, when a patient with essential head tremor lies supine, ensuring maximum relaxation of neck musculature, the head tremor does not necessarily resolve. Jankovic has also noted that with essential tremor of the head, oscillation persists, irrespective of the position of the head (4). The trajectory of tremor is commonly no–no, but may occur in more than one plane of movement. In a recent study by Bain et al., no–no tremor was far more common than yes–yes tremor by a factor of 6:1 (3). In two-thirds of the patients assessed, tremor was intermittent. The frequency of the main component of head tremor in essential tremor, ranges from 2.3 to 6.2 Hz (5). Its frequency is not altered by treatment (6). There appears to be two peak ages for onset of essential tremor: younger than 20 years and in the sixth decade. Most studies suggest the onset of head tremor tends to occur in the latter peak (7).

The diagnosis of essential head tremor relies on the fact that essential tremor is basically a monosymptomatic disorder, and there is an absence of other physical signs. In isolated head tremors, the possibility of dystonia as a cause must always be considered, particularly if there is any abnormal head posture (see later discussion). Approximately 43% of patients with essential tremor will have a history of tremor in a first-degree relative. Inheritance is dominant and fully penetrant (1,2).

It is the authors' views, from clinical observation, that patients with essential head tremor do not respond as well to standard medications as do patients with ET affecting other body parts. It may reflect that a patient, whose hand tremor is 50% reduced by a drug, may be satisfied with the degree of improvement and emphasize the fact to his doctor, whereas a patient, whose head tremor has been reduced by 50%, may still be socially aware of the involuntary movement and, thus, not as satisfied.

Some studies have reported improvements in head tremor with propranolol in doses ranging between 60 and 320 mg daily (8,9). Koller showed a 50% decrease in amplitude of tremor with higher doses of propranolol (6). However, the treatments with the standard drugs for essential tremor (i.e., propranolol or primidone), are usually unsatisfactory in their control of essential tremor of the head. Occasionally, the combination of propranolol and primidone, can have a good therapeutic effects.

It is worth emphasizing what has already been stated, and that is, that head tremor does not in general cause a functional disability, but is a major cause of embarrassment and unhappiness to the afflicted. Indeed, even when treatment does reduce essential tremor, the suppression, objectively, is not usually sufficient to change the distress and embarrassment experienced by the patient. The differential responses of hand and head tremor to the drug primidone, with a better effect on hand tremor, may suggest that there are different underlying pathophysiological mechanisms for tremors affecting different body parts, even in the same patients (5). It is commonly known that patients with essential tremor may improve with alcohol intake, but this, unfortunately, does not predict their response to other drugs (9).

Dystonic Versus Essential Head Tremor

Head tremor may occur in up to 28% of patients with cranial dystonia or torticollis (11). Head tremor may also be the first manifestation of dystonia (12,13). In such patients, dystonia develops subsequent to the development of tremor. In addition to tremor of the head and neck in patients with cervical dystonia, several studies have shown that between 20 and 30% of such patients will have a separate and apparently unconnected tremor of the upper limbs, indistinguishable from that seen in essential tremor (11,13).

Oscillation or tremor that is associated with cervical dystonia can be considered in two types: essential type tremor and dystonic tremor. These can usually be identified clinically and can also be recognized by electromyogram (EMG) studies (14). Essential type tremor of the head in association with dystonia, usually has a higher frequency (i.e., greater than 7 Hz) than does dystonic tremor, with a peak at 5 Hz. Dystonic tremor can be considered to be a component of the dystonia, which is most obviously seen when the patient turns the neck in the direction opposite that of the main dystonic force. It tends to be a somewhat irregular and large-amplitude movement. The ET seen with dystonia of the head and neck behaves independently of the dystonia and is clinically similar to ET occurring without dystonia. With use of the foregoing clinical features, tremor was identified in 60% of all patients with cervical dystonia: 38% were considered to have a dystonic head tremor, and 30% an essential head tremor. A combination of dystonia and ET was seen in 8% (13).

From what has already been stated, the possibility of dystonia as a background cause must be considered in anyone who presents with an isolated tremor of the head. It should be particularly considered in any patient who presents with a head or trunk tremor that can be ameliorated or changed by an alteration in posture—a feature that is characteristic of dystonic movements. For example, head tremor in the primary position may disappear on lateral rotation, on neck extension, or when lying down (12,15). Any patient presenting with an abnormal posture of the head and a tremor must be considered to have a dystonia until proved otherwise.

A diagnostic uncertainty in stating whether an isolated head tremor is due to dystonia or is due to ET, is exemplified in the literature in descriptions of patients with cervical dystonia who have a high proportion of family members with presumed ET (13). Some authors feel that familial ET is frequently associated with dystonia, so that the two disorders may be pathogenically related (13). In a recent study of inherited ET involving 20 indexed cases (all involving three living generations), 71 secondary cases from the families were also studied, as well as the unaffected individuals. No cases of dystonia were encountered (2). This, however, does not rule out the possibility that there is a relation with sporadic ET (nonfamilial) and various dystonic syndromes (2).

There are no specific pharmacological tests that enable us to separate ET from dystonic tremors. The effect of small quantities of alcohol on ET is felt, by many clinicians, to be fairly specific. However, alcohol may improve or relieve the associated head tremor of cervical dystonia in at least 13% of patients (12,13). Changes of tremor attributable to stress may occur equally in essential and dystonic head tremors (16). The effect of propranolol on essential and dystonic head tremor is unpredictable, but it can have an effect on both; thus, it is not specific. Clinical tests that may be of help in distinguishing essential and dystonic head tremor include the effect of *geste antagonistique*, a usually sensory cue that reduces dystonia. Characteristically in torticollis, the patient may obtain relief or a lessening of symptoms on touching the chin lightly with a finger or resting the head against the back of a chair. The alleviation of head tremor with a "geste" may, therefore, be expected to favor a diagnosis of dystonia.

The pathophysiology of cervical dystonia and dystonic head tremor has not been elucidated. Several studies have suggested a primary disturbance in the vestibular system (17). Other studies have concluded that "vestibular hyperactivity" was secondary in some patients with cervical dystonia (18). Studies of Bronstein and Rudge showed a directional preponderance of vestibular nystagmus in a direction opposite that of the chin deviation (17). It was suggested that vestibular abnormality produced a "tonic imbalance in muscle activity both in the neck and the extraocular system." Other studies have implicated the midbrain in the pathogenesis of cervical dystonia (19).

The possible theories underlying the pathophysiology of dystonic head tremor, have to explain why it may be improved by the sensory cue of geste antagonistique. We have recently studied 12 patients with torticollis and geste and assessed two possible physiological abnormalities in this condition: asymmetry of the vestibulo-ocular reflex and impaired recovery of the blink reflex (17,20). With the head in the position of unrestrained torticollis and with the head in the primary position, with the aid of the geste antagonistique there was no consistent change in the asymmetry of the vestibulo-ocular reflex and no uniform change in the recovery of the blink reflex. These unpublished observations suggest that the action of the geste in dystonia, and possibly also in dystonic head tremor, is through pathways that do not primarily affect brain stem interneurons in the region of the fifth or vestibular nucleus.

The pharmacological management of dystonic head tremor is difficult. Sometimes the head tremor may be paroxysmal (lasting minutes to hours) and occurs with only mild features of spasmodic torticollis. Between the episodes the patient may become completely asymptomatic and, thus, may resemble paroxysmal dystonic choreoathetosis. Propranolol or primidone, or a combination thereof, may be worth a therapeutic trial in the management of tremor. It seems, however, that only a few patients with this type of head tremor respond satisfactorily. Indeed, none of the dystonic head or trunk tremors described by Rivest and Marsden, were responsive to propranolol or primidone (12). As in other types of dystonia, anticholinergic drugs, such as trihexyphenidyl, may be effective. However, relatively high doses are usually required for any effect to be seen (21). Side effects are clearly a problem with anticholinergic drugs, but very slow dosage increments may allow the drug to be tolerated. Fahn, in 1983, found the mean dose of trihexyphenidyl to be 41 mg/day (21). Botulinum toxin is becoming the treatment of choice in the management of cervical dystonia with tremor (discussed later).

Head Tremor in Degenerative Disease of the Cerebellum and Cerebellar–Brain Stem Connections

Head tremor is a feature of the involuntary movements of advanced demyelinating disease and cerebellar system degeneration of all types. In such generalized disorders, no clues are given for localization of the lesions responsible for head tremor. Anecdotal clinical observation in a patient with persistent head tremor, occurring as a consequence of a severe migraine attack, has confirmed that a markedly symptomatic head tremor can arise without there being macroscopic central nervous system lesions. In the clinical situation, distinctions should be made between tremor arising from activity within the cervical muscles themselves and oscillations of the head that occur because of passive transmission of involuntary movements arising in the trunk or limbs, which is common in multiple sclerosis. Such passive transmission is likely to occur in a hypotonic patient.

Active tremor of the head is often accompanied by hypertonia; hence, tremor may persist when the head and trunk are supine and fully supported. Some tremors of the head can be "reset or provoked" by external perturbation and may be considered to be due to delayed or enhanced oscillation around long-loop reflexes associating the periphery with cerebellar circuits (22). Midline vermal lesions commonly cause rhythmic tremor of the head or trunk, or both, with a slow (3–4 Hz) predominantly anteroposterior oscillation, usually described as a "titubation" (23).

Many treatments have been advocated for the management of cerebellar tremor, but there seems to be no fundamental change in recommendations since the 1984 review of Legg (24). Isoniazide and acetylcholine precursors, may be helpful in some patients, but they do not have predictable effects. Clearly, in some patients with static or unilateral disease, conventional stereotaxis of permanent stimulation techniques may have a part to play in management.

Head Tremor Associated With Parkinson's Disease

It is well recognized in Parkinson's disease that tremor of the legs, jaw, lower lip, and tongue can occur, in addition to the more classic rest tremor of the hands. It has been well recorded in the literature that head tremor is distinctly *uncommon* and, when present, must suggest a possible alternative diagnosis (4,23). However, it is also recognized clinically that tremor of the chin, tongue, and lips is common in Parkinson's disease, but tremor of the head is rare. This point was emphasized by Charcot himself (25).

Head Tremor (Myoclonic) as Part of Palatal Myoclonus

Typical myoclonus, when affecting the head, closely resembles tremor. In the syndrome of oculopalatolaryngeal myoclonus any associated head myoclonus may be phased-locked to the myclonus of other body parts (15,26).

Head-Nodding and Head Tremor Associated With Congenital Nystagmus

Congenital nystagmus in children may sometimes be associated with compensatory head-shaking, with an improved visual acuity compared with when the head is still. For this deliberate "head-nodding" to improve vision, it is likely that the compensatory vestibulo-ocular reflex (VOR), or dolls-head phenomenon, as a consequence of the head movement, interacts with the nystagmus to lessen its effect.

The following example shows the two ways that this can be achieved. In spasmus nutans, the horizontal pendular nystagmus that impairs visual acuity may be suppressed by the infant typically shaking his or her head from side to side while staring straight ahead at a target. During the head-shaking, the normal compensatory dolls-head eye movements (VOR) are present, and these suppress the nystagmus such that acuity is improved (1,15). This probably reflects an intact oculomotor circuitry, with the VOR overriding pendular nystagmus. The implication of this is that head-shaking is not pathological, but is a learned response to switch off the nystagmus.

In other patients with congenital nystagmus, compensatory head-shaking takes the same pattern as the nystagmus, but is executed in the opposite direction. Although there is little change in the pattern of nystagmus, the eye remains relatively stable in space because the patterns of head movement are more or less a mirror image of the eye movements. This provides a period of relatively stable vision. The VOR is suppressed during this maneuver, but in other circumstances (e.g., with impulsive rotation), the VOR is intact. This again is an example of a central-adapted mechanism (15). In some subjects with congenital nystagmus, there may be an associated involuntary sinusoidal oscillation of the head in yaw, at a frequency similar to the nystagmus cycle, with the result that the subject appears to have a head tremor. Visual acuity is unaffected by the presence or absence of head movement, which is considered to be a form of congenital head tremor (15,26).

Psychogenic Head Tremor

Tremor as the result of a conversional reactional state is recognized, but is rarely encountered. The authors cannot recall the last time a patient's diagnosis was psychogenic head tremor. Anecdotally, in one instance, there was clinical doubt about whether the patient concerned had an organically determined head tremor. However, when assessed, he had a constant frequency of head tremor, which we were not able to emulate ourselves; that is, on attempting to simulate a sinusoidal head tremor of 3–4 Hz, we were able to maintain this regularly for even short periods. Spectral analysis of head tremors invariably show multiple tremor frequencies. In general, psychogenic or hysterical tremor is usually exacerbated when attention is paid to it, and it often disappears when the patient is diverted to another subject. To be strictly sure that tremor is due to a conversion state, remission must occur either with psychotherapy or spontaneously.

Tremor and Neuropathy

Limb tremor may complicate hereditary or acquired demyelinating neuropathy, but we have not seen head tremor with this.

Head Tremor and Vestibular Failure

Patients with head tremor do not complain of oscillopsia because their VORs exactly compensate for the involuntary head movement. This can be confirmed clinically by fundoscopy when, in such asymptomatic patients, the optic disc is noted to be "stable," despite the head tremor. In contrast, if patients with head tremor complain of oscillopsia then it is diagnostic of loss of vestibular function. This state can be easily confirmed on fundoscopy when, because of the absence of vestibular function and a VOR, the optic disc will no longer be stable, but will be seen to be oscillating also. Here, rigid immobilization of the head abolishes the oscillations. In one patient, propranolol (40–120 mg/day) lessened her oscillopsia in association with the subjective dampening of a head tremor.

The eye movement visible in this situation, although compensatory to head movement, is in phase error, as the compensatory mechanisms involving the cervical ocular reflex—pursuit and optokinesis—are less efficient and operate at a longer latency than the VOR. The out-of-phase ocular compensation, visible as optic disc oscillation on ophthalmoscopy, results in visual oscillopsia (12). The clinical distinction from cerebellar disease is clear, with resolution of the visual symptoms with the head immobilized and otherwise normal examination of pursuit and saccadic function in the absence of visible eye nystagmus on simple inspection.

Influence of Head Position on Head Tremor

Rivest and Marsden (12) show a number of possible reasons why head tremor may vary with head position. Thus, the effect of head position in altering head tremor may be due to an alteration in muscle spindle input (which has altered muscle stretch); be due to altered muscle tone (with a change in the contractile force of different muscles when the head is in different positions); be related to the execution of a different motor program; or be due to otolith mechanisms for which tonic firing is dependent on the orientation of the gravity vector (28).

TREATMENT

Drug Treatments

The generally poor pharmacological effect of primidone and propranolol in ET of the head has been mentioned. In a double-blind controlled study, no consistent attenuation of tremor was found with primidone, up to 750 mg/day in divided doses. Importantly, an acute toxic reaction, even to a small initial dose (62.5 mg of primidone), was seen in 6 of 22 patients (5). To reduce this acute toxicity, it may be beneficial to induce hepatic enzymes by prescribing phenobarbitone, 15 or 30 mg three times a day, for some weeks before commencing treatment with primidone.

Rivest and Marsden (12) concluded that, in patients presenting with head or trunk tremors, therapeutic trials of propranolol, primidone, and anticholinergics should always be given.

Botulinum Toxin

Botulinum toxin may be helpful in the management of head tremor, in particular, of an uncomplicated no–no type (12). Dystonic head tremor is said to respond, as well as the positional and postural abnormality of torticollis. Injections for head tremor are into both the splenei and include the sternomastoid, particularly if there is a yes–yes component to the tremor. Effective doses are recommended to be between 1000 and 1200 mouse units (Dysport) or about 240 mouse units (Oculinum). Although approximately 70% of patients with head tremor improve with this therapy, its efficacy in head tremor has not as yet been subject to controlled trials. Side effects relate mainly to dysphagia, but these are usually transient, lasting only 2–3 weeks. They may be lessened by reducing the dose in women with thin necks and reducing or avoiding sternomastoid injections, although this may lessen efficacy (29,30). Jankovic and Schwartz (30) noted, in the course of treating many patients with botulinum toxin, that those patients with dystonic tremor tended to respond better than those with essential tremor.

CONCLUSION

In summary, head tremor usually occurs in clearly defined syndromes that can be diagnosed almost entirely by observing the patient. However, the distinction of essential tremor and dystonic head tremor may sometimes be difficult. Clues pointing toward dystonic head tremor include the abnormal posture, effectiveness of the geste antagonistique, and the influence of changes of head posture on the head tremor. Nevertheless, these features are not necessarily common to all forms of dystonic head tremor, and the distinction between dystonia and essential head tremor may only ensue over the course of time. Despite these diagnostic difficulties, botulinum toxin may be a promising treatment for the alleviation of head tremor of all types.

REFERENCES

1. Findley LJ, Gresty MA. Head, facial and voice tremor. Facial dyskinesias. Adv Neurol 1988; 49:239–253.
2. Bain PG, Findley LJ, Thompson PD, Gresty MA, Rothwell JC, Harding AE, Marsden CD. A study of hereditary essential tremor. Brain (in press).
3. Massi EW, Paulson GW. Essential vocal tremor. Clinical characteristics and response to therapy. South Med J 1985; 78:316–317.

4. Jankovic J. Cranial–cervical dyskinesias: an overview. Facial dyskinesias. Adv Neurol 1988; 49:1–13.
5. Findley LJ, Cleeves L, Calzetti S. Primidone in essential tremor of the hands and head: a double blind controlled clinical study. J Neurol Neurosurg Psychiatry 1985; 48:911–915.
6. Koller WC. Propranolol therapy for essential tremor of the head. Neurology 1984; 34:1077–1079.
7. Mengano A, Di Maio L, Maggio M, Squitieri F, Di Donato M, Barbieri F, Campanella G. Benign essential tremor: a clinical survey of 82 patients from Campania. Acta Neurol 1989; 11:239–246.
8. Tolosa ES, Lowenson RB. Essential tremor treated with propranolol. Neurology 1975; 25:1041–1044.
9. Sweet RD, Blumberg J, Lee, McDowal F. Propranolol in treatment of essential tremor. Neurology 1974; 24:64–67.
10. Koller WC, Biary N, Cone S. Disability in essential tremor: effective treatment. Neurology 1986; 36:1001–1004.
11. Chan J, Brin M, Fahn S. Idiopathic cervical dystonia: clinical characteristics. Mov Disord 1991; 6:119–126.
12. Rivest J, Marsden CD. Trunk and head tremor as isolated manifestations of dystonia. Mov Disord 1990; 5:60–65.
13. Jankovic J, Leder S, Warner D, Schwartz K. Cervical dystonia: clinical findings in associated movement disorders. Neurology 1991; 41:1088–1091.
14. Deuschl G, Heinen F, Kleedorfer B. Clinical and polymyographic investigations of spasmodic torticollis. J Neurol 1992; 239:9–15.
15. Gresty MA, Halmagyi G. Abnormal head movements. J Neurol Neurosurg Psychiatry 1979; 42:705–714.
16. Hughes A, Lees A, Marsden CD. Paroxysmal dystonic head tremor. Mov Disord 1991; 6:85–86.
17. Bronstein AM, Rudge P. Vestibular involvement in spasmodic torticollis. J Neurol Neurosurg Psychiatry 1986; 49:290–295.
18. Huygen PLM, Verhagen WIM, Van Hoof JJM, Horstink MWIM. Vestibular hyperactivity in patients with idiopathic spasmodic torticollis. J Neurol Neurosurg Psychiatry 1989; 52:782–785.
19. Plant GT, Kermode AG, Bonley EPGH, McDonald WI. Spasmodic torticollis due to a midbrain lesion in a case of multiple sclerosis. Mov Disord 1989; 4:359–362.
20. Tolosa ES, Montserrat L, Bayes A. Blink reflex studies in focal dystonia: enhanced excitability of brainstem interneurones in cranial dystonia and spasmodic torticollis. Mov Disord 1988; 3:61–69.
21. Fahn S. High dosage anticholinergic therapy in dystonia. Neurology 1983; 33:1255–1261.
22. Mauritz KH, Schmitt C, Dickgan J. Delayed and enhanced long loop reflexes as the possible cause of postural tremor in late cerebellar atrophy. Brain 1981; 104:97–116.
23. Koller WC, Huber SJ. Tremor disorders of ageing: diagnosis and management. Geriatrics 1989; 44:33–41.
24. Legg N. Treatment of cerebellar tremor. In: Findley LJ, Capildeo R, eds. Movement Disorders: Tremor. London: Macmillan, 1984:377–386.

25. Capildeo R. Parkinson's disease complex. In: Findley LJ, Capildeo R, eds. Movement Disorders: Tremor. London: Macmillan, 1984:285–294.
26. Gresty MA. Stability of the head: studies in normal subjects and in patients with labyrinthine disease, head tremor and dystonia. Mov Disord 1987; 2:165–185.
27. Bronstein AM, Gresty MA, Mossman SS. Pendular pseudonystagmus arising as a combination of head tremor and vestibular failure. Neurology 1992; 42:1527–1531.
28. Mossman S, Cleeves L, Findley LJ. The influence of head position upon head tremor. J Neurol Neurosurg Psychiatry 1993 (in press).
29. Anderson TJ, Rivest J, Stell R, et al. Botulinum toxin treatment of spasmodic torticollis. J R Soc Med 1993 (in press).
30. Jankovic J, Scwartz K. Botulinum toxin treatment of tremors. Neurology 1991; 41: 1185–1188.

34

Tremor Induced or Enhanced by Pharmacological Means

Peter A. LeWitt
Wayne State University School of Medicine
Detroit, Michigan
and Clinical Neuroscience Center
West Bloomfield, Michigan

I. INTRODUCTION

The complexity of tremor as a motor phenomenon is further enhanced by the variety of neurochemical mechanisms that can contribute to tremorogenesis. Tremorous movements are common, although nonspecific manifestations of central nervous system (CNS) toxicity from a number of causes. Substances that impair the electrochemical functions of neuronal membranes, or disrupt cerebello-thalamic circuits can produce tremor along with additional types of neurological impairment. Of hundreds of pharmacological substances active in the CNS, only a few are known to be relatively selective for producing tremor. Certain compounds, such as oxotremorine (1) and harmaline (2), have been especially influential for the investigation of tremorogenesis in animal research. Other classes of drugs producing tremor have been less thoroughly characterized in their actions at the cellular level.

In some instances, tremor occurs as an idiosyncratic response to a drug that does not usually produce such an effect. Examples of this include case reports of tremor induced by trimethoprim–sulfamethoxazale in acquired immunodeficiency syndrome (AIDS) patients (3) or after injection of calcitonin (4). More commonly, the induction of tremor occurs by enhancing physiological tremor. Research into pharmacological means for inducing or enhancing tremor may be informative for discovering new strategies to treat disabilities from several forms of rhythmic, involuntary movements. The search for rational therapy of tremor has unfortunately not been as successful as serendipitous observation, which was the basis for discovery of propranolol and primidone as treatments for essential tremor and amantadine for Parkinsonian tremor. This chapter will review clinical experience with expanding lists of medications known to produce tremor, and will provide an update from previous reviews of this topic (5–8).

II. DRUG-INDUCED PARKINSONIAN TREMOR

Virtually all features of idiopathic parkinsonism can be duplicated by pharmacological disruption of dopaminergic projections to the striatum from the substantia nigra. In animal models as well as in humans, such interventions include depletion of dopamine synthesis and storage by reserpine, tetrabenazine, and α-methyl-*para*-tyrosine. Selective destruction of the nigrostriatal pathways can be achieved with compounds such as 6-hydroxydopamine or 1-methyl-4-phenyl-1,2,3,6-tetra-hydropyridine (MPTP). In humans, the latter substance has produced a tremor at rest which is indistinguishable from that observed in Parkinson's disease (PD) (9).

Medications that block dopamine receptors can produce resting tremor in addition to other parkinsonian features. This tremor tends to show the same body distribution as in idiopathic PD, sometimes asymmetrically. Tremor can occur either acutely or only after months of sustained therapy. Regardless of their age or prior neurological health, all patients treated with neuroleptic medications are susceptible to develop parkinsonism in proportion to the extent of dopaminergic blockade. In addition to tremor at rest, neuroleptic medications can also produce coarse, action-induced or flapping properties (10,11).

Persons affected with idiopathic Parkinson's disease are much more sensitive for neuroleptic medications to exacerbate tremor and other motor deficits, possibly reflecting their marginal dopaminergic neurotransmission in this disorder (12). The full range of parkinsonian clinical features can be produced by neuroleptic medications. Patients vary greatly in the occurrence of parkinsonian features from a neuroleptic dose sufficient to produce an adequate antipsychotic action. There appears to be a great deal of idiosyncracy in the occurrence of parkinsonism, as is true for other phenomena such as dystonic reactions or the emergence of tardive dyskinesia. In part, this may be due to different clinical profiles of neuroleptics relative to receptors mediating dopaminergic and serotonergic neurotransmission (13). The additional property of anticholinergic activity in several classes of neuroleptic drugs may be of clinical significance in their likelihood for producing tremor. Anticholinergic effects may be one reason that thioridazine has a low potency for producing parkinsonism. The atypical neuroleptic clozapine, which is quite effective against parkinsonian tremor, also has prominent central anticholinergic effects (despite its propensity to cause hypersalivation).

The basis for variability in neuroleptic drug action is not well understood. As in the idiopathic disorder, severe bradykinesia, cogwheel-type rigidity, and other stigmata of parkinsonism can be found in individuals who do not manifest any tremor. Another characteristic that distinguishes idiopathic Parkinson's disease from the neuroleptic-induced variety pertains to the incidence of resting tremor. While tremor is commonly an early manifestation of mild parkinsonism, it is unusual for neuroleptic-treated patients to demonstrate resting tremor in the absence of any other parkinsonian features [although this has been reported (14), and I have observed it on several occasions]. Parkinsonian tremor from neuroleptics, as the outcome of postsynaptic dopamine receptor blockade, would be expected to reverse following withdrawal of the medication. However, there have been cases reported of tardive tremor (15) indicating that tremor can persist long after the drug has been cleared, possibly on a self-perpetuating basis.

Tremor in parkinsonian patients can occur in the context of posture maintenance and movement of the arms, resembling the characteristics of essential tremor (including responsiveness to β-adrenergic blocking medications; 16). On occasion, resting or action tremor appears to be enhanced in typical Parkinson's disease patients on a regular basis at the time of peak levodopa concentrations. This unmasking or initiation of tremor has not been characterized as to its mechanism. Conceivably, it might reflect the small rise of norepinephrine synthesis that can follow the administration of levodopa, which is also a precursor for this neurotransmitter. The rise in tremor amplitude when the patients with parkinsonism deal with stressful situations may be a reflection of interaction between noradrenergic mechanisms and parkinsonian rest tremor (17).

Parkinsonian tremor is also unmasked or enhanced by increasing striatal cholinergic tone with physostigmine administration (18). Therapy with other means for increasing CNS cholinergic stimulation, such as intraventricular behaechol infusion, can also bring out resting tremor in individuals who may have latent Parkinson's disease (64). It seems less likely that increased cholinergic tone is a means by which parkinsonian tremor can be produced in nonparkinsonian individuals. Extensive clinical experience in using oral sustained-release physostigmine (Synapton), tacrine (tetrahydroaminoacridine; Cognex), and velnacrine (Mentane; HP-029) has not been associated with reports of tremor occurrence, despite the prominent actions of these compounds in the CNS. One report has argued that the induction of tremor by physostigmine is not a consequence of enhanced central acetylcholine, but rather, of effects on serotonin metabolism (19).

A. Valproate-Induced Tremor

The occurrence of tremor is not a general property of anticonvulsants. Indeed, several anticonvulsants (such as clonazepam, phenobarbital, and primidone) can be useful in treating essential tremor. Phenytoin and carbamazepine are capable of causing involuntary movements of a choreic or dystonic nature, but not tremor (even when toxic doses have produced other aspects of cerebellar toxicity). Valproate can produce a clinically significant degree of tremor (resting, postural, or action) (20,21). The tremor is usually evident within the first month of drug therapy, and it is not related to dose or plasma valproate concentration (22). Recording techniques used in one study showed that 80% of patients treated with valproate had findings typical of enhanced physiological tremor (23). The majority of patients who develop a clinically significant tremor from valproate have responded to propranolol. In some instances, treatment with amantadine or cyproheptadine have lessened tremor (22). The tremor caused by valproate is not associated with the development of additional neurotoxicity, such as parkinsonism or cerebellar dysfunction, nor does it seem to be a permanent outcome.

B. Tremor Induced by Calcium Channel Blockers

Rarely, calcium channel blockers, such as flunarizine and cinnarizine, can induce typical features of parkinsonism, including tremor at rest (24). Flunarizine use has also been associated with enhanced physiological tremor (25). Another calcium channel blocker, nifedipine, has been noted to produce an increase in physiological tremor (26).

C. Amiodarone-Induced Tremor

The class III antiarrhythmic compound amiodarone, a benzofurane derivative, has been associated with a variety of neurological toxicities, including tremor (27–29). Usually, the tremor has affected the hands during action or postural maintenance. It can occur without other types of neurological impairment, such as cerebellar dysfunction. Amiodarone has also been associated with the reversible production of resting tremor and other parkinsonian features (28,30). Another antiarrhythmic compound, procainamide, has also been described to produce tremor (31).

D. Tremor Induced by Medications for Affective Disorders

Along with other types of movement disorder, tremor is a common side effect of lithium carbonate use. Tremor is present, sometimes prominently, in one-third or more of individuals treated with effective psychotropic doses of this drug (32,33). The incidence and severity of lithium-induced tremor are increased among patients with higher intake (34). Tremor is especially likely when the plasma lithium concentration exceeds the upper limit of its usual therapeutic range (e.g., higher than 1.2 mEq/L). Hence, the onset of tremor may be a sensitive indicator for encephalopathy that can accompany an excessive intake of lithium. By reducing lithium dose, tremor may be decreased or eliminated. Another strategy has been to lessen the abruptness of rise in plasma concentrations by use of sustained-release preparations. Administering lithium at bedtime may help minimize the discomforts of tremor, since the rise from each dose to its highest concentration occurs while subjects are asleep (32).

The characteristics of lithium-induced tremor resemble those of physiological tremor. Hence, its mechanism has been assumed to be an enhancement of normal tremorogenesis (35). One clue for this has been the improvement generally encountered following the use of β-adrenergic blockers (36). There has been no systematic study of other medications, such as primidone for lithium-induced tremor, but it has been useful for at least one patient managed by the author. Tremor tends to persist with continued lithium use (37), but may diminish in amplitude over time (33).

Although it can be severe (38), only rarely is the tremor more than a mild manifestations in the hands or, less commonly, in the face. It can be present at rest, but is most evident during action or posture maintenance (39). A hand-written spiral may show jerkiness of somewhat less regularity than commonly encountered with essential tremor. However, lithium-induced tremor should not be considered a mild manifestation of cerebellar dysfunction, since the tremor can be quite prominent without disturbance of gait, eye movements, coordination, or other elements of cerebellar system function. The occurrence of resting tremor may occur together with cogwheel rigidity or slowed movements. These features of parkinsonism have been described to be a rare, reversible outcome of lithium therapy (37,40–42). Long-term lithium therapy has been suspected (43), but not proved to produce an irreversible tremor.

An estimated 10% of patients treated with tricyclic antidepressant medications develop some tremor (44,45). This form of tremor may be an enhancement of physiological tremor. Another possibility is that the effect of the drug in enhancing central noradrenergic mechanisms might be the basis for inducing tremor. There has been limited clinical experience in the therapeutics of tricyclic antidepressant-induced tremor, but it can be responsive to low doses of propranolol (46–49).

An enhancement of physiological tremor can occasionally be a feature of treatment with the broad-potency monoamine oxidase inhibitors (46,48), although not with the selective monoamine oxidase B inhibitors deprenyl (selegiline) or lazabemide (Ro 19-6327).

E. Tremor Induced by Neuroactive Amines and Related Compounds

Compounds enhancing or duplicating the effects of an activated sympathetic nervous system can produce an increase of physiological tremor. Similar to anxiety or stress, isoproterenol administration can enhance both essential and physiological tremor (50,51). These actions appear to be mediated through β-adrenoreceptor mechanisms. Pharmacological experiments have been carried out in which isoproterenol-induced tremor could be blocked with propranolol and other centrally acting β-adrenergic blockers (52,53). Though sympathomimetically induced tremor is thought to be largely central in origin (54), there may also be a peripheral component behind its production (55). A β-adrenergic blocker with prominent intrinsic sympathomimetic activity, pindolol, can produce tremor, presumably because of agonist properties also at β-adrenoreceptors (56). The thermogenic β-3-adrenoceptor agonist BRL 26830A has been reported to produce an enhancement of physiological tremor in humans, possibly through activation of β_2-adrenoceptors (57).

Tremulousness has been described to be a common side effect of treatment for asthma with drugs, such as isoproterenol, terbutaline, and methyl xanthines (aminophylline and theophylline). Sometimes enhanced physiological tremor induced through β_2-adrenoreceptor mechanism can be a dose-limiting side effect (58–60). More commonly, the sense of jitteriness accompanying use of these medications is an outcome of the distress, anxiety, and restlessness that can be produced jointly by an asthmatic attack and the psychic effects of these treatments. The role of methyl xanthines, in particular, has been questioned in their propensity for inducing tremor. Although jittery feelings are part of the cultural legacy of caffeine excess, several studies have not been able to show that this compound produces tremor (61). In one trial, intake of 325 mg of caffeine neither enhanced physiological tremor, nor produced alterations in parkinsonian or essential tremor (62).

Drugs with α-adrenergic effects are not known to induce tremor. Injections of dopamine or epinephrine do not cause tremor on a peripheral basis. Similarly, sympathomimetic drugs with central actions, such as dextroamphetamine, pemoline, and methylphenidate, do not commonly bring on tremor, although physiological tremor may be enhanced.

Two cases of action tremor associated with the start of terfenadine, an H_1-receptor antagonist of the piperidine class, have been reported (63).

REFERENCES

1. Hallberg H, Almgren O. Modulation of oxotremorine-induced tremor by central beta-adrenoceptors. Acta Physiol Scand 1987; 129:407–413.
2. Lamarre Y. Animal models of physiological, essential, and parkinsonian-like tremors. In: Findley LJ, Capildeo R, eds. Movement Disorders: Tremor. London: Macmillan Press, 1984:183–194.
3. Borucki MJ, Matzke DS, Pollard RB. Tremor induced by trimethoprim–sulfamethoxazole in patients with the acquired immunodeficiency syndrome (AIDS). Ann Intern Med 1988; 109:77–78.
4. Conget JI, Vendrell J, Halperin I, Esmatjes E. Widespread tremor after injection of sodium calcitonin. Br Med J 1989, 298:189.
5. Pelnar J. Das Zittern. Berlin: Springer-Verlag, 1913.

6. Brimblecombe RW, Pinder RM. Tremors and Tremorogenic Agents. Bristol (UK): Scientechnica, 1972.
7. Pinder RM. Drug-induced tremor. In: Findley LJ, Capildeo R, eds. Movement Disorders: Tremor. London: Macmillan Press, 1984:445–461.
8. Elble RJ, Koller WC. Tremor. Baltimore: Johns Hopkins University Press, 1990: 134–142.
9. Tetrud JW, Langston JW. Tremor in MPTP-induced parkinsonism. Neurology 1992; 42:407–410.
10. Boshes RA, Oepen G, Handren M. Flapping tremor produced by high-potency neuroleptics. J Clin Psychopharmacol 1991; 11:76–77.
11. Friedman JH. "Rubral" tremor induced by a neuroleptic drug. Mov Disord 1992; 7:281–282.
12. Klawans HL, Weiner WJ. Attempted use of haloperidol in the treatment of L-dopa-induced dyskinesias. J Neurol Neurosurg Psychiatry 1974; 37:427–430.
13. Casey DE. Extrapyramidal syndromes in nonhuman primates: typical and atypical neuroleptics. Psychopharmacol Bull 1991; 27:47–50.
14. Gabellini AS, Martinelli P, Coccagna G. Drug-induced tremor of the tongue. Ital J Neurol Sci 1989; 10:89–91.
15. Stacy M, Jankovic J. Tardive tremor. Mov Disord 1992; 7:53–57.
16. Foster NL, Newman RP, LeWitt PA, Gillespie MM, Larsen TA, Chase TN. beta-Blockade of parkinsonian tremor. Ann Neurol 1984; 16:505–508.
17. Owen DA, Marsden CD. Effect of adrenergic beta-blockade on parkinsonian tremor. Lancet 1965; 2:1259–1262.
18. Duvoisin RC. Cholinergic–anticholinergic antagonism in parkinsonism. Arch Neurol 1967; 17:124–136.
19. Mohanakumar KP, Mitra N, Ganguly DK. Tremorogenesis by physostigmine is unrelated to acetylcholinesterase inhibition: evidence for serotoninergic involvement. Neurosci Lett 1990; 120:91 99.
20. Hyman NM, Dennis PD, Sinclair KG. Tremor due to sodium valproate. Neurology 1979; 29:1177–1180.
21. Schmidt D. Adverse effects of valproate. Epilepsia 1984; 1:S44–S49.
22. Karas BJ, Wilder BJ, Hammond EJ, Bauman AW. Treatment of valproate tremors. Neurology 1983; 33:1380–1382.
23. Karas BJ, Wilder BJ, Hammond EJ, Bauman AW. Valproate tremors. Neurology 1982; 32:428–432.
24. Capella D, Laporte JR, Castel JM, Tristan C, Cos A, Morrales-Olivas FJ. Parkinsonism, tremor, and depression induced by cinnarizine and flunarizine. Br Med J 1988; 297:722–723.
25. Amery WK, Heykants J. Essential tremor and flunarizine. Cephalalgia 1988; 8:227.
26. Topaktas S, Onur R, Dalkara T. Calcium channel blockers and essential tremor. Eur Neurol 1987; 27:114–119.
27. Charness ME, Morady F, Scheinman MM. Frequent neurologic toxicity associated with amiodarone therapy. Neurology 1984; 34:669–671.
28. Palakurthy PR, Iyer V, Meckler RJ. Unusual neurotoxicity associated with amiodarone therapy. Ann Intern Med 1987; 147:881–884.

29. Della Sala S, Marchetti C. Tremor: a possible side effect of prolonged therapy with low doses of amiodarone. Ital J Neurol Sci 1989; 10:219–220.
30. Werner EG, Olanow CW. Parkinsonism and amiodarone. Ann Neurol 1989; 25: 630–632.
31. Rubinstein A, Cabili S. Tremor induced by procainamide. Am J Cardiol 1986; 57: 340–341.
32. Mellerup ET, Plenge P, Rafaelsen OJ. Renal and other controversial adverse effects of lithium. In: Meltzer HY, ed. Psychopharmacology: The Third Generation of Progress. New York: Raven Press, 1987:1443–1448.
33. Schou M, Baastrup PC, Grof P, Weis P, Angst J. Pharmacological and clinical problems of lithium prophylaxis. Br J Psychiatry 1970; 116:615–619.
34. Persson G. Lithium side-effects in relation to dose and to levels and gradients of lithium in plasma. Acta Psychiatr Scand 1977; 55:208–213.
35. Young RR. In: Findley LJ, Capildeo R, eds. Movement Disorders: Tremor. London: Macmillan Press, 1984:127–134.
36. Zubenko GS, Cohen BM, Lipinski JF. Comparison of metoprolol and propranolol in the treatment of lithium tremor. Psychiatr Res 1984; 11:163–164.
37. Kane J, Rifkin A, Quitkin F, Klein DF. Extrapyramidal side-effects with lithium treatment. Am J Psychiatry 1978; 135:851–853.
38. Van Putten T. Lithium-induced disabling tremor. Psychosomatics 1978; 19:27–31.
39. Tyrer P, Lee I, Trotter C. Physiologic characteristics of tremor after chronic lithium therapy. Br J Psychiatry 1981; 139:59–61.
40. Reches A, Tietler J, Lavy S. Parkinsonism due to lithium carbonate poisoning. Arch Neurol 1981; 38:471.
41. Lang AE: Lithium and parkinsonism. Ann Neurol 1984; 15:214.
42. Vestergaard P. Clinically important side-effects of long-term lithium treatment: a review. Acta Psychiatr Scand [Suppl] 1983; 67:11–36.
43. Donaldson IM, Cunningham J. Persisting neurological sequelae of lithium carbonate therapy. Arch Neurol 1983; 40:747–751.
44. Nelson JC, Jatlow PI, Quinlan DM. Subjective complaints during desipramine treatment. Arch Gen Psychiatry 1984; 41:55–59.
45. Baldessarini RJ. Drugs and the treatment of psychiatric disorders. In: Gilman AG, Rall TW, Nies AS, Taylor P, eds. Goodman and Gilman's The Pharmacological Basis of Therapeutics. 8th ed. New York: Macmillan Publishing, 1993:383–435.
46. Evans DL, Davidon J, Raft D. Early and late side effects of phenelzine. J Clin Psychopharmacol 1982; 2:208–210.
47. Kronfol Z, Greden JF, Zis AP. Imipramine-induced tremor: effects of a beta-adrenergic blocking agent. Arch Gen Psychiatry 1983; 44:225–226.
48. Baldessarini RJ. Chemotherapy in Psychiatry: Principles and Practice. 2nd ed. Cambridge, MA: Harvard University Press, 1984.
49. Koller WC, Musa MN. Amitriptyline-induced abnormal movements. Neurology 1985; 35:1086.
50. Teräväinen H. beta-Blockers in isoproterenol-enhanced essential tremor. Acta Neurol Scand 1984; 69:125–127.
51. Aronson JK. Positive inotropic drugs and drugs used in the dysrhythmias. In: Dukes

MNG, ed. Meyler's Side Effects of Drugs. 11th ed. New York: Elsevier Scientific, 1988:333–358.

52. Larsson S, Svedmyr N. Tremor caused by sympathomimetics is mediated by beta adrenoreceptors. Scand J Respir Dis 1967; 58:5–10.

53. Perucca E, Pickles H, Richens A. Effect of atenolol, metoprolol, and propanalol on isoproterenol-induced tremor and tachycardia in normal subjects. Clin Pharmacol Ther 1981; 29:425–433.

54. Abila B, Wilson JF, Marshall RW, Richens A. Differential effects of alpha-adrenoceptor blockade on essential, physiological and isoprenaline-induced tremor: evidence for a central origin of essential tremor. J Neurol Neurosurg Psychiatry 1985; 48:1031–1036.

55. Marsden CD, Foley TH, Owen DA, McAllister D. Peripheral beta adrenergic receptors concerned with tremor. Clin Sci 1967; 33:53–65.

56. Koller WC, Orebaugh C, Larsen L, Potempa K. Pindolol-induced tremor. Clin Neuropharmacol 1987; 10:449–460.

57. Connacher AA, Lakie M, Powers N, Elton RA, Walsh EG, Jung RT. Tremor and the anti-obesity drug BRL 26830A. Br J Clin Pharmacol 1990; 30:613–615.

58. Jenne JW, Valcarenghi G, Druz WS, Starkey PW, Yu C. Comparison of tremor responses to orally administered albuterol and terbutaline. Am Rev Respir Dis 1986; 134:708–713.

59. Tinkelman DG, DeJong R, Lutz C, Spangler DL. Evaluation of tremor and efficacy of oral procaterol in adult patients with asthma. J Allergy Clin Immunol 1990; 85: 719–728.

60. Lipworth BJ, Brown RA, McDevitt DG. Assessment of airways, tremor and chronotropic responses to inhaled salbutamol in the quantification of beta$_2$-adrenoceptor blockade. Br J Clin Pharmacol 1989; 28:95–102.

61. Wharrad WJ, Birmingham AT, Macdonald IA, Inch PJ, Mead JL. The influence of fasting and of caffeine intake on finger tremor. Eur J Clin Pharmacol 1985; 29:37–43.

62. Koller WC, Cone S, Herbster G. Caffeine and tremor. Neurology 1987; 37:169–172.

63. Soto J, Sacristan JA, Alsar MJ, Sainz C. Terfenadine-induced tremor. Ann Neurol 1993; 33:226.

64. Fox JH, Bennett DA, Goetz CG, Penn RD, Savoy S, Clasen R, Wilson RS. Induction of Parkinsonism by intraventricular bethanechol in a patient with Alzheimer's disease. Neurology 1989; 39:1265.

35

Tremor in the Acquired Immune Deficiency Syndrome

Carlos Singer and William J. Weiner
University of Miami School of Medicine
Miami, Florida

I. INTRODUCTION

Neurological complications are reported in up to 40% of clinical surveys of acquired immune deficiency syndrome (AIDS) (1–3). Autopsy-based surveys have found neuropathological involvement in 70–80% of cases (4). One-third of AIDS patients with neurological complications (NC-AIDS) will present to medical attention with the neurological symptoms as the first manifestation of the disease (2,3).

The exact prevalence of movement disorders in the NC-AIDS population has not been adequately studied. In the only available retrospective study, movement disorders were seen in 11% of all cases of NC-AIDS (5).

Tremor in AIDS has been described in three different clinical situations. These include the AIDS dementia complex, cerebral toxoplasmosis, and drug-induced disorders.

II. AIDS–DEMENTIA COMPLEX (HIV ENCEPHALOPATHY)

Dementia is a complication of AIDS characterized by a progressive encephalopathy in which cognitive and motor dysfunction predominate (6). It is thought to be a consequence of a direct effect of the human immunodeficiency virus on the central nervous system (CNS) (6).

This complex is the most frequent neurological complication of AIDS (7). It has been found in at least 17% (54/315) of NC-AIDS cases with CNS involvement (2) and in 36% (18/50) of NC-AIDS cases when both the central and peripheral nervous system involvements are included (1). In a review of 70 autopsied cases with AIDS (6), 46 (65%) suffered from HIV encephalopathy (patients with macroscopic focal nervous system disease or who had suffered from sustained metabolic encephalopathies had already been excluded from the original series of 121 patients).

Although cytomegalovirus (CMV) infection had been thought to be the etiology of the HIV encephalopathy (1), more recent studies have demonstrated that, even in those cases of HIV encephalopathy with postmortem histopathological evidence of CMV infection of the brain, no correlation can be found between these changes and the degree of cognitive and motor disturbance seen in these patients (6).

The spectrum of movement disorders seen in patients with the HIV encephalopathy has not been entirely described. Patients often have motor symptoms, such as postural tremor, bradykinesia, and weakness, early in the course of their disease (8).

Although tremors have been reported in only 5.5% of all cases of NC-AIDS (9), a higher prevalence of tremors has been observed in HIV encephalopathy, in which the tremor may present as an early or late manifestation (8). Twenty-three of 46 patients with HIV encephalopathy (50%) had motor symptoms early in the course of their disease (8), with a "rapid tremor on sustention" seen in 7 patients (7/44). In the late stage of their disease tremor was seen in an additional 13 patients (20/45).

Tremor is frequently associated with other neurological symptoms and signs in cases of NC-AIDS (5,8,10). In one report (5) three of seven NC-AIDS patients with movement disorders were described as having tremor, along with other neurological deficits. Two had a "parkinsonian" tremor. In one of these patients, associated findings included branchial myoclonus, supranuclear ophthalmoparesis, bulbar palsy, and peripheral neuropathy, and in the second patient segmental lower extremity myoclonus was present. The third patient had a postural tremor associated with dystonic posturing of both arms, and mild right hemiparesis [magnetic resonance imaging (MRI) demonstrated a small lesion in left thalamus and posterior internal capsule]. Only in the first patient was an etiological diagnosis made (biopsy proved cerebral Whipple's disease). The latter two patients had elevations of IgG in their cerebrospinal fluid (CSF), of unknown etiology. These two patients may have had HIV encephalopathy. Metzer described a patient with dementia, lower extremity upper motor neuron weakness, torticollis, and a 3- to 5-Hz resting tremor, with rigidity of the upper extremities (11).

We reported a patient with HIV encephalopathy (10) who presented with a postural and kinetic tremor of the right hand, associated with inability to write, clumsiness, and unusual finger posturing (with the thumb curling under the other fingers). Subclinical cognitive impairment was documented at the initial presentation. As the disease progressed, the patient developed bilateral motor impairment, predominantly of the upper extremities (postural and kinetic tremor, bradykinesia, and unusual posturing), hypophonic slurred speech; and facial asymmetry, with hypomimia, suggestive of basal ganglia dysfunction. He did not respond to treatment with zidovudine azidothimidine (AZT) or to trials of benztropine mesylate and levodopa–carbidopa.

Patients with suspected HIV encephalopathy may already have a reversal of T4/T8 ratio in addition to the positive HIV titer. In evaluating these patients, opportunistic CNS infections and lymphoma need to be excluded with imaging procedures (toxoplasmosis, progressive multifocal leukoencephalopathy, lymphoma), serologies (syphilis and toxoplasmosis), and CSF studies including cultures and cytological studies.

Diffuse white matter demyelination, particularly of the centrum semiovale, but also involving the internal capsule, brainstem, and cerebellum, is a prominent neuropathological feature of the HIV encephalopathy (6). There is also prominent involvement of the basal ganglia (6), with foamy macrophages, multinucleated cells, and microglial nodules. This latter feature is probably the cause of the involuntary movements and other extrapyramidal signs described in the HIV encephalopathy. Perivascular and parenchymal infiltrates of lymphocytes and macrophages are frequently seen in white and subcortical gray matters. Foci of coagulation necrosis, with cavitation resembling microinfarcts, may also be noted in some patients.

There have been two patients reported in whom cerebellar ataxia was a prominent component of the HIV encephalopathy (12,13). In neither case is intention or kinetic tremor specifically mentioned. In one patient (13) a subacute cerebellar syndrome (gait unsteadiness, dysarthria, and limb incoordination) was the first manifestation of the disease and was fully developed before cognitive impairment appeared 2 months later. At autopsy loss of Purkinje cells in the cerebellum was found in both patients, as well as the expected pathological findings in the subcortical white matter and basal ganglia.

III. CEREBRAL TOXOPLASMOSIS

Although better known for causing hemichorea–hemiballismus (5,8,14–16), AIDS associated with cerebral toxoplasmosis may also have tremor as one of its features. Rubral tremor has been reported associated with a 1-cm–round enhancing lesion of cerebral toxoplasmosis in the ipsilateral midbrain (17). This patient had a coarse 3- to 4-Hz tremor involving the jaw and proximal and distal muscles of the left upper and lower extremities. It increased in amplitude with posture or intention. Additional findings induced dystonic posturing of the same extremities (noted on review of the videotape), left ptosis, with incomplete eye elevation and adduction, and a right hemiplegia and left gaze preference (the latter secondary to a concurrent large left frontal mass with shift of the midline to the right). Treatment with pyrimethamine and trisulfapyrimidine resulted in radiological, but not clinical improvement.

Parkinsonism, including tremor, associated with toxoplasmal abscesses of the anterior limbs of both internal capsules has also been reported (18). This patient developed marked bradykinesia, tremor, hypophonia, and rigidity, as well as encephalopathic changes within 2 weeks of the onset of symptoms. A clinical description of the tremor was not provided. Treatment with pyrimethamine and sulfadiazine was unsuccessful, and the patient died within 4 months of admission from intercurrent infection.

Additional examples of other movement disorders in toxoplasmosis include unilateral akathisia, associated with a contralateral subthalamic abscess (19), and focal upper extremity dystonia, associated with contralateral lenticular nucleus and thalamic lesions (20). Although in neither patient was tremor present, the potential for such cases to be associated with tremor has to be kept in mind.

IV. DRUG-INDUCED TREMORS

Patients with AIDS may require neuroleptics for the treatment of a variety of psychiatric states, including agitation, delirium, psychosis, and anxiety. Active or prophylactic treatment of *Pneumocystis carinii* pneumonia (trimethoprim–sulfa-methoxazole and pentamidine) is frequently complicated by nausea and vomiting. Antiemetics with dopamine-blocking properties may be used in this setting. In either event, tremors may appear as part of drug-induced parkinsonism or as the neuroleptic malignant syndrome.

The preferential involvement of the basal ganglia by the HIV virus, as exemplified in the HIV encephalopathy may underlie the apparent susceptibility of the AIDS patients—frequently younger than 40—to the extrapyramidal side effects of dopamine-blocking agents (21–27). There have been as yet no large prospective studies addressing this question, and information is based on case reports. Five cases have been reported of AIDS patients developing extrapyramidal reactions secondary to prochlorperazine (21,25,27). Two had parkinsonism, including one with hand tremor. Two patients developed neuroleptic malignant syndrome, and one a dystonic reaction. The patients were all young homosexual men. Their extrapyramidal syndromes developed within 5–10 days of initiation of prochlorperazine. Discontinuation of treatment resulted in reversal of symptoms.

This clinical observation is perhaps comparable with the increased incidence of phenothiazine-induced extrapyramidal syndromes that has been reported in individuals older than 40 in the general population (21). Moreover, side effects caused by prochloperazine, a low-potency phenothiazine, tend to be rare, except in the elderly (21,28,29). In one series, 21 of the 48 cases of drug-induced parkinsonism

(DIP), referred to a geriatric medicine department over a 2-year period, were due to prochlorperazine (28,29). After a mean follow-up of 41 months, 25% of the surviving DIP patients (5/20) developed Parkinson's disease. This may signify that elderly patients who have drug-induced parkinsonism already have a reduced supply of dopaminergic neurons in the substantia nigra and, therefore, are at increased risk of subsequently developing Parkinson's disease (30). Phenothiazines and other dopamine-blocking agents may tip them over into overt parkinsonism or unmask latent idiopathic Parkinson's disease (29).

Susceptibility to drug-induced dystonia has also been described in AIDS patients. Hollander et al. (22) reported patients with AIDS-related *Pneumocystis carinii* pneumonia who had to be treated with metoclopramide as an antiemetic agent and who developed dystonic reactions. It occurred in four of seven such patients at one of their hospitals, a higher incidence than the expected 0.2% in the general population (an additional two patients were found at another institution). The dose had been 20 mg every 6–8 h. They also reported dystonia in 4 of 11 patients who had received low-dose chlorpromazine, in the same clinical situation, over a 1-year period. Although all of these cases consisted of dystonic reactions, future reports of drug-induced parkinsonism could be reasonably forthcoming.

Tremor—rest, intention, or both—associated with apathy or a full-blown cerebellar syndrome has been reported in four AIDS patients affected with *Pneumocystis carinii* pneumonia while receiving trimethoprim–sulfamethoxazole (31). Additional findings included sustained ankle clonus (2/4), rash (2/4) and hallucinations (1/4). The electroencephalogram (EEG), computed tomography (CT) scan, and CSF determinations were unremarkable. Symptom onset occurred within 3–11 days of initiation of treatment, and resolution was within 2–3 days of stopping it. Only one of these patients developed HIV encephalopathy within the ensuing year, arguing against an underlying encephalopathy in the majority of these cases. The mechanism is unknown. Since children with congenital AIDS have been reported with low CSF folate levels and since trimethoprim and sulfamethoxazole affect folate metabolism, the authors postulate a pharmacological aggravation of preexisting folate deficiency.

V. SUMMARY

Tremor, at rest or with intention, can be seen both as an early or late manifestation of the HIV encephalopathy. It is associated with other motor symptoms and signs (dystonia, bradykinesia, myoclonus) and results from direct effect of the HIV virus on the CNS, including the basal ganglia. It does not respond to antiretroviral or symptomatic therapy.

The AIDS patients receiving active or prophylactic treatment for *Pneumocystis carinii* pneumonia may develop iatrogenic rest or intention tremors. Consideration should be given to discontinuation of trimethoprim–sulfamethoxazole or antiemetics before embarking in a costlier workup for infectious etiologies. Similar considerations apply to the use of neuroleptics in this population.

Cerebral toxoplasmosis has been associated with a rubral tremor and a parkinsonian picture in two isolated reports. Treatment with antitoxoplasmosis agents may result in neurological improvement.

REFERENCES

1. Snider WD, Simpson DM, Nielsen S, Gold JWM, Metroka CE, Posner JB. Neurological complications of acquired immune deficiency syndrome: analysis of 50 patients. Ann Neurol 1983; 14:403–418.
2. Levy RM, Bredesen DE, Rosenblum ML. Neurological manifestations of the acquired immunodeficiency syndrome (AIDS): experience at UCSF and review of the literature. J Neurosurg 1985; 62:475–495.
3. Levy RM, Bredesen DE, Rosenblum M. Opportunistic central nervous system pathology in patients with AIDS. Ann Neurol 1988; 23(suppl):S7–S12.
4. Elder GA, Sever JL. AIDS and neurological disorders: an overview. Ann Neurol 1988; 23(suppl):S4–S6.
5. Nath A, Jankovic J, Pettigrew L. Movement disorders and AIDS. Neurology 1987; 37: 37–41.
6. Navia BA, Cho E-S, Petito CK, Price RW. The AIDS dementia complex: II. Neuropathology. Ann Neurol 1986; 19:525–535.
7. McArthur JC. Neurologic manifestations of AIDS. Medicine 1987; 66:407–437.
8. Navia BA, Jordan BD, Price RW. The AIDS dementia complex: I. Clinical features. Ann Neurol 1986; 19:517–524.
9. Berger JR, Moskowitz L, Fischl M, Kelley RE. The neurologic complications of AIDS: frequently the initial manifestation. Neurology 1984; 34(suppl 1):134–135.
10. Singer C, Sanchez-Ramos J, Rey G, Levin B, Weiner WJ. AIDS dementia complex presenting as an unusual unilateral hand tremor, clumsiness and posturing. Ann Neurol 1990; 28:301.
11. Metzer WS. Movement disorders with AIDS encephalopathy: case report. Neurology 1987; 37:1438.
12. Clark GL, Vinters HV. Dementia and ataxia in a patient with AIDS. West J Med 1987; 146:68–72.
13. Graus F, Ribalta T, Abos J, et al. Subacute cerebellar syndrome as the first manifestation of AIDS dementia complex. Acta Neurol Scand 1990; 81:118–120.
14. Navia BA, Petito CK, Gold JWM, Eun-Sook C, Jordan BD, Price RW. Cerebral toxoplasmosis complicating the acquired immune deficiency syndrome: clinical and neuropathological findings in 27 patients. Ann Neurol 1986; 19:224–238.
15. Sanchez-Ramos JR, Factor SA, Weiner WJ, Marquez J. Hemichorea–hemiballismus associated with acquired immunodeficiency syndrome and cerebral toxoplasmosis. Mov Disord 1989; 4:226–273.
16. Martinez-Martin P. Hemichorea–hemiballism in AIDS. Mov Disord 1990; 5:180.
17. Koppel BS, Daras M. "Rubral" tremor due to midbrain toxoplasma abscess. Mov Disord 1990; 5:254–256.

18. Carrazana E, Rossitch E, Jr, Samuels MA. Parkinsonian symptoms in a patient with AIDS and cerebral toxoplasmosis. J Neurol Neurosurg Psychiatry 1989; 52:1445–1447.

19. Carrazana E, Rossitch E, Martinez J, et al. Unilateral "akathisia" in a patient with AIDS and a toxoplasmosis subthalamic abscess. Neurology 1989; 39:449–450.

20. Tolge CF, Factor SA. Focal dystonia secondary to cerebral toxoplasmosis in a patient with acquired immune deficiency syndrome. Mov Disord 1991; 6:69–72.

21. Edelstein H, Knight RT. Severe parkinsonism in two AIDS patients taking prochlorperazine. Lancet 1987; 2:341–342.

22. Hollander H, Golden J, Mendelson T, Cortlan D. Extrapyramidal symptoms in AIDS patients given low dose metoclopramide or chlorpromazine. Lancet 1985; 2:1186.

23. Breitbart W, Marotta RF, Call P. AIDS and neuroleptic malignant syndrome. Lancet 1988; 2:1488–1489.

24. Burch EA, Montoya J. Neuroleptic malignant syndrome in an AIDS patient. J Clin Psychopharmacol 1989; 9:228–229.

25. Swenson JR, Erman M, Labelle J, Dimsdale JF. Extrapyramidal reactions: neuropsychiatric mimics in patients with AIDS. Gen Hosp Psychiatry 1989; 11:248–253.

26. Lazarus A. EPS, NMS, and AIDS [letter]. Biol Psychiatry 1990; 28:551–554.

27. Bernstein WB, Scherokman B. Neuroleptic malignant syndrome in a patient with acquired immunodeficiency syndrome. Acta Neurol Scand 1986; 73:636–637.

28. Wilson JA, Smith RG. Relation between elderly and AIDS patients with drug-induced Parkinson's disease [letter]. Lancet 1987; 2:686.

29. Wilson JA, Primrose WR, Smith RG. Prognosis of drug-induced Parkinson's disease. Lancet 1987; 2:443–444.

30. Stephen PJ, Williamson J. Drug-induced parkinsonism in the elderly. Lancet 1984; 2:1082–1083.

31. Borucki MJ, Matzke DS, Pollard RB. Tremor induced by trimethoprim–sulfamethoxazole in patients with the acquired immunodeficiency syndrome (AIDS). Ann Intern Med 1988; 109:77–78.

36

Psychogenic Tremor

Steven L. Moon and William C. Koller
University of Kansas Medical Center
Kansas City, Kansas

I. INTRODUCTION

Tremors, in addition to being symptoms of neurological disease or merely physiological, may be psychogenic. Gowers (1) noted that tremors frequently accompanied hysteria, and thought them to be intermittent and commonly evoked by movement or excitement. In addition, he noted that they were increased by attention and ameliorated by distraction. Campbell has also described the cessation of functional tremor with distraction (2).

II. CLINICAL MANIFESTATIONS

Cases of psychogenic tremor have been infrequently reported in the literature and, therefore, are rather poorly defined. Koller and colleagues reported 24 patients with psychogenic tremor and documented a number of manifestations that they had in common (3). The cases, once diagnosed, were divided according to classification for psychogenic movement disorders previously established by Fahn and colleagues (4):

1. *Documented*: Symptoms are relieved by psychotherapy, suggestion, or by placebo, or the patient is witnessed as being free of symptoms when left alone supposedly unobserved.
2. *Clinically established*: Movement disorder is inconsistent over time or is incongruent with classic condition, other neurological signs are present that are psychogenic, multiple somatizations are present, and a psychiatric disturbance is present.

3. *Probably psychogenic*: Movements are inconsistent or incongruent with the classic movement disorder, and there are no other features to provide support for such a diagnosis of psychogenicity.
4. *Possible psychogenic*: Suspicious that the movements are psychogenic if an obvious emotional disturbance is present.

Sixteen of the 24 cases of psychogenic tremor were clinically established, and 8 were documented. Probable or possible cases were not included. In addition, appropriate laboratory testing was performed to rule out organic disease when appropriate. A summary of the salient clinical features for this condition is listed in Table 1. The clinical features are frequently atypical, thereby making the tremor unclassifiable as one of the more clearly defined organic tremors. The tremors often have an abrupt onset and, frequently, start bilaterally, in addition to having a nonprogressive course with fluctuating severity. This distinguishes them from other tremor disorders, such as Parkinson's disease and essential tremor, which typically have an insidious onset, begin unilaterally, and commonly increase in severity.

The tremors often had resting, postural, as well as kinetic components. They are typically worst in postural positions and are similar in all positions, another characteristic usually not found in organic varieties. Selective disability, such as being able to write, but only able to draw a tremulous spiral, can also be seen (see Fig. 1 in Ref. 3). The nature of the tremor can be variable, present in a certain position at one time, but absent or different at another. The tremors may increase in frequency when attention is given to them; conversely, their frequency may decrease or even disappear when the patient is distracted. In some instances, the tremor may assume the frequency of a motor task being performed by the other

Table 1   Clinical Features of Psychogenic Tremor

1. Abrupt onset
2. Static course
3. Spontaneous remissions
4. Unclassifiable tremors (complex tremors)
5. Clinical inconsistencies (selective disabilities)
6. Changing tremor characteristics
7. Unresponsiveness to antitremor drugs
8. Tremor increases with attention
9. Tremor lessens with distractibility
10. Responsiveness to placebo
11. Absence of other neurological signs
12. Remission with psychotherapy

hand. The direction of the tremor may change from a supination–pronation orientation to one of flexion–extension. Table 2 lists other factors that, if associated with tremor, also suggest a possible psychogenic etiology.

Tremogram analysis of psychogenic tremors may reveal marked fluctuation in tremor amplitude during the recording, in contradistinction to organic tremors, which tend to fluctuate to a minimal degree during recording. In addition, tremor frequency may also change during a recording, a feature not seen in organic tremor. Reduction in tremor with distraction may be seen on a tremogram (see Fig. 2 in Ref. 3). An exaggeration of physiological tremor by strong voluntary muscle contraction displays synchronous electromyographic (EMG) bursts in opposing muscles that commonly have a frequency of 8–12 Hz (5).

Several psychiatric conditions may include psychogenic tremor as a manifestation. Somatoform disorders (including conversion and somatization syndromes), factitious disorders (such as Münchausen's syndrome), and malingering are some examples (6). Fahn and Williams point out that, as in psychogenic dystonia, it may be difficult to classify these movement disorders into specific psychiatric diagnostic categories (4). For example, it might be difficult to distinguish hysteria from malingering. It should be remembered, however, that some organic movement disorders are often accompanied by psychiatric symptoms. For example, depression may be seen with Parkinson's disease or cranial dystonia, and a variety of psychiatric symptoms may be seen in Huntington's disease.

III. TREATMENT

Pharmacological treatment is not usually effective. Drugs are frequently discarded because of reported toxicity or simply lack of effect. Resolution of an underlying social problem or treatment of a psychiatric illness may result in

Table 2   Other Medical Factors Suggesting Psychogenic Tremor

1. Multiple somatizations
2. Multiple undiagnosed conditions
3. Spontaneous remissions or cures of symptoms
4. Presence of unphysiological weakness or sensory complaints
5. No evidence of disease by laboratory or radiographic procedures
6. Presence of unwitnessed paroxysmal disorders
7. Employed in allied health professions
8. Litigation or compensation pending
9. Presence of secondary gain
10. Presence of psychiatric disease
11. Documented functional disturbances in the past

reduction or cessation of the tremor. In some cases, the tremor may cease abruptly for no known reason. Placebo therapy may result in a dramatic response in other patients. Total cessation of the tremor would be uncharacteristic of organic tremor, but it should be remembered that organic tremor may be reduced by up to 30% with placebo (7). Fahn (8) reported two cases of psychogenic tremor: In one patient, the tremor disappeared after psychotherapy; in the other, initial drug therapy was unsuccessful, but improvement occurred later with psychotherapy.

IV. CONCLUSION

Psychogenic tremor is largely a diagnosis of exclusion. One must remember that organic disease frequently coexists with psychogenic disease and, therefore, a thorough search for the former is needed in all suspected cases. One may feel more secure in the diagnosis if a large number of the foregoing manifestations are present, but this frequently does not occur. Therefore, in this condition, one must frequently accept a certain degree of diagnostic uncertainty, while remaining open to new clinical information as it presents itself.

A diagnosis of "psychogenic" tremor should be made only by a clinician experienced in the assessment of movement disorders.

REFERENCES

1. Gowers WR. Disease of the Nervous System. Philadelphia: Blakiston, Son, & Co, 1988.
2. Campbell J. The shortest paper. Neurology 1979; 29:1633.
3. Koller W, Lang A, Vetere-Overfield B, et al. Psychogenic tremors. Neurology 1989; 39:1094–1099.
4. Fahn S, Williams PJ. Psychogenic dystonia. Adv Neurol 1988; 50:431–455.
5. Clare M, Bishop G. Electromyographic analysis of the physiologic components of tremor. Arch Phys Med Rehabil 1949; 30:559–567.
6. American Psychiatric Association. Diagnostic and Statistical Manual of Mental Disorders. 3rd ed, revised. Washington, DC: American Psychiatric Association Press, 1987.
7. Koller WC. Treatment of essential tremor. In: Marsden CD, Conrad B, Beneche R, eds. Motor Disorders. London: Academic Press, 1987:55–67.
8. Fahn S. Atypical, rare, and unclassified tremors. In: Findley LJ, Capildeo R, eds. Tremor Disorders. London: Macmillan Press, 1984:431–444.

37

Vocal Tremor

Mitchell F. Brin and Andrew Blitzer
College of Physicians and Surgeons
Columbia University
New York, New York

Celia Stewart
New York University
and Columbia University
New York, New York

I. INTRODUCTION

The involuntary, rhythmic, oscillatory movements (1) that affect the distal musculature in patients with tremulous diseases may also affect the muscles of the sound production mechanism and generate rhythmic alterations in pitch and loudness, called *vocal tremor*. Vocal tremor is clinically identified by the phonatory characteristics. Vocal tremor has been described perceptually as "tremulous voice" (2), "wavy voice" (3), or "tremulous, quavering speech" (4), and has been associated with neurological disorders, such as essential tremor, orthostatic tremor (5), Parkinson's disease (6–8), cerebellar ataxia, dystonia (9,10), myoclonus (9,11), motor neuron disease (12,13), or developmental speech and language deficits (14). It may result in rapid decreases and increases in loudness and pitch, or in brief complete phonation stoppages. Intelligibility and rate of speech may be decreased.

Vocal tremor may be the only symptom, or a concomitant symptom, of a neurological disease (2,15,16). The frequency, amplitude, and regularity of vocal tremor may differ among diseases of different neural subsystems (11,17,18). Analysis of vocal tremor may make important contributions to early and differential diagnosis of neurological diseases and, consequently, to treatment decisions.

Teams of researchers and clinicians from speech pathology, otolaryngology, and neurology have contributed to knowledge about vocal tremor.

Various sites have been documented as physiological bases of vocal tremor within the speech mechanism. Whereas the "prime generator" of voice tremor is usually a central nervous system (CNS) disturbance, the phonatory reflection is typically multifactorial, involving a combination of the intrinsic and extrinsic laryngeal muscles; pharyngeal muscles, including any supraglottic structure; and the respiratory support muscles, including those of the diaphragm, chest wall, and abdomen. Critchley suggested that "tremor of muscles of the larynx, lips, tongue and diaphragm may be responsible for quavering speech" (19). Lebrun (17) discounted the diaphragm in contributing to tremulous speech because it is generally relaxed in speech and is not affected by the intension tremor when a subject talks. The muscles that control expiratory air pressure during speech are the external and internal intercostals (20,21), which most probably contribute to the intensity and pitch fluctuations characteristic of voice tremors. Others have supported this view, stating that vocal tremor resulted from changes in subglottal air pressure induced by an action tremor of the respiratory muscles (22), rhythmic activity in the rectus abdominus respiratory muscle (23), and rhythmic fluctuations in contraction of expiratory chest muscles (17). Vertical movement of the larynx (2) and rhythmic abduction (24) and adduction of the vocal folds, and rhythmic reduction of tension of the vocal folds owing to cricothyroid action (24) have been associated with vocal tremor and the accompanying vocal arrests and breaks. Lips, tongue, soft palate, and jaw movements have been reported to contribute to vocal tremor as well (17,24). Passive vibration from gross tremor elsewhere in the body may be reflected in secondary vocal tremor (16,25).

Fundamental frequency (F_0) measures the rate at which the vocal folds open and close. The vibration of the vocal folds is primarily a passive process, resulting from the interaction of subglottal air pressure built up by the respiratory system, and vocal fold stiffness set by the internal laryngeal muscles (26). As a result, both fluctuations of subglottal air pressure and fluctuations of vocal fold stiffness are probable causes of perceptually identified vocal tremor. Because of coupling of larynx and tongue by extrinsic laryngeal muscles, changes in articulatory configurations and precision of movement may result in F_0 modifications that may manifest as tremor. Oscillatory changes of subglottal air pressure sufficient for the generation of vocal tremor can be reflected in speech intensity contours and oscillations in pitch, contributing to a perceptually quavering speech.

Acoustic analysis has been the primary noninvasive method for quantification of vocal tremor. Most acoustic data on vocal tremor have been obtained from visual inspection of oscillographic displays of waveform data (Fig. 1) (2,22), or from graphic level recorder displays of amplitude contours (3,27) of sustained vowel phonation. Consequently, the bulk of acoustic data on vocal tremor includes only visually quantifiable amplitude oscillations, without frequency modulation components.

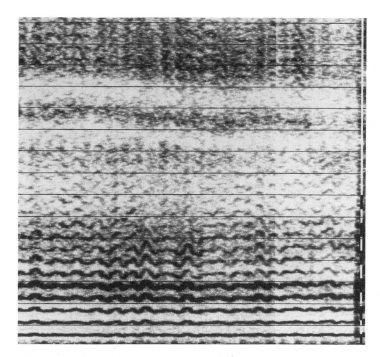

Figure 1 Essential voice tremor: The narrow-band spectrogram of prolonged /a/ shows fluctuations in amplitude with a relatively preserved frequency. The total duration of the recording is 3.5 s. The frequency is continuous throughout the recording. The harmonics are present throughout the frequency range, and the mild aperiodic noise between the harmonics indicates mild breathiness.

Phonatory tremor may cause variations in either frequency (cycle length) or amplitude (cycle height). If the respiratory system were the prime generator of vocal tremor, then one should measure changes in amplitude, rather than frequency. However, variations in frequency are postulated to be associated with laryngeal muscle firing (28,29) and were proposed to contribute to phonatory tremor (18,30). This assertion is supported by the observation that a singer's vibrato results in frequency variations (31).

Researchers have demodulated the acoustic signal into the amplitude and frequency components (18,32) and have applied spectral analysis to the demodulated signals (33,34). The data suggests that vocal tremor may involve oscillations in frequency, in addition to the amplitude oscillations previously reported (18,32,34), and that tremor is a complex waveform comprising a number of components (33,35,36), rather than the single frequency usually measured from oscillographic data. These more precise analyses may facilitate distinctions among tremors accompanying different neurological diseases and contribute to our understanding about underlying physiological bases of vocal tremor within the speech mechanism (37). Recognition that tremor has frequency modulations supports a nonrespiratory muscle contribution to the genesis of tremor.

Quantification of the frequency, amplitude, and regularity of vocal tremor has resulted in various hypotheses about its physiological bases within the speech mechanism (respiratory, phonatory, or articulatory muscle oscillation). Commonly, the frequency of vocal tremor accompanying neurological diseases has been reported to range from 4 to 8 Hz (2,17,22,32), with amplitudes of oscillation ranging widely (2,18,32). Some vocal tremors may be constant (regular) throughout sustained phonation, others may crescendo in amplitude and slow in frequency toward the end of the phonation (2), and others may be too variable and irregular for analysis (18). Reports of normal physiological vocal tremor have been most often in the 8- to 20-Hz range (18), with amplitudes of oscillation of approximately 25% (2).

Electromyography (EMG) has been used to study laryngeal muscle activation in patients with vocal tremor (23,38–40). Ardran (38) documented tremor in the cricothyroid, hyoglossus, and limb muscles of an elderly man with 60 years of symptomatic essential tremor (ET). Tomada examined two patients with voice and limb tremor, and one with isolated voice tremor (23). Acoustically identified vocal tremor was associated with synchronous rhythmic contraction of the cricothyroid and rectus abdominis muscles. Rhythmic vocalis muscle contractions were recorded only in the one subject with isolated voice tremor; the vocalis contractions were synchronous with recordings from the soft palate and rectus abdominis (4–5 Hz). Tremor occurred only on voluntary phonation or expiration, but not during voluntary inspiration or during involuntary respiration (breathing at rest).

Koda, studying eight patients with acoustically obvious tremor, found thyroarytenoid tremor in all patients, at some time during the study (39). Their data suggest that more than one recording may be necessary to document tremor in a muscle tested. The mean thyroarytenoid tremor frequency was 4.7 Hz, with a frequency range of 4.0–5.2 Hz for all laryngeal muscles tested. Tremor frequency was altered by the gestures being performed, such as phonation or respiration, and may be dependent on the level of activation of the motor neuron pool for a particular gesture: 9.0 Hz during inhalation, 6.6 Hz during whisper, 4.7 Hz during exhalation, and 4.9 Hz during phonation. Although muscle signals within patients may have had similar frequencies, usually there were significant delays in the timing of the tremor peaks between muscles, suggesting that the putative central generator modulates each motoneuron pool independently. Activation for different laryngeal gestures appeared to affect the tremor modulations in each motoneuron pool independently too.

Because vocal tremor may be perceptually similar in different neurological

Table 1 Differential Diagnosis of Vocal Tremor/Tremulousness:
Disorders with Rhythmical or Arhythmical Oscillations Involving
Larynx, Palate, Pharynx, Tongue, or Diaphragmatic Muscles

Hyperkinetic conditions
  Essential tremor
  Dystonia
  Ataxia
  Segmental cranial myoclonus
  Vibrato
  Physiological tremor
Bradykinetic conditions
  Parkinson's disease/parkinsonism
  Motor neuron disease (rapid tremor or flutter on vowel prolongation)

---

disorders, there is overlap in classification. Some of the conditions causing vocal
tremor (Table 1) are discussed in the following sections.

II. ESSENTIAL VOICE TREMOR

The appendicular tremor of ET is a rhythmic oscillatory movement of 4–12 Hz,
with variable amplitude (41–44), most commonly caused by reciprocal activation
of antagonistic muscles, although periods of cocontraction may be observed (45).
The frequency of tremor affecting different individuals is quite variable, and there
is overlap with the characteristic frequencies of physiological and parkinsonian
tremors. Therefore, frequency cannot be the sole criterion by which essential
tremor may be distinguished (46).

Essential voice tremor is characterized by quavering intonation, especially
during sustained vowel prolongation, often associated with rhythmic alterations in
loudness and, to a lesser degree, pitch of vowels and continuant consonants (2).
Vocal tremor occurs in approximately 10–20% of patients with essential tremor
(17). It may be the first (2) or only sign of the disease (22,33), or it may accompany
tremors in other body parts (16). Vocal tremor may parallel the onset of other
symptoms, or have a sudden onset and cause rapid deterioration in speech
intelligibility (2,16). It has been reported that vocal tremor is greater with
emotional stress or fatigue (11). Although clinicians (including ourselves, initially)
thought coffee would exacerbate vocal tremor, stable doses do not consistently
worsen appendicular essential tremor (47); our patients with vocal tremor do not
report improvement when coffee is stopped. Pitch breaks (octave breaks to a lower
or higher frequency) and phonation arrests have been reported in certain cases of
essential tremor (15,17) and have been associated with visible vertical oscillations

of the larynx (48), vocal folds, the hyolaryngeal complex, or a combination thereof.

Findley and Gresty found that 11% of ET patients had voice tremor, and only one had vocal involvement in isolation, without signs of ET involving other segments of the body (49). Massey and Paulson identified 26 of 131 (20%) ET patients with voice tremor and 4 of 131 (3%) with it in isolation (27,50). Lou and Jankovic reviewed 350 patients evaluated at one center; 62 (17.7%) had voice tremor and only 1 had voice tremor in isolation (57). Those with voice involvement were equally represented in the early-onset (younger than 30 years) versus late-onset (older than 40 years) groups, those with a family history versus sporadic cases, and those with generally mild versus severe disease. Additional series report voice tremor present in 20% of 194 (52), 19% of 81 (53), and 9% of 35 (54) patients studied.

Pharmacotherapeutic treatment of ET voice tremor has been disappointing, with equivocal results. Alcohol may be of benefit (27), but is not recommended as routine therapy. Some reports show reductions in vocal tremor with propranolol (27,33,50); primidone (55,56); and clonazepam, propranolol, and diazepam, in combination (23). However, Koller's double-blind study (4) showed no significant improvement with propranolol versus placebo, even though one patient had a dramatic improvement with propranolol. In their study, four of six patients had symptomatic hand tremor that was improved with active drug. From this study, and that of Tomada's (23), it is suggested that upper limb tremor is more responsive to pharmacotherapy than voice tremor. In our practice, we, as others have, found limited clinically significant changes in vocal tremor with administration of propranolol (4,43,57), primidone (57–59), or clonazepam (57). Although one report suggested that methazolamide helps patients with essential voice tremor (60), we have not found it to be a particularly useful pharmacological agent.

We have used local injections of botulinum toxin (BTX) in the treatment of essential vocal tremor, with a dramatic benefit noted in our preliminary series. The technique is the same as that used to treat patients with spasmodic dysphonia (61,62). Botulinum toxin is injected percutaneously through the cricothyroid membrane into the vocal folds using electromyographic guidance. For the first treatment, we perform bilateral, low-dose injections of 1.0–2.5 U per vocal fold. With a "percent-of-normal-function" linear rating scale (100% = normal function; 0% = no functional voice), patients had a significant improvement in vocal function (Table 2). The improvement is statistically significant in this open study. Some of the patients required injections of the sternohyoid and sternothyroid muscles to prevent the tremoulous elevation and lowering of the entire laryngeal apparatus. However, injections of these strap muscles can be associated with a higher incidence of dysphagia, particularly if performed without electromyographic guidance.

Table 2 Botulinum Toxin-A For Essential Voice
Tremor ($N = 21$)

	% of Normal function		
	Mean ± SD	Median	Range
Preinjection	35.0 ± 13.2	30.0	25–50
Postinjection	87.5 ± 13.6	87.5	60–100
Pretreatment vs Posttreatment (medians):			
$p = 0.0003$			

III. VOCAL TREMOR, LARYNGEAL DYSTONIA (SPASMODIC DYSPHONIA), AND DYSTONIC TREMOR

Dystonia is a syndrome dominated by sustained muscle contractions that frequently cause twisting and repetitive movements, or abnormal postures that may be sustained or intermittent. Dystonia can involve any voluntary muscle. Dystonic movements can be rapid and repetitive, and tremor may be seen in dystonia affecting a segment of the body.

Idiopathic *spasmodic dysphonia* (SD) and *laryngeal dystonia* (LD) are clinical terms used to describe an action-induced laryngeal movement disorder (63). In 1871, Traube (64) coined the term *spastic dysphonia* when describing a patient with nervous hoarseness. In the early literature, SD has been compared with other focal dystonias, such as occupational writer's cramp (65,66) and oromandibular dystonia (67). The association of SD with dystonia involving other segments of the body is established; many of the phenomenological, clinical, and laboratory features of patients with focal SD are similar to those with more generalized disease (10,68–70). The affliction has been described as though the patient were "trying to talk whilst being choked" (71), or "stuttering with the vocal cords" (72). Although Aronson (73,74) documented that the Minnesota Multiphasic Personality Inventory (MMPI) and psychiatric interviews did not discriminate between patients with SD and those in the normal population, many patients are still referred to psychiatrists for treatment because the correct diagnosis is not made when the patient initially presents for treatment. Patients may be misdiagnosed as having laryngitis, vocal abuse, polyps, gastric reflux, stress-related disorders, or psychogenic.

Two distinct types of SD have been distinguished; *adductor*, caused by irregular hyperadduction of the vocal folds; and *abductor*, caused by intermittent abduction of the vocal folds. Some patients appear to have a combination of the two. Patients with *add*uctor SD exhibit a choked, strained-strangled voice quality, with abrupt initiation and termination of voicing, resulting in short breaks in phonation. Patients with *abd*uctor SD exhibit a breathy, effortful voice quality with abrupt termination of voicing, resulting in aphonic whispered segments of speech. Because many patients with SD present with a tremulous voice, the differential diagnosis between SD caused by ET versus that caused by a dystonic tremor can be difficult.

Dystonic tremors are typically irregular and have a directional preponderance; symptoms are increased when the patient postures the affected body part in a position opposed to the primary dystonic contractions. For instance, patients with torticollis often have a head tremor that can be dampened by placing the head into the preferred posture. Dystonic limb tremor is typically irregular; there is often a preferred posture in which the tremor is less prominent. Many patients with SD have an irregular vocal tremor that can be recorded both acoustically, electromyographically (40), and with accellerometry.

The presence of a postural tremor, caused by dystonia, that resembles ET is elaborated elsewhere in this volume; since Yanagisawa and Goto's report (75), there have been three recent electrophysiological studies examining the relation between dystonia and tremor (76–78). Elble et al. documented that tremor may be seen in limb muscles with abnormal coactivation of antagonistic muscles, rhythmic 5- to 7-Hz bursts of motor unit discharge, and tonic activity in antagonistic muscles (78), supporting the diagnosis of dystonia. Rivest and Marsden reviewed 12 patients who presented with isolated head or trunk tremor (77). Most patients had a slow 2- to 5-Hz tremor and either clinical or pharmacological characteristics suggesting the diagnosis of dystonia rather than ET; some later progressed with clinically obvious dystonia. Jedynak et al. studied tremor in 45 patients with various forms of idiopathic dystonia (76). With electrophysiological methods, they found that dystonic tremor was typically postural, localized, and irregular in amplitude and periodicity, absent during muscle relaxation and frequently associated with myoclonus. They emphasized that, although the tremor that accompanies idiopathic dystonia resembles ET because of its postural character, it is distinguished by its clinical and EMG characteristics. Myoclonus, a feature never seen in ET, may be present in dystonic tremor.

The clinical distinction between primary dystonia causing symptoms of tremor, and the condition of essential tremor, may be difficult in many cases, particularly when a patient presents with symptoms of essential tremor in other body parts (51,79). Discriminating between tremulousness that is due to essential tremor or to dystonia is particularly difficult when studying the voice: (1) the laryngeal muscles of phonation (Table 3), as a whole, are never available for study at complete rest: one or more muscle is contracting at a given moment; (2) in the presence of dystonia, laryngeal muscles cannot twist or turn; the glottic muscles can only adduct or abduct in some inappropriate fashion, including tremor and myoclonus.

In 1966, Ardran and coauthors reported laryngeal spasms, glottal stops, and interrupted speech resulting in dysphonia in one subject of a multiplex family with

Table 3 Intrinsic Muscles of the Larynx

Muscles that open and close the glottis
   Lateral and posterior cricoarytenoids
   Transverse arytenoid (interarytenoid)
Muscles that control tension of vocal ligaments
   Thryoarytenoid
   Vocalis (thicker inferior, medial segment)
   Lateral thyroarytenoid (superior, lateral)
   Cricothyroid
Muscles that alter shape of laryngeal inlet
   Aryepiglottic muscle
   Thyroepiglottic muscle

ET (38). The EMG of the hyoglossus and cricothyroid muscles revealed "fairly regular" tremors of 5–6 and 8 Hz. Tremor studies were not as sophisticated in 1966 as they are currently. A 6-Hz rhythmical tremor was measured in limb muscles. It was their impression that the interruption of voice was due to rhythmic wide separation of the vocal cords. This description suggests that the patient had the phonatory characteristics of abductor spasmodic dysphonia.

At about the same time that Ardran et al. published their study, other studies (73,74,80) were characterizing the clinical features of patients with spasmodic dysphonia, characterized predominantly by strain-strangle, voice stoppages, monopitch, and inappropriately low pitch level. Of 31 patients with a clinical diagnosis of SD, 58% had voice tremor during contextual speech, and 13% had pitch breaks. They also evaluated 26 patients with ET, finding that 100% had tremor on vowel prolongation (/a/), 92% had tremor during contextual speech, 85% had voice stoppages, 100% had strain-strangle dysphonia (either intermittent or constant), and 100% had harshness (Table 4). They recommended that rhythmic voice stoppages were suggestive of an ET etiology whereby there was inappropriate hyperadduction of the vocal cords. Voice tremor in contextual speech was more likely to be heard in ET than in SD. In an earlier study (80) of 34 patients with SD, voice tremor was heard in 18 during contextual speech and on prolongation of the vowel /a/ in 20. However, 6 patients had tremor of the hand or head, suggesting that the etiology may have been ET rather than SD. Regardless, the groups of Aronson and Ardran set the stage for documenting that patients with ET may have glottal stops suggestive of SD, and patients with dystonic larynges may have tremorous speech.

In 1975, it was suggested that "When organic voice tremor becomes sufficiently severe, the range or amplitude of the adductor phases of most or all of the vocal fold tremor cycles is so extensive that the folds momentarily meet in the

Table 4 Characterization of Clinical Features in Patients with ET
or SD

	Incidence (%)	
Factor	ET ($n = 26$)	SD ($n = 31$)
Voice tremor on vowel prolongation (/a/)	100	N/A
Harshness	100	100
Voice Tremor in contextual speech	92	58
Excessively low pitch	92	100
Monopitch	85	100
Regular voice stoppage	77	N/A
Strain-strangle dysphonia	100	100
Intermittent	50	
Constant	50	
Pitch breaks	31	13
Voice stoppages	100	97
Irregular	12	N/A

ET; essential tremor; SD; spasmodic dysphonia; N/A, data not available.
Source: Ref. 74.

midline and seal the glottis, producing a strained or staccato voice arrest" (48).
These characteristics have been misdiagnosed as the voice arrests and adductory
laryngeal spasms accompanying adductor spasmodic dysphonia (71) and, as a
result, essential tremor in certain patients has been misdiagnosed (3). It is
acknowledged that when a patient presents with vocal tremor as a monosymptomatic complaint, the differential diagnosis between ET and SD is difficult. Vocal
tremor has been observed in 30% of a group of patients with adductor spasmodic
dysphonia of unknown origin (81). A comparison between these patient groups
suggests that essential tremor patients have greater regularity in vocal arrests (82)
and vocal tremor than spasmodic dysphonia patients (18,34). Furthermore, it has
been reported that in essential tremor patients, frequency oscillations were more
predominant than amplitude oscillations (18), whereas in spasmodic dysphonia
patients, only amplitude oscillations were observed (83).

    Lebrun et al. studied the tremulous speech of an 84-year-old man with a 60-year
history of limb tremor, and later vocal tremor with glottal breaks (17). Oscillographic recording of a sustained /i/ revealed a 4-Hz rhythmic tremor. He had
intensity and pitch fluctuations in addition to erratic vocal breaks to a lower pitch
and voice arrests. The vocal break to a lower pitch was a sudden and short drop of
F_0. In connected speech, there were also sudden increases in F_0. Lebrun et al.
explained that, if the voice breaks were due to vocal cord hyperadduction, then
there would be an abrupt beginning of the second part of the vowel immediately

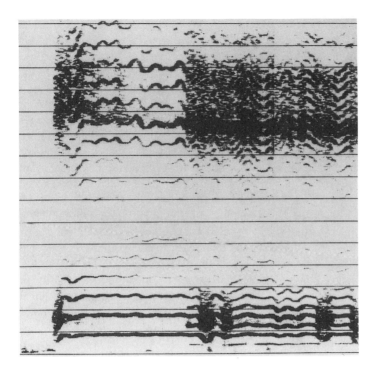

Figure 2 Dystonic tremor: The narrow-band spectrogram of prolonged /a/ shows irregu-lar fluctuations in frequency. The total duration of the recording is 3.5 s. A pitch break is observed at the middle of the recording where the harmonic lines abruptly double in number. The higher harmonics (not present in the parkinsonian patient, Figure 4) are clearly visible, with mild aperiodic noise between the high harmonics indicating minimal breathiness.

after the glottal catch, and the sonagram would have shown a spike corresponding to the forceful opening of the glottis at the end of the spasm (17). Their patient's sonagram showed a smooth, gradual resumption of voice production [*weicher Einsarz*; 84), suggesting a momentary decrease in laryngeal muscle tension (hyperabduction), rather than a laryngospasm (hyperadduction). In contrast with Aronson's experience, Lebrun's patient did not have an excessively low pitch, voice arrests did not occur at regular intervals, nor did they coincide with points of highest pitch. Finally, the patient's speech delivery was approximately half the rate of normal speakers, probably because of a combination of prolongation of normal sounds and short pauses between successive syllables or between words.

It is clear, therefore, that patients with vocal ET can have breaks and hesita-tions in their speech pattern, likely owing to either hyperadduction or hyperabduction of the vocal folds during contextual speech or phonatory tasks. Additional contribution to the choppy speech pattern may come from lingual tremor whereby the tongue beats up against the posterior pharyngeal wall and interrupts airflow. These patients present with the phenomenology of spasmodic dysphonia. In the clinic, we have found that asking the patient to speak or perform tasks with a whisper is often useful because there is less muscle activation, and a subtle tremor may become discernible. It is also evident that patients with dystonic larynges presenting with the phonatory characteristics of SD may have vocal tremor (9,85,86). Acoustic evaluation (Fig. 2) and tremor physiology evaluation may be useful in making the proper diagnosis. It is likely, however, that some patients with isolated phonatory tremor with strain-strangle speech are initially misdiagnosed and sometimes later are correctly categorized (82).

Several authors have noted the association of ET with Parkinson's disease (PD) (87–96) and dystonia (51,76–78, 97–99). Essential tremor has been claimed to be more common in patients with idiopathic torsion dystonia, particularly the focal dystonias, torticollis, blepharospasm, and oromandibular dystonia (51,79,97, 100–102). The clinical similarities of these tremors do not prove identity in nosological or pathophysiological terms. Whether there is a pathophysiological link between these conditions, or whether the tremor simply reflects a motor instability associated with PD and dystonia independently, remains to be established when more specific diagnostic procedures become available.

IV. MYOCLONUS

Myoclonus refers to sudden, brief, shocklike involuntary movements caused by muscular contractions (positive myoclonus) or inhibitions (negative myoclonus, "asterixis") arising from the central nervous system (103–105). Laryngeal involvement can become problematic in patients with myoclonic involvement of the primary laryngeal structures or muscles of respiration. Singulus (hiccup) and palatal myoclonus may cause vocal tremor.

A. Singulus

A common form of myoclonus is singulus or hiccup. Hiccup is an intermittent, abrupt, involuntary contraction of the diaphragm that results in sudden inspiration that is opposed by a closed glottis. It is a segmental, slow rhythmic myoclonus, typically stimulated by peripheral irritation of the diaphragm, more often on the left side. Like other forms of myoclonus, the etiologies may be cortical (brain tumor, meningitis, encephalitis), spinal (tumor, abscess), metabolic (uremia), or peripheral (gastric irritation, pulmonic and thoracic cavity disorders) (106). Experimental electrophysiological studies (107) have demonstrated sudden inspiratory muscle contractions of the diaphragm and external intercostal muscles associated with inhibition of expiratory muscle activity. Glottic closure occurs within 35 ms of the diaphragmatic stimulation. Hiccup frequency decreased with a rise in arterial P_{CO_2}, and increased with its decline. Treatment has included physical maneuvers, such as breath-holding, rapidly drinking liquids, breathing into a bag, and pharmacotherapies, such as baclofen, amyl nitrate, atropine, narcotics, barbiturates, benzodiazepines, and chlorpromazine. Pharyngeal stimulation, usually performed by nasal intubation with a gastric feeding tube, was very effective in one series (108), as was baclofen (109) or noninvasive phrenic nerve stimulation (110) in intractable cases.

B. Palatal Myoclonus

"Branchial" or "oculopalatal" myoclonus refers to myoclonic symptoms affecting cranial structures. Spencer, in 1886, used the term nystagmus for a case of rhythmic synchronous pharyngeal, laryngeal, and ocular movements in a young girl with a presumed tumor. Because of the association of the term "nystagmus" with physiologically and phenomenolocally different eye movements, the term myoclonus was later proposed by Guillain et al. (111) for the syndrome affecting the branchial musculature. When peering into the oral cavity, the movements are characterized by involuntary, usually unconscious, movements of the soft palate and pharynx (112). Further exploration will often document synchronous jerks affecting the eyes, face, palate, larynx (Fig. 3), diaphragm, neck, shoulder, and arm, giving rise to the syndrome of "myoclonies velo-pharyngo-laryngo-oculo-diaphragmatiques" (113).

The pharyngeal movements are most commonly bilateral and symmetric, but can be unilateral, with the palate and uvula being drawn to one side. The rhythmicity nearly always persists in sleep, usually between 1.5 and 3 Hz, with a range of 0.3–100 Hz (112); variation with respiration has been documented (114). Myoclonic jerks can be briefly suppressed in some patients. Once symptoms begin, they are usually lifelong, but may disappear in rare cases (115).

The patient's complaint of clicking in the ears, thought to be due to involvement of the eustachian tube and tensor veli palatini muscle, was noted in the 19th century by Muller and then by Politzer (116). The clicking can often be heard by family and examiners. Laryngeal, palatal, pharyngeal, or diaphragmatic involvement may produce a broken speech pattern, simulating that heard in laryngeal dystonia (117) or slow tremor (see Fig. 3). Examination of the vocal cords often shows slow rhythmic adduction and abduction of the vocal cords at the same timing and frequency as the palatal, pharyngeal, and occasional diaphragmatic contractions. Ventilatory dysfunction has been documented (118).

An anatomical abnormality has been identified in cases of branchial myoclonus: there is enlargement of the inferior olivary nucleus (ION) in the medulla (for review, see Refs. 112,114) these may be seen on magnetic resonance imaging

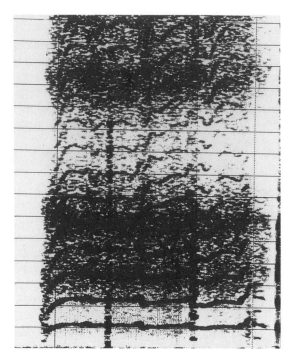

Figure 3 Myoclonic tremor: The narrow-band spectrogram of prolonged /a/ shows abrupt slow regular fluctuations in both frequency and amplitude. The region marked by dotted lines represents 2 s; 3.5 tremor cycles are visible. A cessation of voice production corresponded with the fourth cycle. Aperiodic noise in the high and low middle region indicate excessive breathiness.

(MRI) scans (119). There is gross hypertrophy of the olives, with microscopic evidence of enlarged, vacuolated, bizarre-shaped neurons, and enlarged astrocytes, with prominent thick processes. Associated findings include fibrillary gliosis and demyelination of white matter.

Through anatomical and later histopathological analysis, a specific pathway has been proposed as etiological. The ipsilateral central pontine tegmental tract and contralateral cerebellar dentate nucleus appear to be involved. Guillain et al. proposed a triangular pathway to relate hypertrophic ION degeneration to cerebellar lesions (111). However, it later became apparent that lesions of the olivodentato fibers have not produced symptoms. Trelles (120,121) proposed a pathway from the dentate nucleus to the contralateral ION, later substantiated by Ben Hamida (122) and Lapresle and Ben Hamida (112). The ION hypertrophy is thought to be due to a unique effect of transsynaptic degeneration (123).

Focal palatal myoclonus is usually a minor annoyance; the syndrome is problematic when associated with spread to other muscles. Although usually unresponsive to pharmacotherapy, there have been isolated cases reported who respond to the serotonin precursor, 5-hydroxytryptophan (5-HTP; 124,125), carbamazepine (126), clonazepam (127,128), tetrabenazine (128), and trihexyphenidyl (129,130). Treatment with tenotomy of the tensor veli palatini, stapedius, or tensor tympani muscles, and myringotomy may have a varying degree of success (131).

V. "ATAXIC" OR CEREBELLAR TREMOR

"Coarse voice tremor," (11) or irregular vocal tremor (2) has been reported in patients with cerebellar ataxia. Zemlin reported "galloping" in the phonation of a group of patients with ataxic involvement associated with multiple sclerosis. He associated this with tremors or ataxia of the cricothyroid, vocalis, or thyroarytenoid muscles (132). Ackermann and Ziegler (133) specifically studied one patient with primary autosomal dominant cerebellar atrophy, who had gait difficulty and an audible voice tremor. The frequency of the voice tremor was about 3 Hz, similar to that reported for other cerebellar kinetic and postural tremors (134–137). The primary abnormalities were oscillations of pitch, which contributed to perceptually identified vocal tremor. Speech intensity contours of sustained voiceless fricatives showed no rhythmic modulation, suggesting that the respiratory system did not contribute to tremor, nor was there any abnormality of the spectral characteristics of the fricatives suggesting that the articulators were not tremulous. During sustained phonation, the intrinsic laryngeal muscles were in a state of isometric contraction and rhythmically active, supporting the idea that, in their patient, the "cerebellar" voice tremor is a form of a postural tremor.

VI. VIBRATO

Vocal vibrato in singing is thought to result from undulating or rhythmical modulation in frequency, amplitude, and timber (spectrum) (138,139). Electrically modeled (140), the vibrato rate is the number of frequency changes ("extent") around a set fundamental frequency, over a unit of time. The source of the periodic neural innervation that controls the vibrato rate and extent have not been clearly identified, but may be partly contributed to by changes in the diaphragm, thoracic muscles, extrinsic laryngeal muscles, the vocal folds, or the articulatory muscles (tongue, pharynx) (141). Detailed investigation of singers has revealed that there are perceptually different types of vibrato, including, but not limited to, those due to pitch or flow variations (141). Typical vibrato is 4–7 Hz (142). Pitch vibrato is probably the most common type. It contains a strong variation in periodicity or frequency. It is this variation in periodicity that is perceived primarily as an oscillation in pitch. Flow vibrato is probably due to variation in vocal fold abduction. Synchronous variations in the glottal airflow pulse may have an effect on the perception of loudness, contributing to amplitude vibrato. It is the singer's goal to have a clear tremor, without roughness (rapid random variations in the periods or amplitudes of successive cycles; 140). This is likely best achieved when the vibrato rate is slow ($\leq$ 6 Hz) compared with faster rates ($\geq$ 6 Hz). In addition, greater roughness is perceived with wider extent from the fundamental frequency (140).

VII. ACCENTUATED PHYSIOLOGICAL VOICE TREMOR

Phonation is due to tremor of the vocal apparatus at, or close to a given fundamental frequency. We could not locate any references that discussed exaggerated physiological voice tremor, or rhythmic fluctuations in fundamental frequency under situations when exaggerated physiological tremor may be present.

However, an examination of the speech characteristics of infant utterances has received some attention. An infant's (younger than 9 months old) cry is frequently associated with tremor, which has been termed vibrato in the literature. Instabilities in laryngeal control of the fundamental frequency included tremor (vibrato), acute F_0 shifts, harmonic doubling, and breathiness (143). Infants with laryngeal abnormalities, including infections and congenital disorders (laryngomalacia, vocal cord paresis, subglottic stricture) (144) and cleft palate (145), and those with asphyxia (146) had a higher incidence of vibrato than normal control babies.

VIII. VOICE TREMOR IN PARKINSON'S DISEASE

In addition to the other voice, speech, and language disturbances seen in Parkinson's disease (PD) (8,25,147–164), Logemann et al. reported that 13.5% of a group of patients with PD had tremulousness of speech (25) (Fig. 4). The vocal tremor frequency in patients with PD has been reported in the range of 5–7 Hz (7) and 4–6 Hz (33). This is similar to the tremor frequencies reported in the lip and jaw musculature of parkinsonian patients (35). Vocal tremor in parkinsonian patients has been reported to include both frequency and amplitude oscillations (7), and mainly frequency oscillations (33). Patients with postencephalitic parkinsonism also have tremor in the laryngeal muscles. A quivering of the interarytenoid muscles and the false folds has been associated with the quivering voice quality observed in these patients (165).

Ramig et al. noted that the frequency of vocal tremor in PD (5–6 Hz) is similar to that of vibrato (7). They proposed that these tremors have a similar central generator that, in parkinsonism, is released from suppression by disease and, for singers, is selectively recruited. Izdebski and Dedo proposed (83) that singers are able to inhibit periodic neural signals coming through the recurrent laryngeal nerve to both the glottic adductors and abductors while, at the same time, allowing

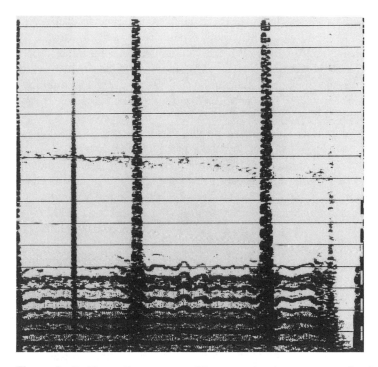

Figure 4 Parkinson disease tremor: The narrow-band spectrogram of prolonged /a/ shows irregular fluctuations in both frequency and amplitude. The total duration of the recording is 3.5 s. In this patient, the irregular tremor increased as time passed. The upper part of the spectrogram shows an absence of higher harmonics and aperiodic breakdown of the harmonics in the middle, suggesting breathiness.

input though the superior laryngeal nerve to the cricothyroid to manifest as frequency modulation. This hypothesis is weakened by the observation that vibrato typically is a frequency oscillation, whereas the vocal tremor in PD has both frequency and amplitude oscillations.

IX. VOCAL "FLUTTER" OF AMYOTROPHIC LATERAL SCLEROSIS

Bulbar amyotrophic lateral sclerosis (ALS) produces a flaccid or spastic dysarthria, with a strained, wet hoarseness; hypernasal resonation; and slow, imprecise articulation (8). When examined, the vocal cords display unilateral or bilateral flaccid weakness, spastic hyperadduction of the false vocal folds, palatal and labial weakness; there may be lingual fasciculations. Carrow et al. examined the speech characteristics of ALS patients and reported that 63% of 79 patients had tremor

(12). Although often undetectable during conversational speech, many ALS patients have a rapid vocal flutter (8,13), which is perceived as a rhythmic, 7- to 10-Hz tremor, and is distinct from tremors perceived in other neurological disorders. In a spectral and demodulation analysis (13), there are both frequency and amplitude modulations of various frequencies and magnitudes. The prominent frequencies spanned a wide range, up to 25 Hz (the maximum analyzed), with most patients' amplitude or frequency peaks between 6 and 12 Hz.

Flutter may be confused with *diplophonia* (the simultaneous perception of two different pitches, thought to be due to each vocal fold vibrating at a different frequency), which may occur in flaccid patients with unilateral vocal fold paralysis or myasthenia gravis. Flutter is not heard in patients with purely spastic, upper motor neuron disorders, suggesting that the tremor is not of central origin. Patients with a peripheral neuropathy can display limb tremor in the 8- to 12-Hz range (166), and patients with a subclinical peripheral neuropathy may display enhanced physiological tremor (167). However, Aronson et al. noted that, on fiberoptic examination of an ALS patient, the pharynx and larynx display rapid tremorous movements of the entire vocal tract, including the vocal folds and supraglottic musculature (13). They proposed that the tremor is a sign of loss of motor units, resulting in intermittent absence of intrinsic laryngeal muscle motor unit firing. In a detailed longitudinal study of one patient with ALS, Ramig et al. found a 4-Hz amplitude and frequency fluctuation in a sustained vowel sound (168). She proposed that the vocal irregularity is based in a respiratory muscle tremor (of unknown etiology) that generates systematic increases in subglottal air pressure or a variation in glottal length.

X. CONCLUSIONS

We recommend a careful neurological and laryngological examination to define the anatomical substrate for tremor in patients presenting with vocal tremulousness. Physiological studies may be helpful in some patients. Appropriate classification may dictate appropriate management and therapy.

ACKNOWLEDGMENTS

This work is supported in part by the Dystonia Medical Research Foundation, DC-01139, NS-26656. Sections of this chapter were based on a prior chapter with Lorraine Ramig (9).

REFERENCES

1. Cohen AH, Rossingnol S, Grillner S. Neural control of rhythmic movements in vertebrates. New York: John Wiley & Sons, 1988.

2. Brown JR, Simonson J. Organic voice tremor: a tremor of phonation. Neurology 1963; 13:520–525.

3. Hartman DE, Overholt SL, Vishwanat B. A case of vocal cord nodules masking essential (voice) tremor. Arch Otolaryngol 1982; 108:52–53.

4. Koller W, Graner D, Mlcoch A. Essential voice tremor: treatment with propranolol. Neurology 1985; 35:106–108.

5. Yokota J, Imai H, Seki K, Ninomiya C, Mizuno Y. Orthostatic tremor associated with voice tremor. Eur Neurol 1992; 32:354–358.

6. Seguier N, Spira A, Dordain M, Lazar P, Chevrie-Muller C. [Relationship between speech disorders and other clinical manifestations of Parkinson's disease]. Folia Phoniatr (Basel) 1974; 26:108–126.

7. Ramig LA, Scherer RC, Titze IR, Ringel SP. Acoustic analysis of voices of patients with neurologic disease: rationale and preliminary data. Ann Otol Rhinol Laryngol 1988; 97:164–172.

8. Aronson AE. Clinical Voice Disorders: An Interdisciplinary Approach. 3rd ed. New York: Thieme, 1990.

9. Brin MF, Fahn S, Blitzer A, Ramig LO, Stewart C. Movement disorders of the larynx. In: Blitzer A, Brin MF, Sasaki CT, Fahn S, Harris KS, eds. Neurological Disorders of the Larynx. New York: Thieme, 1992:248–278.

10. Blitzer A, Brin MF, Fahn S, Lovelace RE. Clinical and laboratory characteristics of focal laryngeal dystonia: study of 110 cases. Laryngoscope 1988; 98:636–640.

11. Aronson AE. Clinical Voice Disorders. New York: Thieme, 1985:52.

12. Carrow E, Rivera V, Mauldin M, Shamblin L. Deviant speech characteristics in motor neuron disease. Arch Otolaryngol 1974; 100:212–218.

13. Aronson AE, Ramig LO, Winholtz WS, Silber SR. Rapid voice tremor, or "flutter," in amyotrophic lateral sclerosis. Ann Otol Rhinol Laryngol 1992; 101:511–518.

14. Amorosa H, von Benda U, Dames M, Schaferskupper P. Deficits in fine motor coordination in children with unintelligible speech. Eur Arch Psychiatry Neurol Sci 1986; 236:26–30.

15. Meeuwis CA, Baarsma EA. Essential (voice) tremor. Clin Otolaryngol 1985; 10:54.

16. Findley L, Gresty M. Head facial and voice tremor. Adv Neurol 1988; 49:239–253.

17. Lebrun Y, Devreux F, Rousseau JJ, Darimont P. Tremulous speech. Folia Phoniatr (Basel) 1982; 34:134–142.

18. Ludlow C, Bassich C, Connor N, Coulter D. Phonatory characteristics of vocal fold tremor. J Phonet 1986; 14:509–515.

19. Critchley M. Observations on essential (heredo–familial) tremor. Brain 1949; 72:113–139.

20. Draper M, Ladefoged P, Whitteridge D. Expiratory pressures and air flow during speech. Br Med J 1960; 1837–1843.

21. Lebrun Y. Sur l'activite des muscules thoraco-abdominaux pendant la phonation. Folia Phoniatr (Basel) 1966; 18:354–368.

22. Hachinski VC, Thomsen IV, Buch NH. The nature of primary vocal tremor. Can J Neurol Sci 1975; 2:195–197.

23. Tomoda H, Shibasaki H, Huroda Y, Shin T. Voice tremor: dysregulation of voluntary expiratory muscles. Neurology 1987; 37:117–122.

24. Ardan G, Kinsbourne M, Rushworth G. Dysphonia due to tremor. J Neurol Neurosurg Psychiatry 1966; 29:219–223.
25. Logemann J, Fisher H, Boshes B, Blonsky E. Frequency and cooccurrence of vocal tract dysfunctions in the speech of a large sample of parkinson patients. J Speech Hear Disord 1978; 43:47–57.
26. Lieberman P, Blumstein SE. Speech Physiology, Speech Perception, and Acoustic Phonetics. Cambridge: Cambridge University Press, 1988:90.
27. Massey EW, Paulson G. Essential vocal tremor: response to therapy. Neurology 1982; 32:A113.
28. Baer T. Investigation of the phonatory mechanism. In: Ludlow CL, Hart MO, eds. Proceedings of the Conference on the Assessment of Vocal Pathology. Rockville: American Speech Hearing Association, 1981:38–47.
29. Larson C, Kempster G. Voice fundamental frequency changes following discharge of laryngeal motor units. In: Titze IR, Scherer RC, eds. Vocal Fold Physiology. Denver: Denver School for Performing Arts, 1985:91–103.
30. Ludlow CL, Naunton RF, Bassich CJ. Procedures for the selection of spastic dysphonia patients for recurrent laryngeal nerve section. Otolaryngol Head Neck Surg 1984; 92:24–31.
31. Shipp T, Izdebski KP. Current evidence for the existence of laryngeal macrotremor and microtremor. J Forensic Sci 1981; 26:501–505.
32. Ramig LA, Shipp T. Comparative measures of vocal tremor and vocal vibrato. J Voice 1987; 2:162–167.
33. Philippbar SA, Robin DA, Luschei ES. Limb, jaw and vocal tremor in Parkinson's patients. In: Yorkston K, Beukelman D, eds. Recent Advances in Clinical Dysarthria. San Diego: College Hill Press, 1991.
34. Hartman DE, Abbs JH. Vishwanat B. Clinical investigations of adductor spastic dysphonia. Ann Otol Rhinol Laryngol 1988; 97:247–252.
35. Hunker C, Abbs J. Physiological analysis of parkinsonian tremors in the oral facial system. In: The Dysarthrias. San Diego: College Hill Press, 1984:69–100.
36. Freund HJ, Dietz V. The relationship between physiological and pathological tremor in physiological tremor, pathological tremor and clonus. In: Desmedt J, ed. Progress in Clinical Neurophysiology. Basel: S Karger, 1978:66–89.
37. Winholtz WS, Ramig LO. Vocal tremor analysis with the vocal demodulator. J Speech Hear Res 1992; 35:562–573.
38. Ardran G, Kinsbourne M, Rushworth G. Dysphonia due to tremor. J Neurol Neurosurg Psychiatry 1966; 29:219–223.
39. Koda J, Ludlow CL. An evaluation of laryngeal muscle activation in patients with voice tremor. Otolaryngol Head Neck Surg 1992; 107:684–696.
40. Blitzer A, Lovelace RE, Brin MF, Fahn S, Fink ME. Electromyographic findings in focal laryngeal dystonia (spastic dysphonia). Ann Otol Rhinol Laryngol 1985; 94:591–594.
41. Critchley E. Clinical manifestations of essential tremor. J Neurol Neurosurg Psychiatry 1972; 35:365–372.
42. Davis CH, Kunkle CE, Durham NC. Benign essential (heredofamilial) tremor. Arch Intern Med 1991; 108–116.

43. Duvoisin RC. Benign essential tremor. In: Rowland L, ed. Merritt's Textbook of Neurology. Philadelphia: Lea & Febiger, 1984:525–526.
44. Marshall J. Pathology of Tremor. In: Findley LJ, Capildeo R, eds. Movement Disorders: Tremor. New York: Oxford University Press, 1984:95–123.
45. Marshall J. Observations on essential tremor. J Neurol Neurosurg Psychiatry 1986; 49:122–125.
46. Findley LJ. Essential tremor: introductory remarks. In: Findley LJ, Capildeo R, eds. Movement Disorders: Tremor. New York: Oxford University Press, 1984: 207–209.
47. Koller WC, Cone S, Herbster G. Caffeine in tremor. Neurology 1987; 37:169–172.
48. Darley FL, Aronson AE, Brown JR. Motor Speech Disorders. Philadelphia: WB Saunders, 1975.
49. Findley LJ, Gresty MA. Head, facial, and voice tremor. In: Jankovic J, Tolosa E, eds. Advances in Neurology. New York: Raven Press, 1988:239–253.
50. Massey EW, Paulson GW. Essential vocal tremor: clinical characteristics and response to therapy. South Med J 1985; 78:316–317.
51. Lou JS, Jankovic J. Essential tremor: clinical correlates in 350 patients. Neurology 1991; 41:234–238.
52. Rautakorpi I, Takala J, Marttila RJ, Sievers K, Rinne UK. Essential tremor in a Finnish population. Acta Neurol Scand 1982; 66:58–67.
53. Larsson T, Sjogren T. Essential tremor: a clinical and genetic population study. Acta Psychiatr Neurol Scand [Suppl] 1960; 144.
54. Longe AC. Essential tremor in Nigerians: a prospective study of 35 patients. East Afr Med J 1985; 62:672–677.
55. Koller WC, Royse VL. Efficacy of primidone in essential tremor. Neurology 1986; 36:121–124.
56. Chakrabarti A, Pearce JM. Essential tremor: response to primidone [letter]. J Neurol Neurosurg Psychiatry 1981; 44:650.
57. Koller WC, Glatt S, Biary N, Rubino FA. Essential tremor variants: effect of treatment. Clin Neuropharmacol 1987; 10:342–350.
58. Hartman DE, Vishwanat B. Spastic dysphonia and essential (voice) tremor treated with primidone. Arch Otolaryngol 1984; 110:394–397.
59. Findley LJ, Gresty MA. Head, facial, and voice tremor. Adv Neurol 1988; 49: 239–253.
60. Muenter MD, Daube JR, Caviness JN, Miller PM. Treatment of essential tremor with methazolamide [see comments]. Mayo Clin Proc 1991; 66:991–997.
61. Brin MF, Blitzer A, Fahn S, Gould W, Lovelace RE. Adductor laryngeal dystonia (spastic dysphonia): treatment with local injections of botulinum toxin (Botox). Mov Disord 1989; 4:287–296.
62. Blitzer A, Brin M. Laryngeal dystonia: a series with botulinum toxin therapy. Ann Otol Rhinol Laryngol 1991; 100:85–89.
63. Brin MF, Blitzer A, Stewart C, Fahn S. Treatment of spasmodic dysphonia (Laryngeal dystonia) with local injections of botulinum toxin: review and technical aspects. In: Blitzer A, Brin MF, Sasaki CT, Fahn S, Harris KS, eds. Neurological Disorders of the Larynx. New York: Thieme, 1992:214–228.

64. Traube L. Gesammelte Beitrage zur Pathologie und Physiologie. 2nd ed. Berlin: Verlag von August Hirschwald, 1871:674.

65. Fraenkel B. Ueber Beschaeftigungsneurosen der Stimme. Leipzig: G Thieme, 1887.

66. Fraenkel B. Ueber die beschaeftigungsschwaeche der stimme: mogiphonie. Dtsch Med Wochenschr 1887; 13:121–123.

67. Gerhardt P. Bewegunggsstoerungen der stimmbaender. Nothnagels Spezielle Pathologie Therapie. Vol. 13, 1896.

68. Jacome DE, Yanez GF. Spastic dysphonia and Meigs disease [letter]. Neurology 1980; 30:349.

69. Marsden CD. Sheehy MP. Spastic dysphonia, Meige disease, and torsion dystonia [letter]. Neurology 1982; 32:1202–1203.

70. Golper LAC, Nutt JG, Rau MT, Coleman RO. Focal cranial dystonia. J Speech Hear Disord 1983; 48:128–134.

71. Critchley M. Spastic dysphonia ("inspiratory speech"). Brain 1939; 62:96–103.

72. Bellussi G. Le disfonie impercinetiche. Atti Labor Fonet Univ Padova 1952; 3:1.

73. Aronson AE, Brown JR, Litin EM, Pearson JS. Spastic dysphonia. I. Voice, neurologic, and psychiatric aspects. J Speech Hear Disord 1968; 33:203–218.

74. Aronson AE, Brown JR, Litin EM, Pearson JS. Spastic dysphonia. II. Comparison with essential (voice) tremor and other neurologic and psychogenic dysphonias. J Speech Hear Disord 1968; 33:219–231.

75. Yanagisawa N, Goto A. Dystonia musculorum deformans. Analysis with electromyography. J Neurol Sci 1971; 13:39–65.

76. Jedynak CP, Bonnet AM, Agid Y. Tremor and other idiopathic dystonia. Mov Disord 1991; 6:230–236.

77. Rivest J, Marsden CD. Trunk and head tremor as isolated manifestations of dystonia. Mov Disord 1990; 5:60–65.

78. Elble RJ, Moody C, Higgins C. Primary writing tremor. A form of focal dystonia? Mov Disord 1990; 5:118–126.

79. Lang A, Quinn N, Marsden CD, et al. Essential tremor [letter; comment]. Neurology 1992; 42:1432–1434.

80. Aronson AE, Peterson HW, Litin EM. Voice symptomatology in functional dysphonia and aphonia. J Speech Hear Disord 1964; 29:367–380.

81. Schaefer SD. Neuropathology of spasmodic dysphonia. Laryngoscope 1983; 93:1183–1204.

82. Aronson AE, Hartman DE. Adductor spastic dysphonia as a sign of essential (voice) tremor. J Speech Hear Disord 1981; 46:52–58.

83. Izdebski K, Dedo HH. Characteristics of vocal tremor in spastic dysphonia: a preliminary study. In: Lawrence V, ed. Transcripts of the 7th Symposium on Care of the Professional Voice. New York: The Voice Foundation, 1979:17–23.

84. Krech M. Sprechwissenschaftlich-Phonetische Untersuchungen zum Gebrauch des Glottisschlageinsatzes in der Allgemeinen Deutschen Hochlautung. Basle: S Karger, 1968.

85. Rosenfield DB, Donovan DT, Sulek M, Viswanath NS, Inbody GP, Nudelman HB. Neurologic aspects of spasmodic dysphonia [see comments]. J Otolaryngol 1990; 19:231–236.

86. Pool KD, Freeman FJ, Finitzo T, et al. Heterogeneity in spasmodic dysphonia. Neurologic and voice findings. Arch Neurol 1991; 48:305–309.

87. Lang AE, Kierans C, Blair RD. Association between familial tremor and Parkinson's disease [letter]. Ann Neurol 1986; 19:306–307.

88. Marttila RJ, Rautakorpi I, Rinne UK. The relation of essential tremor to Parkinson's disease. J Neurol Neurosurg Psychiatry 1984; 47:734–735.

89. Findley LJ, Cleeves L. The relation of essential tremor to Parkinson's disease [letter]. J Neurol Neurosurg Psychiatry 1985; 48:192.

90. Jankovic J. Essential tremor and Parkinson's disease. Ann Neurol 1989; 25:211–212.

91. Meneghini F, Rocca WA, Grigoletto F, et al. Door-to-door prevalence survey of neurological diseases in a Sicilian population. Background and methods. Neuro-epidemiology 1991; 10:70–85.

92. Dupont E. Parkinson's disease and essential tremor: differential diagnostic and epidemiological aspects. In: Rinne UK, Klingler M, Stamm G, eds. Parkinson's Disease. Current Progress, Problems and Management. Amsterdam: Elsevier, 1980.

93. Ivanova Smolenskaia IA. [Clinical variants of essential tremor]. Zh Nevropatol Psikhiatr 1979; 79:291–298.

94. Marttila RJ, Rinne UK. Parkinson's disease and essential tremor in families of patients with early-onset Parkinson's disease. J Neurol Neurosurg Psychiatry 1988; 51:429–431.

95. Cleeves L, Findley LJ, Koller W. Lack of association between essential tremor and Parkinson's disease. Ann Neurol 1988; 24:23–26.

96. Koller WC, Vetere Overfield B, Barter R. Tremors in early Parkinson's disease. Clin Neuropharmacol 1989; 12:293–297.

97. Baxter DW, Lal S. Essential tremor and dystonia syndrome. Adv Neurol 1979; 24:373–377.

98. Jacome DE. Writing tremor myoclonus. Eur Neurol 1988; 28:126–130.

99. Ravits J, Hallett M, Baker M, Wilkins D. Primary writing tremor and myoclonic writer's cramp. Neurology 1985; 35:1387–1391.

100. Couch JR. Dystonia and tremor in spasmodic torticollis. Neurol 1976; 14:245–258.

101. Jankovic J, Ford J. Blepharospasm and orofacial–cervical dystonia: clinical and pharmacological findings in 100 patients. Ann Neurol 1983; 13:402–411.

102. Yanagisawa N, Goto A, Narabayashi H. Familial dystonia musculorum deformans and tremor. J Neurol Sci 1972; 16:125–136.

103. Fahn S, Marsden CD, Van Woert MH. Definition and classification of myoclonus. Adv Neurol 1986; 43:1–5.

104. Young RR, Shahani BT. Asterixis: one type of negative myoclonus. Adv Neurol 1986; 43:137–156.

105. Marsden CD, Hallett M, Fahn S. The nosology and pathophysiology of myoclonus. In: Marsden CD, Fahn S, eds. Movement Disorders. London: Butterworth Scientific, 1982:196–248.

106. Shim CM. Motor disturbances of the diaphragm. Clin Chest Med 1980; 1:125–129.

107. Newsom-Davis J. An experimental study of hiccup. Brain 1970; 93:851–872.

108. Rohr H, Lenz H. Diaphragm paralysis after traumatic injury to cervical spine nerve roots. Acta Neurochir 1960; 8:44–69.

109. Lance JW, Bassil GT. Familial intractable hiccup relieved by baclofen. Lancet 1989; 2:276–277.

110. Aravot DJ, Wright G, Rees A, Maiwand OM, Garland MH. Non-invasive phrenic nerve stimulation for intractable hiccups. Lancet 1989; 2:1047.

111. Guillain G, Mollaret P, Rees A, Maiwand OH, Garland MH. Duex cas de myoclonies synchrones et rythmees velo-pharyngo-laryngo-oculo-diaphragmatiques. Le probleme anatomizue et physiopathologiqque de ce syndrome. Rev Neurol 1931; 2: 545–566.

112. Lapresle J, Ben Hamida M. The dentato-olivary pathway. Somatotopic relationship between the dentate nucleus and the contralateral inferior olive. Arch Neurol 1970; 22:135–143.

113. Guillain G. The syndrome of synchronous and rhythmic palato-pharyngo-laryngo-oculo-diaphragmatic myoclonus. Proc R Soc Med 1938; 31:1031–1038.

114. Dubinsky RM, Hallet M. Palatal myoclonus and facial involvement in other types of myoclonus. Adv Neurol 1988; 49:263–278.

115. Jacobs L, Newman RP, Bozian D. Disappearing palatal myoclonus. Neurology 1981; 31:748–751.

116. Rondot P, Ben Hamida M. Myoclonies du voille et myoclonies squelettiques. Etude clinique et anatomique. Rev Neurol (Paris) 1968; 119:59–83.

117. Doody RS, Rosenfield DB. Spasmodic dysphonia associated with palatal myoclonus. Ear Nose Throat J 1990; 69:829–832.

118. Andrews J, Dumont D, Fisher M, Chausow A, Szidon JP. Ventilatory dysfunction in palatal myoclonus. Respiration 1987; 52:76–80.

119. Yokota T, Hirashima F, Furukawa T, Tsukagoshi H, Yoshikawa H. MRI findings of inferior olives in palatal myoclonus. J Neurol 1989; 236:115–116.

120. Trelles JO. Les ramollissements protuberantiels. These de Medicine, Paris, 1935.

121. Trelles JO. La oliva bulbar. Su estructure, funcion, y patologia. Rev Neuropsiquiatr 1943; 6:433–521.

122. Ben Hamida M. Contribution a l'etude anatomique de couple olivo-dentele. A propos de 13 observations de degenerescence hypertrophique des olives. These de Medicine, Paris, 1965.

123. Barron KD, Dentinger MP, Koeppen AH. Fine structure of neurons of the hypertrophied human inferior olive. J Neuropathol Exp Neurol 1982; 41:186–203.

124. Magnussen I, Dupont E, Prange HA, et al. Palatal myoclonus treated with 5-hydroxytryptophan and a decarboxylase-inhibitor. Acta Neurol Scand 1977; 55: 251–253.

125. Williams A, Goodenberger D, Calne DB. Palatal myoclonus following herpes zoster ameliorated by 5-hydroxytryptophan and carbidopa. Neurology 1978; 28:358–359.

126. Sakai T, Murakami S. Palatal myoclonus responding to carbamazepine [letter]. Ann Neurol 1981; 9:199–200.

127. Gauthier S, Young SN, Baxter DW. [Palatal myoclonus associated with a decrease in 5-hydroxyindole acetic acid in cerebrospinal fluid and responding to clonazepam]. Can J Neurol Sci 1981; 8:51–54.

128. Jankovic J, Pardo R. Segmental myoclonus: clinical and pharmacologic study. Ann Neurol 1986; 43:1025–1031.

129. Jabbari B, Rosenberg M, Scherokman B, Gunderson CH, McBurney JW, McClintock W. Effectiveness of trihexyphenidyl against pendular nystagmus and palatal myoclonus: evidence of cholinergic dysfunction. Mov Disord 1987; 2:93–98.
130. Jabbari B, Scherokman B, Gunderson CH, Rosenberg ML, Miller J. Treatment of movement disorders with trihexyphenidyl. Mov Disord 1989; 4:202–212.
131. Hanson B, Ficara A, McQuade M. Bilateral palatal myoclonus. Pathophysiology and report of a case. Oral Surg Oral Med Oral Pathol 1985; 59:479–481.
132. Zemlin WR, Daniloff RG, Shriner TH. The difficulty of listening to time-compressed speech. J Speech Hear Res 1968; 11:875–881.
133. Ackermann H, Ziegler W. Cerebellar voice tremor: an acoustic analysis. J Neurol Neurosurg Psychiatry 1991; 54:74–76.
134. Mai N, Bolsinger P, Avarello M, Diener HC, Dichgans J. Control of isometric finger force in patients with cerebellar disease. Brain 1988; 111:973–998.
135. Fahn S. Cerebellar tremor: clinical aspects. In: Findley LJ, Capildeo R, eds. Movement Disorders: Tremor. New York: Oxford University Press, 1984; 355–363.
136. Silfverskiold BP. A 3 c/sec leg tremor in a "cerebellar" syndrome. Acta Neurol Scand 1977; 55:385–393.
137. Dichgans J, Mauritz KH, Allum JHJ, Brandt T. Postural sway in normals and atactic patients: analysis of the stabilizing and destabilizing effects of vision. Agressologie 1976; 17:15–24.
138. Horii Y, Hata K. A note on phase relationships between frequency and amplitude modulations in vocal vibrato. Folia Phoniatr (Basel) 1988; 40:303–311.
139. Schultz-Coulon HJ, Battmer RD. [Quantitative evaluation of the vibrato of singers]. Folia Phoniatr (Basel) 1981; 33:1–14.
140. LaBelle JL. Judgments of vocal roughness related to rate and extent of vibrato. Folia Phoniatr (Basel) 1973; 25:196–202.
141. Rothenberg M, Miller D, Molitor R. Aerodynamic investigation of sources of vibrato. Folia Phoniatr (Basel) 1988; 40:244–260.
142. Shonle JI, Horan KE. The pitch of vibrato tones. J Acoust Soc Am 1980; 67:246–252.
143. Kent RD, Murray AD. Acoustic features of infant vocalic utterances at 3, 6, and 9 months. J Acoust Soc Am 1982; 72:353–365.
144. Raes J, Michelsson K, Dehaen F, Despontin M. Cry analysis in infants with infectious and congenital disorders of the larynx. Int J Pediatr Otorhinolaryngol 1982; 4:157–169.
145. Michelsson K, Sirviö P, Koivisto M, Sovijarvi A, Wasz-Höckert O. Spectrographic analysis of pain cry in neonates with cleft palate. Biol Neonate 1975; 26:353–358.
146. Michelsson K, Sirviö P, Wasz-Höckert O. Pain cry in full-term asphyxiated newborn infants correlated with late findings. Acta Paediatr Scand 1977; 66:611–616.
147. Hofman S. Aspects of language in parkinsonism. Adv Neurol 1990; 53:327–333.
148. Johnson JA, Pring TR. Speech therapy for Parkinson's disease: a review and further data. Br J Disord Commun 1990; 25:183–194.
149. Pitcairn TK, Clemie S, Gray JM, Pentland B. Impressions of parkinsonian patients from their recorded voices. Br J Disord Commun 1990; 25:85–92.
150. Ackermann H, Ziegler W, Oertel WH. Palilalia as a symptom of levodopa induced hyperkinesia in Parkinson's disease. J Neurol Neurosurg Psychiatry 1989; 52:805–807.

151. Gath I, Yair E. Analysis of vocal tract parameters in parkinsonian speech. J Acoust Soc Am 1988; 84:1628–1634.
152. Illes J, Metter EJ, Hanson WR, Iritani S. Language production in Parkinson's disease: acoustic and linguistic considerations. Brain Lang 1988; 33:146–160.
153. Ludlow CL, Conner NP, Bassich CJ. Speech timing in Parkinson's and Huntington's disease. Brain Lang 1987; 32:195–214.
154. Robbins JA, Logemann JA, Kirshner HS. Swallowing and speech production in Parkinson's disease. Ann Neurol 1986; 19:283–287.
155. Hartman DE, Abbs JH. The response of the apparent receptive speech disorder of parkinsonism to speech therapy. J Neurol Neurosurg Psychiatry 1985; 48:606.
156. Robertson SJ, Thompson F. Speech therapy in Parkinson's disease: a study of the efficacy and long term effects of intensive treatment. Br J Disord Commun 1984; 19:213–224.
157. Scott S, Caird FI. The response of the apparent receptive speech disorder of Parkinson's disease to speech therapy. J Neurol Neurosurg Psychiatry 1984; 47:302–304.
158. Scott S, Caird FI, Williams BO. Evidence for an apparent sensory speech disorder in Parkinson's disease. J Neurol Neurosurg Psychiatry 1984; 47:840–843.
159. Streifler M, Hofman S. Disorders of verbal expression in parkinsonism. Adv Neurol 1984; 40:385–393.
160. Lang AE, Fishbein V. The "pacing board" in selected speech disorders of Parkinson's disease [letter]. J Neurol Neurosurg Psychiatry 1983; 46:789.
161. Schley WM, Fenton EP, Niimi SM. Vocal symptoms in parkinson's disease treated with levadopa: a case report. Ann Otol 1982; 91:119–121.
162. Logemann J, Fisher H. Vocal tract control in Parkinson's disease: phonetic feature analysis of misarticulations. J Speech Hear Disord 1981; 46:348–352.
163. Critchley EM. Peak-dose dysphonia in parkinsonism [letter]. Lancet 1976; 1:544.
164. Wolfe VI, Garvin JS, Bacon M, Waldrop W. Speech changes in Parkinson's disease during treatment with L-dopa. J Commun Disord 1975; 8:271–279.
165. Ward PH, Hanson DG, Berci G. Observations on central neurologic etiology for laryngeal dysfunction. Ann Otol Rhinol Laryngol 1981; 90:430–441.
166. Shahani BT. Tremor associated with peripheral neuropathy. In: Findley LJ, Capildeo R, eds. Movement Disorders: Tremor. New York: Oxford University Press, 1984: 389–398.
167. Said G, Bathien N, Cesaro P. Peripheral neuropathies and tremor. Neurology 1982; 3234:481–485.
168. Ramig LO, Scherer RC, Klasner ER, Titze I, Horii Y. Acoustic analysis of voice in amyotrophic lateral sclerosis: a longitudinal case study. J Speech Hear Disord 1990; 55:2–14.

38

The Surgical Treatment of Tremor Disorders

Marc S. Goldman and Patrick J. Kelly
Mayo Clinic
Rochester, Minnesota

I. INTRODUCTION

Victor Horsley and R. H. Clarke developed the definitive method of stereotaxy at the turn of the century (1,2), but it was not until 1947 that Spiegel and Wycis performed the first human procedure (Fig. 1). Their prototype instrument was first used to produce dorsal median thalamic lesions for the treatment of psychiatric disorders and later used in the treatment of movement disorders (3,4). In the early 1950s, Guiot and Brion, and Narabayashi developed stereotactic instruments specifically designed for the treatment of movement disorders (Fig. 2) (5,6). Many other stereotactic instruments suitable for surgical treatment of subcortical movement disorders were subsequently developed as interest in this field grew.

A. Historical Perspectives

Movement disorders are a result of disinhibition of a facilitatory loop between the cortex, striatum, globus pallidus, and thalamus (7). Various elements within this loop have served as targets in ablative neurosurgery to abolish specific movement disorders (8–14). Victor Horsley successfully treated athetoid and "spastic movements" of an upper extremity by resection of the precentral gyrus in 1908 (15). In the 1930s, Bucy (16) also treated choreoathetosis and the dyskinesias of Parkinson's disease by extirpation of the motor cortex. Meyers (17) resected the head of the caudate and anterior limb of the internal capsule and, later, interrupted pallidofugal fibers in the ansa lenticularis (ansalotomy) to relieve the tremors of Parkinson's disease. However, this transventricular procedure was associated with

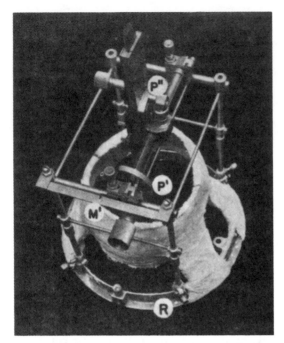

Figure 1 The first stereotactic instrument for human subcortical surgery. (From Ref. 3.)

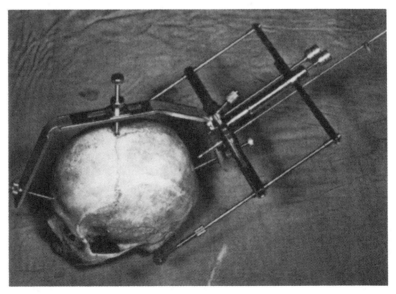

Figure 2 The Guiot stereotactic frame specific for the treatment of movement disorders. (From Ref. 3.)

a 10–15% mortality. Fenelon (18) described a safer subfrontal approach for the placement of lesions in the ansa lenticularis. In 1953, Spiegel and Wycis (4) performed the first stereotactic ansalotomy. Guiot and Brion, Gillingham, and Cooper stereotactically lesioned the origin of the ansa lenticularis and the lenticular fasciculus at the medial segment of the globus pallidus (pallidotomy) Fig. 3) (5,9,12). Bravo and Cooper, and Hassler found that stereotactic lesions of the ventrolateral thalamus (thalamotomy) and thalamic fasciculus in Field H of Forel (campotomy) provided good relief of rigidity and tremor with less operative morbidity (8,19). It was clear that lesions in the basal ganglia and thalamus were effective in treating dyskinesias irrespective of the etiology (20) and extensive stereotactic programs subsequently developed in the mid- to late 1960s (21).

In the 1960s, over 40,000 stereotactic procedures were performed worldwide (21). The most common indication for stereotactic surgery proved to be thalamotomy or pallidotomy for Parkinson's tremor (22). After levodopa was developed in 1968, interest in stereotactic neuroablative procedures for Parkinson's disease all but disappeared, and only a few European centers continued to refine stereotaxy for nonparkinsonian movement disorders (Fig. 4) (23–27). However, interest was resurrected as levodopa treatment failures emerged and stereotactic surgical mortality and morbidity decreased (27–29).

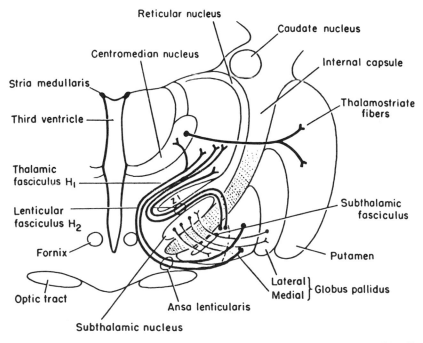

Figure 3 The pallidofugal fiber systems in transverse section. (Courtesy of M. Carpenter, Williams & Wilkins, Baltimore.)

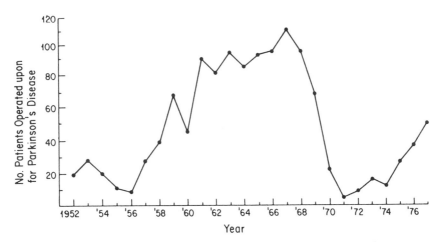

Figure 4   The number of stereotactic thalamotomies per year done at the Hopital Foch in Surenes, France from 1957 through 1977. (From Ref. 3.)

B.   Modern Stereotactic Thalamotomy

Currently, the ventralis lateralis nucleus of the thalamus is the most frequent target for lesion production (Fig. 5) (30). The ventralis oralis posterior (VOP) and ventralis intermedius (VIM) nuclei receive cerebellar afferents and are the most common targets for the treatment of tremor and the ventralis oralis anterior (VOA) nucleus receives pallidofugal afferents and is the most common target for the treatment of rigidity (13,31–34). The VIM nucleus receives kinesthetic input from contralateral muscle receptors that respond to tactile stimulation or joint movement and produce rhythmic bursts of neuronal activity synchronous in phase with the contralateral peripheral tremor (35–40).

Guiot (32) mapped the thalamic nuclei and internal capsule with microelectrodes through an occipital trephine and found that somatotopically arranged evoked activity in the ventralis posterior (VP) nucleus could serve as a guide to placement of a ventralis lateralis (VL) lesion. A somatotopic organization, which reflects the homuncular arrangement of the body in the VP nucleus, is present in the VL nucleus. Destruction of a 3-mm portion of this somatotopically organized nucleus can result in selective and permanent disappearance of tremor, independent of etiology, without detectable sensory or motor disturbances postoperatively (41). The optimal lesioning site is in the VIM nucleus just anterior to the ventralis posterior receptive field corresponding to the contralateral buccal commissure, thumb, and index finger (42). This has proved effective in the treatment of the resting tremor of Parkinson's disease, essential tremor, and the cerebellar intention tremors of multiple sclerosis, severe head injury, and stroke (35). In these tremors, Hitchcock et al. (43) found that immediate symptomatic improvement can be

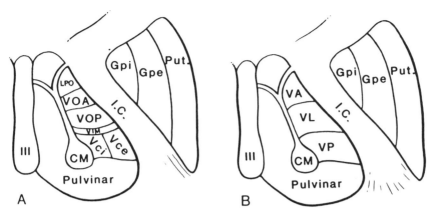

Figure 5 The ventral thalamus in (A) Hassler and (B) Anglo-American terminology. LPO, lateral polaris; VOA, ventralis oralis anterior; VOP, ventralis oralis posterior; VIM, ventralis intermedius; VCi, ventralis caudalis interna; VCe, ventralis caudalis externa; CM, centrum medianum; VA, ventralis anterior; VL, ventralis lateralis; VP, ventralis posterior; IC, internal capsule; GPi, internal segment of globus pallidus; GPe, external segment of globus pallidus; Put, putamen. (From Ref. 2.)

expected in up to 93% and can be maintained, at 4 years, in 55%. Immediate improvement in Karnofsky disability scores has been achieved in 58% and maintained at 4 years in 33%. Wester and Hauglie-Hanssen (28) reported that hemiballismus, the dystonias of cerebral palsy, and dystonia muscularum deformans respond in a good to moderate fashion in 50% of cases at median follow-up time of 24 months.

II. METHOD

A. Surgical Procedure

The target coordinates for neuroablative procedures are first approximated using stereotactic computed tomography (CT) scans, magnetic resonance imaging (MRI) scans, and positive contrast ventriculography, and are precisely localized with neurophysiological recording and stimulation control. The following is the procedure used at our institution (7,44,45).

The patient is placed in a stereotactic head frame, a localization system is attached to the headholder, and a stereotactic CT, MRI, or both, scan is performed (Fig. 6). Five-millimeter slices overlapping at 3-mm intervals are obtained through the region of the third ventricle. A computer resident Schaltenbrand-Wahren stereotactic atlas is scaled to superimpose the individual thalamic nuclei 2.5 mm above and parallel to a line connecting the anterior and posterior commissures

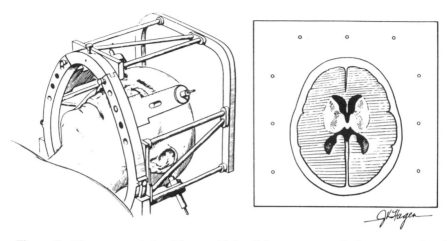

Figure 6   The stereotactic head frame with localizing system attached creates a series of nine marks from which coordinates are calculated. (From Ref. 6.)

(Fig. 7). The ventrolateral nucleus can be targeted on a computer display console, and the stereotactic coordinates calculated.

The patient is then placed onto the operating table and the head frame positioned in a COMPASS arc-quadrant stereotactic frame (Stereotactic Medical Systems, Inc., New Hartford, New York; Fig. 8). Under local anesthesia, a burr

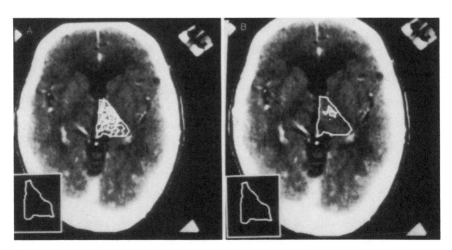

Figure 7   Computer-generated stereotactic atlas superimposes the thalamic nuclei on the stereotactic CT scan. Subnuclei can be selected and targeted. (From Ref. 2.)

hole is made 12 cm posterior to the nasion and 2.5 cm from midline. The foramen of Monro is placed at the system's focal point and a cannula is stereotactically introduced. The ventrolateral nucleus is moved into the focal point, and a positive contrast anteroposterior (AP) and lateral ventriculogram is performed using standard teleradiographic techniques (Fig. 9). On the teleradiographs, the thalamic nuclei are approximated as follows:

A line connects the anterior and posterior commissures (AC–PC line) (Fig. 10a). This is divided equally into thirds (see Fig. 10b), and a perpendicular erected from the midpoint to the floor of the lateral ventricles defines the thalamic height (see Fig. 10c). A parallel from the midpoint of the thalamic height line to a perpendicular from the posterior commissure is drawn (see Fig. 10d). An oblique from a point on this line corresponding to the junction of the middle and posterior thirds of the AC–PC line to the midpoint of the posterior third defines the ventralis posterior (VP) nucleus (see Fig. 10e). A parallel oblique from the junction of the middle and posterior thirds of the AC–PC line defines the VIM nucleus, and a parallel oblique from the midpoint of the AC–PC line defines the ventralis oralis posterior (VOP) nucleus. The preliminary lesion site is 2 mm posterior to and 2.5 mm superior to the AC–PC midpoint (see Fig. 10f). The laterality is 11.5 mm from the lateral wall of the third ventricle. The lesion coordinates in the anterior–posterior, left–right, and superior–inferior planes are adjusted from the computer resident stereotactic atlas approximation. A point 1 mm anterior to the posterior commissure on the AC–PC line and 11.5 mm lateral to the lateral wall of the third ventricle is targeted and a bipolar concentric electrode is directed from the frontal burr hole (46). Cellular "noise" is encountered at the cortex, caudate, dorsal thalamus, and VP nucleus (Fig. 11). The contralateral side of the body is stimulated tactilely or electrically. High-amplitude (150 mV) evoked responses are obtained when stimulating a body part represented by the part of the thalamus in which the electrode lies (Fig. 12). The physiological floor of the thalamus (normally at the AC–PC line) is confirmed as the electrode passes into the medial lemniscal system: the evoked potentials become nonspecific (Fig. 13), and the N14 wave reverses polarity (Fig. 14) (7).

In general, the final target coordinates for the lesion are 2 mm posterior to and 2.5 mm superior to the AC–PC line midpoint and at a laterality established by microelectrode recording. However, the superior–inferior coordinate can be adjusted up or down, depending on the neurophysiological localization of the inferior aspect of the thalamus. For upper extremity tremor, the laterality in the VL nucleus should correspond to the neurophysiologically established laterality of the thumb or index finger in the VP nucleus. For lower extremity tremor, the laterality in the VL nucleus should correspond to the laterality of the fifth digit in the VP nucleus (Fig. 15). Because of the obliquity of the internal capsule and that the somatotopic organization in VOP–VIM is shifted medially relative to VP because of that obliquity, the laterality of the VL nucleus target should be adjusted 1 mm medially

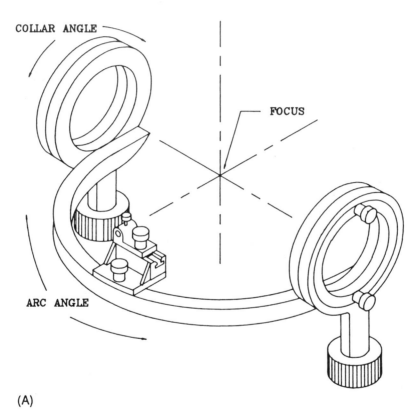

COLLAR ANGLE

FOCUS

ARC ANGLE

(A)

Figure 8 The COMPASS arc-quadrant provides two angular degrees of freedom for trajectories: (A) the arc angle and the collar angle; (B) the arc-quadrant with circular headframe placing target at the focus. (From Ref. 3.)

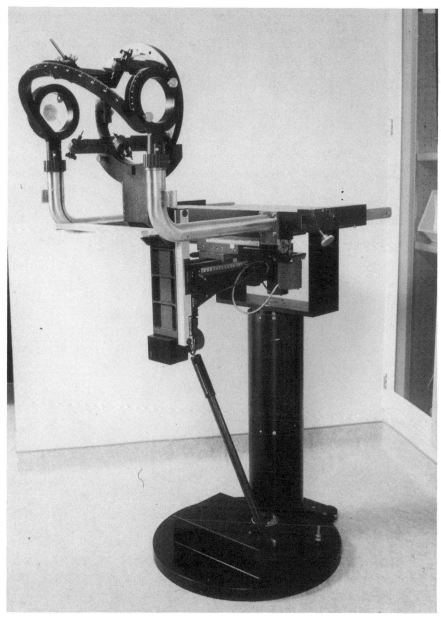

(B)

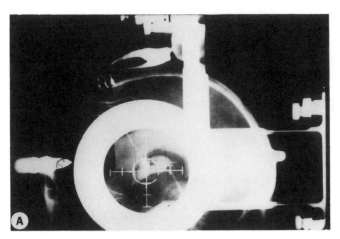

Figure 9   Teleradiographic-positive contrast lateral ventriculogram. (From Ref. 6.)

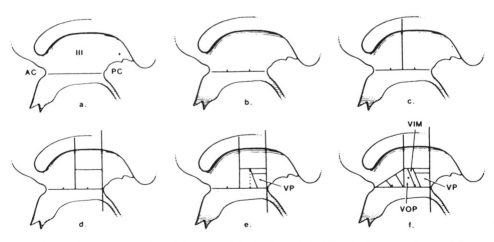

Figure 10   Construction of the ventral thalamic nuclei. AC, anterior commissure; PC, posterior commissure; III, third ventricle; VP, ventralis posterior; VOP, ventralis oralis posterior; VIM, ventralis intermedius. (From Ref. 2.)

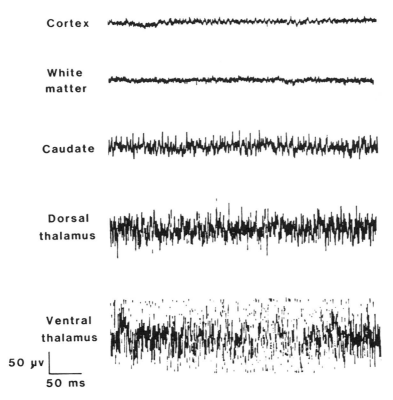

Figure 11 Semimicroelectrode recordings of the cortex, caudate, dorsal thalamus, and ventral thalamus. (From Ref. 3.)

for every 5 mm that the VL target lies anterior to the position of the recording electrode in the VP nucleus (46).

A radiofrequency-lesioning probe (1.6-mm diameter, 3-mm exposed tip) is passed to the target coordinates (Fig. 16). A low-frequency, low-amplitude stimulus will drive the tremor and a high-frequency, high-amplitude stimulus will ablate the tremor in a reversible fashion. The temperature-monitored electrode is heated to 42°C for 60 s to create a temporary lesion. An examination of strength, tremor, coordination, speech, and language is performed. If no untoward effects are discovered, the probe is heated to 70°C for 60 s to generate a 4-mm–diameter and 4.5-mm–long permanent lesion. The probe is allowed to cool to body temperature and withdrawn.

Tremors of low-frequency, high-amplitude, and proximal distribution, such as those typically occurring after stroke or severe head injury, require larger lesions of approximately 200 mm³, whereas tremors of high-frequency, low-amplitude,

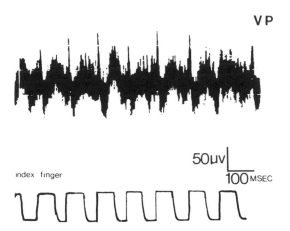

Figure 12 High-amplitude (150-mV)–evoked responses are obtained when stimulating a body part represented by the part of the thalamus in which the electrode lies. (From Ref. 6.)

and distal distribution such as those typically occurring with Parkinson's disease and essential tremor can respond to a coagulation lesion volume as small as 40 mm³ (47).

III. PREOPERATIVE AND POSTOPERATIVE EVALUATION

General neurological examinations performed by the surgical team and an independent neurologist, psychometric evaluations, speech pathology evaluations, and

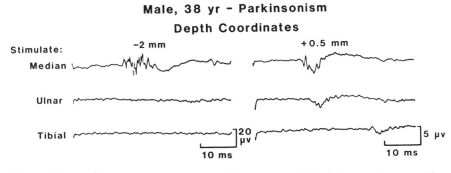

Figure 13 Averaged somatosensory-evoked responses in VP thalamus show specific median nerve response (left). Averaged somatosensory-evoked responses in medial lemniscus show nonspecific response (right). (From Ref. 6.)

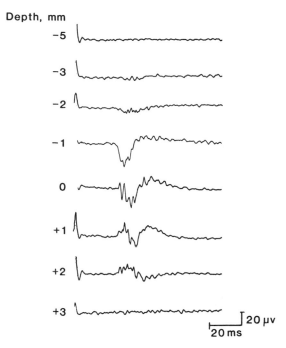

Depth, mm

−5

−3

−2

−1

0

+1

+2

+3

20 µv
20 ms

Figure 14 Serial-averaged median somatosensory-evoked responses with N14 wave polarity reversal at the AC–PC line (electrode depth = 0). (From Ref. 6.)

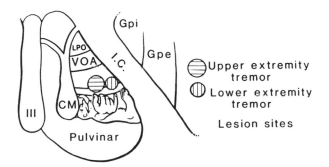

Figure 15 Homuncular representation in VP nucleus and optimal VL lesion sites. CM, centrum medianum; GPe, external segment of globus pallidus; GPi, internal segment of globus pallidus; IC, internal capsule; LPO, lateral polaris; VOP, ventralis oralis anterior; III, third ventricle. (From Ref. 6.)

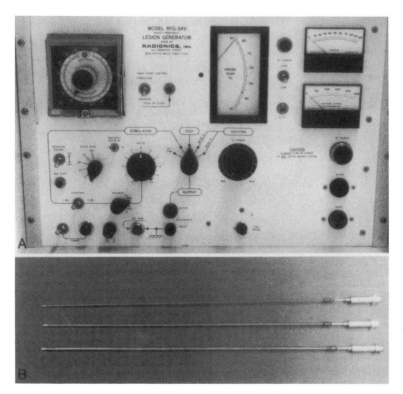

Figure 16   (A) Radiofrequency lesion generator and (B) lesioning probes in 1.1-, 1.6-, and 2.1-mm–diameter sizes. (From Ref. 3.)

neuroradiological scans (CT or MRI) are performed preoperatively and repeated during the first postoperative week. This complete evaluation is repeated again at the patient's first follow-up appointment at 3-months postoperatively, and at successive visits, as circumstances permit. Videotaped documentation of the tremor and selected segments of the neurological examination are performed preoperatively and at each postsurgical evaluation. Tremor is graded on a 4-point scale (0 = none, 4 = severe) for each component: rest, static, action, and terminal accentuation.

Seventy-three patients underwent stereotactic ventrolateralis thalamotomy at the Mayo Clinic from September 1984 to March 1991 for the treatment of medically refractory dyskinesias. Sixty-seven (91.8%) were treated for tremor. These included 42 (62.7%) patients with Parkinson's disease, 8 (11.9%) patients with essential tremor, 14 (20.9%) patients with intention tremor of various etiologies, and 3 (4.5%) patients with other neurodegenerative disorders. The remaining 6 (8.2%) patients were treated for various complex dystonias. These results will be discussed in the following segments.

IV. SPECIFIC INDICATION AND RESULTS

A. Parkinson's Disease

Since the development of levodopa, the role of stereotactic thalamotomy in Parkinson's disease has become less ubiquitous. There are instances for which levodopa proves inadequate or problematic, and surgery becomes an important option. Approximately 15% of parkinsonian patients will have a suboptimal initial response to levodopa, and it is estimated that, of the remaining 85% who demonstrate a good initial response, one-third will lose all benefit over 5 years (48). Patients with severe disease may require dosing up to every 60–90 min and experience bothersome "on–off" phenomena. Large or chronic doses may lead to dyskinesias. Nausea and drowsiness are common side effects and psychological symptoms develop in 15–25% of patients (49). Pre-levodopa era VL thalamotomy relieved tremor in 80–93% and decreased rigidity in 50–90% of parkinsonian patients (20). Although there have been claims that previous levodopa therapy diminishes the effectiveness of VL thalamotomy, recent reports dispute this (50,51).

1. Symptomatic Relief

Immediate symptomatic relief of tremor is achieved in 80–90% of patients (43). Hitchcock et al. (43) showed immediate dramatic symptomatic improvement in 92% of patients. Long-term follow-up studies confirm lasting benefits of thalamotomy in controlling tremor. Nagaseki et al. demonstrated complete or near complete ablation of tremor in 92% of 25 patients at a mean follow-up interval of 6.58 years (52). Tasker found that 82% of patients had no tremor at 2-year follow-up (53). Tremors that do recur, do so in older patients (43) and within 3 months of surgery (54).

2. Functional Improvement

Symptomatic improvement from relief of tremor is not always accompanied by functional improvement in the quality of the patient's life. This is because other symptoms of Parkinson's disease, such as bradykinesia, can be far more disabling than tremor (43). Meyer noted that patients may fail to use treated limbs because of rigidity (55). Not stated in this report, however, is that postoperative limb neglect and dyspraxia can also play a significant role in a patient not using a tremor-free limb. However, Miyamoto et al. (48) were successful in abolishing tremor in 80% of 14 patients and functionally improved 1–2 grades on the Hoehn-Yahr scale in 68% at a mean follow-up interval of 67.8 months. Functional improvement is more likely in those patients who are less disabled (43), whose disease is manifested primarily by tremor, or who have significant asymmetry of symptoms (hemi-parkinsonism) (56). Tremor-dominant Parkinson's patients enjoyed expanded daily activities in 76.2% of 21 cases studied by Narabayashi et al. (56) at 3–8 years postoperatively. In this same series, 57.3% of 68 patients with asymmetric symptoms and 70% of 37 hemiparkinsonian patients enjoyed expanded daily activities at follow-up. There seems to be no clear correlation between the duration of tremor and likelihood of functional improvement following surgery (43).

3. Medical Therapy Following Ventrolateral Thalamotomy

Miyamoto et al. found that 36% of patients were able to discontinue levodopa therapy altogether (48).

4. Other Symptoms

Lesions in the VOA and VOP nuclei can improve rigidity and secondarily improve motor fatiguing (55) and akinesia (56) in approximately 80% of cases. Ventro-lateral thalamotomy can provide protection against the levodopa-induced dyskin-esias of choreoathetosis, dystonia, and ballism in the contralateral-targeted ex-tremity, and it is effective in relieving levodopa-induced limb dyskinesias once manifested (50). Meyer found that voluntary movement in single-handed tasks improved bilaterally after unilateral thalamotomy (57), probably related to bilat-eral diencephalic influence of voluntary proximal muscle movements.

Ventrolateral thalamotomy neither stops the natural progression of Parkinson's disease (58) nor effectively treats midline parkinsonian symptoms. These include oculogyric crises, autonomic changes, difficulties in speech and balance, cogni-tive deficits, and bradykinesia unassociated with rigidity (59). It is an effective treatment in medically refractory tremor-dominant cases, in unilaterally symp-tomatic patients, and in severe levodopa-induced extremity dyskinesias. This represents 10–15% of the parkinsonian population (56).

B. Parkinson's Disease: Mayo Clinic Experience

Fox et al. reviewed the Mayo Clinic's experience with ventrolateral thalamotomy for Parkinson's tremor (54), and their data is updated herein. Forty-two patients with medically refractory resting tremor of Parkinson's disease were referred for stereotactic VL thalamotomies. Forty-one underwent the thalamotomy procedure. Thalamotomy was not performed in one patient with moderately advanced disease owing to transient post-ventriculogram confusion. This, in conjunction with atrophy noted on CT scanning and borderline psychometrics, resulted in the decision not to proceed with thalamotomy. Two of the remaining 41 patients received staged bilateral thalamotomies for bilateral disabling tremor. Table 1 summarizes the clinical characteristics of the patients. The average length of follow-up was 35.7 months (range 25–77 months). There were 11 right and 28 left thalamotomies performed. There were 2 bilateral thalamotomies staged 5 years

Table 1 Clinical Characteristics of 42 Patients Referred for Thalamotomy With Parkinson's Tremor

Pt. no.	Age/ sex	Dominant hand	Side of lesion	Preop tremor[a]	Postop tremor	Intraop. changes	Transient morbidity	Permanent morbidity
1	30/F	R	R	3+	0	None	None	None
2	49/F	R	L	3+	0	None	None	None
2'	50/M	R	R	2,3+	0		Weakness left hand Dyspraxia left hand	None
3	66/F	R	L	3+	3+	None	None	None
4	61/F	R	L	2+	0,1+		Global dysphasia after ventriculogram	None
5	65/F	R	R	3+	0		Weakness left face	None
6	48/F	R	L	4+	0	Speech	See permanent complications; weakness right face	Dyspraxia right arm
7	38/M	L	R	2+	0		Weakness left face	None
7'	42/M	L	L	3,4+	0	Speech	Verbal cognitive dysfunction	Dysarthria
8	54/M	R	L	3+	0		Weakness right face, arm	None
9	66/M	R	L	4+	0		Weakness right arm	None
10	47/F	L	R	3+	0		Weakness left face; dyspraxia left hand; numbness left hand	None
11	62/M	R	L	3+	0	Speech	Hypokinetic dysarthria[b]	None
12	65/F	R	L	3,4+	0		None	None
13	65/M	R	R	3+	0		None	None
14	55/M	R	R	3+	0		None	None
15	41/M	R	R	3+	0		Weakness left face	None
16	62/F	R	L	4+	1,2+		Expressive dysphasia[b]	None
17	52/M	R	L	2,3+	0		None	None
18	69/M	R	L	3,4+	0	Speech	Expressive dysphasia[c] and cognitive dysfunction[c] s/p probe tract hematoma	Expressive dysphasia[c] and cognitive dysfunction[c]

Table 1 Continued

Pt. no.	Age/ sex	Dominant hand	Side of lesion	Preop tremor[a]	Postop tremor	Intraop. changes	Transient morbidity	Permanent morbidity
19	63/M	R	L	3+	0	Speech	None	None
20	64/M	R	L	3+	0	Speech	See permanent complications	Spastic dysarthria
21	56/M	R	R	4+	1,2+		Weakness left arm	None
22	72/M	R	L	2,3+	0	Speech	Weakness right face Hypokinetic dysarthria	None
23	50/M	R	L	2+	0		Weakness right face	None
24	49/M	R	L	3+	0	Speech	Weakness right face	None
25	69/M	R	L	3+	0	Speech	Hypokinetic dysarthria[b]	None
26	61/F	R	L	2,3+	0	Speech	See permanent complications; weakness right hand; numbness right hand; hypokinetic dysarthria	Dyspraxia right arm[a]
27	72/M	R	L	3+	0		Expressive dysphasia[b]; seizure s/p ventriculogram	None
28	53/M	R	L	3+	0		See permanent complications	Hypokinetic dysarthria[b]
29	54/M	R	L	3+	0		Weakness right arm; global dysphasia/delusions	None
30	52/M	R	L	3,4+	0		Disorientation	None

31	69/M	R	L	3+	3+	Speech	Global dysphasia after ventriculogram	None
32	59/M	R	L	4+	0		Abulia[c]	None
33	61/M	R	R	2,3+	0		Disorientation	None
34	34/M	R	L	3+	0	Speech	Weakness right face; hypokinetic dysarthria[b]	None
35	56/M	R	L	4+	0		None	None
36	58/M	R	L	3,4+	0		None	None
37	39/M	R	L	2,3+	0		None	None
38	65/M	R	L	4+	0	Speech	None	Spastic dysarthria
39	64/M	R	L	3,4+	0		None	Spastic dysarthria
39'	65/M	R	R	3,4+	0	Speech	None	Spastic dysarthria[b]
40	66/M	R	Aborted	3+				
41	67/M	L	R	3,4+	0	Speech	None	None
42	58/M	R	R	3+	0		Gait imbalance	None

Transient, less than 3 months; permanent, present at last follow-up.
[a] 4+, severe; 3+, moderate; 2+, mild; 1+, slight; 0, none.
[b] Worsening of preoperative condition, nondisabling.
[c] Disabling to patient.

and 6 months apart. Almost all patients had $+3$ (61.0%) or $+4$ (36.6%) resting tremor preoperatively.

1. Medical Therapy

Carbidopa–levodopa (Sinemet) was used by all but four (9.8%) patients before thalamotomy. These four were unable to tolerate this medication because of associated and disabling gastrointestinal or psychiatric disturbances. Twenty-four (58.5%) were taking Sinemet alone, and 13 (31.7%) were taking Sinemet plus other drugs. The average daily dose of Sinemet was 1200 mg/day. Thirty-four patients had notable side effects from their medications. These included dyskinesias (16 patients), nausea (10 patients), and sedation (4 patients). Ten patients required dosing every 60–90 min for tremor control.

2. Results

At the time of hospital discharge, there was complete (39 patients) or near complete (1 patient) ablation of contralateral tremor in 97.6% of cases. At follow-up, 25–77 months (mean 35.7 months) postoperatively, 39 (95.1%) experienced complete (36 patients) or near complete (3 patients) tremor ablation. In 2 (4.9%) patients, tremor recurred to preoperative levels within 3 months of surgery.

Postoperatively, 9 patients discontinued, and 9 additional patients significantly reduced their intake of antiparkinsonian medicines. Another 14 patients remained on their preoperative dose and schedule, whereas 9 patients ultimately required additional medicines in an attempt to control contralateral tremor or bradykinesia.

3. Morbidity

Of the 43 procedures performed (39 unilateral, 2 staged bilateral), there was no operative mortality, and only one case (2.3%) of significant permanent morbidity: a 61-year-old woman developed contralateral upper extremity dyspraxia following a left-sided lesion that had been extended in the mediolateral plane in an attempt to control severe right upper and lower extremity tremors. Furthermore, careful postoperative neurological, neuropsychological, and speech evaluations revealed that four additional patients (9.3%) experienced mild and nondisabling postoperative side effects: upper extremity dyspraxia in one patient and hypokinetic dysarthria in three patients.

Transient (nonpermanent) postoperative neurological findings occurred in 24 patients (55.8%) following thalamotomy. In most instances, these were worsening of preoperatively noted problems, which included cognitive deficits in 6 (14.0%), hypokinetic dysarthria in 5 (11.6%), lower facial weakness in 10 (23.3%), mild contralateral extremity weakness in 7 (16.3%), and extremity hypesthesia in 2 (4.7%). All patients with transient dysarthrias had undergone left thalamotomy. All of these patients with transient deficits had returned to the preoperative baseline at hospital discharge or when evaluated 3 months following surgery.

C. Essential Tremor

Essential tremor affects over 5 million persons older than 40 years of age in the United States (60). A small percentage of this population possess severe debilitating tremors that are refractory to medical management.

Stereotactic thalamotomy for the treatment of essential tremor was first described in the French literature in 1960. Guiot (61), Wertheimer (62), and Thurel (63) published case reports of tremor (dyskinesie volitionnelle d'attitude) having good results from stereotactic lesions placed in the VL thalamus, VL thalamus and subthalamus, and internal capsule, respectively. Cooper (64), in 1962, treated three cases of "heredofamilial tremor" with stereotactic VL thalamotomy, with good results. Laitinen (65) reported on the surgical treatment of nine patients with essential tremor in 1965: tremor in seven of these improved or resolved with the use of electrocautery or leukotome at various intracranial sites. Adams and Rutkin (66), in 1965, also published a series of 26 tremors treated with stereotactic centrum medianum lesions. Obrador and Dierssen (67) described ten patients with heredofamilial tremor; stereotactic lesions in the VL thalamus and Forel's Field H improved or abolished the tremor in some patients. They were less successful lesioning the globus pallidus, VP thalamus, or red nucleus–midbrain tegmentum. Twelve of 15 patients with essential tremor reported by Blacker et al. (68) experienced sustained tremor relief with stereotactic leukotome VL thalamotomy and subthalamotomies. Bertrand et al., in 1968, described 25 cases of VL thalamotomy for essential tremor, with good results in all (69). Van Manen, in 1974, published a series of 52 hereditary action tremors, 23 of which underwent stereotactic thermocoagulation VL thalamotomies, with immediate ablation in 100% (70). At 3-month follow-up, 22 patients with preoperative serious to moderate tremors experienced no tremor to slight tremor. Ohye et al., in 1982, reported stereotactic VIM thalamotomy for 15 cases of essential tremor with arrest or slight residual in all cases (71). Mohadjer et al. reported good long-term results of stereotactic thalamotomy in the treatment of essential tremor in a large population (104 patients) with long follow-up (mean 8.6 years) (72).

D. Essential Tremor: Mayo Clinic Experience

At the Mayo Clinic, nine stereotactic VL thalamotomies were performed on eight patients for medically intractable debilitating essential tremor. Clinical characteristics of the patients are listed in Table 2. Left thalamotomies were performed on six patients (75%), right thalamotomy was performed on one patient (12.5%), and one patient (12.5%) received staged bilateral stereotactic VL thalamotomies for bilateral tremor. All of the patients were men and the mean age at operation was 46.4 years (range 18–69 years). The mean age of tremor onset was 25.5 years (range 5–60 years), and mean duration of tremor preoperatively was 21.1 years

Table 2 Clinical Characteristics of Eight Patients Referred for Thalamotomy With Essential Tremor

Pt. no.ª	Age/sex	Side of lesion	Family history	Preop tremor	Immediate postop tremor	Follow-up postop tremor	Follow-up interval (mo)	Transient morbidity	Permanent morbidity	Preop disabilityª	Postop disabilityª
1	33/M	L	(?)	+2,3	0	0	1	Hypesthesia		22	4
2	69/M	L	+	+2	0	0	3	Attention deficit	Spastic dysarthria	21	1
3	68/M	L	+	+2,3	0	0+1	3	Attention deficit; spastic dysarthria		21	5
4	44/M	L	+	+2	0	0	50	Ataxic dysarthria		See 4'	See 4'
4'	45/M	R	+	+3	0	+1,2	43	Hypesthesia; extremity dyspraxia	Ataxic dysarthria	19	2
5	22/M	L	+	+2	0	0+1	4				
6	68/M	L	+	+3	0	0+1	8	Anomic dysphasia	Verbal cognitive deficit	22	5
7	18/M	R	+	+3	0	+1	43			20	0
8	51/M	L	+	+2,3	0	0	1	Verbal cognitive deficit		20	0

aʹ, second of staged procedures.

(range 5–55 years). Positive family histories of tremor were present in all cases for whom obtainable (one patient was adopted).

Results

There was complete immediate ablation of the contralateral upper extremity tremor in all nine patients. Follow-up examination (mean 17.3 months) disclosed complete ablation (four patients) or significant amelioration (four patients). Seven patients rated their tremor disability on a modified version of an established rating scale before and after surgery. At mean follow-up interval of 19 months (range 3–50 months), disability was reduced from moderate (15–21) in four and severe (22–28) in three, to absent (0–7) in six, and mild (8–14) in one (Fig. 17).

There was no permanent severe operative morbidity in this group of patients. A mild permanent dysarthria and mild verbal cognitive deficit were found in two patients, respectively. Both underwent left thalamotomies.

E. Intention Tremor

A kinetic tremor caused by dysfunction of the cerebellorubral system was first described by Holmes, in 1904 (73). Denny-Brown (11) coined the term "rubral tremor" referring to a characteristic tremor produced by midbrain dysfunction caused by multiple sclerosis, stroke, severe head injury, tumor, or toxins. This is a 2- to 2.5-Hz, irregular, kinetic tremor that appears weeks to months after injury to the superior cerebellar peduncle, midbrain tegmentum, or posterior thalamus

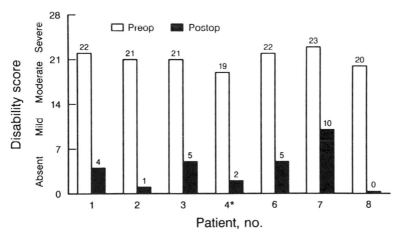

Figure 17 Comparison of preoperative and postoperative disability scores after VL thalamotomy for medically intractable debilitating essential tremor. (Scale modified from Fahn, S, Urban and Schwarzenberg, Inc., Baltimore.)

and is associated with paresis, plastic rigidity, dystonic posturing, and often hemianesthesia. These dyskinesias respond well to VL thalamotomy (74–76).

1. Multiple Sclerosis

Intention tremor is one of the most severe symptoms of multiple sclerosis and the main reason for invalidation (77). There is substantial symptomatic benefit from VL thalamotomy in 73–95% of cases (78–81). Kandel and Hondcarian (77) reported initial symptomatic ablation in 100% of 20 cases, with 50% ablation or substantial improvement of tremor at follow-up, 1–10 years postoperatively. Cooper (82) demonstrated arrest of tremor immediately in 93% of patients and long-term symptomatic improvement in 83% at 5–10 years. However, the long-term functional improvement is not as gratifying owing to the progressive nature of the disease (26). Speelman and Van Manen were able to ablate tremor in 100% of 11 patients with multiple sclerosis at mean follow-up of 1.5 years (81), but disability or arm function status did not improve. Hitchcock et al. were able to obtain initial symptomatic improvement in 100% of cases (43), but initial functional improvement in 33%. Currently, it is reasonable to recommend VL thalamotomy for symptomatic relief of severe intention tremor of multiple sclerosis if present for more than 1 year. One should avoid this procedure in those patients with severe irreversible damage to other systems (i.e., spastic paraparesis), a rapidly progressive form of multiple sclerosis, general poor health, or significant cognitive dysfunction (77,81).

2. Posttraumatic Tremor

It is not uncommon for patients with severe head injury to develop intention tremor as a late complication (83,84) owing to midbrain or cerebellar damage (85). Elevated supratentorial intracranial pressure causes stretching and tearing of the paramedian arteries in the upper brainstem (86,87), producing the characteristic syndrome of spastic hemiparesis, dysarthria, appendicular ataxia, and oculomotor dysfunction (83–85). Typically, a static and kinetic tremor with a myoclonic or hemiballismic component appears at a mean interval of 6 weeks postictus as the ipsilateral hemiparesis improves (84,85). These are poorly responsive to medical management, but may resolve spontaneously within a year.

Iwadate et al. reported excellent symptomatic relief by VL thalamotomy in two of three cases (83). Niizuma et al. (88), Ohye et al. (89), Andrew et al. (75), and Bullard et al. (90), all reported 100% immediate symptomatic improvement in cases of posttraumatic rubral tremor. Richardson described alleviation of tremor by VL cryothalamectomy in 69% of patients (85). Andrew et al. found that 100% of eight cases enjoyed functional improvement, although not always immediately (75). Bullard reported functional improvement, in 82% of patients, that was persistent at follow-up 3 months to 2 years postoperatively (90).

Andrew et al. discovered a transient morbidity rate higher than that of patients with Parkinson's disease or essential tremor (75), and they identified preoperative ataxia, dysarthria, and pseudobulbar palsy as risk factors. Because some posttraumatic tremors resolve spontaneously, he recommended an observation period of 1 year before thalamotomy was to be considered. However, he warned that delay of surgery too long in the young could delay development because of disuse of the affected extremity.

Damage to the cerebellar vermis, hemispheres, and brachium conjunctivum leads to the posttraumatic cerebellar syndrome of extremity tremor, dysarthria, voice tremor, ocular dysmetria, and ataxia, first described by Cantu (91). Gerstenbrand et al. (92) noted that this syndrome followed the apallic state in many (92). Stein et al. found that as appendicular ataxia abated, intention tremor developed (93). Kelly has found VL thalamotomy effective in symptomatic treatment of intention tremor of this etiology (44).

3. Stroke

Mesodiencephalic strokes in the territories of the thalamogeniculate, posteriomedial choroidal, and posteriolateral choroidal arteries result in tremor, myoclonus, chorea, and athetosis in combination with hemianesthesia, hemidysesthesia, hemiparesis, spasticity, hemianopia, delusions, hallucinations, confusion, and altered level of consciousness. Van Manen and Speelman abolished stroke-induced movement disorders in three patients, which persisted at 5 years (94). Niizuma et al. (88) and Ohye et al. (89) reported successful immediate results in a total of 12 patients. They postulated that the larger coagulation volumes required were due to postinfarct nuclear reorganization (95).

4. Tumor

Slowly growing mesencephalic tumors can produce tremor in addition to Parinaud's sign, anisocoria, and elevated intracranial pressure. Maeda et al. (76) reported two cases with this "red nucleus syndrome" who enjoyed immediate tremor ablation after thalamotomy.

F. Intention Tremor: Mayo Clinic Experience

Fourteen patients with secondary intention tremor (multiple sclerosis 5 patients, posttraumatic 4 patients, post infarct 5 patients) were treated by VL thalamotomy. Table 3 lists the clinical characteristics of these patients. There were six males and eight females whose mean age was 37.4 years (range 15–61). Preoperative duration of symptoms was a mean of 11 years (range 10 months to 34 years). Associated symptoms included spastic paresis in eight, diplopia in one, ataxia in six, and cognitive difficulties in one.

There were five right-sided and seven left-sided thalamotomies. Two procedures were aborted: one owing to transient extremity weakness following probe placement and one because of failure to obtain adequate evoked responses required

Table 3 Clinical Characteristics of 14 Patients Referred for Thalamotomy With Intention Tremor

Pt. no.	Age/sex	Side of lesion	Preop tremor	Immediate postop tremor	Follow-up postop tremor	Follow-up interval (mo)	Transient morbidity	Permanent morbidity	Etiology
1	45/F	L	+3	0	+2	3		Worsened ataxic dysarthria	MS
2	41/F	Aborted	+3						MS
3	32/F	L	+4	+1			Worsened ataxic dysarthria		MS
4	43/M	R	+3,4	0	0+1	34			MS
5	48/M	Aborted	+4				Extremity weakness		MS
6	18/F	L	+3	0	+1	17			PT
7	15/M	R	+4	0	0	55	Cognitive dysfunction		PT
8	25/M	L	+2,3	0	+3	20	Worsened dysarthria		PT
9	17/M	L	+2,3	0					PT
10	37/F	L	+4	0	+1	3			CVA
11	61/F	R	+3	0	0	31		Worsened dysarthria	CVA
12	56/M	R	+4	+1	+1	29			CVA
13	56/F	L	+3,4	0	+1	10			CVA
14	72/M	R	+4	0	0	0.5		Died	CVA

MS, multiple sclerosis; PT, posttraumatic; CVA, cerebrovascular accident.

for target localization. In the 12 thalamotomies performed, tremor was immediately completely abolished in 10 (83.3%) and significantly reduced in 2 (16.7%).

Results

Postoperative follow-up (6–55 months; mean 20.3 months) information was available in ten patients.

At follow-up, tremor was completely abolished in three (30%) and significantly reduced in six patients (60%). All of these patients noted marked improvement of their functional ability. Tremor returned and was unchanged from preoperative levels in one patient (10%). Two patients with preoperative ataxic dysarthrias noted worsened, but nondisabling, dysarthria postoperatively. One patient with severe preoperative general medical problems died 2 weeks postoperatively from pulmonary problems unrelated to the surgery.

G. Nonspecific Tremor

Three additional patients suffering from other neurodegenerative diseases underwent VL thalamotomy for resting and intention tremors. Their clinical characteristics are shown in Table 4. Notable are a 45-year-old man with olivopontocerebellar degeneration and a 48-year-old woman with spinocerebellar degeneration. Both experienced complete and immediate ablation of tremor following thalamotomy. At follow-up, the patient with spinocerebellar degeneration is free of tremor 4 months postoperatively. The patient with olivopontocerebellar degeneration died of complications associated with disease progression 18 months postoperatively, but without tremor recurrence. This patient's preoperative ataxic dysarthria was mildly worsened following left thalamotomy. The third patient was a 29-year-old woman with a nonspecific neurodegenerative process characterized by rubral tremor, spasticity, and mild dementia, who received staged bilateral thalamotomies and demonstrated immediate complete ablation of tremor from the right thalamotomy and significant reduction of tremor from the left thalamotomy.

Table 4 Clinical Characteristics of Three Patients Referred for Thalamotomy With Neurodegenerative Disorders

Pt. no.[a]	Age/ sex	Side of lesion	Preop tremor	Immediate postop tremor	Follow-up postop tremor	Follow-up interval (mo)	Transient morbidity	Permanent morbidity
1	29/F	L	+3	+1	0+1	16		
1'	29/F	R	+3	0	0+1	7		
2	48/F	R	+4	0	0	4		
3	45/M	L	+4	0		18		

[a]', second of staged procedures.

H. Dystonia

Dystonias may be idiopathic or secondary, focal or generalized.

1. Overall

Dystonias as a heterogeneous group are improved 25–50% with thalamotomy in one-quarter of cases, and improved more than 50% in one-quarter to one-third of cases (96). Cooper reported mild to marked improvement in various dystonias in 69.7% of 208 patients (97). Gros et al. observed immediate good results in 77% and long-term good results in 33% of 25 cases with various dystonias (98).

2. Focal Dystonias

Andrew et al. reported good relief of focal dystonia in 62% of 27 patients (99). This included 22 cases of spasmotic torticollis. Cooper performed bilateral VL thalamotomy for spasmodic torticollis with a 60–70% success rate (100). Others have combined unilateral thalamotomy with peripheral denervation procedures, yielding good results in 36–73% of patients (101–104).

3. Generalized Dystonias

Cooper found moderate to marked improvement in dystonia in 69.7% of 226 patients with generalized dystonia (97). He also noted that young patients in this category tolerated bilateral thalamotomy better than older parkinsonian patients. Zervas has suggested that unilateral VL thalamotomy plus dentatectomy may avoid the need for bilateral thalamotomy (105). Tasker et al. noted an improvement in limb status in 47% of 20 patients, but postoperative regression in 65% (96). Infantile dystonias respond with immediate good results in 40–70% of cases and in long-term good results in 50–80% (98). Laitinen reported that older patients respond better than younger patients, but this observation was not reproduced by Gros et al. (98). In fact, Gros et al. recommended early surgery to improve motor performance and enhance development.

4. Secondary Dystonias

Tasker et al. reported that tonic and phasic limb movements were reduced in 49% of 29 patients (96). Proximal and neck musculature responded poorly, extremity dexterity did not improve significantly owing to paresis, and postoperative symptom regression occurred in 31%. In 75% of cases, posttraumatic and postinfarction dystonic hemiplegias respond to thalamotomy (85).

5. Prognosis

Cooper claimed that genetic dystonias, dystonias manifesting between ages 9 and 13, dystonias treated between ages 11 and 15, and dystonias in Jewish patients with a positive family history predicted good surgical outcome (97). Tasker et al. found that neck and trunk involvement, three of four extremity involvement, and progressive disease predicted poor surgical outcome (96). There are several problems in assessing benefit from thalamotomy in dystonias. The dystonic population is not homogeneous. There are many etiological factors in secondary dystonias. Idiopathic focal or generalized dystonias may carry different prognoses. Many secondary dystonias and most generalized dystonias are progressive and mask beneficial long-term effects of thalamotomy. Also the dystonic process is complex and the essential target has not been physiologically identified (96).

I. Dystonia: Mayo Clinic Experience

Six cases with complex dystonias (idiopathic focal dystonias in two patients, secondary focal dystonias due to tumor, AVM, and trauma in three patients, and secondary generalized postencephalitic dystonia in one patient) underwent VL thalamotomy. The clinical characteristics are shown in Table 5. There were four males and two females (mean age 24.3 years, range 13–33). Preoperative duration of symptoms was a mean of 10.7 years (range 5–17). Types of movement disorders included dystonic postures in four, hemiballismus in two, chorea in two, myoclonus in one, torticollis in one, and tremor in two patients. Associated symptoms included paresis in three, pseudobulbar palsy in one, and ataxia in one. There were five right-sided and one left-sided thalamotomies.

Results

In the six thalamotomies performed, the targeted extremity dystonia was immediately and completed ablated in all. However, long-term follow-up, obtained in all six patients (1–64 months, mean 19.8 months postoperatively) revealed that the targeted dystonia was totally ablated in only three (50%), greatly improved in one (16.7%), but had returned and was unchanged from preoperative level in two (33.3%). Analyzed in other ways, good results were obtained in two of two idiopathic dystonias and two of four secondary dystonias. Also, good results were obtained in three of five focal dystonias and in the treated extremity of the patient with generalized dystonia. One patient with an idiopathic focal dystonia showed a mildly worsened ataxic dysarthria and nondisabling verbal cognitive deficit 13 months postoperatively.

J. Cerebral Palsy

Patients with cerebral palsy suffer from paretic and spastic limbs, involuntary movements, disturbances in vision or hearing, abnormal speech or language, seizure disorders and, sometimes, mental retardation (106,107). Stereoencephalotomy for the dyskinesias, rigidity, and spasticity of cerebral palsy has been used since the 1950s (108), but analyses of results were difficult because of the variety of movement disorders present and their varied pathophysiological mechanisms (109). Cooper felt that cerebral palsy patients were poor surgical candidates owing to diffuse CNS abnormalities and mental retardation (110). However, Narabayashi

Table 5 Clinical Characteristics of Six Patients Referred for Thalamotomy With Dystonia

Pt. no.	Age/ sex	Side of lesion	Type of dystonia	Classification of dystonia	Immediate result	Follow-up result	Follow-up interval	Transient morbidity	Permanent morbidity
1	33/M	R	Extremity myoclonus	Idiopathic focal	0	0	1		
2	20/M	R	Extremity dystonic	Secondary focal (tumor)	0	As preop	59		
3	23/F	L	Extremity dystonic posture	Secondary generalized encephalitis	0	0	64		
4	13/F	R	Hemiballismus	Secondary focal (AVM)	0	0	56		
4'	16/F	R	Choreoathetosis	Secondary focal (AVM)	0	0	20		
5	27/M	R	Chorea, kinetic tremor	Idiopathic focal	0	0	13	Extremity dyspraxia	Worsened ataxic dysarthria Verbal cognitive deficit
6	30/M	R	Extremity dystonic posture	Secondary focal (trauma)	0	As preop	66		

', second of staged procedures; 0, abolition.

and Kubota reported improvement in choreoathetosis and dystonias in 78% of selected patients (111). Broggi et al. reported fair to considerable symptomatic improvement in 96.9% of 33 patients (109). Hemiparetics fared better than tetraparetics: 85.6% of hemiparetics displayed functional improvement in all areas, whereas tetraparetics improved symptomatically, but not functionally. Tremors respond well and tend not to recur. Large excursion dyskinesias respond well immediately, but tend to regress to some degree. The response of dystonias is unpredictable. Spasticity does not respond well to VL thalamotomy in these patients. Acquired traumatic cerebral palsy dyskinesias respond less well than acquired embolic or neoplastic cerebral palsy dyskinesias or congenital cerebral palsy dyskinesias (109). Because postoperative physical therapy is essential in developing new patterns of movement, perseverance and IQ are important determinants of functional improvement (107,112).

K. Miscellaneous Movement Disorders

Choreoathetosis was first treated surgically by Horsley, in 1909, with resection of the precentral gyrus (15). Mundinger et al. reported initial improvement with VL thalamotomy in 97%, and long-term fair to good results in 50% of patients (113). Hemiballismus after stereotactic thalamotomy, subthalamic hemorrhage, or infarct, if not spontaneously remitting, can be treated with VL thalamotomy with effectiveness in 50–60% of cases (96,110). Myoclonias without electroencephalographic correlates respond well in 70% of patients (114). Primary writing tremor, a rare form of essential tremor, was ablated by Ohye et al. in three patients (115). Idiopathic oromandibular and buccolingual dyskinesias were almost completely relieved by Narabayashi et al. in two patients (116). Mimura et al. have reported a case of tremor with thalamic pain syndrome ablated with VL thalamotomy (117). Dyskinesias of Huntington's chorea have been treated in the past, but predictable progressive neurological deterioration deems stereotactic thalamotomy unrewarding in the patients (100).

V. COMPLICATIONS OF THALAMOTOMY

A. Overview

Cooper and Stellar found postoperative deficits a transient phenomenon in 0.3–13.1% of patients (118), and it is probably related to perilesional edema (119). Tasker et al. found transient deficits in 25.3% and permanent deficits in 8% of 75 cases undergoing VIM thalamotomy for Parkinson's tremor (27). Complications are associated with improperly placed lesions, but can also be associated with correctly placed lesions. In the latter group these associated complications are more frequently seen in patients with advanced disease.

B. Complications Associated with Improperly Placed Lesions

Lesions too lateral cause dysfunction in the posterior limb of the internal capsule and hemiparesis; lesions too posterior cause ventralis posterior nucleus dysfunction and contralateral hemihypesthesia or dysesthesia; lesions too inferior cause subthalamic nucleus dysfunction and hemiballismus; and lesions too medial, especially if bilateral, cause forniceal dysfunction and cognitive deficits (7). Morbidity in stereotactic neuroablative procedures was greatly reduced with the development of reversible trial lesion instrumentation, physiological recording and stimulation techniques that allowed identification of nuclear structures, and stereotactic CT guidance. These made practical small, precise lesions, thereby reducing morbidity (120).

The first stereotactic lesions were performed by wire leukotome (Fig. 18), later modified by Obrador (121). Cooper experimented in the production of reversible lesions. He first utilized procaine injection and the compression inflatable balloon cannula, but later developed the cryocannula to produce physiological neuronal inhibition at temperatures of 0–19°C and permanent lesions at temperatures less than −30°C (122). Radiofrequency lesioning probes were introduced by Aronow (123) and proved to be a practical, reproducible, and safe method of lesioning. Lesion size is determined by probe diameter, length of exposed tip, and temperature.

In 1963, Albe-Fessard developed microelectrodes that enabled precise target localization by neurophysiological recording and stimulation techniques (124). Individual variability in the location of subcortical structures relative to midline radiological landmarks increases as one moves from midline (125). Postmortem studies have demonstrated a wide scatter of stereotactic lesions around intended target sites (126). Early stereotactic surgeons compensated for localization inac-

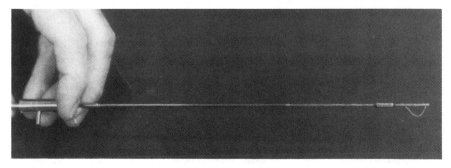

Figure 18   Wire leukotome. (From Ref. 3.)

curacies by producing larger lesions that carried greater risk of untoward effects (7). Stereotactic CT guidance provided a renaissance in stereotactic procedures and afforded accurate localization of subcortical structures (127).

C. Complications Associated with Well-Placed Lesions

1. Speech and Language Deficits

Speech and language can be reproducibly altered by electrical stimulation of the ventralis lateralis nucleus (128,129). Dysarthrias are generally transient, non-debilitating deficits that occur in up to two-thirds of thalamotomies. Those infrequent permanent dysarthrias usually occur after dominant thalamotomy (130). Dominant VL thalamotomy leads to a transient language disturbance in 13.1% of cases (131). These are characterized by dysphasias with perseveration, intrusion of extraneous words, and impairment of expressive and receptive verbal capacities (132,133). In some series, those at risk were identified using intraoperative dichotic listening techniques (134)

2. Cognitive Deficits

Ventrolateral thalamotomy can produce transient cognitive deficits in 10% and mild permanent cognitive deficits in 10–15% of patients (135,136). Dominant VL thalamotomy may lead to mild verbal memory and learning difficulties, and nondominant VL thalamotomy may lead to mild visual–spatial memory and learning difficulties. Both may be ultimately related to a specific deficit in attention (137–140).

Velasco et al. found that 2.5% of 316 cases undergoing unilateral thalamotomy developed neglect in use of the contralateral extremities with indifference to this fact (141). Hassler noted decreased spontaneous contralateral arm swing, without focal sensory or motor deficits in some patients undergoing unilateral VL thalamotomy (142). Patients at risk demonstrated subcortical atrophy, with increased third ventricle width. They postulated that midline thalamic nuclear atrophy in a patient receiving thalamotomy critically decreases reticulothalamocortical projections engaged in selective attention, thereby precipitating neglect (142). Interestingly, Vilkki reported asymptomatic hemi-inattention in visual searching in 21 patients 5–10 days after receiving a unilateral VL thalamotomy for tremor (143). Nondominant thalamotomy resulted in contralateral visual hemi-inattention, and dominant thalamotomy resulted in bilateral hemi-inattention.

3. Other Deficits

Other postoperative deficits are infrequent. Yasui et al. found the slight cerebellar signs of dysmetria and hypotonia in 8.6% of patients receiving VIM thalamotomy (144). Mild gait and balance disturbances may be seen if dentatothalamic projections are disrupted. One may be able to demonstrate transient hypokinesia in the contralateral side.

D. Risk Factors

Waltz et al. found that of 154 patients receiving thalamotomy for Parkinson's tremor, mortality increased from 1.3% to 3% for those older than aged 70 (145). Wester and Hauglie-Hanssen (28) noted permanent untoward effects of thalamotomy only in those patients older than aged 66 who receiving dominant hemisphere lesions ($0.05 > p > 0.02$). If preoperative significant cognitive dysfunction or cerebral atrophy exist, there is increased risk of significant cognitive morbidity associated with thalamotomy (136).

Hypertensive patients have an increased risk of hemorrhage into the operative site (146). Patients with dyskinesias of multiple sclerosis and cerebral palsy receiving thalamotomy suffer higher complication rates when compared with patients with Parkinson's disease or essential tremor ($0.01 > p > 0.001$) (81,107). This is probably related to multifocal cerebral abnormalities present preoperatively. There is also concern that stereotactic thalamotomy may provoke relapse in multiple sclerosis patients (81).

E. Bilateral Procedures

Bilateral thalamotomy carries increased risk of postoperative confusion and disorientation and may produce dysarthria, hypophonia, or dysphagia in up to 30% of patients unless staged 3 months to 2 years apart (59,147). In an attempt to avoid this risk, Benabid (148) has performed VL thalamotomy on the most-disabled side and implanted long-term VIM stimulators on the less-disabled side with encouraging results.

VI. CONCLUSIONS

Modern methods for VL thalamotomy that include the institution of imaging studies along with neurophysiological localization techniques result in improved target localization and excellent control of tremor. However, contemporary patients with parkinsonian tremor are usually more seriously affected by the general symptoms of the disease than in series gathered in the pre-L-dopa era. One must bear in mind that, in patients with degenerative conditions, such as Parkinson's and demyelinating disease, lesions are being created in a diseased and, in some cases, marginally functioning brain. Controlling tremor by thalamic lesions increases the risk of reduced neurological function. In most cases this risk is directly related to the patient's general neurological condition preoperatively. Therefore, in considering thalamotomy in older and more disabled patients with tremor, the physician must weigh the benefit of cessation of tremor against the untoward effects of the procedure. In the vast majority of patients, these untoward effects such as hypokinetic dysarthria are neither disabling nor really bothersome to the patient who is grateful to be relieved of tremor. In most patients tremor relieved by thalamotomy is abolished on a long-term basis. Therefore, earlier consideration of thalamotomy in patients with tremor as the primary manifestation of their disease seems more reasonable, than recommending this procedure later on in the course of the disease when other symptoms are evident, the patient is more debilitated, and the risk of surgery is much higher. Nonetheless, less affected and younger patients with tremor alone do much better and have fewer postoperative side effects than older patients with bradykinetic symptoms. In all cases, however, careful preoperative patient selection and accurate subcortical localization are of paramount importance in achieving a satisfactory postoperative result.

REFERENCES

1. Clarke RH, Horsley V. On a method of investigating the deep ganglia and tracts of the central nervous system. Br Med J 1906; 2:1799–1800.
2. Horsley V, Clarke RH. The structure and function of the cerebellum examined by a new method. Brain 1908; 31:45–124.
3. Spiegel EA, Wycis HT, Marks M. Stereotactic apparatus for operations on the human brain. Science 1947; 106;349–350.
4. Spiegel EA, Wycis HT. Ansotomy in paralysis agitans. Arch Neurol Psychiatry 1954; 71:598–614.
5. Guiot G, Brion S. Traitement des mouvements anormaux par la coagulation pallidale. Technique et resultants. Rev Neurol (Paris) 1953; 89:578–580.
6. Narabayashi H. Stereotactic instrument for operation on the human basal ganglia. Psychiatr Neurol Jpn 1952; 54:669–671.
7. Kelly PJ, Ahlskog JE, Goerss SJ, Daube JR, Duffy JR, Kall BA. Computer-assisted stereotactic ventralis lateralis thalamotomy with microelectrode recording control in patients with Parkinson's disease. Mayo Clin Proc 1987; 62:655–664.
8. Bravo GJ, Cooper IS. A clinical and radiological correlation of the lesions produced by chemopallidectomy and thalamectomy. J Neurol Neurosurg Psychiatry 1959; 22:1–10.
9. Cooper IS. Chemopallidectomy. Science 1955; 121:217.
10. Cooper IS, Poloukhine N. Chemopallidectomy: a neurosurgical technique useful in geriatric parkinsonians. J Geriatr Soc 1955; 3:839–859.
11. Denny-Brown D. The Basal Ganglia. London: Oxford University Press, 1962.
12. Gillingham FJ. Small localized surgical lesions of the internal capsule in the treatment of the dyskinesias. Confin Neurol 1962; 22:385–392.
13. Gillingham FJ, Kalyanaraman S, Donaldson AA. Bilateral lesions in the management of parkinsonism. J Neurosurg 1966; 24:449–453.
14. Torres M, Cooper IS, Poloukhine H. Effects of lesions in the putamen on involuntary movements and rigidity in Parkinson's disease. J Am Geriatr Soc 1956; 4:1309–1319.
15. Horsley V. The Linacre Lecture on the function of the so-called motor area of the brain. Br Med J 1909; 2:125–132.
16. Bucy PC. Cortical extirpation in the treatment of involuntary movements. Res Publ Assoc Res Nerv Ment Dis 1942; 21:551–595.

17. Meyers R. The modification of alternating tremors, rigidity and festination by surgery of the basal ganglia. Res Publ Assoc Res Nerv Ment Dis 1942; 21:602–665.
18. Fenelon F. Essais de traitment neurochirurgical du syndrome parkinsonien par intervention direct sur les voies extrapyramidales immediatement sous-striopallidales (anse lenticulaire). Communication suivie de projection du film d'um des operes pris avant et apres l'intervention. Rev Neurol (Paris) 1950; 83:437–440.
19. Hassler R. The influence of stimulations and coagulations in the human thalamus on the tremor at rest and its physiopathologic mechanism. In: Proceedings of the 2nd International Congress of Neuropathology. Part II. Amsterdam: Excerpta Medica Foundation, 1955:637–642.
20. Zager EL. Neurosurgical management of spasticity, rigidity, and tremor. Neurol Clin 1987; 5:631–647.
21. Nashold BS Jr. Stereotactic neurosurgery: the present and future. Ann Surg 1970; 36:85–93.
22. Guiot G, Derome P, Jedynak P. Permanence des indications de la chirurgie stereotaxique dan le treblement parkinsonien et certain mouvements anormaux rebelles. Ann Med Intern 1975; 126:295–296.
23. Andrew J, Rice Edwards JM, Rudolf N de M. The placement of stereotactic lesions for involuntary movements other than in Parkinson's disease. Acta Neurochir [Suppl] 1974; 21:39–47.
24. Bertrand C, Molina-Negro P, Martinez S. Stereotactic targets for dystonias and dyskinesias: relationship to corticobulbar fibers and other adjoining structures. Adv Neurol 1979; 24:395–399.
25. Cooper IS. Dystonia: surgical approaches to treatment and physiologic implications. In: Yahr MD, ed. The Basal Ganglia. New York: Raven Press, 1976:369–383.
26. Krayenbuhl H, Yasargil MG. Relief of intention tremor due to multiple sclerosis by stereotaxic thalamotomy. Confin Neurol 1962; 22:368–374.
27. Tasker RR, Siqueira J, Hawrylyshy P, Organ LW. What happened to VIM thalamotomy for Parkinson's disease? Appl Neurophysiol 1983; 46:68–83.
28. Wester K, Hauglie-Hanssen E. Stereotaxic thalamotomy—experiences from the levodopa era. J Neurol Neurosurg Psychiatry 1990; 53:427–430.
29. Van Manen J, Speelman JD, Tans BW. Indications for surgical treatment of Parkinson's disease after levodopa therapy. Clin Neurol Neurosurg 1984; 86:207–212.
30. Laitinen LV. Brain targets in surgery for Parkinson's disease. Results of a survey of neurosurgeons. J Neurosurg 1985; 62:349–351.
31. Bertrand C, Hardy J, Molina-Negro P. Optimum physiological target for the arrest of tremor. In: Gillingham FJ, Donaldson A, eds. Third Symposium on Parkinson's Disease. Edinburgh: Churchill Livingstone, 1969.
32. Guiot G, Hardy J, Albe-Fessarh D. Delimitation precise des structures souscorticales et identification des moyaux thalamiques chez l'homme par l'electrophysiologie stereotaxique. Neurochirurgie 1962; 5:1–18.
33. Narabayashi H, Ohye C. Importance of microstereoencephalotomy for termor alleviation. Appl Neurophysiol 1980; 43:222–227.
34. Taren J, Guiot G, Derome P, Trigo J. Hazards of stereotaxic thalamectomy. J Neurosurg 1968; 19:173–182.

35. Narabayashi H. Stereotactic VIM thalamotomy for treatment of tremor. Eur Neurol 1989; 29(suppl 1):29–32.

36. Narabayashi H. Tremor: its generating mechanisms and treatment. In: Vinker PJ, Bruyn GW, Klawans HL, eds. Handbook of Clinical Neurology. Vol. 5. Amsterdam: Elsevier, 1986:597–607.

37. Ohye C. Anatomy and physiology of the thalamic nucleus ventralis intermedius. In: Ito M, et al., eds. Integrative Control Functions of the Brain. Tokyo: Kodansha, 1978:152–163.

38. Ohye C. Neurons of the thalamic ventralis intermedius nucleus—their special reference to tremor. Adv Neurol Sci 1985; 29:224–231.

39. Ohye C, Saito A, Fukamachi A, Narabayashi H. An analysis of the spontaneous rhythmic and nonrhythmic burst discharges in the human thalamus. J Neurol Sci 1974; 22:245–259.

40. Ohye C, Shibazaki T, Hirai T, Wada H, Hirato M, Kawashima Y. Further physiological observations on the ventralis intermedius neurons in the human thalamus. J Neurophysiol 1989; 61:488–500.

41. Ricchcrt T. Long-term follow up results of stereotaxic treatment of extrapyramidal disorders. Confin Neurol 1962; 22:356–363.

42. Kelly PJ, Derome P, Guiot G. Thalamic spatial variability and the surgical results of lesions placed with neurophysiologic control. Surg Neurol 1978; 9:307–315.

43. Hitchcock E, Flint GA, Gutowski NJ. Thalamotomy for movement disorders: a critical appraisal. Acta Neurochir [Suppl] 1987; 39:61–65.

44. Kelly PJ, Principles of stereotactic surgery: instrumentation and procedural aspects. In: Youmans JR, ed. Neurological Surgery. 3rd ed. Philadelphia: WB Saunders, 1990:4183–4226.

45. Kelly PJ. Tumor Stereotaxis. Philadelphia: WB Saunders, 1991.

46. Kelly PJ. Microelectrode recording for the somatotopic placement of stereotactic thalamic lesions in the treatment of parkinsonian and cerebellar intention tremor. Appl Neurophysiol 1980; 43:262–266.

47. Hirai T, Miyazaki M, Nakajima H, Shibazaki T, Ohye C. The correlation between tremor characteristics and the predictive volume of effective lesions in stereotaxic nucleus ventralis intermedius thalamotomy. Brain 1983; 106:1001–1018.

48. Miyamoto T, Bekko H, Moriyama E, Tsuchida S. Present role of stereotactic thalamotomy for parkinsonism. Retrospective analysis of operative results and thalamic lesions in computed tomograms. Appl Neurophysiol 1985; 48:294–304.

49. Adams RD, Victor M. Principles of Neurology. New York: McGraw-Hill, 1981.

50. Kelly PJ, Gillingham FJ. The long-term results of stereotaxic surgery and L dopa therapy in patients with Parkinson's disease. A 10-year follow-up study. J Neurosurg 1980; 53:332–337.

51. Broggi G, Giorgi C, Servello D. Stereotactic neurosurgery in the treatment of tremor. Acta Neurochir 1987; 39:73–76.

52. Nagaseki Y, Shibazaki T, Hirai T, et al. Long-term follow-up results of selective VIM-thalamotomy. J Neurosurg 1986; 65:296–302.

53. Tasker RR. Tremor of parkinsonism and stereotactic thalamotomy. Mayo Clin Proc 1987; 62:736–739.

54. Fox MW, Ahlskog JE, Kelly PJ. Stereotactic ventrolateralis thalamotomy for medically refractory tremor in post-levodopa era Parkinson's disease patients. J Neurosurg (in press).

55. Meyer CH. Parkinsonism: if surgery is necessary, can it help spontaneous movement and motor fatiguing? Acta Neurochir 1980; 54:149–155.

56. Narabayashi H, Maeda T, Yokochi F. Long-term follow-up study of nucleus ventralis intermedius and ventrolateralis thalamotomy using a microelectrode technique in parkinsonism. Appl Neurophysiol 1987; 50:330–337.

57. Meyer CH. Bilateral improvement in involuntary movement after unilateral diencephalic lesions for parkinsonism. Appl Neurophysiol 1981; 44:345–354.

58. Scott RM, Brody JA, Cooper IS. The effect of thalamotomy on the progress of unilateral Parkinson's disease. J Neurosurg 1970; 32:286–288.

59. Krayenbuhl H, Wyss O, Yasargil M. Bilateral thalamotomy and pallidotomy as treatment for bilateral parkinsonism. J Neurosurg 1961; 18:429–444.

60. Hubble JP, Busenbark KL, Koller WC. Essential tremor. Clin Neuropharmacol 1989; 12:453–482.

61. Guiot G, Brion S, Fardeau M, Bettaie BA, Molina P. Dyskinesie volitionnelle d'attitude supprimee par la coagulation thalamocapsulaire. Rev Neurol (Paris) 1960; 102:220–229.

62. Wertheimer P, Bourret N, Lapraz C. A propos d'un cas de dyskinesie volitionnelle d'attitude trait par leucotomie thalamique et sous-thalamique. Rev Neurol (Paris) 1960; 102:481–486.

63. Thurel R, Nehlil J, O'Keefe P. Resultats de la coagulation de la voie pyramidale dans la capsule interne sur un tremblement d'action, statique et cinetique. Rev Neurol (Paris) 1960; 103:77–79.

64. Cooper IS. Heredofamilial tremor abolition by chemothalamectomy. Arch Neurol 1962; 7:129–131.

65. Laiten F. Stereotactic treatment of hereditary tremor. Acta Neurol Scand 1965; 41:74–79.

66. Adams JE, Rutkin BB. Lesions of the centrum medianum in the treatment of movement disorders. Confin Neurol 1965; 26:231–236.

67. Obrador S, Dierssen G. Observations on the treatment of intention and postural tremor by subcortical stereotactic lesions. Confin Neurol 1965; 26:250–253.

68. Blacker HM, Bertrand C, Martinez N, Hardy J, Molina-Negro P. Hypotonia accompanying the neurosurgical relief of essential tremor. J Nerv Ment Dis 1968; 147:49–55.

69. Bertrand C, Hardy J, Molina-Negro P, Martinez SN. Tremor of attitude. Confin Neurol 1969; 31:37–41.

70. Van Manen J. Stereotactic operations in cases of hereditary and intention tremor. Acta Neurochir [Suppl] 1974; 21:49–55.

71. Ohye G, Hirai T, Miyazuki M, Shibazaki N. VIM thalamotomy for the treatment of various kinds of tremor. Appl Neurophysiol 1981; 45:275–280.

72. Mohadjer M, Georke H, Milios E, Etou A, Mundinger F. Long-term results of stereotaxy in the treatment of essential tremor. Stereotact Funct Neurosurg 1990; 54–55:125–129.

73. Holmes G. On certain tremors in organic cerebral lesions. Brain 1904; 27:327–375.
74. Beckovic SF, Bladin PF. Rubral tremor: clinical features and treatment of three cases. Clin Exp Neurol 1984; 20:119–128.
75. Andrew J, Fowler CJ, Harrison MJG. Tremor after head injury and its treatment by stereotactic surgery. J Neurol Neurosurg Psychiatry 1982; 45:815–819.
76. Maeda T, Kondo T, Ohye C, Narabayashi H. Physiologically controlled VIM thalamotomy for red nucleus syndrome: report of two cases. Appl Neurophysiol 1979; 42:310–311.
77. Kandell GI, Hondcarian OA. Surgical treatment of the hyperkinetic form of multiple sclerosis. Acta Neurol 1985; 7:345–347.
78. Arsalo A, Hanninen A, Laitinen L. Functional surgery in the treatment of multiple sclerosis. Ann Clin Res 1973; 5:74–79.
79. Cooper IS. Neurosurgical alleviation of intention tremor of multiple sclerosis and cerebellar disease. N Engl J Med 1960; 263:441–444.
80. Riechert T, Richter D. Stereotaktische operationen zur behandlung des tremors der multipele sklerose. Schweiz Arch Neurol Neurochir Psychiatr 1972; 111:411–416.
81. Speelman JD, Van Manen J. Stereotactic thalamotomy for the relief of intention tremor of multiple sclerosis. J Neurol Neurosurg Psychiatry 1984; 47:596–599.
82. Cooper IS. Relief of intention tremor of multiple sclerosis by thalamic surgery. JAMA 1967; 199:689–694.
83. Iwadate Y, Saeki N, Namba H, Odaki M, Oka N, Yamura A. Post-traumatic intention tremor—clinical features and CT findings. Neurosurg Rev 1989; 12(suppl 1):500–507.
84. Kremer M, Russell WR, Smythe GE. Mid-brain syndrome following head injury. J Neurol Neurosurg Psychiatry 1947; 10:49–60.
85. Richardson RR. Rehabilitative neurosurgery: posttraumatic syndromes. Stereotact Funct Neurosurg 1989; 53:105–112.
86. Andrew J, Fowler CJ, Harrison MJG, Kendall BE. Post-traumatic tremor due to vascular injury and its treatment by stereotactic thalamotomy. J Neurol Neurosurg Psychiatry 1982; 45:560–562.
87. Tomlinson BE. Brain-stem lesions after head injury. J Clin Pathol 1970; 23(suppl 4):154–165.
88. Niizuma H, Kwak R, Ohi T, Suzuki J, Saso S. Three cases of red nucleus syndrome treated by stereotactic thalamotomy. Appl Neurophysiol 1979; 42:311–312.
89. Ohye C, Hirai T, Miyazaki M, Shibazaki T, Nakajima H. VIM thalamotomy for the treatment of various kinds of tremor. Appl Neurophysiol 1982; 45:275–280.
90. Bullard DE, Nahsold BS Jr. Stereotaxic thalamotomy for treatment of posttraumatic movement disorders. J Neurosurg 1984; 61:316–321.
91. Cantu RC. Transient traumatic cerebellar dysfunction: a report of a syndrome. Int Surg 1969; 52:392–394.
92. Gerstenbrand F, Lucking CH, Peters G, Rothemund E. Cerebellar syndromes as sequelae of traumatic lesions of upper brainstem and cerebellum. Int J Neurol 1970; 7:271–278.
93. Stein DG, Rosen JJ, Butters N, eds. Plasticity and Recovery of Function in the Central Nervous System. New York: Academic Press, 1974.

94. Van Manen J, Speelman JD. Thalamotomy for tremor after a vascular brainstem lesion. Acta Neurochir [Suppl] 1987; 39:70–72.

95. Ohye C, Shibazaki T, Hirai T, Kawashima Y, Hirato M, Matsumura M. Plastic change of thalamic organization in patients with tremor after stroke. Appl Neurophysiol 1985; 48:288–292.

96. Tasker RR, Doorly T, Yamashiro K. Thalamotomy in generalized dystonia. Adv Neurol 1988; 50:615–631.

97. Cooper IS. 20-year followup study of the neurosurgical treatment of dystonia musculorum deformans. In: Eldridge R, Fahn S, eds. Dystonia. Adv Neur 1976; 14: 423–452.

98. Gros C, Frerebeau PH, Perez-Dominguez E, Bazeir M, Privat JM. Long term results of stereotactic surgery for infantile dystonia and dyskinesias. Neurochirurgia 1976; 19:171–178.

99. Andrew J, Fowler CJ, Harrison MJG. Stereotactic thalamotomy in 55 cases of dystonia. Brain 1983; 106:981–1000.

100. Cooper IS. Neurosurgical treatment of the dyskinesias. Clin Neurosurg 1977; 24: 367–390.

101. Bertrand C, Molina-Negro P, Martinez SN. Combined stereotactic and peripheral surgical approach for spasmodic torticollis. Appl Neurophysiol 1978; 41:122–123.

102. Colbassani HJ, Wood JH. Management of spasmodic torticollis. Surg Neurol 1986; 25:153–158.

103. Hassler R, Dieckman G. Stereotactic treatment of different kinds of spasmodic torticollis. Confin Neurol 1970; 32:135–143.

104. Mundinger F, Riechert T, Disselhoff J. Long term results of stereotactic treatment of spasmodic torticollis. Confin Neurol 1972; 34:41–46.

105. Zervas N. Long-term review of dentatectomy in dystonia musculorum deformans and cerebral palsy. Acta Neurochir [Suppl] 1977; 24:49–51.

106. Guidetti B, Fraioli B. Neurosurgical treatment of spasticity and dyskinesia. Acta Neurochir [Suppl] 1977; 24:27–39.

107. Speelman JD, Van Manen J. Cerebral palsy and stereotactic neurosurgery: long term results. J Neurol Neurosurg Psychiatry 1989; 52:23–30.

108. Spiegel EA, Wycis HT. Effect of thalamic and pallidal lesions upon involuntary movements in choreoathetosis. Trans Am Neurol [A] 1950; 75:234–237.

109. Broggi G, Angelini L, Bono R, Giorgi C, Nardocci N, Franzini A. Long term results of stereotactic thalamotomy for cerebral palsy. Neurosurgery 1983; 12:195–202.

110. Cooper IS. Involuntary Movement Disorders. New York: Hoeber Medical Division, Harper & Row, 1969.

111. Narabayashi H, Kubota K. Reconsideration of ventrolateral thalamotomy for hyperkinesias. Prog Brain Res 1966; 21:339–349.

112. Ohye C, Miyazaki M. Hirai T, Shibazaki T, Nagaseki Y. Stereotactic selective thalamotomy for the treatment of tremor type cerebral palsy in adolescence. Child Brain 1983; 10:157–167.

113. Mundinger F, Riechert T, Disselhoff J. Long-term results of stereotactic operations on extrapyramidal hyperkinesia (excluding parkinsonism). Confin Neurol 1970; 32:71–78.

114. Wycis HT, Spiegel EA. Campotomy in myoclonia. J Neurosurg 1969; 30:708–713.
115. Ohye C, Miyazaki M, Hirai T, Shibazaki T, Nakajuma H, Nagaseki Y. Primary writing tremor treated by stereotactic selective thalamotomy. J Neurol Neurosurg Psychiatry 1982; 45:988–997.
116. Narabayashi H, Tokochi F, Nakajima Y. Idiopathic oromandibular dyskinesia treated by Vo complex microstereotactic thalamotomy. Appl Neurophysiol 1985; 48: 309–314.
117. Mimura Y, Bekku H, Miyamoto T, Ohmoto T, Nishimoto A. VL thalamotomy for the treatment of tremor in patients with thalamic syndrome. Appl Neurophysiol 1976–77; 39:199–201.
118. Stellar S, Cooper IS. Mortality and morbidity in cryothalamectomy for parkinsonism: a statistical study of 2868 consecutive operations. J Neurosurg 1968; 28: 459–467.
119. Tomlinson F, Kelly PJ, Jack CR Jr. Sequential magnetic resonance imaging following stereotactic radiofrequency ventralis lateralis thalamotomy. J Neurosurg 1991; 74: 579–584.
120. Kelly PJ. Contemporary stereotactic ventralis lateralis thalamotomy in the treatment of parkinsonian tremor and other movement disorders. In: Heilbrun MP, ed. Stereotactic Neurosurgery. Vol. 2. Concepts in Neurosurgery. Baltimore: Williams & Wilkins, 1988:133–148.
121. Obrador SA. A simplified neurosurgical technique for approaching and damaging the region of the globus pallidus in Parkinson's disease. J Neurol Neurosurg Psychiatry 1957; 20:47–49.
122. Cooper IS, Gioino G, Terry R. The organic lesion. Confin Neurol 1965; 26: 161–177.
123. Aronow S. The use of radiofrequency power in making lesions in the brain. J Neurosurg 1960; 17:431–438.
124. Albe-Fessard D, Arfel G, Guiot G. Activities electriques caracteristique de queques structures cerebrales chez l'homme. Ann Chir 1963; 17:1185–1214.
125. Brierley J, Beck E. The significance in human stereotactic brain surgery of individual variation in the diencephalon and globus pallidus. J Neurol Neurosurg Psychiatry 1959; 22:287–298.
126. Smith MC. Localization of stereotactic lesions confirmed at necropsy. Br Med J 1962; 1:900–906.
127. Brown RA. A computerized tomography–computer graphics approach to stereotactic localization. J Neurosurg 1979; 50:715–720.
128. Guiot G, Hertzog E, Rondet P, et al. Arrest or acceleration of speech evoked by thalamic stimulation in the course of stereotactic procedures for parkinsonism. Brain 1961; 84:363–369.
129. Ojemann GA, Ward AA. Speech representation in ventrolateral thalamus. Brain 1971; 94:669–680.
130. Bell DS. Speech functions of the thalamus inferred from the effects of the thalamotomy. Brain 1968; 91:619–638.
131. Waltz JM, Riklan M, Stellar S, Cooper IS. Cryothalamectomy for Parkinson's disease. A statistical analysis. Neurology 1966; 16:994–1002.

132. Ojemann GA. Brain organization for language from the perspective of electrical stimulation mapping. Behav Brain Sci 1983; 6:189–230.

133. Ojemann GA. Language and the thalamus: object naming and recall during and after thalamic stimulation. Brain Lang 1975; 2:101–120.

134. Hugdahl K, Webster K, Asbjrnsen A. The role of the left and right thalamus in language symmetry: dichotic listening in Parkinson patients undergoing stereotactic thalamotomy. Brain Lang 1990; 39:1–13.

135. Rossitch E, Zeidman SM, Nashold BS, et al. Evaluation of memory and language function pre- and post-thalamotomy with an attempt to define those patients at risk for postoperative dysfunction. Surg Neurol 1988; 29:11–16.

136. Shapiro DY, Sadowsky DA, Henderson WG, et al. An assessment of cognitive function in post-thalamotomy Parkinson patients. Confin Neurol 1973; 35:144–166.

137. Almgren PE, Andersson AL, Kellberg G. Long term effects of verbally expressed cognition following left and right ventrolateral thalamotomy. Confin Neurol 1972; 34:162–168.

138. Kocher J, Siegfried J, Perret E. Verbal and nonverbal learning ability of Parkinson patients before and after unilateral ventrolateral thalamotomy. Appl Neurophysiol 1982; 45:311–316.

139. Vilkki J. Effects of thalamic lesions on complex perception and memory. Neuropsychologia 1978; 16:427–437.

140. Vilkki J, Laitinen LV. Effects of pulviotomy and ventrolateral thalamotomy on some cognitive functions. Neuropsychologia 1976; 14:67–78.

141. Velasco F, Velasco H, Ogarria C, Olvera A. Neglect induced by thalamotomy in humans: a quantitative appraisal of the sensory and motor deficits. Neurosurgery 1986; 19:744–751.

142. Hassler R. Thalamic regulation of muscle tone and the speed of movements. In: Purpura DP, Yahr MD, eds, The Thalamus. New York: Columbia University Press, 1966:419–436.

143. Vilkki J. Visual hemi-inattention after ventrolateral thalamotomy. Neuropsychologia 1984; 22:399–408.

144. Yasui N, Narabayashi H, Kondo T, Ohye C. Slight cerebellar signs in stereotactic thalamotomy and subthalamotomy for parkinsonism. Appl Neurophysiol 1976–77; 39:315–320.

145. Waltz JM, Aristizabal G, Riklan M, et al. Results of cryothalamectomy for parkinsonism in patients over 70. Am Geriatr Soc 1967; 15:1–8.

146. Ojemann GA, Ward AA Jr. Abnormal movement disorders. In: Youmans JR, ed. Neurological Surgery. Vol. 6. Philadelphia: WB Saunders, 1982:3821–3857.

147. Matsumoto K, Shichijo F, Fukami T. Long-term follow-up review of cases of Parkinson's disease after unilateral and bilateral thalamotomy. J Neurosurg 1984; 60:1033–1044.

148. Benabid AL, Pollak P, Louveau A, Henry J, deRougemont J. Combined (thalamotomy and stimulation) stereotactic surgery of the VIM thalamic nucleus for bilateral Parkinson disease. Appl Neurophysiol 1987; 50:344–346.

Index

About the Editors

Leslie J. Findley is a Consultant Neurologist at the Regional Centre for Neurology and Neurosurgery at Oldchurch Hospital and Harold Wood Hospitals, Essex, United Kingdom; and an Honorary Senior Lecturer at the Institute of Neurology, London, United Kingdom. The cofounder of the International Tremor Foundation, Dr. Findley is a Fellow of the Royal College of Physicians and the Royal Society of Medicine (U.K.). The author or coauthor of more than 150 professional papers, he is currently Chairman of the Parkinson Disease Society of the United Kingdom and a member of the Association of British Neurologists, the American Academy of Neurology, the Movement Disorder Society, and the American Neurological Association. Dr. Findley received the M.B.ChB. degree (1968) and the M.D. degree (1988) from the University of Sheffield, United Kingdom.

William C. Koller is a Professor in and Chairman of the Department of Neurology, and a Professor of Pharmacology at the University of Kansas Medical Center, Kansas City. A Fellow of the American Academy of Neurology and a member of the American Neurological Association and the Movement Disorder Society, Dr. Koller is the coauthor, editor, or coeditor of several books, including the *Handbook of Parkinson's Disease, Second Edition* and (with George Paulson) *Therapy of Parkinson's Disease, Second Edition* (both titles, Marcel Dekker, Inc.). He is also the editor of the Neurological Disease and Therapy series (Marcel Dekker, Inc.) and the author or coauthor of over 200 journal articles. Dr. Koller received the M.S. (1971) and Ph.D. (1974) degrees in pharmacology, and the M.D. degree (1976) from Northwestern University Medical School, Chicago, Illinois.